T0229111

Office-Based Endovascular Centers

Office-Based Endovascular Centers

KRISHNA M. JAIN, MD, FACS
Clinical Professor
Surgery
Western Michigan University Homer Stryker M.D. School of Medicine
Kalamazoo, United States

ELSEVIER

Office-Based Endovascular Centers
ISBN: 978-0-323-67969-5
Copyright © 2020 Elsevier Inc. All rights reserved.

No part of this publication may be reproduced or transmitted in any form or by any means, electronic or mechanical, including photocopying, recording, or any information storage and retrieval system, without permission in writing from the publisher. Details on how to seek permission, further information about the Publisher's permissions policies and our arrangements with organizations such as the Copyright Clearance Center and the Copyright Licensing Agency, can be found at our website: www.elsevier.com/permissions.

This book and the individual contributions contained in it are protected under copyright by the Publisher (other than as may be noted herein).

Notices

Practitioners and researchers must always rely on their own experience and knowledge in evaluating and using any information, methods, compounds or experiments described herein. Because of rapid advances in the medical sciences, in particular, independent verification of diagnoses and drug dosages should be made. To the fullest extent of the law, no responsibility is assumed by Elsevier, authors, editors or contributors for any injury and/or damage to persons or property as a matter of products liability, negligence or otherwise, or from any use or operation of any methods, products, instructions, or ideas contained in the material herein.

Publisher: Cathleen Sether
Acquisition Editor: Good Gabbedy
Editorial Project Manager: Sara Pianavilla
Production Project Manager: Poulouse Joseph
Cover Designer: Alan Studholme

3251 Riverport Lane
St. Louis, Missouri 63043

ELSEVIER Book Aid International
Working together to grow libraries in developing countries
www.elsevier.com • www.bookaid.org

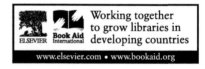

List of Contributors

Sam Ahn, MD, FACS, MBA
Vascular Management Associates
Los Angeles, CA, United States

Jose I. Almeida, MD, FACS, RPVI, RVT
Founder
Miami Vein
Voluntary Professor of Surgery
Division of Vascular and Endovascular Surgery
University of Miller Miami School of Medicine
Miami, FL, United States

Charles E. Ananian, BS, DPM
Co Medical Director Amputation Prevention Center Beverly Hospital
Montebello, CA, United States
President New Hope Podiatry Group
Los angeles, CA, United States

Enrico Ascher, MD, FACS
Chief of Vascular and Endovascular Surgery
NYU Langone Hospital – Brooklyn
Brooklyn, NY, United States
Professor of Surgery
NYU Langone Hospital – Brooklyn
New York University
Brooklyn, NY, United States

Asad Baig, MD
Chief Resident
Nassau University Medical Center Radiology
East Meadow, NY, United States

Jessica L. Bailey-Wheaton, ESQ
Health Capital Consultants
St. Louis, MO, United States

Laura D. Bauler, PhD
Assistant Professor
Department of Biomedical Sciences
Western Michigan University
Homer Stryker M.D. School of Medicine
Kalamazoo, MI, United States

John Blebea, MD, MBA
Professor and Chair of Surgical Disciplines College of Medicine Central Michigan University
Saginaw, MI, United States

Jon Bowman, MD
The Vascular Experts
Darien, CT, United States

Jeffrey G. Carr, MD, FACC, FSCAI
Medical Director- Outpatient Endovascular and Interventional Society National Registry
Medical Director- Tyler Cardiac and Endovascular Center
Tyler, TX, United States

Jesse Chait, BS
Medical Student
Division of Vascular Surgery
NYU Langone Hospital-Brooklyn
Brooklyn, NY, United States

Paramjit "Romi" Chopra, MD
Associate Professor of Radiology, Radiology
Rush University
Chicago, IL, United States
Chairman
MIMIT Health
Chicago, IL, United States

Rafael Santini Dominquez, MD
University of Maryland School of Medicine
Division of Vascular Surgery
Baltimore, MD, United States

Adbelhamid Elfaham, PhD
Director
Medical Physics & Radiation Safety Officer
Maimonides Medical Center
Brooklyn, New York, United States

Paul J. Gagne, MD
The Vascular Experts
Darien, CT, United States

Daniel R. Gorin, MD, FACS
Southeastern Vascular
Hyannis, MA, United States

Anil Hingorani, MD
Associate Clinical Professor
Department of Surgery
New York University Langone - Brooklyn
Brooklyn, NY, United States

Motahar Hosseini, MD
University of Maryland School of Medicine
Division of Vascular Surgery
Baltimore, MD, United States

Azher Iqbal, MD
Medical Director
Vascular Interventional Associates at Buffalo Vascular Care
Buffalo, NY, USA
Clinical Assistant Professor of Radiology SUNY Buffalo, Buffalo, NY, USA

Krishna Jain, MD, FACS
Clinical Professor Surgery
Western Michigan University Homer Stryker MD School of Medicine
Kalamazoo, MI, United States

Shikha Jain, MD
Assistant Professor
Physician Director of Media Rush University Cancer Center
Hematology Oncology
Rush University Medical Center
Chicago, IL, United States

Nicholas D. Jurkowitz, BA, JD
Fenton Law Group
LLP
Los Angeles, CA, United States
Partner
Litigation/Transactional/Regulatory Fenton Law Group
Los Angeles, CA, United States

Elias H. Kassab, MD, FACC, FSCAI, FACP, FASA, RPVI, FAHA, FSVM
Clinical Assistant Professor of Medicine, WSU
President and CEO of Dearborn Cardiology President and CEO of Michigan Outpatient Vascular Institute Dearborn
Michigan, United States

Matthew Keuten, JD
Honigman LLP
Detroit, MI, United States

Ali Khalifeh, MD
University of Maryland School of Medicine
Division of Vascular Surgery
Baltimore, MD, United States

Hwa Kho, PhD, MBA
Vascular Management Associates
Los Angeles, CA, United States

Taras Kucher, MD
The Vascular Experts
Darien, CT, United States

Andrea N. Lee, JD
Honigman LLP
Detroit, MI, United States

Anna Leyson-Fiel, BSN, RN, CCRC
Clinical Research Manager
Michigan Outpatient Vascular Institute
Dearborn, MI, United States

Edward G. Mackay, MD
Medical Director Vascular Surgery Vein and Circulatory Specialists
Palm Harbor, FL, United States

Nicolas J. Mouawad, MD, MPH, MBA, FSVS, FRCS, FACS
McLaren Bay Heart & Vascular
McLaren Bay Region
Bay City, MI, United States

Khanjan H. Nagarsheth, MD, MBA, FACS
University of Maryland School of Medicine
Division of Vascular Surgery
Baltimore, MD, United States

Deepak Nair, MD, MS, MHA, RVT, FACS
Chief of Vascular Surgery
Associate Professor of Surgery
Sarasota Memorial Hospital
Florida State Medical School
Sarasota, FL, United States

Albert Pavalonis, DO
Vascular Surgery
NYU Langone Hospital-Brooklyn
Brooklyn, NY, United States

Alexandra De Rivera, JD
Fenton Law Group
LLP
Los Angeles, CA, United States

Sean P. Roddy, MD
Professor of Surgery
Albany Medical College
Albany, NY, United States

Bhagwan Satiani, MD, MBA, DFSVS, FACHE, FACS
Division of Vascular Diseases & Surgery
The Ohio State University
Columbus, OH, United States

Maxim E. Shaydakov, MD, PhD
Department of Surgery
Central Michigan University College of Medicine
Saginaw, MI, United States

Jeff Smith, JD
Honigman LLP
Detroit, MI, United States

David C. Sperling, MD, FSIR
Vice Chair
Associate Professor of Radiology
Strategy and Development
Department of Radiology
Columbia University Irving Medical Center
New York, NY, United States

Sunita Srivastava, MD
Assistant Professor of Surgery
Massachusetts General Hospital
Boston, MA, United States

Bob Tahara, MD, FSVS, FACS, RVT, RPVI
Director Vascular & Endovascular Surgery
Allegheny Vein & Vascular
Bradford, PA, United States

Magean Whaley, RN
Vascular Management Associates
Los Angeles, CA, United States

Todd A. Zigrang, MBA, MHA, FACHE, CVA, ASA
Health Capital Consultants
St. Louis, MO, United States

Biography

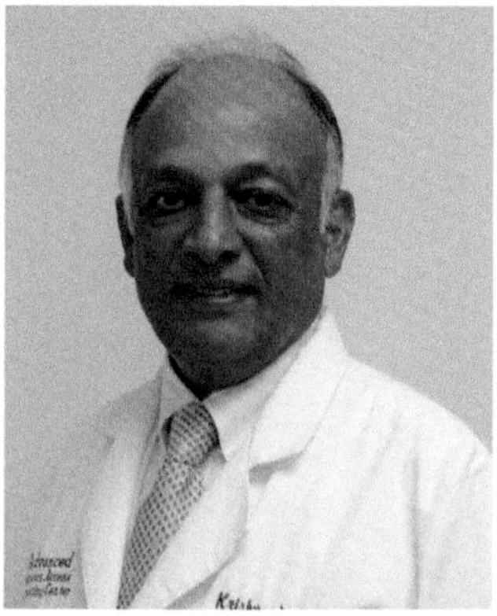

Dr Krishna Jain graduated from Maulana Azad Medical College, Delhi, India, followed by a residency and fellowship at UMDNJ, Newark, New Jersey. In his illustrious career, he has served as the chief of surgery and vascular surgery at Borgess Medical Center, Kalamazoo, Michigan, and the president of Paragon Health. He is a clinical professor of surgery at the Western Michigan University Homer Stryker School of Medicine. He is a founding member of the Outpatient Endovascular Interventional Society and the South Asian American Vascular Society. He has served in leadership roles in several surgical organizations. He is an internationally recognized expert in the field of office-based endovascular centers and has authored numerous papers and chapters in books on the topic.

Acknowledgment

The majority of my original ideas come into my head during long showers. I announce these wonderful ideas to my wife. She usually shoots them down very quickly, as many of the ideas are impractical. This time, it was different. After an unusually long shower, I announced to Poonam that I was going to write a book about office-based endovascular centers. She knows I am passionate about this particular subject and to my surprise she said, "That is a great idea and you should do it." The next challenge I foresaw would be talking to my children. However, they also were very supportive. My son Muneesh had just finished writing a book and Shikha, my daughter, even offered to contribute a chapter. Shakthi, my son in law, felt that the book was very timely and needed. I could not have finished writing several chapters and editing this book without the enormous support of my family. I am very thankful to them.

A book with multiple authors cannot be completed without the conviction and support of many other experts in the field. All the authors contributing to this publication have very busy practices and lives. I offer my sincere thanks to them for taking the time out of their busy lives to contribute to the book.

Contents

CHAPTER 1

Introduction: Changing Healthcare Delivery Models

KRISHNA JAIN, MD, FACS

There was a time when barbers were the healthcare providers to local citizens. We have come a long way, driven by advances in technology and drug discovery. The challenge continues, as we try to identify a healthcare delivery model that provides quality care at an optimal price. Society has reached a point where the people and the government are demanding balance between healthcare expenditure, quality, and value. Changes in the marketplace are driven by Centers for Medicare and Medicaid Services (CMS), since the government accounts for the largest individual share of healthcare expenditures[1]. This book provides a road map for the latest innovation in healthcare delivery systems: the "office-based endovascular center" (OEC). The CMS predicts annual healthcare costs in 2020 will be $4.64 trillion dollars, which represents nearly 20% of the US gross domestic product. Since medical inflation consistently outpaces the general inflation, CMS continues to look at ways to provide excellent healthcare for Medicare and Medicaid recipients at affordable prices. One of the ways it is trying to balance quality and fiscal responsibility is by shifting care from hospital settings (inpatient and outpatient) to ambulatory settings (surgery centers and physician offices). Let us look at the journey healthcare delivery has taken to reach at the point where we are today.

In 1756, the College of Philadelphia (now the University of Pennsylvania) offered the first medical training in the colonies. The American Medical Association (AMA) was formed in 1847 as a membership organization to protect the interest of its members, medical providers. In 1901, the AMA was reorganized by county and state. In 1904, the Council on Medical Education was created to establish standards for medical education. By 1910, 70,000 physicians, half the practicing doctors, had joined the AMA.[2] This was the beginning of organized medicine. Doctors were no longer expected to provide free service for all hospital patients, and railroads became the leading industry to develop an employee medical program.[2,3]

In the 1920s, medical reformers emphasized the cost savings value of medical care outweighed the potential loss of wages due to sickness.[4] The relatively higher cost of medical care was a new and dramatic development, especially for the middle class.[2] Physicians' incomes grew and it became a prestigious profession. General Motors signed a contract with Metropolitan Life to insure 180,000 workers. The Social Security Act was passed in 1935, which omitted health insurance. Against the advice of insurance professionals, Blue Cross began offering private coverage for hospital care in dozens of states.[2] During World War II, wage and price controls were placed on American employers.[2] To compete for workers, companies began to offer health benefits, giving rise to the employer-based system in place today.[2,4] In 1947, the Blue Cross Commission was established to create a national doctors network. By 1950, 57% of the population had hospital insurance. At present around 90% of population has health insurance.[3]

In the 1950s, the price of hospital care doubled. At the start of the decade, healthcare expenditure was 4.5% of gross national product.[2] In the early 1960s, those outside the workplace, especially the elderly, had difficulty affording insurance.[4] Over 700 insurance companies sold health insurance. Concern about a "doctor shortage" and the need for more "health manpower" led to federal measures to expand education in the health professions.[2] In 1965, President Lyndon Johnson signed Medicare and Medicaid into law. In the subsequent decades, healthcare costs escalated rapidly due to multiple factors which included unexpectedly high Medicare expenditures, rapid inflation in the economy, expansion of hospital expenses and profits, changes in medical care including a greater use of technology, and new medications.[4] In response to a

Office-Based Endovascular Centers. https://doi.org/10.1016/B978-0-323-67969-5.00001-0
Copyright © 2020 Elsevier Inc. All rights reserved.

call for affordable quality outpatient surgical care, hospitals in California and Washington, DC, started providing ambulatory surgical care.

Anesthesiologists Reed and Ford[5] opened the first surgicenter on February 12, 1970. Several other centers opened across the United States soon after that.[6] In 1971, the AMA began endorsing outpatient surgery under general and local anesthesia as an option for selected procedures and patients. In 1973, the American Society of anesthesiologists developed a list of nine guidelines published in "Guidelines for Ambulatory Surgical Facilities."[6]

In 1982, Medicare approved payment for approximately 200 procedures that could be performed in the ambulatory surgery center (ASC).[6] In 1987, Medicare modified the ASC list to use specific CPT (current procedural terminology) codes and expanded the list to include 1535 procedures. In 1988, the number of ASCs in the United States reached a milestone of 1000 centers and using the information from a 1986 cost survey of ASCs, Medicare implemented a new payment system for ASCs, which continues to be the basis for ASC payments today.

Further innovation in delivery of care occurred in 2005. The deficit reduction act authorized CMS to pay for endovascular procedures performed in the office. This was an attempt to further move the cost-intensive technology—driven procedures to a less expensive site of service. The regulations to provide invasive treatment in the office were much less stringent as compared to the ASC. In 2008, Medicare modified the reimbursement rates to encourage more efficient outpatient use of peripheral vascular intervention.

Medicare pays ASCs for a bundle of facility services primarily linked to the outpatient prospective payment system (OPPS), which Medicare uses to pay for most of the services provided in hospital outpatient departments (HOPDs).[7] Services covered under both an ASC and OPPS are paid at a lower rate in the ASC than in the OPPS system. To maintain budget neutrality in 2018, the ASC's relative weight was reduced by 10.1% below the relative weight in the OPPS. For most procedures covered under the ASC system, the payment rate is the product of its relative weight and a conversion factor. In 2018, the conversion factor for ASC's was set at $45.58 as compared to the OPPS conversion factor of $78.64. The conversion factor was started in 2008 at a lower rate than OPPS and has remained at a lower level ever since. CMS uses a different method to determine payment rates for procedures that are predominantly performed in physicians' offices.[7] CMS sets the rates to prevent migration of office-based procedures from physicians' offices to ASCs for financial reasons. Medicare beneficiaries can have more than 3500 different procedures performed in an ASC and account for approximately 30% of the care provided in an ASC.[7] In 2011, more than 5300 ASCs in the United States performed 23 million surgeries annually.[6] Currently there are more ASCs than acute care hospitals.

The Hill—Burton Act was passed in 1946 to regulate the number of medical facilities. In 1964, New York became the first state to enact a statute granting the state government power to determine whether there was a need for a new hospital or nursing home before it was approved for construction.[8] In 1974, the National Health Planning and Resources Act required all 50 states to have CON laws to qualify for federal funding. All states except Louisiana enacted the law. In 1987, this federal law was repealed, and 12 states terminated their programs.[8] Currently, 35 states have a CON requirement, while three states have some variation of it.[7] A certificate of need is not required prior to opening an office endovascular center as this is considered an extension of practice.

Our OEC, also referred to as an office-based laboratory (OBL) or access center, opened in 2007. We published the initial data from our practice in a paper titled "Future of Vascular Surgery is in the Office."[9] There are probably between 600 and 700 hundred labs being operated by vascular surgeons, interventional cardiologists, interventional radiologists, and interventional nephrologists. It is difficult to know the exact number since these centers can work independent of any certification. This number is an estimate presented at various national meetings. Interventional nephrology is a new specialty created to meet the needs of OECs since initially the bulk of cases performed in the centers was related to dialysis access. At present, almost all endovascular procedures except carotid stenting and endovascular repair of an aortic aneurysm can be performed in the OEC. These procedures are reimbursed by CMS and almost all private insurance companies. Since there is no federally mandated certification required for an OEC and there is no peer review, it is obligatory for the center to follow the same practice guidelines as followed in the more structured hospitals and ASCs. It took more than 40 years for ASCs to exceed the number of acute care hospitals. With increasing number of procedures that can be performed in an OEC, there may be more than 2000 centers in the next 10 years.

This book has been written with the intent of providing the reader the basics of opening an OEC. We have tried to cover all aspects of opening and running a center. This book should not be used as a substitute for proper business planning including obtaining relevant legal opinions..

REFERENCES

1. https://www.cms.gov/research-statistics-data-and-systems/statistics-trends-and-reports/nationalhealthexpenddata/nhe-fact-sheet.html.
2. PBS-healthcare. crisis: healthcare timeline. *Public Broadcast Syst*; 2019. https://www.pbs.org/healthcarecrisis/history.htm.
3. Stewart C. Timeline: history of changes (and battles) in American healthcare. *Dayt Dly News*. March 10, 2017.
4. Griffin J. The history of healthcare in America. *JP Griffin Gr*. 2017.
5. Ford JL, Reed WA. The surgicenter. An innovation in the delivery and cost of medical care. *Ariz Med*. 1969;26(10):801–804. http://www.ncbi.nlm.nih.gov/pubmed/5345881.
6. Advancing surgical care. History of ASCs. *Ambul Surg Cent Assoc*. https://www.ascassociation.org/advancingsurgicalcare/asc/historyofascs.
7. MedPac. *Ambulatory Surgical Center Services Payment System*; 2018. Washington, DC www.medpac.gov.
8. Cauchi R, Nobel A. Con-certificate of need state laws. *Natl Conf State Legis*; 2019. http://www.ncsl.org/research/health/con-certificate-of-need-state-laws.aspx.
9. Jain KM, Munn J, Rummel M, Vaddineni S, Longton C. Future of vascular surgery is in the office. *J Vasc Surg*. 2010. https://doi.org/10.1016/j.jvs.2009.09.056.

CHAPTER 2

State Regulations

DEEPAK NAIR, MD, MS, MHA, RVT, FACS

As medical procedures have migrated out of hospital settings and into physician offices, states have passed regulations for office-based surgeries. State agencies have historically regulated hospitals and ambulatory surgery centers (ASCs) via licensure and certificate of need (CON) requirements. Physicians performing office procedures had been exempted from similar state oversight. As the volume and complexity of in-office procedures increased, guidance regarding the appropriateness of certain procedures, necessary equipment, and qualifications for performing the surgeries became necessary. Professional societies are now developing guidelines for these sites of service. Private organizations, also, have established standards for accreditation of facilities that perform in-office surgeries. The trend for increasing regulation will mirror the increasing trend to perform these procedures in the outpatient setting.

States have broad powers over the performance of medical procedures through their departments of health and medical boards. This allows the state to respond, as issues develop in this burgeoning care setting. However, states' licensing requirements vary in terms of their regulation. For example, formal accreditation is voluntary in many states, but required in some others if deeper levels of anesthesia are to be used. States also may use voluntary guidelines or position statements if no law exists. Many states also look to accreditation agencies to provide oversight and also reduce the burden on state government. Private organizations such as the Accreditation Association for Ambulatory Health Care (AAAHC), American Association for Accreditation of Ambulatory Surgery Facilities (AAAASF), and the Joint Commission (TJC) have stepped in to provide this role.[1] Most states exempt offices from regulation if only local or topical anesthesia is used. Despite the variability in licensing requirements by states, common themes have emerged[1]:

- Federal, state, and local laws and codes must be followed.
- Procedural rooms should provide oxygen, suction, resuscitation equipment, and medications for emergencies.
- Equipment must be maintained and inspected per manufacturer's specifications.
- Adequately trained personnel should be present (i.e., basic life support, etc.).

As we discuss classifications of office-based surgery, it is important to clearly describe the terms that make references to them. Levels I–III describe surgical complexity and are often used by many state medical boards. Class A–C refers to the level of anesthesia required as termed by the American College of Surgeons ("Guidelines for Optimal Ambulatory Surgical Care and Office-based Surgery.")[2,3]

Level I Surgery	Level II Surgery	Level III Surgery
Minor surgical procedures performed under topical, local, or regional block anesthesia not involving drug-induced alteration- of consciousness, other than minimal sedation utilizing preoperative oral anxiolytic medications	Minor or major surgical procedures performed in conjunction with oral, parenteral, or intravenous sedation or under analgesic or dissociative drugs	Procedures that require deep sedation, general anesthesia, or major nerve blocks and support of bodily functions

Office-Based Endovascular Centers. https://doi.org/10.1016/B978-0-323-67969-5.00002-2
Copyright © 2020 Elsevier Inc. All rights reserved.

Class A	Class B	Class C
Topical and local anesthesia with or without oral or intramuscular preoperative sedation	Oral, parenteral, or intravenous sedation or analgesic or dissociative drugs to perform minor or major surgical procedures	General or regional block anesthesia and support of vital bodily functions for major surgical procedures

States differ in their regulation of office-based surgeries. Some have very strict laws, while some have none at all. A review of all 50 states and their laws on facilities performing office-based surgeries was performed. In this chapter an explanation of each state's view on the topic will be detailed. Key differences in state statutes and novel ideology will be highlighted. The following review is not meant to be a comprehensive description of each state's regulatory stance on office-based surgery, but rather a view on regulations in general on the topic. References to individual state mandates will be provided when applicable. If you are planning to open an office-based endovascular center (OEC), you should study the state regulations in detail and possibly get a healthcare attorney's advice.

ALASKA

In Alaska, the state medical board has not issued guidelines or policies nor has a position on office-based surgery in general. There is no law that regulates office-based surgeries. Alaska does, however, license and certify ambulatory surgery centers (ASCs) in the state.

ALABAMA

Alabama has a law that regulates facilities performing office-based procedures (r. 540-X-10-.06).[4] This statute includes specific instructions and recommendations based on the level of anesthesia. Annual registration is required for offices performing procedures with moderate or deeper sedation. Alabama's law also clearly states that at least one practitioner who is current in their ACLS training must be immediately and physically available until the last patient is discharged from the facility. Alabama also has reporting requirements as part of its law. Reporting to the Alabama Board of Medicine is required within three business days for all deaths, transfers to the hospital, any patient requiring CPR, surgical site infection (deep wound infection), or unscheduled hospitalization related to the office surgery. The state law also requires written policies and procedures including an Emergency Care and Transfer Plan and an Infection Control Policy.

ARIZONA

Arizona's statute (R4-16-701-707) is one of the most comprehensive regarding office-based surgery.[5] It requires reporting and registering even in cases that involve minimal sedation. They define minimal sedation as a drug-induced state during which a patient responds to verbal commands with unaffected respiratory and cardiovascular functions. Cognitive function and coordination are allowed to be impaired. The state law also requires that every patient be provided a "patients' rights policy" before surgery. Arizona also states unequivocally that the physician is to be physically present in the room where office-based surgery is performed while the procedure is performed. Furthermore, after the procedure and until the patient's postsedation monitoring is complete, Arizona law clearly states that a physician is physically to be at the office and sufficiently free of other duties to respond to an emergency. A receipt of discharge instructions also needs to be clearly documented.

ARKANSAS

Arkansas also has a law (R. 060.00.1-35) that regulates office-based procedures, but only the ones that require deep sedation.[6] Though not as restrictive as many other states in their statutes for office procedures, they do require a transfer agreement with a specified medical care facility and a requirement that all physicians performing any office-based surgery have admitting privileges at that specified facility.

CALIFORNIA

California Business and Professions Code 2216[7] and 2240[8] as well as California Health and Safety Code 1248[9] are laws that apply to regulation of office-based procedures in that state. California, unlike other states, requires two staff members to be present at all times until the patient is discharged; at least one must be a physician or have current certification in ACLS. California also allows for proceduralists, that cannot get admitting privileges due to their professional classification or other administrative limitations, to do procedures in the office, provided they have a transfer agreement with others who do have admitting privileges. They further require that cases that involve transfer to a facility, be subject to peer review by that facility to determine any inappropriateness of care delivered at the transferring center. The review outcome will be reported. Physicians must agree to cooperate with this process. California also mandates a system for quality assessment and improvement. Each licensee who performs procedures in the office facility must also be peer reviewed at least every 2 years with recommendations for quality improvement and education.

COLORADO

Colorado has no law regulating facilities that perform office-based surgery. Their state medical board has some guidelines but more general and nebulous than most other states. The ones they do have mostly apply to ASCs.[10]

CONNECTICUT

Connecticut General Statute 19a-493a,b,c[11] regulates outpatient surgical facilities. They exempt offices from regulation if the facility has no designated operating room or surgical area, bills no facility fees to third-party payers, administers no deep or general anesthesia, and performs only minor surgical procedures incidental to the work performed in that facility.

DELAWARE

Delaware is vague when referring to office-based surgery in its two codes that refer to this site of service (Delaware Code title 16 122[12] and Delaware Administrative Code 4408-2.0[13]). Any office procedure that requires any level of sedation triggers regulation. Facilities are excluded from regulation if it is already licensed as another class of healthcare facility specifically a hospital, freestanding birthing center, freestanding surgical center, or freestanding emergency center.

DISTRICT OF COLUMBIA

In the District of Columbia, DC Statutes 44-501 through 44-504[14] are meant to govern office-based surgeries. Interestingly, the Mayor is granted subjective powers to determine and define the classification of a facility. Furthermore, the Mayor makes the final determination of whether a facility is subject to regulation via determination of whether a provision is contextually appropriate or inappropriate for the given entity. It is also unusual in that the regulation is not based on the level of anesthesia provided like in most states, but rather indirectly by the complexity of the procedure or the degree of patient risk. Interestingly, no procedures have yet been defined.

FLORIDA

Florida continues to be one of the most active states in the nation in its activity and prescience in regards to office-based surgery regulation. Work of the Office Surgery Subcommittee within the Florida Department of Health has led to regulation (Florida Administrative Code r. 64B9-9.009)[15] that is much more patient centered than facility or provider centric. Florida's statute begins with the "Golden Rule" of office surgery: "Nothing … relieves the surgeon of the responsibility for making the medical determination that the office is an appropriate forum for the particular procedure(s) to be performed on the particular patient."[15]

Much of the regulatory language has specific requirements and instructions regarding cosmetic surgery procedures. This is due to the disproportionate number of adverse events and disciplinary action that emanated from office-based cosmetic procedures over the past three decades in Florida. Florida's law regulates facilities that perform office-based procedures utilizing moderate or higher levels of sedation. Florida is unique in that it has requirements regarding specific levels of nursing staff based on the level of sedation.

It is the only state to specifically address percutaneous endovascular intervention in its law. In the statute, percutaneous endovascular intervention is "defined as a procedure performed without open direct visualization of the target vessel, requires only needle puncture of an artery or vein followed by insertion of catheters, wires, or similar devices which are then advanced through the blood vessels using imaging guidance. Once the catheter reaches the intended location, various maneuvers to address the diseased area may be performed which include, but are not limited to, injection of contrast for imaging; treatment of vessels with angioplasty, atherectomy, covered or uncovered stents, intentionally occluding vessels or organs (embolization); and delivering medications, radiation, or other energy using laser, radio frequency, or cryotherapy."[15] The law goes on to define major blood vessels as "a group of critical arteries and veins including the aorta, coronary arteries, pulmonary arteries, superior and inferior vena cava, pulmonary veins, and any intracerebral artery or vein."[15] The Board of Medicine, in its wisdom, adopted the Standards of the American Society of Anesthesiologists for Basic Anesthetic Monitoring[16] instead of developing its own criteria. Florida law also has strict risk and quality review protocols that are required. Quarterly review and analysis of quality and risk must be done at all facilities that perform office-based procedures. The statute is also prescriptive in its minimum medication requirements (Table 2.1) based on the level of office surgery. These medications need to be onsite and readily available.[15]

TABLE 2.1
Medication Requirements Based on the Level of Office Surgery in Florida.

Level I Office Surgery	Level II Office Surgery	Level III Office Surgery
Atropine 3 mg	Adenosine 18 mg	All medications required in Level II office surgery
Diphenhydramine 50 mg	Albuterol 2.5 mg with small volume nebulizer	Dantrolene 720 mg (if halogenated anesthetics or succinylcholine used)
Epinephrine 1 mg in 10 mL	Amiodarone 300 mg	
Epinephrine 1 mg in 1 mL vial, three vials total	Atropine 3 mg	
Hydrocortisone 100 mg	Calcium chloride 1 g	
	Dextrose 50%; 50 mL	
	Diphenhydramine 50 mg	
	Dopamine 200 mg minimum	
	Epinephrine 1 mg in 10 mL	
	Epinephrine 1 mg in 1 mL vial, three vials total	
	Flumazenil 1 mg	
	Furosemide 40 mg	
	Hydrocortisone 100 mg	
	Lidocaine 100 mg (appropriate for cardiac administration)	
	Magnesium sulfate 2 g	
	Naloxone 1.2 mg	
	Beta-blocker	
	Sodium bicarbonate 50 mEq/50 mL	
	Paralytic agent (appropriate for use in rapid sequence intubation)	
	Vasopressin 40 units	
	Calcium channel blocker	
	Intralipid 20% 500 mL solution (if nonneuraxial regional blocks are performed)	

Ongoing changes to the statute are always in progress. Most notably, in Florida, there is pressure to require facilities to demonstrate financial responsibility when deemed at fault. For example, current Florida law does not require cosmetic surgery clinics to have medical liability insurance. Many office surgery facilities are owned by nonphysician investors who often are not liable when things go wrong.

GEORGIA

The state of Georgia has no law in place to regulate office-based surgery. However, the Georgia Composite Medical Board has issued guidelines for office-based anesthesia and surgery.[17] There are recommendations in their guidelines that are of particular interest and are original; Georgia's guidelines encourage obtaining accreditation and demonstrating "truth in advertising" by presenting credentials, education received, specialty board certification, and proficiency evaluations in any form of advertising and having them readily available in writing to all patients.[17]

HAWAII

Hawaii has no laws that regulate office-based surgery. The state is unique in its relative silence regarding the matter. It may be due to decreased penetrance of outpatient and office-based surgeries in the state. There are only 22 registered freestanding outpatient surgical facilities on these islands, with two of them not affiliated with Medicare.[18]

IDAHO

Idaho, also, has no regulatory statutes on office-based surgery. Their ASC regulations are mainly dependent on federal guidelines. ASCs are only federally certified in the state of Idaho.

ILLINOIS

Illinois law (Illinois Statute 5/3, Illinois Administrative Code 77 205.110[19]) does not specifically regulate office-based surgery. It does have language that regulates ambulatory surgical treatment centers, which it defines as any facility that primarily performs office-based procedures (i.e., more than 50% of the activities at the location are procedural).[19] This seems to immediately categorize offices that mainly perform office surgeries into an ASC; along with this categorization comes very stringent regulation. Illinois is one of the few states in which the percentage of procedures performed at the site triggers regulation rather than the level of anesthesia or type of procedure.

INDIANA

Indiana has specific laws (844 Indiana Administrative Code 5-5-20[20]) that govern the performance of office-based procedures. These statutes require accreditation. Indiana law allows for a transfer agreement with another practitioner who has admitting privileges or an emergency transfer agreement with a nearby hospital in lieu of admitting privileges by the proceduralist. It is the only state to require agreements with local emergency medical services (EMS), and for these agreements to be renewed annually.[20] Regulation does not apply to facilities limiting themselves to procedures requiring only local anesthesia, superficial nerve blocks, or minimal sedation and anxiolysis.

IOWA

Iowa, like Idaho, has neither regulation nor guidelines for office-based surgery. It also does not license surgical centers. Iowa has just over 26 Medicare-certified ASCs that are inspected once every 3 years, but there are many more that are not part of the Medicare system and thus do not get tracked or monitored by the federal government.[21]

KANSAS

Kansas has a specific statute (Kansas Administrative Regulations 100-25-3[22]) that regulates office-based surgeries. The statute is in line with most of the other states' prescriptions and guidelines. Kansas law does state that any office procedure extending more than 4 h beyond the planned duration is reportable to the Kansas Board of Medicine. It also is unique in its stated restriction of lidocaine injection to not exceed 7 milligrams per kilogram of body weight. This also applies to tumescent anesthesia.[22]

KENTUCKY

Kentucky, like Georgia, has no laws regulating office-based procedures, but does have a formal guideline in the form of a "Board opinion related to office-based surgery."[23] This document offers standard guidelines that are in line with many other states' statutes. The guidelines are notable in their unequivocal mandate "that a physician only" may perform procedures and anesthesia services,[23] which are not in line with most other state guidelines and statutes that allow for advanced practice providers to provide these services. The Kentucky guidelines also include a useful "Sample Patient Bill of Rights"[23] that may be a good reference for those looking to adopt such a document.

LOUISIANA

The state of Louisiana has laws (Louisiana Administrative Code 46:XLV, Chapter 73[24]) that regulate facilities performing office-based surgery. It includes definition of "reasonable proximity" of a facility that a patient may be transferred to: "a distance of not more than 30 miles or one which may be reached within 30 min for patients 13 years of age and older and a distance of not more than 15 miles or one which can be reached within 15 min for patients 12 years of age and under."[24] The Louisiana code regulates only facilities that provide moderate or greater levels of sedation. It is one of the only states to exempt regulation if the facility is State or Federally run, or if accredited by TJC, the Joint AAAASF, or the AAAHC. Mandated reports to the state include unplanned readmissions and death of the patient within 30 days of surgery after a procedure in an office-based facility. Louisiana also requires a continuous log by calendar date of all procedures with patient identifiers, type and duration of each procedure.[24]

MAINE

Maine offers no rules or guidelines for office-based surgery.

MARYLAND

Maryland is an interesting state in regards to how it handles statutes (Maryland Code Health Occupations 14-404 (41)[25]; Maryland Code Regulations 10.12.03.01; Maryland Code Regulations 10.12.03.02[26]) for office-based surgeries. It only regulates performance of cosmetic surgeries using moderate or greater sedation in the office. Other surgical procedures performed in the office are free of specific requirements other than standard Board of Medicine requirements for practitioners unrelated to site of service.

MASSACHUSETTS

Massachusetts has no law regulating office-based surgical procedures but does have the most comprehensive set of guidelines by any state. They were created by the Massachusetts Medical Society's Task Force on Office-Based Surgery.[27] They are based on the American Society of Anesthesiologists Guidelines for Office-Based Anesthesia (2008 edition)[28] and the South Carolina Medical Association's Office-Based Surgery Guidelines (which were adopted by the South Carolina Board of Medical Examiners[29]). It is comprehensive and well thought out in its construction and recommendations.

MICHIGAN

Michigan offers guidelines for sedation for in-office procedures but has no laws to regulate office surgery. The Michigan Quality Improvement Consortium periodically updates its "In-Office Use of Sedation" document.[30] It addresses and recommends accreditation, careful patient selection, informed consent, quality improvement, education, hospital affiliation, and appropriate monitoring and resuscitation.

MINNESOTA

Minnesota has administrative rules that regulate outpatient surgical centers (Minnesota Administrative Rules Chapter 4675[31]) but not office surgery.

MISSISSIPPI

Mississippi law (Mississippi Code 30-17-2635[32]) regulates office-based surgery in the state. Any facility performing Level II or Level III office-based surgery must register with Mississippi State Board of Medical Licensure. Mississippi requires physicians performing office-based surgery to document board certification or board eligibility by a board approved by the American Board of Medical Specialties or American Board of Osteopathic Specialties. If the procedures are "outside the physician's core curriculum," credentialing must be applied through the Mississippi State Board of Medical Licensure and reviewed by a multispecialty board appointed by the Executive Director.[32] Other requirements are similar to other states with laws regulating office-based surgeries.

MISSOURI AND MONTANA

Missouri and Montana have regulation for ambulatory surgical centers through its Department of Health and Senior Services and Department of Public Health and Human Services, respectively, but no guidance specifically for facilities performing in-office surgeries.

NEBRASKA

Nebraska has neither regulations nor guidelines regarding office surgery or anesthesia.

NEVADA

Nevada has statutes (Nevada Rev. Statute Ann. 449.435–436[33]) that govern the performance of office procedures if performed under moderate or greater levels of sedation. The law is of particular interest for its strict and broad definition of conscious sedation. It defines conscious sedation as a minimally depressed level of consciousness produced by pharmacological or nonpharmacological means. It does exempt office surgery facilities that administer a medication to relieve the patient's anxiety or pain and if the dosage given does not induce a controlled state of depressed consciousness. Nevada law is also prescriptive in its requirement for accreditation by a national organization that is approved by its Board of Medicine.[33]

NEW HAMPSHIRE

New Hampshire has no set of guidelines nor laws regarding office-based surgery or anesthesia. However, it does have a Code of Administrative Rules for ambulatory surgical centers.[34]

NEW JERSEY

New Jersey is among the states with the most detailed set of codes (New Jersey Administrative Code 13:35-4A.4–15[35]) that regulate facilities performing office-based surgeries in the nation. They are comprehensive and instructive in their guidance on the performance of office-based surgery. Any office procedure that uses moderate or greater levels of sedation triggers the statute. Any complications within 48 h of surgery need reporting back to the state. However, the statute later states that any incident related to surgery which results in a patient death, observation in the hospital for over 24 h, or untoward event as defined by the New Jersey Administrative Code 13:35-4A.3[35] needs to reported to the New Jersey State Board of Medical Examiners. State law is specific regarding privileging. Anyone performing office surgery must be credentialed to do the same procedure by a hospital. If not credentialed in the hospital, application to do the procedure must be made to the State Board to seek Board-approved privileges. The same requirement exists for administering or supervising anesthesia (i.e., the provider must be privileged by a hospital to provide the particular anesthesia service, or obtain Board-approved privileging from the state). A transfer agreement with a hospital within 20 min of the office is needed. This agreement must be posted, according to the law, in the office. New Jersey is prominent and very particular in its requirement that only patients with an American Society of Anesthesiologists (ASA) physical status classification of I or II are appropriate candidates for an office surgery. The state also requires at least eight Category I or II hours of continuing medical education in any anesthesia services, including conscious sedation every 3 years.[35]

NEW MEXICO

New Mexico does not license facilities that perform office-based procedures. It does regulate ASCs.

NEW YORK

New York Public Health Law 230-d[36] is responsible for the regulation of office-based surgery. The law calls for accreditation (by agencies determined by the commissioner), adverse event reporting (any patient death within 30 days), transfer to hospital within 72 h of office-based surgery, unscheduled hospital admission for longer than 24 h within 72 h of the office-based surgery, or any other serious or life-threatening event.[36]

NORTH CAROLINA

North Carolina has no laws that regulate facilities that perform office-based surgeries, but does have a position statement on the matter by the North Carolina Medical Board.[37] The guideline is in line with most state statues on office-based surgeries.

NORTH DAKOTA

North Dakota does not have statutes that govern the performance of office-based surgery in the state. It also has no stipulations for ambulatory surgical centers other than the need for certification by CMS to participate in the Medicare/Medicaid program.

OHIO

Ohio has a law (Ohio Administrative Code 4731-25-07[38]) in place that regulates the performance of office-based surgeries. The law is notable for its detail in declaring that physicians shall not perform on more than one patient at the same time if a procedure requires sedation or analgesia, or more simply put, only one patient may be actively operated on at a time. The law is also unique in its mention of podiatrists and specific limitations in regards to that specialty in regards to office-based surgeries. Ohio law also requires 20 h of category I continuing medical education relating to the delivery of anesthesia services every 2 years. Accreditation is required by law.[38]

OKLAHOMA

Oklahoma does not have laws dictating performance of office-based surgeries. The Oklahoma State Board of Medical Licensure and Supervision published guidelines for office-based surgery.[39] The guidelines are among the least restrictive and most general ones in the nation. Despite this, Oklahoma proclaims loudly in the guidelines a warning to those performing office-based procedures:

... wants physicians to be aware that compared with acute care hospitals and licensed ambulatory surgical facilities, office operatories currently have little or no regulation, oversight or control by federal, state or local laws. Therefore, physicians must satisfactorily investigate areas taken for granted in the hospital or ambulatory surgical facility such as governance, organization, construction and equipment, as well as policies and procedures, including fire, safety, drugs, emergencies, staffing, training and unanticipated patient transfers.[39]

OREGON

Oregon Administrative Rules 847-017-0010 and 847-017-0035[40] regulates facilities that perform office-based surgeries. Oregon's requirements are dependent on the level of surgery. Level I surgeries require the physician to have basic life support (BLS) certification and the rule encourages continuing medical education in the field of office-based surgery and in the anesthetic services being provided. For performance of Level II surgeries, Board certification or eligibility are required. Fifty hours of continuing medical education relevant to the Level II surgical procedure to be performed in the office-based facility may be done in lieu of the requirements for board certification/eligibility. For Level III procedures, the proceduralist must have staff privileges to perform the same procedure in a hospital or ASC, maintain board certification/eligibility, and be certified in ACLS. Oregon also requires accreditation for facilities where Level II or Level III office-based surgeries are performed.[40]

PENNSYLVANIA

Pennsylvania has laws (Pennsylvania Code 551.2[41]) that regulate office-based surgical procedures that require moderate or greater sedation (i.e., Class B or Class C). Pennsylvania's statute does apply to office-based endovascular labs in that it specifically states the law is triggered in physician offices if there is a "distinct part used solely for outpatient surgical treatment on a regular and organized basis." Pennsylvania's well-thought-out law is comprehensive in its identification, acceptance, and guidelines for all providers who may be involved in office-based surgery, from surgeons to student nurses. It, like some others states, limits operating time to 4 h, and also recommends no more than a total of 4 h of directly supervised recovery. This recovery time stipulation may influence the use of closure devices in endovascular procedures. There is leeway given in the statute for exceeding the time if the patient's condition demands care beyond the 4-hour limit or if the additional time could not have been anticipated prior to the procedure. It is important to note that the law specifically forbids any office-based surgery that "directly involve major blood vessels." The terms "directly" and "major blood vessel" are certainly subject to interpretation and too vague.[41] This has created a major confusion among the current owners of office endovascular centers and the interventionalists who want to open a new center. Pennsylvania also requires policies to be in place regarding preventative maintenance, infection control, disaster preparation, quality assurance, and peer review of physicians.

RHODE ISLAND

Rhode Island Laws and Codes (Rhode Island General Laws 23-17-4; 31-4, and Rhode Island Code R 3: 2.0)[42] are particular in many of their requirements for facilities performing office-based surgery. The state requires accreditation by the TJC, AAAASF, or the AAAHC. Rhode Island has Continuity of Care Short Form (www.healthri.org) that must be filled out in the case of any transfer of patients to a hospital or emergency care facility from the physician office. Key events that must be reported to the state in Rhode Island in relation to office-based procedures include hospital admission within 72 h of discharge, extension of the procedure beyond 4 h, death of the patient within 30 days, or any incident reported to the malpractice carrier. Rhode Island is one of the very few states to require the person doing an office-based surgery to have current surgical privileges for the same or similar class of procedures at a nearby hospital.[42]

SOUTH CAROLINA

South Carolina has a statute (South Carolina Ann. Reg. 81-96[29]) devoted to the issue of office-based surgery. Level I office surgery is excluded from regulation only if no sedation other than a "preoperative minimal oral anxiolysis of the patient" is given.[29] The state's requirements for the facilities performance improvement program are the most stringent in the nation for office-based surgery. Periodic review must be done at least every 6 months and must be peer reviewed by physicians not affiliated with the same practice. Accreditation is required by one of the agencies approved by the South Carolina Board of Medical Examiners. In addition to the TJC, AAAHC, and AAAASF, the state allows for accreditation by Healthcare Facilities Accreditation Program (HFAP), a division of the American Osteopathic Association.[29] South Carolina's well-thought-out law has been the model for many other states laws and guidelines for office-based surgery statutes.

SOUTH DAKOTA

South Dakota has no law or guideline for facilities performing office-based surgeries. South Dakota does not regulate ASCs in the state either. Only 18 ASCs in the state are Medicare-certified.

TENNESSEE

Tennessee has a dedicated statute for office-based surgery (Tennessee Code Ann. 63-6-221[43]). It regulates all facilities performing office-based surgeries with moderate or greater levels of sedation. The law is unique in its mandate that the "surgical suite may not be shared with other practices or other physicians."[43] Reporting to the state is mandatory for any death as a result of office-based surgery within 72 h, unplanned readmission within 72 h if the admission is related to the surgery, and performance of the wrong surgical procedure, wrong patient, or wrong site of surgery. Tennessee also requires the use of objective criteria (Post Anesthesia Recovery or Aldrete Score[44]) to determine when a patient is medically ready to be discharged. The law also requires transfer to a hospital if the patient cannot be discharged safely within 12 h of the initial administration of anesthesia. Tennessee also requires hospital staff privileges for individuals performing office-based surgery. Tennessee does not require accreditation.

TEXAS

Texas Administrative Code 192.1–2[45] provides regulations for facilities that perform office-based surgeries. It does not apply if the facility is operated by a governmental (state or federal) entity or accredited separately by TJC, AAAHC, or AAAASF. The state includes Level I procedures in its governance under the law if the total dosage of the local anesthetic exceeds 50% of the recommended safe dose during the procedure.[45] It is the only state to (potentially) regulate a Level I procedure.

UTAH

Utah has no law that regulates facilities performing office-based surgeries. It does, however, have a statute that governs freestanding ambulatory surgical centers (Rule R432-500).[46]

VERMONT

Vermont has no law that regulates facilities performing office-based surgeries. Independent ASCs, of which Vermont has only one, are not regulated either. There is increasing progress within the state government to establish regulation for these ASC facilities. Senate bill (S.73) is being introduced in 2019.[47]

VIRGINIA

Virginia Administrative Code 85-20-310[48] and 320[49] regulates facilities performing office-based surgeries in the state. The state requires 4 h of continuing education in topics related to anesthesia every 2 years if not using an anesthesiologist or certified registered nurse anesthetist. The law also requires that the procedural consent form should specifically state the board certification or board eligibility of the doctor performing the procedure. It goes onto require a statement that the doctor performing the surgery is not board-certified nor board eligible if applicable. The surgical consent form also must indicate if the surgery is elective or medically necessary. It is the only state to have such a requirement for disclosures in the informed consent form. Reporting to the state is required for deaths within the immediate 72 h postoperative period. Virginia does not require accreditation.

WASHINGTON

Washington's Administrative Code 246-919-601 regulates facilities performing office-based surgeries via its mandates on analgesia and anesthesia administration in office-based settings.[50] Level 1 procedures are excluded from regulation. Washington does require accreditation by TJC, AAAHC, AAAASF, or CMS. The statute does not directly address specific types of surgical procedures.

WEST VIRGINIA

West Virginia has no rule that regulates facilities performing office-based surgeries. West Virginia also does not regulate ASCs in the state. There are only nine Medicare-certified ASCs in West Virginia.

WISCONSIN

Wisconsin has no rule regulating facilities performing office-based surgeries. ASCs are not licensed nor require a COM in Wisconsin.

WYOMING

Wyoming has no rule regulating facilities performing office-based surgeries. It does license ASCs in the state.

Physicians performing procedures in the OEC should know their state's position on the matter. There is great heterogeneity among states in the regulatory process. Future federal regulation affecting this site of service is unlikely. However, further state regulation is inevitable. Stakeholders are advised to read their respective state's statutes or positions on in-office surgeries and adhere to what is prescribed. Often the organization (i.e., State Medical Board, Accreditation organization) responsible for regulation will provide clarification of the process and procedures. If there are questions, medical specialty specifications and scope of practice as defined by the state are key components to note when looking for licensure or accreditation. Finally, as this is a developing area in patient care, future revisions to the statutes and guidelines are bound to happen. It is important to stay informed and cognizant of changes to be able to run a successful office-based endovascular center.

REFERENCES

1. Schmalbach CE. Patient safety and anesthesia considerations for office-based otolaryngology procedures. *Otolaryngol Clin North Am.* 2019;52(3). PIP:S0030-6665(19) 30010-30016.
2. *Guidelines for Office-Based Anesthesia.* Schaumburg (IL): American Society of Anesthesiologists Ambulatory Surgery Care Committee; 2009. Available at: http://www.asahq.org/quality-and-practice-management/standards-guidelines-and-related-resources/guidelines-for-office-based-anesthesia.
3. Patient Safety Principles of Office-Based Surgery. American College of Surgeons. Available at: www.facs.org/education/patient-education/patient-safety/office-based surgery.
4. Office-Based Surgery. Alabama Board of Medical Examiners Administrative Code Chapter 540-X-10. Available at: http://www.alabamaadministrativecode.state.al.us/docs/mexam/540-X-10.pdf.
5. Office-Based Surgery. Arizona Department of Health Services. Available at: https://azmd.gov/Forms/Files/MD_AAC_Title-4_Chapter-16_Article-7_OfficeBasedSurgery_20180328.pdf.
6. Regulation 35 Office-Based Surgery. Arkansas State Board of Health. Available at: https://www.armedicalboard.org/Professionals/pdf/REGULATION%2035%20Office-based%20Surgery.pdf.
7. Article 11.5. Surgery in Certain Outpatient Settings [2215-2217]. Chapter 5. Medicine [2000-2525.5] Division 2. Healing Arts [500-4999.129]. Business and Professions Code. California Law. Available at: https://leginfo.legislature.ca.gov/faces/codes_displayText.xhtml?lawCode=BPC&division=2.&title=&part=&chapter=5.&article=11.5.
8. Article 12. Enforcement [2220-2319]. Chapter 5. Medicine [2000-2525.5] Division 2. Healing Arts [500-4999.129]. Business and Professions Code. California Law. Available at: http://leginfo.legislature.ca.gov/faces/codes_displaySection.xhtml?lawCode=BPC&sectionNum=2240.
9. Chapter 1.3. Outpatient Settings [1248-1248.85]. Division 2. Licensing Provisions [1200-1797.8]. Health and Safety Code. California Law. Available at: http://leginfo.legislature.ca.gov/faces/codes_displaySection.xhtml?lawCode=HSC&sectionNum=1248.2.
10. Ambulatory Surgery Center. Business Licensing Database. Colorado Office of Economic Development and International Trade. Available at: https://www.colorado.gov/oed/industry-license/10IndDetail.html.
11. Connecticut General Statute 19a-493a,b,c. Chapter 368v* Health Care Institutions. Available at: https://www.cga.ct.gov/current/pub/chap_368v.htm.
12. Delaware Title Code16-122 Powers and Duties of the Department of Health and Social Services. Delaware Code Title 16 Health and Safety. Local Boards of Health; Health Programs. Chapter 1. Department of Health and Social Services. Subchapter II. Powers and Duties Generally; Regulations and Orders. Available at: http://delcode.delaware.gov/title16/c001/sc02/index.shtml.
13. Delaware Title Code 16-4408. Facilities that Perform Invasive Medical Procedures. Delaware Administrative Code Title 16. Health Systems Protection. Available at: http://regulations.delaware.gov/AdminCode/title16/Department%20of%20Health%20and%20Social%20Services/Division%20of%20Public%20Health/Health%20Systems%20Protection%20(HSP)/4408.shtml.
14. Health-Care and Community Residence Facility, Hospice and Home Care Licensure Act of 1983, (DC Law 5-48, DC Official Code 44-501-504). Available at: https://dchealth.dc.gov/sites/default/files/dc/sites/doh/publication/attachments/Health_%20Care_and_Community_%20Residence_%20Facility_Hospice_%20Home_%20Care_%20License_%20Act_%20of_%201983_%20DC_%20Law_%205_48.pdf.
15. Standard of Care for Office Surgery. 64B8-9.009. Standards of Practice for Medical Doctors. Florida Administrative Code & Florida Administrative Register. Available at: https://www.flrules.org/gateway/readFile.asp?sid=0&tid=20550243&type=1&file=64B8-9.009.doc.
16. Standards for Basic Anesthetic Monitoring. American Society of Anesthesiologists. Last amended October 28, 2015 (original approval October 21, 1986). Available at: https://www.asahq.org/standards-and-guidelines/standards-for-basic-anesthetic-monitoring.
17. Office-Based Anesthesia and Surgery Guidelines. Georgia Composite Medical Board. Available at: https://medicalboard.georgia.gov/sites/medicalboard.georgia.gov/files/imported/GCMB/Files/OBS%20Guidelines.pdf.
18. Ambulatory Surgery Centers (Freestanding Outpatient Surgical Facilities). State of Hawaii Department of Health,

Office of Health Care Assurance. Available at: http://health.hawaii.gov/ohca/medicare-facilities/ambulatory-surgery-centers-freestanding-outpatient-surgical-facilities/.

19. Ambulatory Surgical Treatment Center Licensing Requirements. Illinois Administrative Code Title 77: Public Health, Chapter I: Department of Public Health, Subchapter b: Hospital and Ambulatory Care Facilities, Part 2015 Ambulatory Surgical Treatment Center Licensing Requirements. Available at: http://www.ilga.gov/commission/jcar/admincode/077/07700205sections.html.
20. Standards of Professional Conduct and Competent Practice of Medicine. 844 Indiana Administrative Code 5-1-5. Available at: http://www.in.gov/legislative/iac/T08440/A00050.PDF?.
21. Ambulatory Surgery Centers. Available at: https://dia-hfd.iowa.gov/DIA_HFD/StreamPDF?cmd=showPDF&dir=entBooksDir&delete=no&doc=EntBook29.
22. Requirements for Office-Based Surgery and Special Procedures. Kansas Administrative Regulations 100-25-3. Kansas State Board of Healing Arts. Available at: https://www.kssos.org/pubs/KAR/2009/5_100_100_Board_of_Healing_Arts_2009_KAR_Vol_5.pdf.
23. Board Opinion Relating to Office-Based Surgery. Kentucky Board of Medical Licensure. Available at: https://kbml.ky.gov/board/Documents/Board%20Opinion%20Office%20Based%20Surgery.pdf.
24. Physician Practice; Office-Based Surgery. Louisiana Administrative Code 46:XLV. Chapter 73. Department of Health and Hospitals, Board of Medical Examiners. Available at: http://www.lsbme.la.gov/sites/default/files/documents/Notices%20of%20Intent/NOI%20and%20NOA/NOA/MD%20Office%20Based%20Surgery%20NOA%20Nov%2011%202014.pdf.
25. Maryland Health Occupations Code 14-101 (2013). Health Occupations Title 14. Physicians. Subtitle 1. Definitions; General Provisions. Available at: https://dhr.maryland.gov/documents/Licensing-and-Monitoring/Maryland%20Law%20Articles/RCC/HEALTH%20OCCUPATIONS%20Title%2014%20Physicians.pdf.
26. Cosmetic Surgical Facilities. Code of Maryland Regulations, Title 10. Maryland Department of Health. Part 3. Subtitle 12. Adult Health. Chapter 10.12.03. Available at: http://mdrules.elaws.us/comar/10.12.03.
27. Office-Based Surgery Guidelines. Massachusetts Medical Society. Available at: http://www.massmed.org/Physicians/Legal-and-Regulatory/Office-Based-Surgery-Guidelines-(pdf)/.
28. Guidelines for Office-Based Anesthesia. American Society of Anesthesiologists. Available at: https://www.asahq.org/~/media/sites/asahq/files/public/resources/standards-guidelines/guidelines-for-office-based-anesthesia.pdf.
29. Office-Based Surgery. Department of Labor, Licensing and Regulation, State Board of Medical Examiners. Chapter 81, Article 9.7. Available at: https://www.scstatehouse.gov/coderegs/Chapter%2081.pdf.
30. In Office Use of Sedation. Michigan Quality Improvement Consortium Guideline. Available at: http://mqic.org/pdf/mqic_in_office_use_of_sedation_cpg.pdf.
31. Outpatient Surgical Centers. Minnesota Administrative Rules. Chapter 4675. Available at: https://www.revisor.mn.gov/rules/4675/.
32. Part 2635: Chapter 1 Surgery/Post-operative Care. Practice of Medicine. Mississippi Secretary of State. Available at: http://www.sos.ms.gov/ACCode/00000291c.pdf.
33. Medical facilities and other related entities. *Nevada Rev Statute Ann.* 449:435–436. Available at: https://www.leg.state.nv.us/NRS/NRS-449.html.
34. Rules for Ambulatory Surgical Centers. New Hampshire Code of Administrative Rules. Available at: https://www.dhhs.nh.gov/oos/bhfa/documents/he-p812.pdf.
35. Surgery, Special Procedures, and Anesthesia Services Performed in an Office Setting. New Jersey Administrative Code Title 13, Law and Public Safety Chapter 35, Board of Medical Examiners. Available at: https://www.njconsumeraffairs.gov/regulations/Chapter-35-Board-of-Medical-Examiners.pdf.
36. Office-Based Surgery. New York State Department of Health, Public Health Law 230-d. Available at: https://www.health.ny.gov/professionals/office-based_surgery/law/docs/230-d.pdf.
37. Office-Based Procedures. North Carolina Medical Board Position Statement. Available at: https://www.ncmedboard.org/resources-information/professional-resources/laws-rules-position-statements/position-statements/office-based_procedures.
38. Accreditation of Office Settings. Ohio Administrative Code, 4731 State Medical Board, Chapter 4731-25 Office Based Surgery. Available at: http://codes.ohio.gov/oac/4731-25-07.
39. Guidelines for Office-Based Surgery and Other Invasive Procedures. Oklahoma State Board of Medical Licensure and Supervision. Available at: http://www.okmedicalboard.org/download/306/Office+Based+Surgery.htm.
40. Office-Based Surgery. Oregon Medical Board, Chapter 847, Division 17. Available at: https://secure.sos.state.or.us/oard/displayDivisionRules.action?selectedDivision=3884.
41. General Information. The Pennsylvania Code, Chapter 55. Available at: https://www.pacode.com/secure/data/028/chapter551/chap551toc.html.
42. Surgical Procedures – General Provisions. Rhode Island General Laws. Title 23 – Health and Safety, Chapter 23–17 – Licensing of Health-Care Facilities, Section 23-17-49. Available at: https://law.justia.com/codes/rhode-island/2017/title-23/chapter-23-17/section-23-17-49/.
43. Office-Based Surgeries. Tennessee Code Title 63 Professions of the Healing Arts, Chapter 6 Medicine and Surgery, Part 2 General Provisions 63-6-221. Available at: https://law.justia.com/codes/tennessee/2010/title-63/chapter-6/part-2/63-6-221/.
44. Ead H. From Aldrete to PADSS: reviewing discharge criteria after ambulatory surgery. *J Perianesth Nurs.* 2006;21:259.

45. Office-Based Anesthesia Services. Texas Administrative Code Title 22 Examining Boards. Part 9 Texas Medical Board. Chapter 192. Available at: https://texreg.sos.state.tx.us/public/readtac$ext.ViewTAC?tac_view=4&ti=22&pt.=9&ch=192&rl=Y.
46. Freestanding Ambulatory Surgical Center Rules. Utah Administrative Code, Rule R432-500. Available at: https://rules.utah.gov/publicat/code/r432/r432-500.htm.
47. S.73 An Act Relating to Licensure of Ambulatory Surgical Centers. Vermont General Assembly 2019–2020 Session. Available at: https://legislature.vermont.gov/bill/status/2020/S.73.
48. Office-Based Anesthesia. Virginia Administrative Code, Title 18. Professional and Occupational Licensing, Agency 85. Board of Medicine, Chapter 20. Regulations Governing the Practice of Medicine, Osteopathic Medicine, Podiatry, and Chiropractic. Available at: https://law.lis.virginia.gov/admincode/title18/agency85/chapter20/section310/.
49. General Provisions. Administrative Code, Title 18. Professional and Occupational Licensing, Agency 85. Board of Medicine, Chapter 20. Regulations Governing the Practice of Medicine, Osteopathic Medicine, Podiatry, and Chiropractic. https://law.lis.virginia.gov/admincode/title18/agency85/chapter20/section320/.
50. Safe and Effective Analgesia and Anesthesia Administration in Office-Based Surgical Settings. Washington Administrative Code, Title 246, Chapter 246-919, Section 246-919-601. Available at: https://app.leg.wa.gov/wac/default.aspx?cite=246-919-601. Accessed March 15, 2019.

FURTHER READING

1. Report of the Special Committee on Outpatient (Office-Based) Surgery. Federation of State Medical Boards. Available at: http://www.fsmb.org/advocacy/policies.
2. Aspen State Regulation Set: T 2.00 Ambulatory Surgical Centers. Health Facilities Certification & Licensing ASPEN: Regulation Set (RS). Available at: http://dhss.alaska.gov/dhcs/Documents/hflc/PDF/Forms/ASC%20State%20ASPEN%20Reg%20Set.pdf.

CHAPTER 3

Legal Issues

MATTHEW KEUTEN, JD • ANDREA N. LEE, JD • JEFF SMITH, JD

Legal considerations are important to the establishment and operation of office-based endovascular center (OEC). Not surprisingly, these issues are complex and quickly changing, and due care is important to ensure that an OEC is properly formed and operated on an ongoing basis in accordance with federal and state laws and regulations. This chapter is intended to (1) serve as an outline of some of the most important laws that must be considered when owning and operating an OEC and (2) address some of the common legal questions that arise in relation to OECs. It is critically important that all practices contemplating or providing services through an OEC consult with healthcare counsel on the specific legal and compliance issues that may apply to the particular circumstances of the OEC enterprise.

DISCLAIMER

This chapter is provided for general informational purposes only. It is not provided in the course of and does not create or constitute an attorney-client relationship, it does not constitute legal advice and should not be considered legal advice, and it is not a substitute for obtaining legal advice from a qualified attorney. You should consult your own attorney to advise you on your particular situation.

LEGAL FRAMEWORK: GENERALLY

Owners and operators of OECs must navigate a complicated framework of federal and state fraud and abuse laws and corporate law when conducting business. Business arrangements where remuneration passes between patient referral sources are highly regulated and can lead to significant civil and criminal penalties. The most common laws and bodies of law that are implicated by OECs are the following, which are described in this chapter in more detail:

- *The Stark Law.* The federal Physician Self-Referral Prohibition (the "Stark Law") is a series of technical Medicare rules that prohibit a physician from making referrals for certain designated health services payable by Medicare to an entity with which he or she (or an immediate family member) has a financial relationship, unless an exception applies.[1]
- *The Anti-Kickback Statute.* The federal Anti-Kickback Statute (the "AKS") is a criminal statute, which makes it a criminal offense to knowingly and willfully offer, pay, solicit, or receive any remuneration to induce or reward referrals of items or services reimbursable by a federal healthcare program.[2]
- *The Corporate Practice of Medicine.* The Corporate Practice of Medicine doctrine is a state law principle that generally prohibits nonlicensed individuals from being owners of a for-profit company organized to practice medicine.
- *Fee Splitting.* State fee-splitting laws generally prohibit physicians from sharing their professional fees with nonprofessionals.

THE STARK LAW

Prohibited Conduct and Penalties

The Stark Law prohibits (1) a physician from making referrals for certain designated health services ("DHS") payable by Medicare to an entity with which he or she (or an immediate family member) has a financial relationship, unless an exception applies, and (2) the entity receiving the referral from submitting claims to Medicare for those referred services.[3] A physician's practice is a DHS entity when furnishing DHS so the referral prohibition applies to referrals within a physician's own practice and could implicate internal referrals from a practice physician to their OEC if the referral is for DHS.

The Stark Law is a "strict liability" law, meaning that a party's intent to incentivize referrals is not required to violate the law.[4] A Stark Law violation can arise from an arrangement that does not actually influence physician referrals, where the parties did not know or should have known that the claims were in violation of the Stark Law, and involves services that were medically necessary.[5]

Office-Based Endovascular Centers. https://doi.org/10.1016/B978-0-323-67969-5.00003-4
Copyright © 2020 Elsevier Inc. All rights reserved.

Penalties for violating the Stark Law can be severe. Any person that presents or causes to be presented a bill or a claim for a service that such person knows or should know is a service for which payment may not be made under the Stark Law is subject to a civil money penalty of not more than $15,000 for each such claim submitted.[6] Additionally, any physician or entity that enters into an arrangement that the physician or entity knows or should know has a principal purpose of circumventing the Stark Law is subject to a civil money penalty of not more than $100,000 for each such arrangement.[7] Further, the Secretary of the Department of Health and Human Services ("HHS") is authorized to exclude any person, organization, agency, or other entity from participation in the Medicare and/or Medicaid programs for a Stark Law violation which results in civil monetary penalties.[8]

Violations of the Stark Law may also serve as a basis for whistleblower *qui tam* or governmental suits under the federal False Claims Act.[9] Violations of the False Claims Act are penalized with treble damages plus civil penalties of up to $10,000 per false claim, in addition to the penalties incurred for a Stark Law violation.[10]

Application of the Stark Law to OECs

To determine whether the Stark Law applies to an OEC, you must first determine whether the OEC does not furnish procedures that are classified as DHS, the Stark Law referral prohibition does not apply to the OEC.

DHS is broadly defined and includes a long list of medical services.[11] With regard to the services typically provided by an OEC, the most likely category of DHS that applies is "radiology and certain other imaging services." Fortunately, CMS maintains and annually updates a list of Current Procedural Terminology ("CPT")/Healthcare Common Procedure Coding System Codes that identify all radiology and imaging services that are DHS ("DHS Code List").[12] To date, many of the services traditionally provided by OECs do not fall within a DHS category and, therefore, many OEC are not subject to the restrictions of the Stark Law.[13] However, each OEC must compare the services it furnishes against the current year's DHS Code List. If the OEC does not furnish procedures that are classified as DHS, the Stark Law referral prohibition does not apply. If an OEC does furnish DHS, the OEC's operations must meet one of the Stark Law exceptions to avoid liability. The two most commonly used exceptions are the "in-office ancillary services" exception and the exception for "physician services."[14]

The prohibition on referrals under the Stark Law does not apply to in-office ancillary services ("IOAS").[15] The IOAS exception is routinely relied on by physician offices that furnish and bill Medicare for DHS, but the exception is very detailed and technical and an arrangement must meet *all* requirements of the exception for the claims generated under the arrangement to not be in violation of the Stark Law. The IOAS exception has requirements related to (1) who may perform the DHS, (2) where the DHS may be performed (e.g., same building or centralized building), (3) who may bill for the DHS, and (4) notice that must be given to patients for certain DHS.[16] Additionally, multiphysician practices may only rely on the IOAS exception if they meet the Stark Law definition of a "group practice," which is additionally onerous.[17] Therefore, while the IOAS exception is useful, compliance with the exception requires meticulous planning and safeguarding.

Similar to the IOAS exception, the prohibition on referrals under the Stark Law does not apply to physician services that are furnished (1) personally by another physician who is a member of the referring physician's group practice or is a physician in the same group practice as the referring physician; or (2) under the personal supervision of another physician who is a member of the referring physician's group practice or is a physician in the same group practice as the referring physician, provided that the supervision complies with all other applicable Medicare payment and coverage rules for the physician services.[18] Thus, like the IOAS exception, one of the keys to satisfying the physician services exception is meeting the Stark Law's definition of a "group practice."

Given the detailed and technical requirements of the IOAS and physician services exceptions and the "group practice" definition, the path of least resistance is to avoid performing DHS services at the OEC and remaining outside the scope of the Stark Law. For OECs that furnish DHS, careful consideration must be given to the available Stark Law exception, which will impact how the OEC can be structured and operated (e.g., who can perform the OEC services, where can the OEC services be performed, and who can bill for the OEC services). Although the Stark Law is not likely to be an insurmountable hurdle for most OECs, caution must be taken when analyzing the requirements and how they will apply to a particular OEC's legal and operational structure.

THE ANTI-KICKBACK STATUTE

Prohibited Conduct and Penalties

Although the AKS has many parallels to the Stark Law, the AKS is focused on "purposeful" arrangements involving offering, soliciting, or receiving remuneration (broadly defined as anything of value) to generate referrals for items or services payable by any federal healthcare program.[19] At its core, the AKS is intended to protect patients from inappropriate medical referrals or recommendations by healthcare professionals who may be unduly influenced by financial incentives.[20]

The AKS makes it illegal to knowingly and willfully offer, pay, solicit, or receive any remuneration to induce, or in return for, referrals of items or services reimbursable by a federal healthcare program.[21] Prohibited remuneration includes cash payments, bribes, and rebates, whether made directly or indirectly, in cash or in kind.[22] The AKS is broadly drafted and establishes penalties for individuals and entities on both sides of the prohibited transaction.[23] The penalties include imprisonment and substantial civil and criminal penalties, as well as the possibility of exclusion from federal health programs.[24] An AKS violation is, by statute, also a false claim under the False Claims Act.[25]

Because of the breadth of the AKS, the Office of Inspector General, US Department of Health and Human Services (the "OIG"), has promulgated certain "safe harbors" that protect arrangements that would otherwise potentially implicate the AKS. If each element of the safe harbor is met, the arrangement is statutorily exempt from prosecution.[26] Unlike the Stark Law's exceptions (which are mandatory), the AKS's safe harbors are voluntary. If an arrangement falls outside of safe harbor protection, the conduct is not per se illegal because the AKS is an intent-based statute. Rather, the arrangement is judged on a case-by-case basis to determine if the parties "knowingly and willfully" solicited, offered, received, or paid remuneration to induce or reward a referral under a federal healthcare program.

Application of the AKS to OECs: Multispecialty Practices

A common OECarrangement that implicates the AKS is a multispecialty practice that makes payments to nonprocedure performing physicians (e.g., primary care physicians or nephrologists) in relation to their referrals to the OEC, such as a dividend paid as a return on an investment interest in the OEC. The potential exposure relates to the possibility that underlying payments to the referring physicians are not legitimate returns on investment, but rather disguised prohibited payments that are made with improper intent to incentive the nonprocedure performing physician to send referrals to the OEC. Fortunately, the AKS has an available safe harbor to address these concerns.

The AKS "investment in group practices" safe harbor protects returns on investment interests, such as a dividend or interest income, made to a group practitioner investing in his/her own group practice if the following four standards are met:

- The equity interests in the practice or group must be held by licensed healthcare professionals who practice in the practice or group;
- The equity interests must be in the practice or group itself, and not some subdivision of the practice or group;
- Revenues from ancillary services, if any, must be derived from "in-office ancillary services" that meet the definition of such terms in the Stark Law (described above); and
- In the case of group practices, the practice must (1) meet the "group practice" definition in the Stark Law (described above) and (2) be a unified business with centralized decision-making, pooling of expenses and revenues, and a compensation/profit distribution system that is not based on satellite offices operating substantially as if they were separate enterprises or profit centers.[27]

Although not all OECs must comply with the Stark Law (specifically, those OECs that do not furnish DHS), the Stark Law's IOAS exception and definition of a "group practice" are incorporated into the AKS "investment in group practices" safe harbor. Specifically, to meet the safe harbor, the practice must derive revenue from ancillary services from "in-office ancillary services" as defined in the Stark Law and meet the Stark Law's definition of a "group practice." OEC models that do not comply with these safe harbor requirements may be subject to additional scrutiny. Thus, any OEC that is structured outside of the safe harbor must be subject to careful risk analysis with respect to compliance with the AKS.[28]

It is important to remember that failure to satisfy an AKS safe harbor does not mean that the arrangement is illegal. Arrangements that fall outside of safe harbor protection are evaluated on a case-by-case basis to determine if the requisite intent exists for the arrangement to constitute a violation of the AKS. And, there are any number of legitimate reasons as to why an arrangement may fall outside of a safe harbor and still be legal. For example, assuming the state corporate law permits such an arrangement, it is possible that a multispecialty practice operating an OEC could have a nonphysician owner and otherwise operate in a permissible manner under the AKS. In that scenario, the multispecialty practice would not meet the "investment in group practices" safe harbor because of the nonlicensed equity owner, provided that any payments made to nonprocedure performing physicians where not made with improper intent, no violation of the AKS would exist.

Application of the AKS to OECs: management arrangements

Another way an OEC may implicate the AKS is through the use of a management services arrangement. Many physician practices lack the knowledge, time, and resources to establish an OEC on their own. In turn, these practices affiliate with management companies that have the requisite expertise to stand up and manage an OEC for their practice. While this is generally viewed as a legitimate and market practice, these arrangements are not without risk and can present exposure under the AKS if not structured properly.

The OIG has expressed long-standing concerns about certain complex contractual arrangements that the OIG has labeled "contractual joint ventures."[29] According to the OIG, a "contractual joint venture" is a "questionable contractual arrangement where a healthcare provider in one line of business (hereafter referred to as the 'Owner') expands into a related healthcare business by contracting with an existing provider of a related item or service (hereafter referred to as the 'Manager/Supplier') to provide the new item or service to the Owner's existing patient population... The Manager/Supplier not only manages the new line of business, but may also supply it with inventory, employees, space, billing, and other services. In other words, the Owner contracts out substantially the entire operation of the related line of business to the Manager/Supplier—otherwise a potential competitor—receiving in return the profits of the business as remuneration for its... referrals."[30]

The OIG views contractual joint ventures as problematic under the AKS because "by agreeing effectively to provide services it could otherwise provide in its own right for less than the available reimbursement, the Manager/Supplier is providing the Owner with the opportunity to generate a fee and a profit. The opportunity to generate a fee is itself remuneration that may implicate the anti-kickback statute [and is not protected by any available anti-kickback safe harbor.]"[31] Such an arrangement is potentially harmful because it could "(1) distort medical decision-making, (2) cause overutilization, (3) increase costs to the federal healthcare programs, and (4) result in unfair competition by freezing out competitors unwilling to pay kickbacks."[32]

Based on the current state of the OIG guidance, any that will be operated pursuant to a management arrangement should be reviewed by legal counsel to determine that it does not violate the AKS. While management arrangements are commonplace in the industry, there is increased risk associated with such arrangements and due care should be taken to eliminate all avoidable exposure.[33]

THE CORPORATE PRACTICE OF MEDICINE

In addition to the federal prohibitions and penalties described above, the question of how the OEC is to be organized as a legal entity and who may permissibly own an OEC involves an analysis of state laws, some of which specifically address the requirements for how a professional medical practice may be incorporated or formed, and others of which address the requirements for that practice to lawfully provide and bill for patient services.

The Corporate Practice of Medicine ("CPOM") doctrine is a state law principle that generally prohibits a business entity from practicing medicine or employing a physician to provide professional medical services. Many states have a CPOM prohibition, and the scope of the prohibition varies greatly from state to state. CPOM prohibitions can be found in different forms of state law, including under statute and applicable rules and regulations and court and Attorney General opinions.

CPOM prohibitions are generally intended to prohibit arrangements by which a nonphysician will share in the fees charged by a physician for medical services. In many states, the owners (shareholders or members) of a professional entity (PC, PLLC, or other entity allowed under state law to engage in the practice of medicine) must *all* be licensed to practice medicine.[34] Underlying CPOM is the concern that nonphysicians may influence patient care decisions based on profit motives, and that medical care decisions should be left solely to licensed professionals. Consequently, states with CPOM laws generally prohibit nonphysicians from employing physicians, or nonphysicians from joining with physicians in the ownership of a medical practice.

OECs must ensure compliance with all applicable CPOM laws that apply to the OEC in its state(s) of organization and operation. For example, similar to medical practices, the state in which the OEC is operating may not permit the OEC to be owned by an individual who is not a licensed physician. One way to potentially shortcut any burdensome analysis and achieve compliance is to establish an OEC as part of an existing medical practice, which assumes, however, that the original medical practice was properly organized under state law. It is worth noting, however, that compliance with corporate law does not equate to compliance with healthcare regulatory requirements and care must be taken to address the full range of these issues when considering how an OEC should be organized.

FEE SPLITTING

In addition to CPOM laws, many states have laws which prohibit or criminalize the division of patient fees between physicians, or a physician and a nonphysician. These laws, which are commonly referred to as "fee-splitting" laws, are generally akin to the AKS insofar as they are intended to stop the improper payment for referrals between physicians or other individuals or entities. Like CPOM prohibitions, fee-splitting laws can be found in different forms of state law including licensure statutes, case law, and anti-kickback laws.

Fee-splitting laws are commonly implicated when OECs are managed by a management services organization in exchange for a percentage of revenue. When utilizing a management arrangement, particular care must be taken with regard to structuring the management fees in consideration of state fee-splitting laws, which vary greatly. For example, New York law prohibits physicians from splitting their fees with individuals not licensed to provide healthcare services. The implementing regulation expressly sets forth that "[t]his prohibition shall include any arrangement or agreement whereby the amount received in payment for furnishing space, facilities, equipment or personnel services used by a professional licensee constitutes a **percentage** of, or is otherwise dependent upon, the income or receipts of the licensee from such practice [.]"[35] In contrast, Michigan's fee-splitting laws are not as broad and do not expressly prohibit, nor have they been interpreted by the Michigan judiciary or the Attorney General to prohibit, percentage-based compensation models.[36]

The wide variance in fee-splitting laws necessitates the need for any OEC being operated pursuant to a management arrangement to be reviewed by experienced local counsel to review the arrangement from the perspective of the state laws in which the OEC operates.

SUMMARY

A well-organized and efficient OEC facility can be a great enhancement to the practice of vascular medicine. Through proper planning and implementation, potential legal and regulatory hurdles can be minimized or avoided, while at the same time facilitating the practice's utilization of the OEC resources for the benefit of its patients.

ENDNOTES

1. 42 U.S.C. § 1395nn.
2. 42 U.S.C. § 1320(a)-7b(b).
3. 42 U.S.C. §§ 1395nn(a)(1), (g)(1). The Stark Law does not directly apply to Medicaid, but it does prohibit federal Medicaid subsidies from being used by the state to reimburse referrals that would be prohibited under Medicare. 42 USC § 1396b(s). Additionally, the Stark Law allows states to establish their own self-referral laws, and many states have done so in a variety of ways.
4. 42 U.S.C. § 1395(a).
5. 42 C.F.R. § 411.353(c)(2).
6. 42 U.S.C. § 1395nn(g)(3)
7. 42 U.S.C. § 1395nn(g)(4); 42 C.F.R. § 1003.102(b)(10).
8. 42 U.S.C. §§ 1395nn(g)(3), (g)(4); 42 C.F.R. § 1001.901.
9. 31 U.S.C. § 3729(a).
10. 31 U.S.C. § 3729(a); 28 C.F.R. § 85.3(a)(9); 42 U.S.C. § 1320a–7a.
11. DHS includes the following services, when payable, in whole or in part, by Medicare: (1) clinical laboratory services; (2) physical therapy, occupational therapy, and outpatient speech-language pathology services; (3) radiology and certain other imaging services; (4) radiation therapy services and supplies; (5) durable medical equipment and supplies; (6) parenteral and enteral nutrients, equipment, and supplies; (7) prosthetics, orthotics, and prosthetic devices and supplies; (8) home health services; (9) outpatient prescription drugs; and inpatient and outpatient hospital services. 42 C.F.R. § 411.351.
12. Centers for Medicare and Medicaid Services, *Code List for Certain Designated Health Services (DHS)* (last updated November 23, 2018) https://www.cms.gov/Medicare/Fraud-and-Abuse/PhysicianSelfReferral/List_of_Codes.html.
13. When compared against a list of CPT codes for Interventional Cardiology, Peripheral Intervention, and Rhythm Management procedures published by the Boston Scientific Corporation, none of the procedures appeared on the CMS DHS Code List.

14. 42 C.F.R. § 411.355(b). There is also an exception to the definition of a "referral" under the Stark Law for self-referred or self-performed services. 42 U.S.C. 1395nn(h)(5)(A); 42 C.F.R. 411.351. A "referral" under the Stark Law has a detailed regulatory definition: "the request by a physician for, or ordering of, or the certifying or recertifying of the need for, any designated health service for which payment may be made under Medicare Part B, including a request for a consultation with another physician and any test or procedure ordered by or to be performed by (or under the supervision of) that other physician." 42 C.F.R. 411.351. A physician does not make a "referral" under the Stark Law, and the Stark Law is not implicated, *when the physician personally performs the DHS he or she has ordered*. The personal performance does not extend to the physician's employees, independent contractors, or group practice members.
15. 42 U.S.C. § 1395nn(b)(2).
16. 42 C.F.R. § 411.355b.
17. A "group practice" is defined as a single legal entity, with at least two physician members, which operates as a unified business, where each physician member furnishes substantially the full range of patient care services that the physician routinely furnishes through the joint use of shared office space, facilities, equipment, and personnel, where "substantially all" (at least 75%) of the total patient care services provided by group members are furnished through the group, billed under the group's billing number, and with receipts for those services being treated as receipts of the group. 42 U.S.C. § 1395nn(h)(4)(A).
18. 42 U.S.C. § 1395nn(b)(1).
19. 42 U.S.C. §1320a-7b.
20. See, e.g., OIG Special Fraud Alert: Laboratory Payments to Referring Physicians (June 24, 2014).
21. 42 U.S.C. § 1320a–7b.
22. See, e.g., Office of Inspector General, Roadmap for New Physicians: Fraud & Abuse Laws (last accessed April 10, 2019) https://oig.hhs.gov/compliance/physician-education/01laws.asp.
23. 42 U.S.C. § 1320a–7b(b)(1).
24. 42 U.S.C. §§1320a–7b(a)-(g).
25. 42 U.S.C. §1320a–7b(g); 42 C.F.R. § 1001.951
26. 42 C.F.R. § 1001.952
27. 42 C.F.R. § 1001.952(p).
28. OECs would also be well advised to structure their arrangements for physicians that provide services to the OEC, either as employees or independent contractors, to fall within the AKS "bona fide employee" or "personal services" safe harbors. However, payments to owners that constitute a return on investment would need to qualify under the investments in group practices or investment interests safe harbor.
29. 68 Fed. Reg. 23148 (Apr. 30, 2003). The Special Advisory Bulletin is also available on the OIG's web page at http://oig.hhs.gov/fraud/docs/alertsandbulletins/042303SABJointVentures.pdf.
30. *See* The Special Advisory Bulletin is also available on the OIG's web page at http://oig.hhs.gov/fraud/docs/alertsandbulletins/042303SABJointVentures.pdf.
31. 68 Fed. Reg. at 23150.
32. 68 Fed. Reg. at 23148.
33. As it relates to potential risks, see, e.g., OIG Advisory Opinion No. 11-03 (April 14, 2011).
34. State law may require that the physician be licensed in the state in which the entity is formed or conducting business.
35. 4 N.Y. Comp. R. & Regs. Tit. 8 § 29.1.b (**emphasis added**).
36. In Michigan, "[d]ividing fees for referral of patients or accepting kickbacks on medical or surgical services, appliances, or medications purchased by or in behalf of patients" is an "unethical business practice" that may result in a licensed health professional being subject to disciplinary proceedings. Mich. Comp. Laws § 750.428. Additionally, under the Michigan Penal Code, "[a]ny physician or surgeon who shall divide fees with or shall promise to pay a part of his or her fee to or pay a commission to any other physician or surgeon or person who calls him or her in consultation or sends patients to him or her for treatment or operation, and any physician or surgeon who shall receive any money prohibited by this section, is guilty of a misdemeanor punishable by imprisonment for not more than 6 months or a fine of not more than $750.00." Mich. Comp. Laws § 750.428.

CHAPTER 4

Business Plan

HWA KHO, PHD, MBA • SAM AHN, MD, FACS, MBA

The benefits of having an office-based endovascular center (OEC) have become obvious to many physicians: greater financial rewards and control over their time for the physicians and greater satisfaction for the patients. However, while many OECs have indeed become very successful, there are many others that have failed or are struggling to stay afloat. There are many reasons why OECs fail. Some of the reasons have to do with physicians not fully understanding the intricacies of running an OEC. There is no way to eliminate all the risks of starting a new OEC but formulating a sound business plan before embarking on the venture will help physicians understand, anticipate, and avoid problems down the road.

The business plan does not have to be very elaborate, but it should address two crucial areas—financial viability and a road map for managing the OEC. It needs to demonstrate, using assumptions that are as realistic as possible, the financial viability of the OEC. This will help set realistic expectations and marshal adequate resources for the venture. Second, even if the financial prediction is promising, the physicians need to have a plan to manage the business so that it can realize the financial rewards. It is very easy to overlook this part and underestimate the amount of work and organization it takes to run a successful OEC.

FINANCIAL CONSIDERATIONS

Predicting Revenue

In order to predict revenue, we need to know the type and mix of procedures, the volume, the payer mix, and average reimbursements. Many times, a physician's "gut" estimate of the number of cases they can do in an OEC turns out to be quite different in practice. That is because there are many not-so-obvious constraints and limitations on what procedures can be done in the OEC in a practice.

What kind of procedures will the physicians do?

First of all, regardless of profitability, the physicians need to know the kind of procedures the physicians anticipate doing in the OEC. Are these procedures, in fact, allowed to be done in the OEC? The Medicare Fee Schedule generally provides a good guide as a first pass. If Medicare allows a higher fee differential for a given CPT code in an office setting (Place of Service 11), as is the case of the majority of endovascular procedures, that indicates that Medicare expects that procedure may be done in an OEC, and implicitly, that the standard of care allows the procedure to be done in the OEC. In some case, the Medicare Fee Schedule will also clearly indicate Medicare does not expect a procedure to be performed in an OBL, such as carotid stenting and endovascular repair of an abdominal aortic aneurysm. In many cases, Medicare does not explicitly disallow a procedure to be performed in an OEC, but the absence of a higher differential fee for the OEC setting makes these procedures not financially viable to be done in the OEC.

Unfortunately, Medicare is not the final arbiter of which procedures may be performed in an OEC. In some cases, states may have additional restrictions on which kind of procedures may be performed in an OEC. Physicians need to check with their state restrictions or other licensure requirements for the kind of procedures they intended to do. In certain states, some private insurance companies may pay for the procedure to be performed in the office while Medicare does not and vice versa.

Office-Based Endovascular Centers. https://doi.org/10.1016/B978-0-323-67969-5.00004-6
Copyright © 2020 Elsevier Inc. All rights reserved.

What is the payer mix and what are the procedures profitable enough to do?

Not every procedure that can be done in the OEC is worth doing in the OEC. The payment has to be high enough to cover supplies, labor, and overheads. Most vascular OECs will have a high percentage of Medicare patients, and fortunately, Medicare publishes its fee schedule online and it is relatively easy to calculate Medicare payments. Most commercial payers' fees are close to Medicare's and will depend on your negotiated contracts with them.

Practices with a lot of Medicaid patients will have to be particularly careful to make sure that they will not be operating at a loss. Medicaid rates vary from state to state but are generally lower than Medicare rates. In many states, for certain CPT codes, they may be so much lower that they do not even cover the cost of supplies. The physicians will have to analyze the payments by CPT codes and may have to exclude certain cases from the OEC based on financial viability. Similarly, the physicians will have to analyze other major payers in their payer mix and see if the contracted rates are financially viable for the procedures they intend to do.

Even if the contracted rates seem to be financially viable, physicians need to determine if the payers will allow their patients to be treated in the OEC. Many HMOs/IPAs (Independent Physician Association) are reluctant to authorize treatments in the OECs even though their contracts do not explicitly exclude OECs. The reason is that most IPAs are financially responsible only for the physician fee component of their members' treatments, and the health plans cover the facility component. Since the facility fee is rolled into the physician fee in the OEC, the IPAs end up paying a much higher fee to the physicians when the patient is treated in the OEC as compared with the patient receiving treatment in an ASC or hospital outpatient department. For example, if the procedure is done in the OEC, the IPA may have to pay $15,000 for a lower extremity revascularization, whereas if the member had the procedure done in the hospital that fee would have been split between the IPA and the health plan. The IPA may have to pay $1000 only to the physician for the professional fee, and the hospital will bill the member's health plan for the facility fee. Unfortunately, the IPAs, and not the health plans, control where the patient may receive treatment and they have little incentive to authorize treatment in the OEC. For physicians with a significant number of HMO patients in their practice, this economic reality will drastically limit the number of cases they can do in the OEC.

What is the volume?

Going through the exercises described above will help the physicians refine the volume of procedures that are allowed and financially viable to do in the OEC. They will probably not be starting with this number, so the business plan needs to allow for a realistic ramp up in volume over a period of time. You should look at the CPT codes for the procedures you are planning to do in the OEC, billed by the practice in the last 12 months and create a proforma based on 50% of these numbers.

What is the case mix?

The volume of procedures by itself is not sufficient to get a good estimate of revenue. A fistulogram pays much less than a lower extremity revascularization with stent and atherectomy. So, it is important to estimate the case mix and calculate the average payment for each category of cases. In calculating the payment for a sample case, bear in mind that almost all payers apply a multiple procedure discount rule, i.e., they pay 100% of the most expensive surgical CPT code and 50% for the next surgical code. Some added procedures carried out simultaneously may not be paid at all.

With the information as outlined, the number of procedures, types of procedures, average payment per procedure for each type, one should be able to make a reasonably good prediction of revenue collection and create a proforma. If you are applying for a loan, the bank will require the proforma. You still need to calculate the expenses.

Operating Expenses

The major operating expenses will be the following:

Supplies

For a busy practice, supplies and other disposables will be the biggest operating cost (Chapter 7). The cost of supplies is usually bundled into the reimbursements for OEC procedures and cannot be billed separately. The cost of supplies could range from a few hundred dollars for a diagnostic angiogram to several thousand dollars for a revascularization procedure using atherectomy device and stent. In general, the cost of supplies ranges from 15% to 40% of reimbursement depending on the type of procedure and how frugally the physician manages devices. For a more accurate estimate of the total cost of supplies, estimate the cost for each type of case from the case mix.

Staffing

Staffing is the other major component of operating costs. The bare minimum staff consists of:

- Nurse Manager
- Circulating and Recovery Nurse(s)
- Scrub Tech(s)
- X-ray Tech(s)
- Medical Assistant(s)

The nurse manager role is to oversee the day-to-day clinical operations of the endovascular suite, enforce policies and procedures, and oversee compliance with federal and state regulations covering operation of the intervention suite. In a small practice, this role could be played by one of the physicians. However, in a busy practice, it is essential to have one person, ideally a nurse, be dedicated full time to this role. A registered nurse is required to provide care or supervise care in the recovery area. If the physician is providing the conscious sedation, a registered nurse will be required to monitor the patient and administer drugs during the procedure.

In addition to the clinical staff, the practice may need to hire additional clerical and administrative staff to help with the increased workload needed to support the operations of the OEC, such as ordering and managing supplies, coding and billing. An alternative to hiring and training new employees is to outsource some of these functions to third parties.

Some of these positions could be part-time or per diem, especially when the OEC is just starting. If this is a totally new practice, the usual practice staff—Office Manager, schedulers, receptionists, and clerical assistants will also have to be hired. In a typical midsize OEC, staffing costs could run between $40K and $60K per month.

If the practice hires physicians on a fixed salary, those costs have to be included in the business plan as well. We discuss physician compensation in more detail below.

Rent and utilities

Rent and utilities are fixed cost and will typically be about $10K–$30K/month depending on the location. Cost of build out will be reflected in the rent. Most leasing companies will want at-least a 5 year lease.

Equipment leases

The total cost of the equipment in the OBL will range from $500K to $1M. However, much of this will probably be financed through loans or leases so that the practice does not have to bear this expense all at once but spread it over several years.

In using leases to obtain equipment, it is important for the physicians to understand the difference between two types of leases—capital lease and operating lease. A capital lease operates like a loan. It will require more cash outlay every month, but the lessee will have the right to buy the equipment for less than fair market value, typically $1, at the end of the lease. An operating lease is similar to renting the equipment. At the end of the lease term, the lessor maintains ownership of the equipment, and the physicians will have to get a new lease, buy the equipment at fair market value, or get replacement equipment.

Only the interest payment and depreciation of the equipment is considered an operating expense in a capital lease. In an operating lease, the full monthly lease payment is considered an operating expense and no depreciation on the equipment may be taken. The physicians may want to consult an accountant to decide which type of lease is more advantageous in their particular financial situation. The main thing for the physicians to understand is that capital lease requires more cash outlay every month but they get to keep the equipment at the end of the lease, whereas the operating lease requires less cash outlay but they will either have to buy the equipment at fair market value or get a new lease. One of the advantages of a capital lease is that the cash outlay for equipment will end once the equipment has been paid off after the first few years and profit margin of the lab will improve.

Outside services

Other miscellaneous items and services such as hazardous waste, utilities, disposal, linen service, accreditation fees and consultations, added insurance cost, attorney and accounting fees, could also add up to another $5–$10K/month.

Setup Costs

Build-out

A major cost of setting up the OEC is the build-out. Building out a new space can be very expensive, bearing in mind that it is not just the cost of construction, but also architect's fee, possibly attorney's fee, permits, and so on. Depending on the starting point, reconfiguration of an existing space or a major renovation, the cost could range from a hundred thousand to over a million dollars. A power generator should be included in the build out to provide electrify if there is a power failure. One needs to pay special attention to the cost of build-out as it can easily get out of hand. In a leased space the leaser may be able to share in some part of the cost of build-out.

Equipment

The basic equipment for the intervention suite includes the following:

(i) Fluoroscopy unit
(ii) Imaging table
(iii) Backup power supply
(iv) Defibrillator
(v) Crash cart
(vi) Anesthesia cart
(vii) Ultrasound scanner
(viii) Patient monitors
(ix) Stretchers
(x) Sterilizer
(xi) IV stands
(xii) Stainless steel tables
(xiii) Lead aprons
(xiv) Bovie
(xv) Power injector
(xvi) OR lights

The most expensive equipment will be the fluoroscopy unit. A mobile unit is less expensive than a fixed unit and should be adequate for most practices. A new C-arm and imaging table with the appropriate resolution and vascular software package will cost around $300K–$500K. Other items include patient monitors, stretchers, crash cart, power injector, and ultrasound scanners. Purchasing refurbished equipment will reduce the cost but maintenance may be costlier, and if the equipment is down for any substantial period it could result in significant revenue loss.

Supplies

The practice needs to set up an initial stock of supplies. The kind of supplies will depend on the type of cases and the physicians' personal preferences for different devices for various procedures. If there are multiple physicians in the practice, they should develop a consensus about the use of various devices. The OEC is not a hospital and cannot afford to have individual physician preference for each procedure. The OEC should have 1–2 weeks of supplies on hand. Some items may be obtained on a consignment basis. The practice does not pay for consigned items until they are used. Depending on the anticipated volume, the initial cost of supplies will range from $100K to $300K.

Information Technology (IT)

Information technology should not be overlooked—it is essential to have the ability to manage an OEC efficiently (Chapter 7). IT expenses for electronic health records/practice management system, inventory management system, email services, telecommunication services, etc. could easily add up to $5-$10K/month depending on the number of physicians as license fee for electronic health records is usually based on number of users. Software and IT services for the most part can be expensed as part of the monthly operating costs. The setup cost is for connectivity. The facility needs to be adequately wired and connected to the Internet—and needs hardware such as servers, network routers, computers, and tablets. Staff and physicians need to have adequate and easy access to computers. The setup cost would be in the range of $20k–$40k.

Working capital

Although not strictly a setup cost, the practice should set aside or arrange for enough funds for working capital for at least 3–6 months of operations. The volume will probably be low initially and take time to ramp up, and even when everything is working smoothly, it takes 1–3 months for payments to start coming in for the procedures done in the OEC. There are fixed expenses that have to be paid regardless of whether the OEC is fully utilized or not and the practice does not want to be caught in a cash crunch.

MANAGEMENT

In an OEC, physicians have full ownership of patient safety. The stakes are higher than doing surgery in a hospital where there may be other resources to fall back on. Managing an OEC is much like managing a small surgery department in a hospital and a small business at the same time. It requires a level of knowledge of regulatory requirements and compliance, revenue cycle management, business management, and organization that most practices normally do not have. It is important for physicians to think ahead and plan how they would run the OEC or get outside help.

Management Company

One solution is to hire an experienced management company to help run the OEC. The management company can help develop the business plan and implement it. The company can train the staff on appropriate policies and procedures and help obtain accreditation. It can oversee the coding and billing or do the billing for OEC. Among other things, it can help with marketing and provide ongoing training. If the practice decides to manage the OEC itself, then it needs to make sure it has the administrative staff who will have the expertise to carry out these tasks. It may need to recruit additional staff and provide them with ongoing training.

Accreditation

Unlike ASC, CMS does not require any special licensure or accreditation for OEC. Some states may require accreditation, and physicians should check with their states. However, it is good practice to seek accreditation with a national accreditation organization such as the Joint Commission, AAAHC, or AAAASF even if the practice is not required to do so. Having outside validation of the quality of the OEC is not just good for marketing but also helps to maintain a culture of quality and compliance which is crucial for patient safety and the longevity of the OEC.

Coding and Billing

The practice should seriously consider outsourcing its coding and billing to a billing company that is experienced in billing for endovascular procedures in the OEC. Endovascular procedures could be very challenging to code. A single case could involve dozens of codes with complex coding rules. The coding process is typically a bottleneck in getting the claims out quickly. An OEC is expensive to maintain and the practice's cash flow could get into trouble very quickly if collection was denied or delayed because of poor coding and billing. Over coding and under coding are both illegal and can result in fines. Medicare and most major payers take at least 3 weeks to pay a clean claim after they have received it. It is imperative to code the procedures fully and correctly, with adequate documentation for optimal reimbursement and to submit the claim as quickly as possible.

The risk of using in-house coders and billers is that most practices cannot afford to hire sufficiently skilled coders and billers, provide them with continuing education or keep them current with industry development, or have a sufficiently large pool of employees to mitigate against a key employee leaving or taking time off. Often, when a key coder or biller is absent, the revenue cycle grinds to a halt and collection suffers. Outsourcing to a good billing company would mitigate against these problems.

Physician Compensation

Physician compensation is an often-overlooked topic, but implementing an appropriate formula for physician compensation is hugely important to the success or failure of the OEC. There is no one right (magic) formula for every practice. The compensation formula will depend on the ownership of the practice. All the physicians may be owners, some may be employees, or some are employees now but will become owners in the future. However, there are three critical aspects the formula should address:

(i) At least part of it should be based on productivity, so that physicians are rewarded for their work.
(ii) It should incentivize physicians to contain costs.
(iii) It should be perceived as fair to all the physicians.

The physician compensation formula can be a powerful tool to align all the physicians' interests in building a productive and financially successful OEC, and it is well worth it to put a lot of thought into it. Otherwise successful OECs have failed for misaligned compensation schemes or physician conflicts over compensation.

Cost of capitol

The practice may have to borrow money to start the OEC. The interest rates and term of the loan should be carefully negotiated and accounted for while developing the business plan. A heavy debt load can negatively impact the OEC.

Proforma

Once the practice has calculated the expected revenue, fixed cost, operating expenses, need for working capital, and projected growth, a proforma can be created. It is important to have a proforma which is based on facts and conservative projections rather than emotions and best-case scenarios. The financial institutions and leasing companies will need it to finance the project.

CONCLUSION

Building a new OEC can be a very rewarding endeavor for the physician practice and for patients. It is a major project that will reshape how the practice works. With the rewards also comes greater risks, both financial and professional. Building a sound business plan before beginning the process will help to provide more realistic expectations of the rewards as well as the risks, and set out a road map for mitigating against some of the potential potholes down the road. This chapter points out some of the most important issues to consider in the business plan.

CHAPTER 5

Building Plan

HWA KHO, PHD, MBA • SAM AHN, MD, FACS, MBA • MAGEAN WHALEY, RN

Building out an office-based endovascular center (OEC) is an expensive and time-consuming project, and it is critical to get it right because the practice will be stuck with it for a long time. Below, we go over some of the most important things to consider for the OEC.

ZONING AND PERMITS

Make sure that the intended location is zoned and permitted for operating an OEC. Getting the zoning law changed or getting a new permit is costly and takes a very long time. It is usually not worth it to look at locations that are not already appropriately zoned for an OEC. Since it is an extension of practice it may be easier to get the permit than getting permit for an ambulatory surgery center.

Certificate of Need (CON) usually does not apply to OEC but the practice should check if it does in their state as well for other licenses or permits required by the local city or state. Fig. 5.1 below shows states with some form of CON laws (in blue).

LOCATION

The OEC should ideally be situated within 5 miles or 15 min of a major hospital in case of an adverse event, and a patient needs to be urgently transferred to a hospital. Though this should rarely happen, it is, nevertheless inevitable that over the course of time in the life of the OEC, complications will occur, and when they do, it is crucial that patients can be transported to a hospital in a timely manner.

It should be easy for patients to reach, and, especially in metropolitan areas, have adequate and convenient parking for patients when they arrive. A ground floor location is desirable, with a separate emergency entrance for ambulance personnel. If it is on an upper floor, make sure the elevators are big enough to accommodate stretchers. Depending on the type of your practice it may be desirable to have OEC close to dialysis centers and/or wound care clinics.

SPACE

Procedure Room

The more space that can be allocated to the procedure room, the easier it will be to configure the space to work efficiently for the physicians and staff. When you have the performing physician, scrub technician, circulating nurse, X-ray technician, anesthesiologist or certified registered nurse anesthetist, the patient, the C-ARM, the laser machine, anesthesia cart, and bunch of other machines in the room, it can get crowded very fast. It should be at least 600 sf but preferably larger so that there is space for storing devices and other disposables for easy access during a procedure. If a room is used exclusively for vein ablation procedures it may be smaller than the main procedure room. Number of procedure rooms will depend on the projected volume of cases and number of physicians working in the OEC.

The walls will normally need to be lead-lined. The requirement for lead-lining depends on a number of factors, including occupancy of the space behind the wall, size of the room, radiation pattern and power of the C-ARM, and the procedure volume or radiation time. The practice should consult with a medical physicist to determine if lead lining is needed. It also depends on state board of health regulations. In general, it is advisable to lead line the walls.

The floor of the room may need to be reinforced to support the weight of the C-ARM and other machines such as the laser machine. This is especially an issue to bear in mind if the room is not located on the ground floor. Make sure that there are enough power outlets with the right voltage and current for the machines to be used in the room. There is usually no special HVAC requirement for an OEC but for the comfort of the procedure room staff and the patient, provide for adequate air conditioning to keep the room cool. The room can feel very warm for the physicians and staff with heavy lead aprons in a crowded area under the OR lights. There should preferably be a separate temperature control for the procedure room so that the

Office-Based Endovascular Centers. https://doi.org/10.1016/B978-0-323-67969-5.00005-8
Copyright © 2020 Elsevier Inc. All rights reserved.

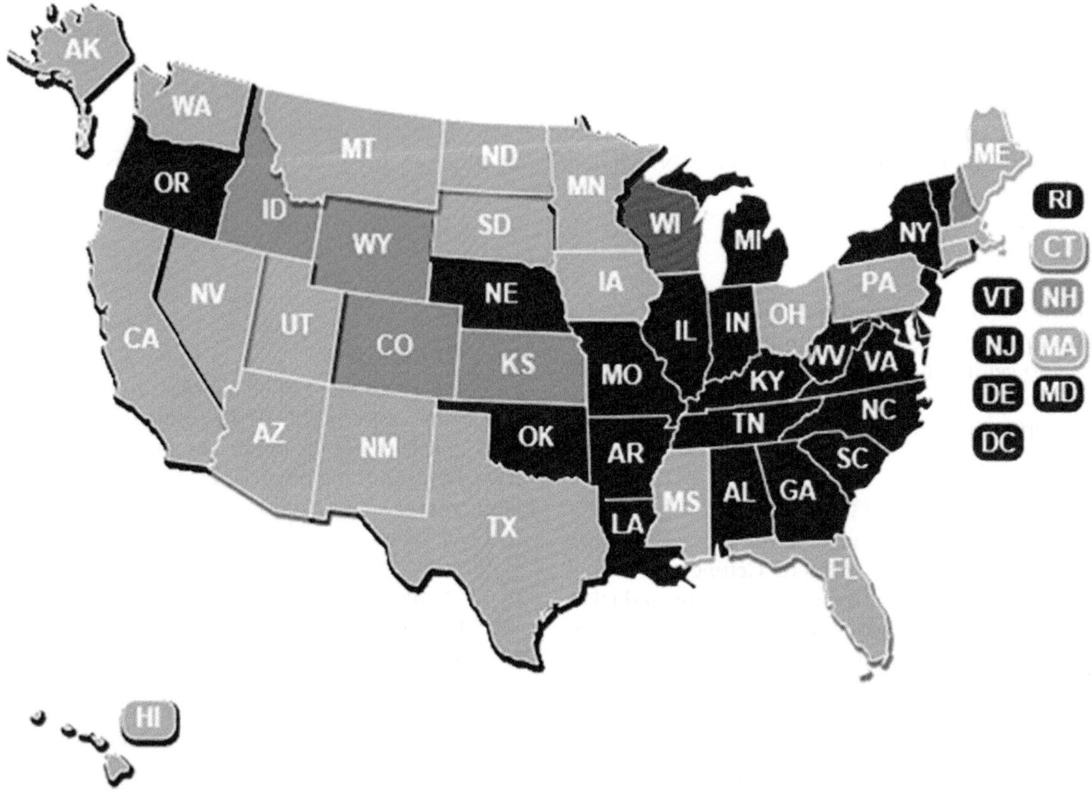

FIG. 5.1 States with some form of Certificate of Need laws (in blue). (Source: National Conference of State Legislatures.)

temperature there can be controlled independently of the rest of the facility. The machines may also be temperature sensitive.

Preop and Recovery Rooms

The sizes of the preop and postop areas depend on how many beds are to be placed there. It should be at least 100 sf for one bed or 80 sf each for multiple beds with space on the wall for mounting patient monitors and space to install curtains around the beds for privacy. In addition to that, allocate some space for a nursing area in the recovery room and space for an attendant, usually a family member, to sit with the patient.

Clean Room and Dirty Room

The clean room and dirty room should be at least 100 sf each. The clean room will be used for storing clean linens and clean supplies. The dirty room is for procedure room trash and hazardous waste.

Storage Area

Some supplies can be stored in the procedure room and clean room but usually more space is needed for storage. It is easy to underestimate the amount of storage space needed when the OEC is fully functional. Wall spaces should be utilized efficiently with built-in cabinets. A separate storage room(s) capable of accommodating large boxes, gas tanks, miscellaneous equipment, wheelchairs, etc. will be needed. They will probably take up another 200 sf of space. There should also, preferably, be a dedicated area for receiving supplies so that the staff can keep track of new deliveries and they are not mixed with older inventory items before they are logged in.

Changing Room and Locker Area

An often-overlooked area is a place for staff and patients to change clothes and keep their valuables. It is good practice to provide patients with a secure locker where they can keep their belongings, including jewelry, when they are being treated in the procedure room.

Other

In addition, of course, the OEC will need spaces for reception area, exam rooms, patient and staff bathrooms, break room, and work areas or offices for staff

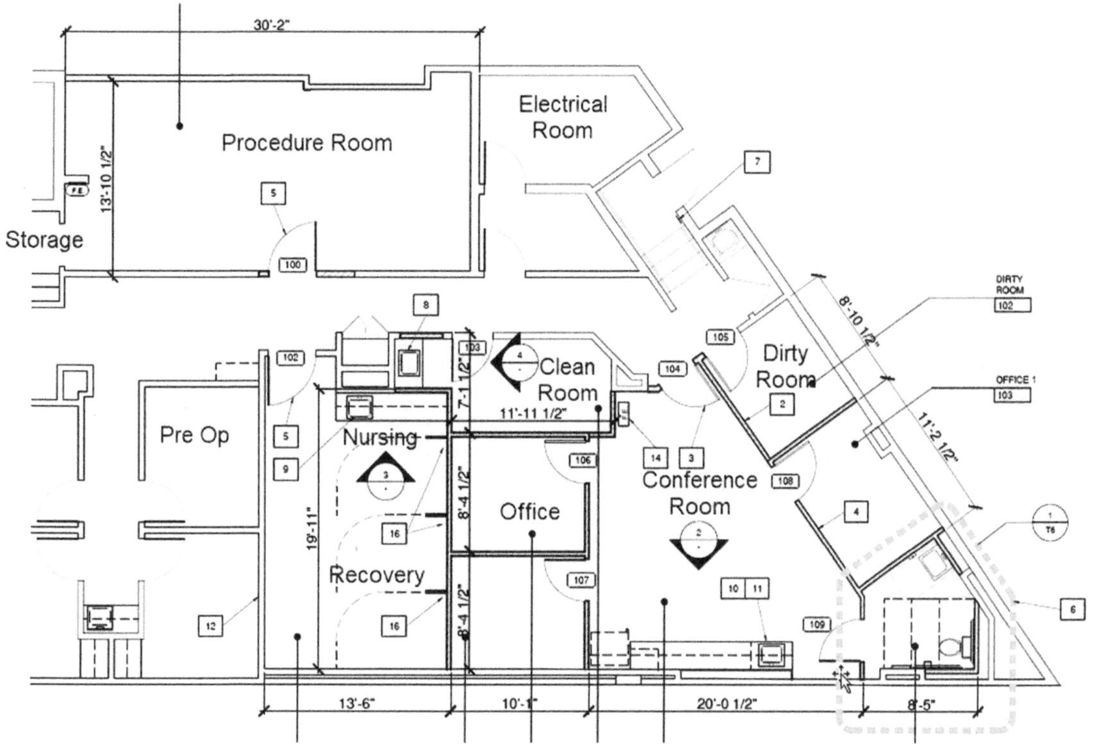

FIG. 5.2 Layout of an existing office-based endovascular center.

and physicians. If a noninvasive vascular lab is needed, it would need at least about 150 sf at the minimum and more if it needs to accommodate more than one patient at a time. Since the OEC is an extension of the office practice the spaces for various functions can be shared with the office, e.g., break room, billing area, bathrooms, etc.

Fig. 5.2 below shows the layout of an existing OEC (the reception area is not shown). It is not meant to represent the optimal layout but rather to show the typical components of a working OEC.

Backup Power

Backup power is needed for the procedure room, recovery room, and emergency exit lights. Unlike a hospital, an OEC does not have to have backup power to stay fully operational for an extended period of time. It just needs to have enough power to safely terminate any procedure, and to evacuate patients safely, if necessary. A battery-based UPS (uninterruptible power supply) that kicks in automatically when the main power fails is usually the most efficient and cost-effective way to provide for backup power. The battery should be sized to provide adequate power to the most critical devices in the procedure room so that the physician can safely terminate the procedure. Normally, this is about 30 min to 1 h of operation.

LAYOUT AND PATIENT FLOW

The practice will need to consider how patients flow through the facility, and plan for adequate clearances with regards to doors and corridors bearing in mind that patients may be on stretchers from the preop room to the procedure room and from the procedure room to the recovery room. The practice also needs to plan for nonambulatory patients arriving and departing the facility in wheelchairs and access for emergency vehicles.

Another consideration is patient privacy. The space should be laid out to provide as much privacy to each patient as possible. This includes things such as curtains in the preop and postop areas if the patients share the same rooms, and a separate exit for patients after their procedures, if the location allows. In an OEC preoperative area and post operative area can be shared.

WORKING WITH ARCHITECTS AND CONTRACTORS

It is very important to select an architect who has experience in medical buildings, especially in office-based surgery offices. They will be able to guide you through what works in other practices and know about regulations that you may not be aware of, such as placement of eye wash stations. If the architect has limited experience, it is worthwhile hiring a consultant to review the plan. Similarly, with contractors, there are many small details that may not be specified in the plans, such as which type of locks should be used on which doors, that having an experienced contractor who understands these things will make the building project go more smoothly and painlessly. The contractor should have familiarity with the permitting process in your city. Many times, a project is delayed because of permitting and inspection issues. A contractor who understands the red tape in your municipality will greatly help.

Building an OEC usually takes longer and costs more than the contractor's projection, and you will need to build in some buffer in the project time line and the budget. If you are planning to build a brand-new building for your practice and the OEC, the project, will obviously take much longer and will be much more expensive. It is important to plan the patient flow in your practice if you are expanding your current office to accommodate an OEC. Unexpected issues will arise and interruptions and delays are almost inevitable. Be patient, it will eventually be completed and it will be worth the effort.

CHAPTER 6

Capital Equipment

KRISHNA JAIN, MD, FACS

Opening an office-based endovascular center (OEC) will require a number of large pieces of equipment, or capital equipment.[1,2] Capital equipment includes items of considerable value (>$5000.00) that have a lifetime of greater than 1 year. These items will include imaging equipment such as a C-ARM, ultrasound machine, surgery table, and power injector (Table 6.1). In addition, there will be items that are required to run an OEC that are of lesser value and may not qualify as capital equipment, such as wheelchair, and storage shelves, etc. (Table 6.1). The most expensive part of the capital equipment is the imaging equipment. This is the workhorse of the OEC that will help determine the success of the center. The operators should purchase equipment that they are most comfortable with. The center will also have to decide if the equipment is bought new, used, or refurbished. While new equipment will have the latest technology, least chance of breakdown, the best manufacturer's warranty, it will also be the most expensive. Refurbished equipment could be refurbished by the manufacturer or by a third party. If the equipment is refurbished by the manufacturer it will have some period of warranty. Third-party refurbishers may or may not offer warranty. It would be cheaper than the new equipment. Used equipment is least desirable since the chances of breakdown would be significant. However, it is the cheapest option. The equipment can be purchased or leased. A typical lease lasts for 5 years with or without a buyout option at the end of the lease.

IMAGING

When buying imaging equipment one has to consider the cost, ease of use, space requirement, the technology, and versatility of the equipment.[3] The machine should provide adequate imaging for the planned procedures. The system should be intuitive thereby decreasing the number of steps. Since more complicated cases are being performed in this setting, the cooling system should be adequate to avoid overheating during a long procedure. The imaging system should become part of the workflow by facilitating export of images to the picture archiving and communication system (PACS) and send data to the electronic medical record (EMR). Any redundant steps should be eliminated. Besides the type of technology, one has to consider the pros and cons of C-ARM versus a fixed system.

C-ARM

A C-ARM requires less space, is mobile, uses less power, can be moved from room to room, and is cheaper than fixed imaging system. Some states do not require lead-lining of the room if there is only one machine and more than one room is used for imaging. The room requirements in terms of square feet and ceiling height are less stringent for the C-ARM than the fixed system. A C-ARM can be run on single-phase power with a 3-KVA uninterruptible power supply. This results in significant savings in power usage as compared with a fixed system. The C-ARM unit can be used for peripheral arterial and venous cases, dialysis access–related cases, embolization, ports and catheters, pacemaker lead placement, and pain-related procedures. Additionally, it is easier to do certain procedures using a C-ARM as compared with a fixed system. For example, it is easier to move the C-ARM to perform dialysis access procedures. However, there are procedures that cannot or should not be performed using a C-ARM, such as coronary angioplasty for a complex lesion. In certain circumstances, coronary angiograms and intervention can be performed using C-ARM but if the center is planning to offer these procedures on a routine basis, a fixed system may better serve the patient's needs. In obese patients, fixed system may provide better image quality. There are other technological advances in the fixed systems that may be helpful in complex cases, such as complex coronary procedures or during embolization to treat endoleaks after endovascular repair of an aortic aneurysm.

Office-Based Endovascular Centers. https://doi.org/10.1016/B978-0-323-67969-5.00006-X
Copyright © 2020 Elsevier Inc. All rights reserved.

TABLE 6.1
Office-Based Lab Equipment List.

IN THE LAB
C-ARM/fixed overhead system
Radiation protection shield
Radiolucent table
Power injector
Ultrasound machine for vessel access
Monitoring equipment
Overhead surgical light
Intravascular ultrasound
Arm boards
Portable oxygen tanks
Suction machine
Laryngoscope
Rolling stand for monitor
Step stool with handle for the patient
Procedure table for instruments
Mayo stand
Kick bucket
Catheter and wire storage cart
Linen hamper for waste
Cautery
Atherectomy device
Surgical instruments
IV pole
PREOPERATIVE AND POSTOPERATIVE AREA
Wheelchair
Reclining chair
Beds/Stretcher
Automated external defibrillator
Crash cart
Patient monitors
Overbed table
Nurse stool
Chair for family
Portable suction with battery
Laryngoscope
Stethoscopes
Handheld doppler
IV pole
MISCELLANEOUS
Furniture
Computers
Blanket warmer
Autoclave
Lead aprons
Lead apron storage rack
Protective hats
Protective glasses
PACS
Emergency generator
Storage racks
Data collection software
Electronic medical records
Narcotic box
Trash cans (UL fire rated)
Wire rack storage carts for storage area
EQUIPMENT FOR VENOUS CENTER
Radiofrequency ablation machine/laser machine
Pump

Flat Panel Detector

C-ARM manufacturers have gradually moved away from image intensifiers to flat panel system. Four major C-ARM manufactures offer flat panel technology on their systems. Flat panel detectors have improved contrast resolution, while image intensifiers have better spatial resolution.[4] Flat panel detectors cause less radiation exposure and have higher detective quantum efficiency (DQI) compared with image intensifiers.[5] Flat panel detectors provide a square image as compared with the round image provided by an image intensifier. This gives up to 60% more information to the operator. The operator also has more room to maneuver as the large cannister-shaped image intensifier is eliminated. The flat panel detectors have limited image degradation over a longer period of time as compared with image intensifiers. When the image intensifier is used and magnification is needed, it reduces field of vision. This is not a concern while using flat panel detector. The flat panel detector also produces better resolution and is not affected by magnetic distortion. The dynamic range of a flat panel detector is greater than an image intensifier and issues such as burnout (blooming) and blackout (saturation into black) are of less concern. The artifacts caused by this technology can be corrected by software and hardware changes while the image intensifier suffers from various artifacts that include pincushion, vignetting, and S distortion.

When deciding on a C-ARM various factors need to be taken into account:

Image quality: It is important to have images with rich detail and contrast to make appropriate decisions. The operator may be working on different vessels in different parts of the body including the heart. The C-ARM technology should adapt to these anatomic areas to provide the best image quality. Ideally, the machine should be able to do no-mask motion-tolerant subtraction resulting in digital subtraction angiography to visualize the runoff vessels in an extremity.

Patient size: The C-ARM should be able to provide quality images for all sizes of patients, but for extremely obese patients, fixed systems may be a better option. Obesity is a growing problem, thus hardware and software purchased for the OEC should provide quality images in obese patients.

Image resolution: As the vascular interventions are being carried out in infrapopliteal vessels with greater frequency, it is critical to have good resolution. It should be easy to differentiate between the guidewire, catheter, and the vessel in the extremity.

CO_2 angiography: Contrast-induced nephropathy causes significant morbidity and mortality. To avoid this complication, CO_2 angiography is being used more frequently.[6] The C-ARM should be able to provide good image quality when CO_2 is used as a contrast agent.

Radiation exposure: It is critical that the C-ARM provide quality images with minimum possible radiation exposure to the patient, operator, and the staff. The complexity of cases treated in the OEC is increasing, resulting in longer cases, thus it is prudent to look for a machine that would give least amount of radiation while producing quality images.[7]

Cooling: As the duration of cases, as well as, the number of cases performed per day is increasing, it is important to make sure that the machine does not get overheated and has adequate cooling system in place.

Footprint and safety: The footprint of the machine becomes very important if the space in the interventional suite is limited. There should be enough room left for other equipment and the team to be able to move freely. The machine should be small enough to be used from both sides of the table. The flat panel detector and joysticks should have built-in features to avoid collision of the detector with operators. If the center also functions as an ambulatory surgery center on certain days, then the space requirements for the ambulatory center should be adhered to.

Monitors: Most monitors are housed on a mobile cart. The monitors should have touch screens for ease of use. In some rooms a boom may serve the needs better. Booms can be floor or ceiling mounted. In ceiling-mounted booms, the wiring goes into the ceiling. With floor-mounted booms the wiring is in the back of the unit. The hardware is in the back of the unit rather than being housed in a closet outside of the OR. Booms should be placed so that the monitor can be visualized from either side of the table.

Cardiac use: Traditionally, cardiac procedures are performed using fixed systems. Cardiac arrhythmia–related cases could be easily performed using the C-ARM designed for peripheral cases. CMS has approved reimbursement for several codes for coronary angiography in ambulatory surgery centers. In the future, codes for intervention may be approved. If the center plans to offer these services, a versatile C-ARM may be useable for some of the cases in this category.

Configuration of a fixed system: The system can be floor mounted or ceiling mounted.[8] Floor-mounted systems are supported by a pedestal base with motorized vertical motion. In the ceiling-mounted systems, a support column is required which can obstruct view. However, it provides more transverse and axial movement as compared with the floor-mounted system. Added reinforcement of the ceiling and a higher ceiling is required for the ceiling-mounted system. If laminar flow is required the suspension rails may block the laminar flow.

Decision-Making

Ultimately the center needs to purchase imaging equipment that would be efficient, durable, user-friendly, and cost-effective. Several factors need to be considered before a decision is made. The system should be able to meet the caseload of the OEC and provide adequate imaging. It should not overheat. It should have high DQI. Higher DQI machines provide images with reduced radiation risk to the patient, operator, and the support staff. While considering the cost of the machine, several other factors should be taken into account. These factors include cost of buying or leasing the machine, annual maintenance contract, expected life of the machine, installation cost, energy consumption per month, and ease of upgrade. The machine should be able to work with the PACS the center is planning to purchase. If the types of cases change in the future, the machine should be versatile enough to meet the needs for software and hardware upgrades. It is also important to have timely support for the system. If the machine is down, it has significant impact on revenue. The company should also provide comprehensive on-site training to the operators at the center.

Service Agreement

It is crucial to have a service agreement with the provider of the imaging equipment. The center cannot afford to lose days of revenue or opportunities to provide appropriate patient care. Usually with the purchase of new equipment, the first year of service is included in the price of the equipment. After that there will be an annual fee to maintain the equipment and repair it if needed. The agreement should include preventive maintenance service as well as less than 24 h on-site service. In case of machine malfunction, it is preferable to have on-site service in less than 8 h. When purchasing the equipment, it is important to know the track record of the company for after-sales service in your geographic area.

POWER INJECTOR

Medrad's founder, M. Stephen Heilman, MD, an emergency room physician, saw a coronary arteriogram during the early 1960s and immediately realized the need for better tools to deliver contrast media. He teamed up with Mark Wholey, MD, who had visited Sweden and had trained with some of the pioneers of angiography in the early 1960s. Together, they invented and developed the first flow-controlled angiographic injector in Dr Heilman's home outside of Pittsburgh, Pennsylvania. The Heilman-Wholey Injector[9] was commercialized in 1967, and was initially distributed by Picker X-ray Company and manufactured by the new company, Medrad, Inc.

Interventionalists use power contrast media injectors to achieve opacification of vessels for diagnostic procedures, which require high flow, high volume, fixed-rate injections delivered with relatively high pressures. These injectors are commonly used for aortograms, ventriculograms, and runoff studies. There are certain issues that need to be addressed while using a power injector, including potential for damage to the vessels, catheter whipping, or chance of air embolus. Power injectors that address these issues are now available. New injector systems have been developed to inject contrast in variable mode at low flow rates and low pressures for small vessels, and fixed mode at high flow rates and high-pressure injections for larger vessels like aorta and peripheral arteries. The systems also have an air management system with fluid level sensing and gross air detection and a bolus sharpness feature. Various systems also offer variable-rate contrast delivery systems for precision and control. Systems that capture, store, and retrieve data produced by the injector, such as flow rate and volume injected, are very useful. These data can be used for budgeting and tracking of contrast utilization. The biggest trend in power injector technology is to have systems that make full use of the existing contrast supply in an effort to reduce contrast dose. New injector systems also integrate with EMRs and PACS. Syringeless power injectors have emerged recently as they provide several advantages such as user-friendliness, high efficiency, and minimum wastage of contrast media. The Joint Commission does not allow the reuse of unused doses from single-use syringe injectors. This option gives the center the opportunity to use contrast media efficiently. Most of the published work in this field relates to contrast enhanced CT scanning. In a study by Colombo et al. the "syringeless system power injector was found to be more user-friendly and efficient, minimizing contrast wastage and providing similar contrast enhancement quality compared with the dual-syringe injector, with comparable contrast-enhanced CT examination quality."[10]

IMAGING TABLE

Imaging tables have a carbon-based tabletop to facilitate imaging. The price of the table will greatly depend on the movement capability of the table. The table can move up and down, have lateral tilt, offer Trendelenburg position, and slide horizontally and vertically. Motorized movements improve ease of use and efficiency, but also cost more. Motorization is a luxury that can be done without due to budgetary issues without impacting the quality of the procedure. Another factor to consider is the mobility of the table in case the table needs to be moved for proper positioning of the C-ARM. Table pads need to be radiolucent and of appropriate thickness. As the patients are becoming larger in size, the weight limit of the table needs to be greater than 450 pounds. In the past, many tables had a weight limit of 300 pounds; it is preferable to buy a new table but a manufacturer-refurbished table could suffice if it has adequate warranty. All mechanical things break down at certain point, thus it is important to have an appropriate after-sale service contract. Preventive maintenance should also be conducted at appropriate intervals. The company representative should provide training for all users. It is not necessary to buy the most expensive table, but is important to ensure that the table will meet the requirements of the procedures being planned.

IMAGING TABLE ACCESSORIES

Depending on the table the center buys, some accessories will be required. There may be additional cost for these products. These accessories include arm boards, which could be table mounted or slide under the pad. If they are table mounted, clasps will be required to attach the arm boards to the table. Other accessories include extensions, radiation shields, restraint straps, gel pads, and other positioners. There may also be a need for an anesthesia screen depending on the operator preference.

PICTURE ARCHIVING AND COMMUNICATION SYSTEM

Picture archiving and communication system (PACS) uses medical technology to securely store and digitally transmit images and reports. This eliminates the use of manual files and physical storage systems.[11] The digital images can be stored off-site in a server and retrieved as and when needed using a computer, workstation, or a mobile device from anywhere. This is particularly important for the OEC because if the patient shows up in the hospital for any reason the physician has to be able to access the images and reports to provide optimum care to the patient. If the patient has undergone multiple procedures in the OEC using the PACS, progression of the disease can be easily documented and used in providing further care.

The center should use a PACS to store all the ultrasound images as well as the images produced during the intervention and associated reports. "PACS has four major components: hardware imaging machines; a secure network for the distribution and exchange of patient images; a workstation or mobile device for viewing, processing and interpreting images; and electronic archives for storing and retrieving images and related documentation and reports."[12] Use of a PACS has multiple benefits that include removing the need for hard copies, allowing remote access, integration with the EMR, and an improved workflow. Most PACS used by the OEC are cloud based. It is crucial to have a reliable fast Internet connection to be able to use the cloud-based PACS efficiently. The cloud service should be HIPPA compliant. The interface between the C-ARM, ultrasound machine, EMR system, and the PACS should be seamless. In a hybrid system, primary images and reports can be kept at the center while the backup is stored in the cloud.

ULTRASOUND EQUIPMENT FOR VESSEL ACCESS

Increasing age, female gender, obesity, and larger thigh circumference have been associated with increased incidence of bleeding complications. Ultrasound-guided vessel entry can help reduce the incidence of these complications.[13,14] The center may have an ultrasound machine that can be used to perform all the diagnostic tests. A smaller, cheaper ultrasound machine specifically designed for vessel access may be used. The procedure is performed using broadband high-resolution linear array transducers generally providing frequencies between 7.5 and 12 MHz. Higher frequency is used for more superficial vessels, and lower frequencies are better for deeper vessels. Small-footprint probes are preferable. A hockey stick–shaped probe is helpful for tibial artery access. Color flow imaging may be helpful in differentiating arteries from veins. Sterile probe covers are needed for all access procedures. Needles with echogenic characteristics help in entering small vessels.

RADIATION PROTECTION

As the number and complexity of procedures increases, radiation exposure to the operator and the team increases. An effort needs to be made to provide maximum protection to the patient and everyone in the room.[15] Traditionally, the team members wear a lead apron or a skirt and a vest along with a neck collar, lead-lined cap, lead gloves, and lead glasses. The thickness of lead in the lead gown determines the protection it provides. A lead gown with 0.25 mm thickness attenuates 66% of the beam at 75 kVp, and 1 mm attenuates 99% of the beam at same kVp. To protect the patient, the fluoroscopic unit must not produce X-rays unless a barrier is in position to intercept the entire cross-section of the useful beam. The fluoroscopic imaging assembly must be provided with shielding to minimize the scatter from the fluoroscopic unit. This shielding needs to be purchased. A radiation shield around the table protects the team from radiation exposure.

The Zero-Gravity radiation protection system by TIDI Products (Neenah, Wisconsin)[16] consists of lead protection hanging from a monorail so there is no weight born by the operator. Use of this system will require appropriate space to accommodate the device. Due to space limitations, it may not always be possible to use the system. It is also more expensive compared with the traditional use of lead aprons.

SURGICAL LIGHT

Two different light sources are needed in an endovascular suite. The surgical light is used to illuminate the entire operating room table. The light must not interfere with head heights or movement of other equipment like C-ARM or monitors. It also should not create glare or reflections. It is used for the initial part of the endovascular procedure when the vessel is being accessed and later when the procedure has been completed. Usually only one surgical light is needed. In procedures that require an incision as with insertion of a port, the light will be needed throughout the procedure. If desired the lights can have built in camera and video capability. Endovascular interventions can be carried out using ambient light; however, the ambient lights should be dimmable. If the center is using a ceiling-mounted fixed imaging system, there needs to be careful planning for lights since a centrally mounted surgical light will not be possible. Some of the existing rooms that are converted into a radiological procedure room may have short ceiling height usually of 8 feet. This should be taken into account before buying the light. The ceiling may need to be raised.

INTRAVASCULAR ULTRASOUND

Intravascular ultrasound (IVUS) is essential for managing deep venous obstructive disease. It can also be useful in managing arterial disease and in dialysis access management (Chapter 16). The equipment used for IVUS is usually supplied by the company on a contract basis. The cost of using the equipment is usually determined by the number of cases performed using the machine at the center as it is tied to overall catheter use.

ATHERECTOMY DEVICES

There are four broad types of atherectomy devices: orbital, directional, rotational, and laser. The center may choose to use one or two atherectomy devices. It is not cost-effective to use all the devices. These devices use various means to decrease the plaque load. The equipment necessary to use these devices is typically brought to the center by the company on a contract basis. Most centers do not buy this equipment. Some devices may not need capital equipment.

VENOUS ABLATION

If the center is planning to provide venous ablation services a decision will need to be made to determine the modality to be used at the center. The equipment needs will depend on the mechanism being used for ablation such as radiofrequency ablation, laser ablation, nonthermal, nontumescent procedure using glue (cyanoacrylate-based medical adhesive), mechanochemical, or chemical method. Capital equipment will be needed for radiofrequency ablation and laser ablation. This is covered in Chapter 29.

ELECTRONIC MEDICAL RECORD

If expanding the services at an existing private practice to include OEC, the office may already have EMR for normal operations. The same EMR may be expanded to the OEC. However, the existing EMR may not be able to record the complex procedures being performed in the OEC. The center may have to purchase a new EMR for the center, but it is mandatory that the new EMR be integrated in the old system for seamless flow of information (Chapter 8).

In addition to the major equipment that needs to be purchased, several smaller items need to be purchased (Table 6.1). While creating a business plan the budget should reflect the purchase of all items. The need may also change in the future as the center grows and meets the demands of future innovations.

REFERENCES

1. Jain K.M., Development and successful operation of an outpatient vascular center. In: Sidawy A., Bruce P., eds. *Rutherford's Vascular Surgery and Endovascular Therapy 9th Edition*. Elsevier (Chapter 198); 2552–2562.
2. Moore W., ed. Building an outpatient interventional suite. In: *Moore's Vascular and Endovascular Surgery. A Comprehensive Review 9th Edition*. Elsevier [chapter 67] 1009–1017.
3. What to expect in a cath lab: 360 degree video. *Hear Matters*.
4. Seibert JA. Flat-panel detectors: how much better are they? *Pediatr Radiol*. 2006;36(suppl 14):173–181. https://doi.org/10.1007/s00247-006-0208-0.
5. Holmes DR, Laskey WK, Wondrow MA, Cusma JT. Flat-panel detectors in the cardiac catheterization laboratory: revolution or evolution – what are the issues? *Catheter Cardiovasc Interv*. 2004. https://doi.org/10.1002/ccd.20166.
6. Sharafuddin MJ, Marjan AE. Current status of carbon dioxide angiography. *J Vasc Surg*. 2017;66(2):618–637. https://doi.org/10.1016/j.jvs.2017.03.446.
7. Mahajan A, Samuel S, Saran AK, Mahajan MK, Mam MK. Occupational radiation exposure from C arm fluoroscopy

during common orthopaedic surgical procedures and its prevention. *J Clin Diagn Res.* 2015;9(3):RC01–4. https://doi.org/10.7860/JCDR/2015/10520.5672.
8. Schueler BA. The AAPM/RSNA physics tutorial for residents general overview of fluoroscopic imaging. *RadioGraphics.* 2000;20(4):1115–1126. https://doi.org/10.1148/radiographics.20.4.g00jl301115.
9. Heilman MS, Wholey MH. A new angiographic injection system. *Br J Radiol.* 1967;40(474):469–470. https://doi.org/10.1259/0007-1285-40-474-469.
10. Colombo GL, Bergamo Andreis IA, Di Matteo S, Bruno G, Mondellini C. Syringeless power injector versus dual-syringe power injector: economic evaluation of user performance, the impact on contrast enhanced computed tomography (CECT) workflow exams, and hospital costs. *Med Devices Evid Res.* 2013;6:169. https://doi.org/10.2147/MDER.S51757.
11. Choplin RH, Boehme JM, Maynard CD. Picture archiving and communication systems: an overview. *RadioGraphics.* 1992;12(1):127–129. https://doi.org/10.1148/radiographics.12.1.1734458.
12. Charles M, DelVecchio A, Sutner S. PACS (picture archiving and communication system). In: *RSNA 2017 conference coverage and analysis.* 2017.
13. Troianos CA, Hartman GS, Glas KE, et al. Guidelines for performing ultrasound guided vascular cannulation: recommendations of the American Society of Echocardiography and the Society of Cardiovascular Anesthesiologists. *J Am Soc Echocardiogr.* 2011;24(12):1291–1318. https://doi.org/10.1016/j.echo.2011.09.021.
14. Kalish J, Eslami M, Gillespie D, et al. Routine use of ultrasound guidance in femoral arterial access for peripheral vascular intervention decreases groin hematoma rates. *J Vasc Surg.* 2015;61(5):1231–1238. https://doi.org/10.1016/j.jvs.2014.12.003.
15. Chambers C E, Fetterly K A, Holzer R, et al. Radiation safety program for the cardiac catheterization laboratory. *Catheter Cardiovasc Interv.* 2011;77(4):546–556. https://doi.org/10.1002/ccd.22867.
16. Haussen DC, Van Der Bom IM, Nogueira RG. A prospective case control comparison of the ZeroGravity system versus a standard lead apron as radiation protection strategy in neuroendovascular procedures. *J Neurointerv Surg.* 2016;8(10):1052–1055. https://doi.org/10.1136/neurintsurg-2015-012038.

CHAPTER 7

Supplies

HWA KHO, PHD, MBA • SAM AHN, MD, FACS, MBA

Supplies are one of the top two expenditures in the office-based endovascular center (OEC); the other is payroll. Good supply management is critical to both the clinical and financial success of the OEC. The difference between a successful or a failed intervention could hinge on whether the OEC has the right device when the physician needs it; whether the OEC is profitable or not may hinge on what was paid for supplies and how they were managed.

WHAT AND HOW MUCH TO STOCK?

It is expensive and operationally very challenging to stock a large array of devices in all different sizes in anticipation of the physician's need during an intervention. From a business perspective, it is desirable to tie up as little capital as possible by keeping a low inventory level, while clinically, it is desirable to keep as much inventory at hand as possible in case something is needed.

Preferences for the type and model of devices can vary widely from physician to physician. Physicians need to convey clearly to the Inventory Manager which devices they absolutely need and must have at all times, including devices which they might very rarely use but would need in an emergency, such as an expensive covered stent. It is important for the physicians to get involved in these discussions as they know best what they need and feel most comfortable with. Physicians in a group should also try to agree on the same manufacturers where possible to reduce the diversity of devices that need to be stocked and also to get to the best possible pricing deals from the vendors.

Consignment arrangements, where the OEC does not have to pay for the devices until it actually uses them, may be used to widen the selection of devices available to the physicians without incurring any upfront costs. However, if they are frequently used devices, it may work out cheaper to purchase them upfront.

The par value should be set so that there are 1–2 weeks of needed supplies at any time. There is usually no need to maintain a larger inventory than that. Most devices can be delivered within a few days of ordering. However, the practice should try to avoid rush orders which incur higher shipping costs. And the practice should, where possible, try to consolidate orders to save on shipping charges; ordering small quantities at high frequency can incur shipping costs which quickly add up to become significant amounts. Sales tax and shipping charges are those expenses that are very easy to overlook. In any case, there will inevitably be hiccups in the supply chain and having a 1–2 weeks' buffer will help to mitigate against such hiccups. It is also good practice for the Inventory Manager to preview upcoming cases to make sure that the devices that are needed will be available Table 7.1.

TABLE 7.1
below shows a list of some common devices and supplies for an OEC.

DEVICES AND SUPPLIES
PTA Balloons (various diameters, balloon lengths, shaft lengths, material, and wire systems)
Stent (various diameters and lengths, shaft lengths, materials, and designs)
Guide wires (various diameters, lengths, stiffness, distal tips, and materials)
Sheaths (various diameters, lengths, shapes, material, and designs)
Catheters (various shapes, various diameters, lengths, stiffness, and materials)
IVUS Catheter (various imaging diameters, lengths,)
Atherectomy catheter (various diameters, lengths, crossing profiles)
Embolization Coil (various coil diameters and lengths, materials)
Snares

Continued

Office-Based Endovascular Centers. https://doi.org/10.1016/B978-0-323-67969-5.00007-1
Copyright © 2020 Elsevier Inc. All rights reserved.

Micopuncture Set
Closure Devices
Drapes
Equipment Covers
Gowns
Procedure Packs
Medications (various types)
IV solutions
IV tubing
Needles

PRICING

Since devices can be very expensive, their costs could help decide the kind of procedures that can be done in the OEC. Profit margin for each procedure is heavily dependent on the cost of the devices used during the procedure. The ability to negotiate a good price for devices has a big impact on the OEC's bottom line.

OECs usually have some leverage to negotiate a better price than the list price. The most effective leverage is volume. It is to the physicians' advantage to try to consolidate their supplies to as few manufacturers as possible to leverage their volume discount. The busier the OEC, the easier it is to get a bigger discount and improve profitability. The OECs with only one or two physicians who are not very busy are at a big disadvantage and may struggle to be profitable.

Manufacturers sometimes offer bulk purchase discounts. The discounts may seem very attractive and they may, indeed, be a good deal. However, the OEC should do a careful analysis. Some of the things to consider are when is the payment due and can the OEC really afford to have a big chunk of its capital tied up in inventory? What is the expiry date of the devices and will the OEC be able to use all the devices before the expiry date? Will the manufacturer exchange the devices if they expire? Does the OEC have the space to store the devices bought in bulk? If the manufacturer will not exchange the expired devices and there is good chance that some of them will expire before they can be used, the deal may not be worth it.

Some manufacturers may also offer a discount in return for a fixed monthly payment, say $10,000.00, for all or a range of their products. The manufacturer will balance bill the OEC if it consumes more than $10,000.00 worth of supplies or refund the OEC if it consumes less on a quarterly basis. The problem with these kinds of deals is that it is very hard to know exactly how much each individual item costs. The manufacturers tend to roll up all the individual items into a consolidated line item, and consequently, it is hard to hard to know if, indeed, the deal was advantageous to the OEC.

The contracts with the vendors should be reviewed on annual basis to make sure that they remain competitive. There is no company which can supply all the products to the lab. The center will have to deal with multiple vendors. The practice should not be afraid to move to a new vendor if it results in significant savings to the lab. Some of the physicians may not want to do it because of device preference or personal relationship with the company representatives. Profitability of the center should override any of these underlying factors preventing migration to a different vendor.

EXPIRATION DATE

The OEC needs to keep a watchful eye on the expiration dates for each type of item and the exchange policy of the manufacturer if it expires or is close to expiring. The Inventory Manager has to make sure that items nearing the expiration date are used first. If a $1000 stent expired and the manufacturer will not give one in exchange for it, the OEC just lost $1000. The expired items could easily add up to tens of thousands of dollars a month if the Inventory Manager is not careful. In hospital operating rooms, it is a common occurrence and surgeons have no control over it, but in the self-financed OEC it can have significant impact on profit margins.

INVENTORY MANAGEMENT SOFTWARE

Ensuring the OEC is adequately stocked at all times is a full-time job in a busy practice. This is a job that is very difficult to do without having a good information technology (IT) system in place to manage the inventory. The IT system should be able to check in supplies, track usage, and report on what is in the inventory in real time. It should be able to identify items that fall below set par levels so that those items can be replenished in a timely basis. It should be able to alert the Inventory Manager on expiring and expired items.

Additionally, and very importantly from the business perspective, the IT system should be able to itemize the supplies used for each case and the total cost of the supplies for that case. This information is essential to monitor costs and providing feedbacks to the physicians on the costs of their choice of devices and the cost of each procedure.

The OEC needs to appoint one or more people to manage the inventory and invest in a good inventory management system. A hospital-based practice may not need those employees or software, but they are vital to the operation of an OEC.

KEEPING SUPPLIES COST DOWN

Working in a hospital, many physicians do not know or care about the cost of the devices they use. For an OEC to be successful, it is imperative that physicians become very cognizant of the devices they use and how much they cost. They need to become cost-efficient without, of course, jeopardizing patient care. The best way to educate the physicians is to provide them with information on the costs of supplies for the cases they perform. Having an inventory management software that can track every item used in a procedure and its cost is essential to achieve this. With an inventory management software, the procedure room staff can track every item used by, typically, scanning in its barcode. At the end of a case, they can print out a list and the cost of the items used which they can then present to the physician to review. Providing physicians with this real-time feedback is a very effective way of educating them and changing the culture of indifference to the cost of supplies.

STORAGE SPACE

Adequate and appropriate space for organizing and storing supplies is important. Supplies should be organized so that particular items are easy to find. Manufacturers will sometimes provide free storage carts which are useful. Keep supplies in a secure area. A small item may cost several thousand dollars, and the OEC cannot afford to have items misplaced or stolen.

Also, a separate and clearly designated area for receiving new deliveries before they are logged in or processed into the inventory management system is highly desirable. This is to prevent new deliveries from being inadvertently used before they can be logged in.

CLOSING THE LOOP ON ORDERS

Finally, and very importantly, the practice must have a process in place to ensure that their orders are fulfilled as they were placed. Were the ordered supplies delivered? Orders are sometimes fulfilled in different batches and it is easy to lose track of the original order. Are the prices correct? Is the OEC being billed for the right devices, the right quantity at the right price? Without a good process in place, the practice will have no way of ensuring that what it is paying for is what it gets.

Managing supplies should not be an afterthought in planning for an OEC. It is critical to the success of the OEC. Physicians need to be engaged in the process and understand pricing and the implications of any deals with the vendors. There should be a good process in place, staff have to be allocated for supplies management and be trained, and the practice needs to provide them with effective tools to carry out their jobs. The contracts with the vendors should be reviewed on annual basis to make sure that they remain competitive.

CHAPTER 8

Data, Analytics, and Information Management for the Office-Based Endovascular Centers

PARAMJIT "ROMI" CHOPRA, MD

INTRODUCTION

Office-based endovascular centers (OECs), also variably known as the office-based lab (OBLs), outpatient endovascular interventional suite (OEIS) or outpatient endovascular interventional center (OEIC), has emerged out of the necessity to provide cost-effective care that is better, faster, and cheaper for the patient and more satisfying and financially viable for the physicians providing the care. Most office-based centers are run as a small- to medium-size business; however as larger health system and multispecialty groups expand into providing patient care in the outpatient space, in the office-based endovascular centers and/or the ambulatory surgery center (ASC), they will deploy larger enterprise systems. OECs and ASCs are expanding into cardiac procedures including the performance of percutaneous coronary angiograms, rhythm management, and other areas such as interventional oncology, spine interventions, among others.

THE CASE FOR AN INFORMATION AND DATA CENTRIC APPROACH

"Amazonification"[1] of our world has raised the patient's (consumer) expectations around the delivery of their healthcare.

The patient as the stakeholder demands as core values improved awareness, better engagement, and a personalized experience with their healthcare team; and as the outcome of this engagement, the patient expects increased survival rates, good clinical outcomes, and improved quality of life.

As healthcare providers, we are expected to provide excellent delivery of care with improved efficiency and efficacy. The expected outcomes consist of reduced hospitalization rates, efficient and successful treatments, and optimum use of existing resources cost effectively. To ensure that the patient has the best clinical outcome and patient engagement experience, we must ensure that the right information is available to the right people, at the right time, to make the right decisions.

To succeed in today's era of healthcare with decreasing reimbursements, increasing competition, expanding technology, consumerism, and demand for value-based care, the providers and managers of the OEC need to be adept at data management and analytics. We will need actionable insight into all the data we collect almost in real time to have excellent outcomes and financial viability. Data is power.

One hears a lot about the analogy between data and oil. "Data are the New Oil."[2]

The information and data technology we use is the "combustion engine," the data are the "oil", and the operators of the OEC are the "spark." When the combination of these three elements occurs, we get controlled powerful energy. The engine alone, the oil or the spark alone will not produce any energy. The oil alone with the spark can cause uncontrolled energy (an explosion).

In my personal observation, world class organizations like Amazon and Costco, have six pillars that support their viability and success: (1) Excellence of product or services; (2) excellent customer service; (3) excellent employee satisfaction; (4) fiscal responsibility—adding value for the customer and the organization; (5) constant innovation and finally, (6) systems to sustain the above five pillars. To achieve this kind of success we need excellent data management and analytics to get the right information to the right people, at the right time, to make the right decisions.

Running an OEC is running a small business, which often goes through three stages: infancy (start-up mode), expansion stage (installation of systems and a

Office-Based Endovascular Centers. https://doi.org/10.1016/B978-0-323-67969-5.00008-3
Copyright © 2020 Elsevier Inc. All rights reserved.

lot of lessons learned along the way), and finally a state of maturity with mature systems and processes.

It is essential to avoid the "Garbage In, Garbage out," phenomenon. The quality and form of the data entered are extremely crucial. Structured data lend themselves easily to analysis and analytics; however, entering structured data can be challenging. Dictations and notes are unstructured data and do not lend themselves to analysis and often lay in the graveyards of massive volumes of data within electronic health records (EHR) and other systems.

Regulatory agencies, payers, and patients (consumers of the services we provide) are demanding interoperability and communications between the various organizations and individuals who provide the care. As operators of the OEC, we can only use data systems that are available to us.

Big Data in Healthcare

In addition to the internal data that we collect, there is a massive amount of external and consumer data relating to the patient care that are available. There are data regarding other providers, revenue cycle data, social media, and social determinants. Payers such as Medicare provide revenue cycle data in the public domain regularly. Understanding data on social determinants of health, such as income, educational level, and employment, can help focus efforts to improve community health.[3]

We often hear of "big data," which is the reality and the world we live in, and we continue to consume constantly on a daily basis in all aspects of our lives. Big data from Medicare and various registries is routinely used to publish articles in peer-reviewed journals and makes the basis of decisions being made by the clinicians and administrators alike. OEC needs to live in this reality. Local storage is often inadequate, inefficient, and ineffective. In the long run, cloud storage of the EHR, PACS (picture archival and communications system), and data warehousing is the emerging and long-term viable solution. Big data is often described with the four Vs: Volume, Variety, Velocity, and Veracity. Others add Variability, Value, and Visualization to compile the seven Vs of big data. All of these adjectives are applicable even to a reasonably small OEC in the new era of healthcare. Capture, storage, curation, transfer, search, sharing, analysis, reporting, and visualization of all these data can be very challenging. Adoption of a proper and established model is highly recommended so that the OEC can grow from the minimally viable center to a mature established system.

Analytics is the **discovery and communication of meaningful patterns in data**. Analysis and analytics are often confused. There is a fine line between the two. Analysis is a way to interpret the data and derive meaningful insights from the data. An example would be the use of a tool or other spreadsheet applications like Microsoft Excel to plot the graph, pivot chart to delve into the subject of interest. Analytics, however, involves statistical tools and techniques with "business acumen" to bring out the hidden patterns and stories from the data that can be utilized to improve the efficiency of the organization, increase profitability, and improve clinical outcomes.

Healthcare Analytics Adoption Model[4]

Healthcare industry is following the path of other industries and is repeating the same trend of computerization and data analysis. This process has three phases. Phase 1 is the specific collection of transaction-based workflows such as the electronic health records. Phase 2 consists of sharing data between the different organizations and involved Health Information Exchanges (HIE). In Phase 3, the data analysis is carried out and this requires large repositories of data, also becoming known as "Big Data." The same pattern of adoption evident in the overall healthcare industry is now evident in different healthcare organizations and is vital in the OEC for providing effective care, and for meeting all other financial and nonfinancial objectives.

Healthcare organizations are drowning in data, and a healthcare analytics adoption model has been proposed and implemented by many. This model provides a road map for organizations to measure their own progress toward adopting analytics systems in their own practice. This also provides a framework for evaluating products from the multitude of vendors that exist in the marketplace. Regardless of the size of the operations, it is essential to look at the data and information management to achieve success.

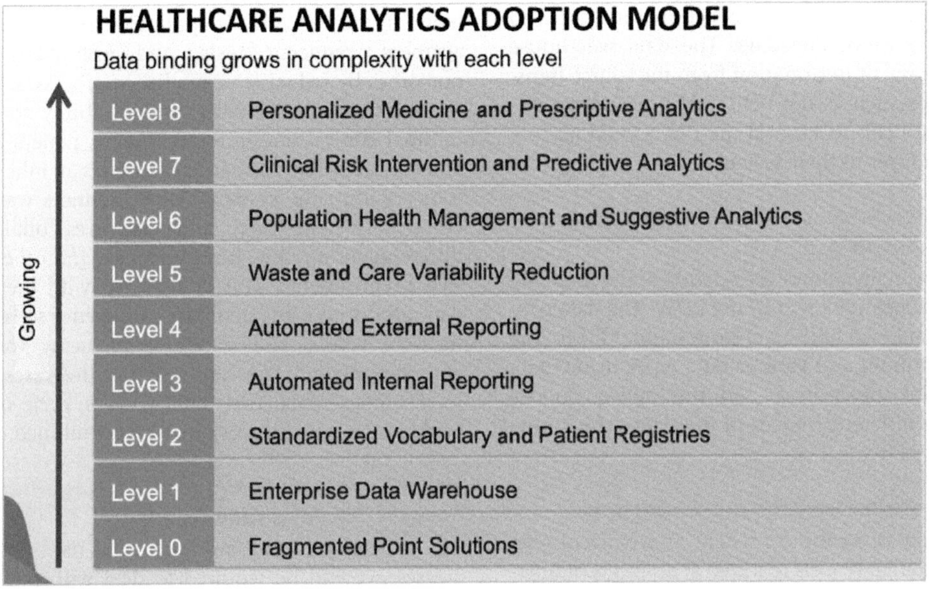
HEALTHCARE ANALYTICS ADOPTION MODEL
Data binding grows in complexity with each level
Growing
Level 8
Personalized Medicine and Prescriptive Analytics
Level 7
Clinical Risk Intervention and Predictive Analytics
Level 6
Population Health Management and Suggestive Analytics
Level 5
Waste and Care Variability Reduction
Level 4
Automated External Reporting
Level 3
Automated Internal Reporting
Level 2
Standardized Vocabulary and Patient Registries
Level 1
Enterprise Data Warehouse
Level 0
Fragmented Point Solutions

This model is not a linear model and multiple organizations may be at different stages, and within each level, they may be in different stages of maturity. In the OEC, it is vital to be at least up to level 3 or 4 to meet the minimum requirements of being successful in this domain. At level 5, the wastage in the center can be diminished or eliminated resulting in improved profit margin.

Level 0—Fragmented Point Solutions

At this level, the organization has multiple fragmented point solutions. The systems are inefficient with inconsistent versions of the truth. Internal and external reporting are cumbersome, challenging, expensive, and difficult for the managers and leaders. Most OECs and smaller healthcare organizations are stuck and remain stuck at this level. They often hope and pray that the EHR, PACS, or revenue cycle and billing vendor will magically solve this problem. At this level, the patient engagement, practice management, EHR, PACS, and billing and revenue cycle systems exist and operate in different silos. None of these entities talk to each other and lack interconnectivity of the data. Data are not shared with each other. At this level, the organization is without any governance, and the quality and the value of the data are extremely low.

Some OECs argue that they are small businesses with limited resources and that they can still do the internal and external reporting listed in level 3 and level 4. However, this is achieved with increased difficulty and at high cost to the center. This fragmented, expensive approach cannot be scaled and cannot reach the upper levels of this model, which would be required for value-based care as demanded by payers and the society. Value-based care is here to stay and will become the method used to pay for services provided by the practice and the OEC.

Level 1—Enterprise Data Warehouse

The very first level is to establish an enterprise data warehouse (EDW). The EDW is a system used for reporting and data analysis and is considered a core component of business intelligence. There are central repositories of integrated data from one or more disparate sources that can store historical and current data in a single location.

This requires the organization to collect and integrate all the core data content from its different systems. It is imperative that the vendor chosen for the EMR and PACS should allow this capability. The main source of the data is cleansed, transformed, cataloged, and made available for use by managers and other business professionals. The definition of EDW is often expanded to include business intelligence tools to extract, transform, and load data into the repository, and tools to manage and retrieve metadata. The data warehouse maintains a copy of information from the source transaction systems such as the EHR, PACS, RCM systems and often the EHR, RCM, and the PACS vendors provide this as a layer in their systems.

Level 2—Standardized Vocabulary and Patient Registries

This level essentially allows the relating and organizing of the core data content within the EDW. The data content in the data warehouse are now standardized. The naming, definition, and various data types in the data warehouse are streamlined, and this allows queries across all the different sources of the data, which now reside in this EDW.

Level 3—Automated Internal Reporting

This level focuses on the consistent and efficient production of internal reports required at all levels of operation and management of the OEC. Often physicians and other managers will be able to conduct "self-service" analytics based on interactive dashboards to meet their requirements at their level of management.

This is a crucial stage with "Automated Internal Reporting" provided to the key people in the organization to make the right decisions at the right time. Based on this level, the reports that are provided are reliable, available on demand, consistent, and accurate. This minimizes wasteful effort and redundancy within the organization. The end users receive the information on which they can act reliably, consistently, and accurately.

Level 4—Automated External Reporting

This level allows for "Automated External Reporting" whether it be to registries, payers for value-based care and risk sharing, etc. This level focuses on production of reports required for external needs such as medical registries for benchmarking and requirements for MIPS, disease registries, accreditation, compliance regulatory, and specialty society databases. OECs will most likely be subjected to accreditation requirements and will need to provide quality data to maintain the accreditation status. This is already happening in various states. They will also need to submit quality data to receive payments from the Center for Medicare and Medicaid services (CMS) and other commercial payers.

Level 5—Waste and Care Variability Reduction

This level allows for operation and systems improvement. In the OEC, this is applicable to inventory management, reducing costs, and improving clinical outcomes by reducing variability in processes. The success of OEC model relies on the ability to provide optimal clinical care in a safe, timely, patient-friendly, and cost-effective manner. This implies an inherent efficiency within the systems, which reduces waste, provides consistent care, and improves quality that differentiates an OEC from hospitals and other expensive environments. This is achieved with the help of data produced using analytics. Adherence to best practices, protocols, and standards; reducing variability; and minimizing waste are essential processes. At this level, clinical data, cost data, revenue cycle data and evidence-based registries can all be combined.

Level 6—Population Health Management and Suggestive Analytics

As "value-based" care and "financial risk" sharing increases, we will be required to deal with populations which will require Population Health Management and Suggestive Analytics. The medical practice that is part of an "accountable care organization" shares the financial risk and reward that is tied to clinical outcomes.

Level 7—Clinical Risk Intervention and Predictive Analytics

At this level, patients are flagged in registries who are unable or unwilling to participate in care protocols and proposed interventions. The data content expands to include home monitoring data, long-term care facility data, and protocol-specific patient reported outcomes.

Level 8—Personalized Medicine and Prescriptive Analytics

This is an advanced level where the motives for the analytics expand to wellness management, physical and behavioral functional health, and mass customization of care. The capability expands to include natural language process of text, prescriptive analytics, and interventional decision support. This stage is useful when the medical practice performing procedures in the OEC is part of a risk sharing group and is managing a population of patients and increased utilization of services will lead to lower revenues and income levels.

Value of the Data Versus Difficulty

The value of the outcome of data analytics correlates with the difficulty of the process. It also moves linearly from "information to optimization." As the value of the data analytics increases, the cost, challenge, and difficulty also increase.

Descriptive analytics: At the very left lower end of the chart is "Descriptive Analytics." This describes or summarizes the raw data that can be interpreted, and attempts are made to answer the question "What happened?"

Diagnostic analytics: As we move linearly to the right, analytics is performed to answer the question—" Why it happened?" It is used to determine the cause of occurrences, whether it be clinical, operational, or financial.

Predictive analytics: the process uses statistical algorithms along with the use of data, machine learning, deep learning, and other techniques to identify what is the possibility of a future outcome based on the historical data. This is used to understand and identify trends, understand patients, and improve clinical outcomes. This can also drive strategic decision-making and also predict behaviors within the organization and in dealing with patients. Predictive analytics provides further insight into "What" will happen.

Prescriptive analytics. This often is the final and the most difficult aspect of analytics. It attempts to provide foresight into how we can make certain things happen and answers questions about what actions should be taken based on the data. Prescriptive analytics provides foresight into "how can we make it happen!"

Electronic Medical Records for the Office-Based Center

Electronic Health Record (EHR), also called the Electronic Medical Record (EMR), and often used interchangeably, received it first real validation in an Institute of Medicine's (IOM) report in 1991.[5]

The EMR has become the core technology and is the center of patient care provided today. Process workflow for patient care is built into the EMR and drives the efficiency and viability of the organization. The information can be accessed from anywhere at anytime and by all the required individuals including the patient. The EMR is intended to meet the triple aim of "Quality, Safety, and Efficiency." The EMR should make running your practice simpler, more efficient, and focused on patient care. EMRs are mandated today, and it is nearly impossible to function without one.

Hundreds of EMR systems are available on the market, and choosing one is not an easy task. Once chosen, the proper installation and training of the staff to use the software to its maximum potential are critical to its success. Integration of the workflow processes of the practice with the EMR is vital and often leads to frustration, increasing inefficiencies and economic loss within the practice. This is contrary to what was expected. Introduction of EMR in the practice is resulting in early retirement of senior physicians and one of the leading causes of physician burnout.

Choosing an EMR for your OEC

To begin with, start by seeking a vendor and software that is suited to and has been established within your specialty and the OEC. It may be better to choose a cardiovascular or specialty-specific EMR based on the size of the practice and specialty. However, it becomes very important that EMR is capable of managing data from other procedures as they are added. For example, interventional radiologists, vascular surgeons, interventional cardiologist have expanded into performing uterine fibroid embolization, spine procedures, embolization for cancer treatment, etc. Ideally in today's world, EMR should be housed in the "cloud" as software as a service allowing you to access your system from anywhere and at any time. The EMR must be secure (meet all HIPPA requirements), connect with other systems while being economical and scalable.

The process starts with the documentation of care provided, and the software must allow for intuitive charting. Several Artificial Intelligence (machine learning and deep learning) systems are now enabling voice to interact with your EMR to document the encounter. EMRs have a practice management component which should help you manage business side of the practice. This deals with patient scheduling, nonclinical interactions with the patients, billing and coding, etc. EMR and the practice management component should work seamlessly.

Almost all systems should enable you to e-prescribe and help you meet regulatory requirements such as Medicare Access and CHIP Reauthorization Act of 2015 (MACRA).[6] They must permit you to easily order labs and imaging studies and connect seamlessly with your PACS system. It is also important to have a patient portal so that the patient can have access to their health data and have ability to communicate with the physician and the office staff for relevant clinical issues.

Procedure Documentation and Image Management PACS

OECs are essentially catheterization labs or interventional labs in the outpatient setting. Physicians using the electronic systems are required to document and manage the process of performing the procedures: recording, storing, and communicating the images and reports of the procedures performed.

Often these are described as cardiovascular information systems (CVIS) and cardiac PACS. These reporting systems allow procedural reporting and connect to the overall EMR. Often ultrasound imaging for peripheral arteries and veins, echocardiogram, ECG, and cath-lab hemodynamics are combined together and stored in the EMR in the aggregate as the cardiovascular patient data.

It is crucial to avoid dependence on paper and film, and utilize structured reporting for ultrasound, cardiac, peripheral, and other invasive procedures. All procedural information must be easily entered in a structured format so that all of this is available for analysis and submission to registries. The voice dictation system should be integrated, and ultimately the system should allow for scalability and accommodation for future growth as the office-based center grows and/or other locations are added. Ultimately, the system must help streamline the center's workflow and improve operational performance. Report generation, communication, and archival must be easy and meet the regulatory documentation requirements to assist your center to be in compliance. All the information must be available anytime, anywhere, securely, and on any device. If the analytics system and or electronic data warehouse is not yet established, submission of data directly from the CVIS should be possible to meet the requirements imposed by CMS and other regulatory agencies.

It is important for the practice to meet the requirements imposed by Merit-Based Incentive Payment System (MIPS). The process is complicated and changes from year to year. However, the energy expended to fully understand and meet the requirements is crucial. With the help of an EMR if all the requirements are met the practice can see its revenues rise by an effective 18% compared with a practice that does not. It is a budget neutral process so that the losers effectively pay for the winners. Penalties for nonparticipation grow from 4% in 2017 to 9% in 2020. The figure displays the math effectively.[7]

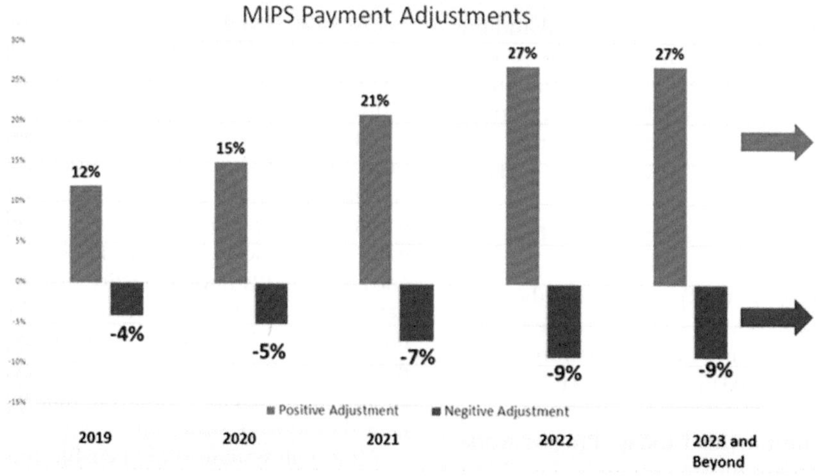

Integration of Inventory Management

In an OEC, where complex and peripheral arterial and venous procedures are performed, the cost of the inventory is substantial and a major portion of the cost of the procedure. This CVIS system should allow tracking of the inventory and possibly have it integrated with the system and allow for the data to be sent into the electronic data warehouse and be made available for further analysis and analytics as needed.

Revenue cycle management which includes coding, billing, and collections of payment from patients and payers is a very complex process and very dependent on the EMR, and the CVIS to provide accurate information for coding billing and collections operations. It is ideal to have the cloud-based clinical workflow and revenue cycle management systems integrated so that appropriate coding of the procedure, billing, and collection functions can all be performed seamlessly and efficiently.

The technology is changing at a rapid pace. Most physicians and clinical staff are not well versed in the technological advances. The payers, regulatory agencies, and the society in general are demanding data to make decisions that will impact the practice of medicine and OEC. An OEC that learns to use the evolving technology and benefit from it will survive and do well. The OEC can ignore these advances at its own peril.

REFERENCES

1. Amazonification of Healthcare. Publicis https://www.visualcapitalist.com/amazonification-healthcare/.
2. *Data-Driven Business Transformation: How to Disrupt, Innovate and Stay Ahead of the Competition*. Peter Jackson, Caroline Carruthers.
3. Sources for Data on Social Determinants of Health. Centers for Disease Control and Prevention, Social Determinants of Health https://www.cdc.gov/socialdeterminants/data/index.htm.
4. Healthcare Analytics Adoption Model: A Framework and Roadmap (white paper) Dale Sanders, President of Technology; David Burton, MD, Senior Vice President.
5. Entitled "The Computer-Based Patient Record: An Essential Technology for Health Care" (www.nap.edu).
6. Centers for Medicare and Medicaid Services. What is MACRA https://www.cms.gov/Medicare/Quality-Initiatives-Patient-Assessment-Instruments/Value-Based-Programs/MACRA-MIPS-and-APMs/MACRA-MIPS-and-APMs.html.
7. Understanding Medicare Access and CHIP Reauthorization Act of 2015 (MACRA), Merit-Based Incentive Payment System (MIPS) and Alternative Payment Models (APM's), Thomas Sullivan. (https://www.policymed.com/2016/02/understanding-medicare-access-and-chip-reauthorization-act-of-2015-macra-merit-based-incentive-payment-system-mips-and-a.html).

CHAPTER 9

From Hospital Employed Model to Independence

KRISHNA JAIN, MD, FACS

When the residency and fellowships are finished, the next step may the hardest one to take. The next step could possibly decide the financial security, happiness, and fulfillment for rest of the life. There is no national match system to place the physician at a certain institution. A decision needs to be made where one will like to raise the family, have professional satisfaction and financial security. There will be various job opportunities to choose from. The choices include solo private practice, single specialty group practice, multispecialty group practice,[1] hospital employment, joining a hospital owned physician group, academic practice, and working for the industry. Few years ago, the main choice used to be between academic practice versus private practice. Now, because of the changing healthcare system, hospital-based or hospital-affiliated employment has become much more popular than other models. The administrative burden, changing, and in most cases decreasing reimbursement, the cost of running a practice, and the increasing regulatory burden have all contributed to physicians either leaving an existing practice to join the hospital or starting their carriers in the hospital employment. Satiani[2] found that younger physicians were more likely to join hospital employment.

In a recent survey,[3] AMA found that employed physicians outnumbered the self-employed physicians, 47.4% to 45.9%. "In the aggregate, 34.7% of physicians worked either directly for a hospital or in a practice at least partly owned by a hospital in 2018, up from 29.0% in 2012." This shift in employment has significant implications for physicians, patients, and the healthcare system. The physicians lose clinical autonomy in treating patients. Government and private insurance policies increasingly favor integrated health systems in the belief that the cost of providing care will go down and outcomes will improve. However, it is not true. Employed physicians perform more services in a hospital outpatient department (HPOD) setting than independent physicians.[4] This increases costs to the Medicare program and financial responsibility for patients.

In 2016, Avalere released a study in collaboration with Physicians Advocacy Institute,[5] documenting the differential in Medicare payment for services performed in HOPD and physician office settings. For the three types of services studied—cardiac imaging, colonoscopy, and evaluation and management services—Medicare paid more for services provided in a HOPD setting than in a physician-owned office. The increased integration of the hospitals and physician resulted in more than $3.1 billion in increased costs from 2012 to 2015. Medicare paid $2.7 billion more for these services, while the beneficiaries faced $411 million (27%) more in financial responsibility. Because the hospital is able to collect more revenue for the same services provided in the private practice, the hospital system is able to reimburse the physician more than what they can expect to earn in a private practice. This results in new physicians being offered higher starting salaries and practicing physicians getting paid higher salary in hospital employment as compared with the ones they were making in the private practice. Once the site differential is eliminated by CMS, the advantage hospitals have in paying higher salary will disappear.

The hospital employment does provide a steady, guaranteed income, though it may be tied to some productivity formula. There is no hassle of negotiating contracts with payers, and usually one does not have to build a practice. The patients come from within the hospital system. The practice expenses are covered. Vacation days are fixed. Despite the security of a hospital, many physicians leave hospital employment. Why do the physicians leave hospital employment? There are various reasons. There is usually no appreciation of

Office-Based Endovascular Centers. https://doi.org/10.1016/B978-0-323-67969-5.00009-5
Copyright © 2020 Elsevier Inc. All rights reserved.

excelling as a physician. There is very little support for intellectual growth and challenge. The continued medical education is tied to vacation days, and the money allocated for this activity is miniscule. There is minimal to no support for joining professional organizations. The staff the physician is forced to work with is not of physician's choosing. In Dr Drummond's[6] view, there are three main reasons which make physicians leave the hospital employment: (1) toxic culture, (2) flawed decision-making process, (3) unacceptable immediate supervisor behavior. In private practice, the physician is his/her own boss, has the opportunity to build a respectable and trusted business. Physician can choose the people to associate with, can help patients in need, can increase revenue by offering different services, has the decision-making power, and has better control over time management.

Once the physician has decided to leave the hospital employment and become independent, there has to be proper planning. First of all, the physician needs to look at the signed contract with the hospital for the restrictive covenant clause. If the clause is reasonable then the hospital will enforce it and win. If the clause is unreasonable the hospital will probably fight it anyway, since they have deep pockets and force you to move because of the expense of litigation. Depending on the availability of other physicians in the same specialty the hospital may want you to stay and have a mutually agreed upon separation. It will take several months to set up a new practice. You have to select a date to start the practice. This will usually be few days to weeks after the current hospital contract expires. Based upon the current contract, you may have to give appropriate timely notice to the current employer.

It is important to have sound legal and accounting advice. This is the time to make a business plan with a start-up budget, working capital, etc. The plan will guide you through the process of starting the practice. It will also be required by the financial institution if you are looking to get a loan to start the practice. Organization structure will need to be decided. Is it going to be a professional corporation or be structured as a different legal entity. The name of the practice needs to be decided and checked to make sure it is available to be used in the state you are going to practice. A budget needs to be created for capital equipment and smaller items needed to furnish the space. Depending on personal savings, and short-term loans from family and friends you may not need a loan from the bank. In all likelihood you will have to apply for a loan from a financial institution.

Location: Once the decision has been made to leave the hospital employment, the first and foremost a decision needs to be made about the location of the practice. When considering location, various factors need to be addressed. One of the important considerations is the geographical area where the physician and the family want to spend most of their active lives. This should be the place where you would like to raise your family. The local competition should be carefully looked at. If there is a need for your services it will be a lot easier to set up a practice. If the local physicians are employees of the local hospital system you may get the patients initially because there is a need you are fulfilling. However, in due course the hospital is likely to get their own specialist and cut you out of the referrals. Hospital-employed physicians are usually required to refer patients within the healthcare system. The exception is if the patient wants to go out of the system and see you. This is frowned upon and you cannot build your practice based on an occasional patient. Next you have to look at a physical place to practice. The space requirement will depend on the kind of services you plan to offer and plan for growth. If the plan is to provide noninvasive ultrasound, office-based endovascular center (OEC), ambulatory surgical services, and wound care, there should be enough space to provide these services. All the services may not be provided at the beginning of the practice, but may be added as the practice grows. If there is enough space, it will avoid a move in the future. The space that is not being used can be left undeveloped to cut down on the leasing expense. If the plan is to grow from one person practice to a larger practice, it should be kept in mind while looking for space. Provision should be made for physician extenders. Once the lease has been negotiated, the space needs to be designed and finished based on the vision of the practice. Usually it is much better to rent than build your own building when starting a new practice. Once the building is finished it will also need outdoor and indoor signs.

Credentialing: Various insurance agencies will need you to submit paperwork to be credentialed by them so that you can receive payment for the services provided. None of these companies with entertain the application unless you have obtained the Medicare number. Medicare enrollment application[7] for physicians and nonphysician practitioners (Form CMS-855I) is used by individual physicians or nonphysician practitioners to initiate the Medicare enrollment process or to change their Medicare enrollment information. If you are planning to move to a different state, you will need state medical license which can take a few months depending on the state. You may also need to make sure that your DEA license is current if you need to apply for state narcotic license. Applications for credentialing need to be submitted in a timely manner so that there is no delay, otherwise you will not be able to receive reimbursement for the services provided. The process can take several months. If you are staying in the area where you are currently employed the wait may be less since you already have a history with the insurance company.

Hospital privileges: If you are staying in the same hospital system where you are currently employed, you do not have to worry about hospital privileges. However, if you are moving to a different location you have to apply for hospital privileges. Make sure you fill out the application properly and include all the procedures you plan to perform with supplemental support for the more recent procedures that you may not have done in your training. Many hospitals have gone to a two-step process. First step is the completion of preliminary application. Once, it is approved, then only you are asked to fill the application that will ultimately give you privileges to practice in the hospital. It can take several months to get privileges. Make sure all the documentation is complete and all the recommendation letters arrive to the credentialing committee in a timely manner. You will get provision privileges, and depending on the hospital bylaws you may get permanent privileges after 1 or 2 years of satisfactory practice in the hospital.

Insurance: There are various insurances that need to be bought to protect yourself, employees, and the practice.

Professional Liability Insurance: Before you are granted hospital privileges, the hospital will want to make sure that you have this kind of insurance. There may be a minimal requirement by the hospital that you have to meet. There are two types of insurances, claims made and occurrence. Claims made are cheaper but will need a tail coverage in case you decide to leave your practice. In certain circumstances, like disability, death, and retirement the tail coverage may not be required. It depends on the policy. Occurrence policy covers all claims made at any time when the occurrence policy was in effect at the time of the injury. These tend to be more expensive than claim-made policies. When buying the policy, you want to be sure that the insurance company cannot settle a lawsuit without your consent.

Property Insurance: This insurance covers both the physical building of the practice and personal properties like office furnishings, inventory, computers, etc. Even if the office space is leased, this insurance is necessary.

Workers Compensation Insurance: In all states except Texas, an employer must have workers compensation insurance, depending on the number of hired employees. This insurance pays for medical care and replaces a portion of lost wages for an employee who is injured at work. In case of employee's death as a result of the injuries the insurance company will compensate the employee's family.

Business Interruption Insurance: This insurance covers income lost due to a disaster-related closing of a business or due to the need for structural rebuilding of the practice. This insurance can be combined with the property insurance under a business owner's policy.

Practice Overhead Insurance: This insurance covers office expenses like utility bills, rent, salaries, taxes, other office costs, etc. if you are temporarily out of the office due to a disability.

Life Insurance: It offers a death benefit to your appointed beneficiaries. Term life insurance is very cheap to buy. Some of the financial institutions will demand an insurance policy before they approve a sizable loan for the practice.

Disability Insurance: This insurance is quite often ignored but is very important to have. In case you cannot practice the only thing you have trained for, you need money to live. Disability insurance can provide that. The disability insurance usually provides a portion of the income that was received by you during active practice. Some insurances will pay even if you are able to practice clinical medicine but not able do procedures.

Cyber Theft Insurance: In the digital age we live in, this insurance has taken increasing importance. There have been several examples, where cyber thieves have stolen patient data and demanded ransom to release data or publish the data violating HIPAA. These thieves can also steal financial data from your computers.

Regulatory Compliance: There are various regulations that need to be adhered to. These include OSHA, HIPAA. There may be a need to get a person in the office to be the compliance officer. Penalties for violating HIPAA are severe. Local, state, and federal compliance guidelines must be identified and implemented. There needs to be total compliance at all times.

Financial Planning: The practice needs to open a checking account and get credit card machines. A financial policy is required that includes payroll, accounts payable, accounts receivable, budgeting, operations, and internal controls. Financial policy is required to keep the practice healthy. A fee schedule needs to be developed based on Medicare allowable charges. The billing can be internal or outsourced to a reliable billing and collection agency with strong ethics. The practice should buy HCFA forms, purchase CPT and ICD—10 books—and obtain Medicare and Medicaid billing manuals.

Electronic Medical Record (EMR): There is no choice but to have electronic medical records. It is important to have the right EMR for the office which should be easy to use, intuitive, and efficient. This should support the practice. Every EMR is not suited for vascular practice. Since the plan is to have an OEC, the EMR should work as well in OEC as in the practice. It should be able to produce structured operative notes. It may be advisable to have an EMR that interacts with the hospital EMR, where you have privileges.

Practice Management Software. It is crucial to have easy to use, efficient software for scheduling, billing and coding, and collections. The software should provide analytic capabilities to be able to assess the practice on a regular basis. The software should also easily interact with the EMR. It should have the capability to help with inventory control.

Communication: It is important to have reliable, efficient telephone system in the office. There may or may not be a need for answering service and paging service since these can be automated.

Office Staff: First and foremost, it is important to have a competent office/business manager. This should be the first hire for the practice. Working with the manger, rest of the team can be hired. Every employee should be cross-trained to fulfill multiple functions. You cannot afford to have the hospital mentality, "Only Mary knows how to do it." You do not need to have full complement of the staff on the first day of practice. You need to have the right staff. You will need a front desk person who can also help with billing and collection. There will be a need for a registered nurse supported by medical assistants. Once the practice matures, there may be a need for physician extenders like nurse practitioners and physician's assistant. Each state has its own rules that govern the scope of practice for nurse practitioners and physician assistants. There are strict billing guidelines when the services are provided by physician extenders. If the billing is kept in house, at least one biller will be required. For the ultrasound machine, at least one certified vascular ultrasound tech will be needed. Some of these employees will also help in the OEC as and when it is opened. Business manger should oversee the practice as well as OEC. There should be no hesitation in terminating an employee if the person is not competent or a team player.

Equipment: The office will need various equipment and supplies to run (Table 9.1). The disposable supplies will include bandages, gauze, adhesive tape, disposable suture/staple removal kits, antibiotic cream, ace wraps, disposable gloves, sterile gloves, Unna boots, etc.

TABLE 9.1
Equipment Needed for the Office.

DOCTOR'S OFFICE
Desk, chair, two visitor chairs, computer, phone, filing cabinet, floor mat, waste paper basket, wall pictures, book shelf
BUSINESS MANGER
Desk, chair, two visitor chairs, computer, phone, filing cabinet, floor mat, waste paper basket, wall pictures, white board, clock
RECEPTION AND FRONT DESK
Exam table, stool for doctor, two visitor chairs, computer, waste basket, OSHA-approved receptacle for biological waste, sharps container, pamphlet/magazine rack, weighing scale, blood pressure instrument, handheld doppler, wall pictures, glove box holder, paper holder
BILLING
Computer, printer scanner, telephone, two chairs, filing cabinet, waste basket, wall pictures
ULTRASOUND ROOM
Ultrasound machine, machine to perform segmental pressures and wave form analysis, plethysmograph, etc., gel warmer, stretcher, computer, telephone stool for the technician, two chairs, waste paper basket, wall pictures, glove box holder, paper holder
NURSES' AREA
Computer, phone, printer scanner, chairs, waste basket, filing cabinet, locked narcotic supply cabinet, wall pictures

Running the Office: There should be policies and procedures and employee manual for the employees to follow (Chapter 10). There should be procedures created for bank deposits, appointment schedule, collection policy, assessing account receivable, account payable policy, monthly financial analysis, bill adjustment guidelines, monthly staff meetings, and employee evaluation.

Marketing: Marketing is not advertising. Physician is his or her own best marketeer. It is important for the physician to look professional and act professional at all times. The first step is to have a logo for the practice and create business cards. In today's digital age the value of a website cannot be underestimated. The marketing can be tailored to digital media, print media, audiovisual media, and personal contact. It is described in greater detail in Chapter 20.

Office-Based Endovascular Center: It is usually a mistake to start the OEC at the same time as opening the practice. OEC is capital intensive and needs to have steady flow of patients to be profitable. If the physician is able to leave the hospital employment and be able to practice in the same hospital then it may be feasible to start the lab simultaneously with the practice. Almost always the hospital will not let the departing physician contact existing patients. This is usually written in the separation agreement. However, the physician can advertise in various media to inform the patient about the new practice location and that the practice is accepting new patients. In case the practice is opening in a new location, the practice should be mature enough to support an OEC. A new pro forma needs to be created to look at the feasibility and profitability of an OEC. If the practice is not busy enough, there will be a temptation to do unnecessary procedures which is obviously unacceptable.

Business Consultant: All the steps needed to start the practice and the OEC can be taken by the physician independent of using management companies. However, it is time-consuming and many steps need to be taken to be compliant, profitable, and have work life balance. It may be advisable to use a company that specializes in opening the practice and OEC for a period of time. A reputable company in the long run will be cost-effective because the practice and OEC will open in timely manner and costly mistakes will be avoided.

Conclusion: In a survey conducted by Geneia,[8] 51% of physicians in independent or working in the physician-owned practice talked negatively about their job as compared with 69% working for hospitals or corporations. By opening a private practice, the physician is investing in his/her future. This can bring happiness and joy. The physicians can treat the patients to the best of their ability without interference and reap financial and emotional rewards. If they want to provide more charity care they can do so, without anyone's permission. The private practice also needs certain managerial skills which can be obtained by taking business courses or by heeding the advice of other colleagues or professionals like attorneys and accountants. For an interventionalist, opening an OEC along with the practice can make the practice profitable.[9]

REFERENCES

1. Wixon CL, Jain KM, Satiani B. Single-specialty versus multispecialty vascular surgery group model. *J Vasc Surg*. 2013. https://doi.org/10.1016/j.jvs.2012.12.045.
2. Satiani B. Health care update: hospital employment or private practice? *Perspect Vasc Surg Endovasc Ther*. 2013; 25(3–4):46–52. https://doi.org/10.1177/1531003513510952.
3. *Employed Physicians Outnumber Self-Employed*. American Medical Association. https://www.ama-assn.org/press-center/press-releases/employed-physicians-outnumber-self-employed.
4. *Hospital-Employed Physicians Drain Medicare*. https://www.modernhealthcare.com/article/20171114/NEWS/171119942/hospital-employed-physicians-drain-medicare.
5. Physicians Advocacy Institute. *Updated Physician Practice Acquisition Study: National and Regional Changes in Physician Employment*; February 2018. www.physiciansadvocacyinstitute.org.
6. *Why Employed Physicians Quit*. https://www.thehappymd.com/blog/bid/328289/why-employed-physicians-quit.
7. *Medicare Enrollment for Physicians, Non-Physician Practitioners and Other Health Care Suppliers. Information About Enrolling in the Medicare Program*. http://www.cms.hhs.gov/MedicareProviderSupEnroll.
8. Geneia | Independent Docs Happier. http://marketing.geneia.com/2018/independentdocshappier.
9. Jain KM, Munn J, Rummel M, Vaddineni S, Longton C. Future of vascular surgery is in the office. *J Vasc Surg*. 2010. https://doi.org/10.1016/j.jvs.2009.09.056.

CHAPTER 10

Policies and Procedures

KRISHNA JAIN, MD, FACS

The policies and procedures that are established at an office-based endovascular center (OEC) will establish the culture, principles, rules, and guidelines for the organization. These policies will provide a vision for employees of the long-term goals of the organization, as well as the fine details of day-to-day practice. The policies and procedures will guide all decisions and actions that occur in the practice. Policies cover what employees can expect from the organization, e.g., employee benefits; what the center expects from employees, e.g., code of conduct, proficiency, confidentiality agreements; and what patients can expect from the OEC. Procedures provide the frame work for the implementation of the policies, by providing a step-by-step guide for every function of the center. Every policy and procedure should be reviewed, signed, and dated. Updates to policies and procedures should be tracked. This chapter will discuss major categories of policies and procedures that should be developed for an OEC, including policies and procedures that are focused on employees, patients, operative procedures, and facility management. In the limited space we have in this chapter it is not possible to describe each element in detail, but we have provided a number of examples in each section of the chapter. It is important to adhere to the procedures as outlined in the manuals for certifications as well as for the safety of the employees and patients.

PHYSICIAN TRAINING

Physicians should be adequately trained in the procedures they are performing. As the new procedures are developed the physician should undergo proper training before performing these procedures at the center. All physicians working in the OEC should be advanced cardiovascular life support (ACLS) certified.

EMPLOYEE-RELATED POLICIES AND PROCEDURES

A list of potential topics to be addressed in the handbook is listed below; however, the center should modify this list to meet their needs.

Policy: All employees will work as a team to provide the best possible care to the patients coming to the OEC.

Procedure: Every employee should be given a handbook that explains in detail the policies and procedures of the center. Most policies of the office apply to all employees of the OEC, as the OEC is an extension of the clinical practice.

I. Introduction to Facility
II. Employment Relationship
III. Commitment to Equal Opportunity
IV. Employee Classifications
V. Introductory Period
VI. Performance Appraisals and Salary Scales
  A. Anniversary Date
VII. Work Schedules
  A. Recording Work Hours and Absences
  B. Overtime Hours
VIII. Corporate Standards
  A. Attendance
  B. Computer Use
  C. Confidentiality
  D. Dress Code and Personal Hygiene
  E. Drug and Alcohol Use
  F. Employee Conduct

Office-Based Endovascular Centers. https://doi.org/10.1016/B978-0-323-67969-5.00010-1
Copyright © 2020 Elsevier Inc. All rights reserved.

G. Employee Safety
H. Ethical Business Conduct
I. Food and Drinks
J. Inspection of Premises
K. Licensing and Certification
L. Personal Property
M. Personnel Information
N. Resolution of Employee Concerns
O. Sexual and Other Unlawful Harassment
P. Smoking
Q. Solicitation and Distribution
R. Telephone Usage
S. Termination
T. Transfers within "Facility Name"

IX. Benefits
A. Educational Assistance
B. Holiday Pay
C. Insurance
D. Leaves of Absences
1. Family and Medical Leave
2. Funeral
3. Jury Duty
4. Military Duty Leave
5. Personal Leave
E. Malpractice and Employee Liability Coverage
F. Paid Time Off
G. Pension/Profit Sharing Plans
H. References
I. Uniforms
J. Workers' Compensation

X. Acknowledgment: _____signed by the employee_____

Below is an example of the employee related policies and procedures relating to dress code and procedure attire.

Dress Code and Procedure Attire

Purpose: The human body is a major source of microbial contamination in this environment; therefore, scrub clothing is worn to promote a high level of cleanliness and hygiene within the semisurgical and office environment. When wearing your uniform anytime, you are representing the company with the expectation that you will be suitably attired and groomed. A good clean appearance bolsters your own poise and self-confidence, which greatly enhances a positive impression to others.

Policy: Employee needs to dress to appear professional and dress appropriately to prevent infection.

Procedure: Royal Blue scrubs (the color to be decided by the center) with white embroidered writing on upper left chest to include logo of the practice, employee name, and center name. White lab coats, white or royal blue scrub jackets are allowed. Writing should be in black with a royal blue logo on white jackets. Dedicated shoes should be worn daily. Shoe covers must be worn by any staff member entering the procedure room in street shoes. Shoe covers are provided. Jewelry is permitted except when doing sterile procedures in which rings, watches, and or bracelets should be removed. Fingernails should be kept short, clean, natural or freshly manicured. Artificial nails should not be worn if scrubbing for a procedure. If scrubbed and assisting the interventionalist, you should wear sterile gown, sterile gloves, hat, mask and safety goggles.

PATIENT-RELATED POLICIES AND PROCEDURES

It is of utmost importance in providing appropriate care to patients for the office to maintain an accurate patient record (Fig. 10.1).

Appointment Status Change

Policy: Document changes in a patient's appointment status and inform the OEC scheduler.

Procedure: The receptionist will be responsible for notifying the scheduler regarding the change in a patient's appointment. The scheduler will contact the patient and document in the patient's chart the cancellation if patient does not want to have the procedure or wants it on a different date. The scheduler will notify the physician of the change in appointment status. The scheduler will document the reason for change in status. The scheduler will make two attempts to contact the patient or the emergency contact person on the telephone and if that fails patient will receive written notification. If the appointment was canceled because of inability of the patient to see a specialist's consultation requested by OEC physician, the office staff will facilitate this appointment.

Preprocedure Patient Assessment

Policy: Patient will have appropriate preprocedure assessment to prevent complications and have an optimal outcome.

Procedure: The assessment needs to be performed and documented (Fig. 10.2).

TODAY'S DATE:

PATIENT'S NAME: **DOB:**

SCHEDULE FOR PHYSICIAN (name):

PROCEDURE:

DIAGNOSIS

☐ fluoroscopy	☐ Lab Slip for PT / PTT, BUN / Creatinine
☐ Power Injector	☐ NPO
☐ U/S needed	☐ Moderate Sedation

ORDER

☐ Hydration	☐ Dye Allergy Prep

STOP

☐ Coumadin 4 days	☐ Plavix 7 days

If contrast given hold Glucophage 48 hours after procedure then order: ☐ Creatinine / GFR

VENOUS CENTER PROCEDURE

Indications for Surgical Treatment for Varicose Veins: (check all that apply)

☐ Periodic leg elevation	☐ Avoidance of Prolonged Mobility
☐ Superficial vein thrombosis	☐ Non-Healing skin ulceration
☐ Hemorrhage	☐ Stasis Dermatitis
☐ Refractory Dependent Edema	

BILLING AUTHORIZATION

☐ Insurance	☐ Authorization # called	☐ No Authorization needed
☐ Authorization Confirmation # obtained	☐ Record in Patient's chart	☐ Unauthorized Procedure

☐ Patient called about unauthorized procedure

☐ Doctor Schedule	☐ NP Schedule
☐ RN Schedule	☐ PA Schedule
☐ Call to Patient	☐ Letter to Patient

SCHEDULER'S NOTES:

SPECIAL REQUEST:

Is patient on dialysis: ☐ Yes ☐ No	If yes what days? M T W T F S	Location:

FIG. 10.1 Example of a patient record.

CONTRAST ALLERGY PREP given / taken per protocol? ☐ yes ☐ no Initials: - ____________

Medications taken today? ____________ ___

Do you take Coumadin or Plavix? ☐ yes ☐ no If yes, last time taken: ____________

Consent signed: ☐ yes ☐ no **Pulses:** Lt DP ______ Rt DP ______ Lt PT ______ Rt PT ______ N/A ______

Vital Signs: T ________ P ________ BP ________ SPO2 ________ CBG ________

IV: solution / location / rate / time / amount: ____________ Started by: ____________

GFR ________ Creatinine ________ BUN ________ PT ________

INR ________ PTT ________ Cap Refill ________ Neuro ________

Is patient currently having pain? ☐ yes ☐ no Level / Location / Treatment: ____________

Pre-Procedure Medication / Sedation:					
TIME	**MEDICATION**	**STRENGTH**	**AMT GIVEN**	**ROUTE**	**GIVEN BY**

Pre Procedure Counts: **W:** ______ **H:** ______ **N:** ______ **B:** ______ **Counted by:** ______

Room start time: ______ Local injected: ______ Dressing time: ______ Room end time: ______

Surgeon: ____________ Fluoroscopy Time: Min: ________ Sec: ________

Room Staff: ____________ ________

Diagnosis: ____________ ________

Procedure: ____________ ________

Micro incisions: ☐ N/A or R ________ L ________ Length of GSV / LSV treated: ________ cm

Laser settings: W ______ ______ Total Pulses: ______ Total Energy: ______ Total Time: ________ in Pulse Mode

MEDICATION	**STRENGTH**	**AMT ON FIELD**	**AMT GIVEN**	**ROUTE**	**GIVEN BY**
Hep Saline	5,000u / 500cc	cc	cc		
Contrast:	1% / 8.4%	cc	cc		
	mg/ml	cc	cc		

FIG. 10.1 cont'd.

Time	B / P	P	02	Pain	Notes

Post Procedure Counts: **W:** ______ **H:** ______ **N:** ______ **B:** ______ **Counted by:** ______

Counts Correct? ☐ yes ☐ no If 'no' MD notified @ ____________ X-Ray Ordered? ☐ yes ☐ no

Results: ____

Time	B / P	P	02	Pain	Notes

Post procedure instructions given to Pt: ☐ yes ☐ no Post op appointment made? ☐ yes ☐ no

Discharg e to care of: ____

CHART		
INITIALS	NAMES	TITLES

FIG. 10.1 cont'd.

Moderate Sedation

Sedation/analgesia

Definition:

The use of drugs such as narcotics, barbiturates, sedative-hypnotics, and benzodiazepines may be used with the intent to lessen the awareness of the patient during surgery, noninvasive or invasive procedures. Because the depth of sedation is a continuum, it is not always possible to predict how an individual will respond to the agent administered. Levels of sedation/anesthesia are defined as follows:

A. **Minimal sedation (aka anxiolysis)**: A drug-induced state during which patients respond normally to verbal commands.

B. **Moderate sedation/analgesia (aka conscious sedation)**: A drug-induced depression of consciousness during which patients respond purposefully to verbal commands, either alone or accompanied by light tactile stimulation.

C. **Deep sedation/analgesia**: A drug-induced depression of consciousness during which patients cannot be easily aroused but respond purposefully to repeated or painful stimulation.

D. **Anesthesia**: Consists of general anesthesia and spinal or major regional anesthesia. It does not include local anesthesia. General anesthesia is a drug-induced loss of consciousness during which patients are not arousable, even by painful stimulation.

Purpose: To provide safe patient management during the use of sedation analgesia.

Equipment: Operating room crash cart, EKG monitor and cables, automatic external defibrillator (AED), blood pressure monitor and cuff, O_2 saturation monitor and finger probe, operating room table safety strap, arm boards, full oxygen tank, 15 Lpm regulator and key, IV Pole, laptop computer with patient records, and procedure template.

Instruments: None

Supplies: EKG stickers and printer paper, fentanyl, versed, syringes, needles, alcohol swabs, O_2 nasal canula tubing, ambu bag, tubing and mask, Narcan, romazicon,

Policy: Patient will have appropriate pre procedure assessment to prevent complications and have optimal outcome
Procedure: The following assessment needs to be performed and documented

Patient Name: ________________________ Date: ____________

☐ Allergies reviewed

☐ NPO Status reviewed

☐ H & P reviewed

☐ Patient re-evaluated immediately prior to procedure / sedation

☐ Site marked

INFORMED CONSENT:

☐ Risks, benefits, complications, and alternatives explained, questions answered, and patient / family accepted plan for sedation.

PRE-PROCEDURE PHYSICAL ASSESSMENT:

	WNL	Other (Specify)
Mouth & Throat	☐	☐
Lungs & Chest	☐	☐
Heart	☐	☐

☐ No previous sedation / anesthesia problems (including family history)	☐ Head and Neck obesity
☐ History of apnea / snoring	☐ Dentures / Loose Teeth (circle)
☐ History of Glaucoma	☐

ASA CLASSIFICATION:

☐ 1 – Healthy Patient	☐ 2 – Mild Systemic Disease
☐ 3 – Severe Systemic Disease without functional limitation	☐ 4 – Severe Systemic Disease that is a constant threat to life

CIRCLE ONE: MALLAMPATI AIRWAY CLASSIFICATION:

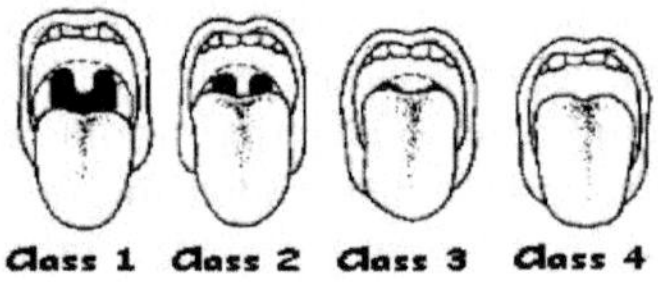

PLAN FOR SEDATION:

☐ Anxiolysis	☐ Moderate Sedation

MEDICATION:

☐ Fentanyl	☐ Versed

Physician Signature: ________________________ Date: ____________

Physician Print Name: ________________________

FIG. 10.2 Pre procedure patient assessment form.

Policy: The center will provide anesthesia and sedation to carry out the procedure in a safe manner.

Procedure

1) A physician is required to be present on site before administration of IV medication for moderate and deep sedation and analgesia. Only licensed practitioners who are trained and proven to be competent in professional standards and techniques to administer pharmacologic agents to predictably achieve desired levels of sedation and to monitor patients carefully in order to maintain them at the desired level of sedation and, when necessary, to rescue them from deeper than desired levels of sedation.
   a. The practitioner administering moderate IV sedation must be qualified to rescue patients from deep sedation and must be trained to manage a compromised airway to provide adequate oxygenation and ventilation.
2) Verify NPO status of patient. Patients should not have anything to eat or drink after midnight, the night before procedure, except for allowed AM meds with a small sip of water. If there is insulin-dependent diabetic and NPO, patient should only take ½ of their AM insulin dose. Oral diabetic medication should be held.
3) Obtain informed consent.
4) A heart and lung assessment must be performed immediately before administration of sedation and documented in the medical record by the physician.
5) A preprocedure Aldrete score (Table 10.1) will be recorded on the patient's medical record.
6) A "time out" must be observed just prior to administration of sedation and a second Aldrete score as well as a sedation level will be determined and recorded by the RN.
7) The patient will be continuously monitored and reassessment will be documented every five (5) minutes until the procedure is completed. This will include vital signs (EKG, oxygen saturation, heart rate, respirations, and blood pressure). The patient's sedation level and Aldrete score will be recorded every 15 min or prior to giving more sedation medication PRN. Any untoward reactions or sudden/significant changes in monitoring parameters are to be immediately reported to the physician.
   a. Drug reversal agents will be at the bedside.
   b. Cart with lifesaving drugs and airway will be at bedside.
8) Sedation and analgesia monitoring may not be discontinued without a physician's order.
9) Documentation of the Aldrete score (Table 10.1) must be completed upon admission to recovery. Before discharge, Aldrete score must be equal to or greater than the preop baseline score.
10) Patient monitoring may be discontinued when the patient meets the following criteria.
   a. Patients must be alert and oriented unless mental status was initially abnormal and then a return to baseline is acceptable.
   b. When reversal agents are utilized the patient must be monitored for 1 h postprocedure.
   c. No procedural complications exist.
   d. Pain is controlled with baseline analgesics.
   e. Neuro/sensation is at baseline.
11) Medications used to provide analgesia and sedation is listed in Table 10.2.

Patient and Family Education

Policy: Both the patient and family members should be provided with information describing the planned procedure and potential alternatives to the planned procedure.

Procedure: For individual procedure provide the following information to the patient and family.

Endovascular intervention procedure

Policies and procedures should be developed for each procedure being conducted at the center. These documents should be reviewed and updated periodically as needed. The procedure for an angiogram is detailed below.

Angiogram

Your procedure is scheduled for________________at________________.

Your arrival time is________________.

1. **Labs**: Kidney function and blood clotting time are necessary prior to having this procedure done. Patients on dialysis will not need to have kidney function labs drawn.

2. **If you are a diabetic**: Please check your blood sugar prior to coming in on the day of your procedure. If you take insulin to manage your diabetes, take only half your regular dose of insulin the morning of your procedure. If you are on Glucophage (Metformin), and/or Glucovance, stop these medicines the morning of your procedure and for 48 h after your procedure. At that time you will need to have your blood drawn again to see if it is safe to restart these medicines.

3. **Medicines**: You may take blood pressure medications on the morning of your procedure. You may take those medications with a small sip of water. If you are unsure which of your medications is prescribed to regulate blood pressure, please contact our office.

You are on blood thinner and follow the instruction given by us to stop the blood thinner at appropriate time.

4. **Contrast dye allergy preparation**: *If you have any allergy to shellfish, iodine, or contrast dye*, you will receive a prescription for a medicine to be taken orally before coming for the procedure. Medication will also be given via the intravenous route.

5. You may not have anything to eat or drink after midnight before your procedure. You may take blood pressure medication with a small sip of water.
6. Bring a driver/support person with you. You must have someone stay with you for 24-hour after the procedure. If you cannot confirm that you will have an attendant, the procedure will be canceled. Bring your insurance card(s).
7. The average procedure lasts about 1–2 h. You should plan for your discharge approximately 1–4 h after your procedure. If your surgeon feels it is important for you to be monitored longer you may need to stay in the hospital overnight (this is extremely rare but is possible).

If you have any questions or concerns, please contact our office

Advance directive: Though it is extremely rare for a person to have a life-threatening event, it is advisable to have a copy of advance directive in the office. It may also be subject to state and federal laws.

Informed consent

***This is only a sample. You may have a consent drawn up by your attorney.*

Consent for procedure

Physician:________________________________

The above physician has told me that I have the following condition:

Condition:________________________________

and has recommended the following procedure:

Procedure:________________________________

To be completed by the patient, or in certain instances or procedures, the designee listed below:

Designee:________________________________

I have been informed by the above named physician of the nature and purpose of the procedure, the risks involved, the possible consequences, the possibility of complications, and other alternative methods of treatment. I also understand that all surgical procedures involve risks, such as severe allergic reaction, loss of blood, infection, blood clot, stroke, pulmonary embolism or death. I have received information regarding specific complications and risks related to the procedure above and have reviewed them. Understanding all of these risks, I consent to submit to the procedure identified above. I recognize that during the course of the procedure unforeseen conditions may necessitate additional or different procedures than the one described above and I consent to any additional or different procedures besides the one above described as deemed necessary by my physician. I acknowledge that no guarantees or assurances have been made to me concerning the result or outcome of the above operation or procedure.

I authorize (clinic name) and its entities to provide care in connection with the above described procedure. I have placed no limitations on the manner in which this procedure may be performed (or the medications or materials to be used), except as follows:

____

____

____

(No limitations unless otherwise note.)

I acknowledge and understand that *(clinic name)* and its entities are teaching facilities, and as such, the above procedure and/or associated medical services may be performed with the assistance of medical students, or students in other healthcare disciplines, or observed by other physicians, or healthcare students in training, as deemed appropriate by the attending surgeon.

I consent to have the method of my examination, treatment, and/or procedure studied, reported, photographed, observed, recorded, and published, so long as my identity is kept confidential for the purposes of marketing or education. Any identifying marks in the photos (such as tattoos or birthmarks) will be removed or obscured.

I have read, or have had read to me upon request, the above consent. I have understood them and have had the opportunity to ask questions of the physician or his representatives, and have has those questions answered to my satisfaction.

If female: Are you or could you be pregnant?

□ Yes □ No □ Unsure

If no: LMP: (mm/dd/yyyy) N/A: (reason: Surgically Sterile, Menopause, etc.)

Patient's signature: ______________________________

Patient's printed name: ______________________________
(or legal representative and relationship)

Date: ______________________________

If person other than patient is signing:

Patient is unable to sign for him/herself because: ______________________________

____

____

____

Witness : ______________________________ Date : ______________

Extremity verified and marked **by patient/legal representative as above**, if applicable, with a pen or marker:

□ Yes □ No

Patient's Initials: ______________________

Patient confidentiality: At all times patient confidentiality should be maintained. In the recovery area when several patients are recovering one needs to be extra careful in discussing patient condition with the patient and family.

Correct Patient, Procedure, and Site Verification

Preprocedure patient preparation

Policy: Ensure that all patients are prepared for their upcoming procedure.

Procedure: To make sure all tests, labs, chart notes, and preprocedural preparations, such as NPO status, IV start, IV hydration, change of clothing, preop medications, etc. are addressed ahead of time to keep the procedure and physician running on time and with the fewest delays possible and ensure patient safety.

Equipment: Gurney, IV pole, visitor chair, bedside table, over bed table. Vital sign monitor with blood/pressure, pulse, temperature, and O_2 saturation. Doppler, O_2 cart with regulator and key, blood glucose monitor, surgical clipper watch or clock with a second hand, ultrasound machine, emergency crash cart, AED, blanket warmer.

Supplies: Patient chart, procedure paperwork such as consent and procedure chart notes, clipboard, prescription pad, medicine prescription pad, lab order slips, med cups, water, apple juice, temperature probe covers, patient gown, IV solutions in various types and amounts, IV tubing, IV extension tubing, angiocatheters in assorted sizes, tourniquet, IV dressings, EtOH swabs, clipper blade, poly backed gurney sheet, pillow ×2, pillow cases, draw sheet, doppler gel, urinary catheter kits—straight catheter/Foley, bed pans, urinals, nonsterile gloves, sterile gloves, nasal canula, oxygen tank with cart and key, CBG, cuvettes/lancets, tape, sharpie permanent marker, patient gown, patient slippers, bandage scissors.

Medications: Oral glucose replacement, regular insulin, heparin lock solution, D5W 1000cc, D5 0.45% NaCl, 0.9% NaCl 250cc, 500cc, and 1000cc, 8.4% sodium bicarbonate 50 mL vials, 2% nitroglycerine ointment, vicodin 5/500, valium 5 mg **or** 10 mg, clindamycin 300 mg tabs **or** cephalexin 500 mg tabs, diphenhydramine 50 mg IV or PO, Solu-Cortef 100 mg IV or 32 mg PO, fentanyl 50mcg/2 mL, versed 2mg/2 mL, Romazicon 0.2 mg, Narcan 0.1 mg, Atropine 0.3–1.2 mg, clonodine 0.1 mg tabs, and all ACLS emergency medications per ACLS recommendations.

Pre procedure planning: The surgeon orders a procedure, discusses risks and benefits with patient, and decides on a sedation plan. The surgeon completes a surgery form noting any needed labs, tests, and prescriptions. The surgery order is sent to billing to get insurance authorization, and then it is sent to the scheduler to put on the surgery schedule. A follow-up appointment is also made at this time. The patient is contacted regarding the date and time of the procedure (enter specific preprocedure info here for every type of case), and preprocedure instructions are reviewed. Medications such as blood thinners, oral antidiabetic medications, insulin, dye allergy medicines, and mucomyst are specifically addressed. Appropriate preprocedure information will also be mailed to the patient by the surgery scheduler. Center staff will call the patient 7–10 days before their procedure to confirm that all necessary testing was completed and to give preprocedure instructions regarding NPO status, when to arrive, medications to take or hold, stockings. Center staff will get results from lab work/tests and based on results instruct patient on arrival time. Any problems are dealt with and resolved at this time. The day before the procedure, all needed procedure papers, like the consent, procedure note, are pulled and filled out as completely as they can be and placed on a clipboard in order of patient arrival for the following day. If electronic health records are being used then the information should be entered in the patient's electronic chart. On the day of the procedure the patient arrives and is checked in at the front desk. Demographics are updated in the computer. The front desk notifies the center staff that the patient is here and they are brought back to the preprocedure area. If IV sedation is planned per surgeon, NPO status is verified, and a presedation examination note is completed by the surgeon while in preoperative area. If patient is diabetic their blood sugar is checked and documented on the procedure record along with any medications taken that morning. If NPO after midnight for IV sedation then only half the normal amount of insulin should be taken in the morning of surgery, and oral diabetes medications are held. The consent is read and signed by the patient or read to the patient at the patient's request. The appropriate extremity is marked with pen by the patient if procedure is to be done on one particular side/extremity. Vital signs are taken and patient can change into a vest or gown. Physical assessment is completed and documented per procedure record and procedure planned. Any abnormal vital signs or other abnormal observations are reported to the RN and MD. After the consent is signed, all questions are answered, and any allergies noted, oral preprocedure medicines including sedatives and antibiotic can be given. Any shave prep, pulses located, IV start, vein mapping, or other preparation will be done at this time. Once IV is started, any needed allergy prep medications can be given. If patient is diabetic, capillary blood sugar will be checked on admit and every 2 h after for duration of stay, or PRN, until discharge. When it is time for the procedure, the family will be escorted to the main waiting room. The patient will then be taken via wheelchair, gurney, or ambulation with assistance to the procedure room for the procedure.

____________________________ ____________________________

Reviewed By Review Date

TABLE 10.1
Aldrete Score.

Color	2 Pink 1 Pale, dusky, ruddy, other 0 Cyanotic
Respiratory	2 Breathing with no distress 1 Impaired, respiration, nasal O_2 0 Apneic, requires ventilation
Circulatory	2 B/P and pulse stable 1 B/P and pulse labile 0 Unable to palpate
Consciousness	2 Fully awake 1 Arousable to stimuli 0 Not responsive
Activity	2 Gait steady 1 Extremity movement on command/ able to dangle w/o dizziness 0 No extremity movement

Operative Procedure and Postprocedure Angiogram

Policy: Patient should have the procedure conducted in a safe manner.

Procedure: Employees responsible for the conduct of the procedure should follow following steps.

Check supplies

Angiography pack Instrument

Pack: two nonperforated towel clips, one hemostat, one mosquito forceps

4 French Mini-Stick Kit

0.035 glidewire 180 cm length

Ultrasound probe cover

4 French Sidearm Sheath (10 cm)

4 French 65 cm Contra Catheter

For power injector: Syringe, multiple patient line, display sheath cover, hand controller, single patient line, hand controller sheath cover (only if more

TABLE 10.2
Medications Used for Sedation.

Generic	Brand	Class	Usual Adult Dose	Reversal Agent
Midazolam	Versed (IV)	Anxiolytic/Sedative	**1–2 mg IV** increments **(over 20–30 s)** Max 10 mg	Flumazenil (Romazicon)
Flumazenil	Romazicon	Benzodiazepine antagonist	**0.2 mg IVP over 15 s** Repeat in 1 min intervals up to 1 mg	n/a
Fentanyl	Sublimaze	Analgesic	**25–50 mcg/dose-slow IVP**, increase by 25–50mcg/dose to a max of 3mcg/kg	Naloxone (Narcan)
Naloxone	Narcan	Opioid antagonist	**0.1 mg IVP** may repeat in 2–3 min intervals up to max of 1 mg	Note: Naloxone has a shorter duration of action than most opiates. Continued monitoring is required and possible redosing.
Diphenhydramine	Benadryl	Antihistamine/ antiemetic	**10–50 mg IVP** q 2–3 h	n/a
Atropine		Vagolytic	**0.3–1.2mg IVP repeat q 4–8 h PRN**	n/a

Note: There are synergistic effects on respiratory depression and sedation when using a benzodiazepine along with a narcotic.

than one scheduled angiogram for the day), 250cc bag normal saline, 500cc bottle Visipaque 320 mg/mL.

(List physician glove sizes)

Medication

Lidocaine 1% = 5cc

Bicarb 8.4% = 5cc

500cc of heparinized NaCl in bowl on sterile table

Visipaque 320 mg/mL start with 20cc purged from power injector on back table

Preprocedure

RN and/or medical assistant. Fill out top portion of consent form, refer to last dictation. Patients need to read and sign consent. Nurse or MA will cosign consent.

Obtain vital signs including respirations and record on procedure form, if patient is diabetic, check blood glucose at time of admit, every 2 h during stay and upon discharge. Report any abnormalities. Place oxygen on patient at 2 L per nasal cannula if oxygen saturation is below 94%. *Verify whether patient has discontinued blood thinners and all other medications besides blood pressure medications. If the patient has taken any medications besides BP meds then obtain further orders from MD. List medications taken on form.*

Obtain patient's weight in kilograms preprocedure.

Remind the surgeon to perform preprocedure assessment and fill out and sign assessment form and mark the site prior to giving conscious sedation medication.

If physician has chosen to give **medication for conscious sedation** ***verify patient was NPO at midnight,*** held all AM medications besides blood pressure medications, and took ½ the dose of AM insulin if patient is diabetic and normally takes insulin.

If GFR <60 inform physician of lab value and follow physician's orders for hydration and calculate the maximum dye that could be used during the procedure. Physician may prefer to cancel the procedure. The following website can be used to calculate amount of allowable contrast that can be used safely in patients with decreased kidney function http://radclass.mudr.org/content/maximum-allowable-contrast-dose-adults-calculator-macd.

Administer PO medications if the procedure is being performed without moderate sedation. If moderate sedation is planned only antibiotic should be given orally with a sip of water.

- Antibiotic—Cephalexin (Keflex) 500 mg, one capsule, if the patient is allergic to penicillin administer: clindamycin (Cleocin) 300 mg, one capsule
- Pain medication—Vicodin 5/325 mg, one tablet, if patient is allergic to vicodin, administer Tylenol 3 (300mg/30 mg) or Ultram (50 mg)
- Sedative—Valium 5 or 10 mg, one tablet depending on age and size of patient

Patients should change into a gown and be given a blanket. Place a sheet and under pad on the gurney. Assist the patient's transfer to the gurney.

Patient needs a shave preparation of both groins if they have not already done this at home before arriving. Use handheld Doppler to mark bilateral dorsalis pedis and posterior tibial arteries at ankle level.

RN will perform IV placement and start hydration orders as directed per protocol:

GFR ≥60: 500 mL 0.9% NaCl IV to be infused over 1 h prior to IV contrast administration then decrease IV rate to 250 mL per hour during procedure; postprocedure keep IV rate at 250 mL per hour for up to 2 h postprocedure or at the discretion of the MD.

GFR <60: 500 mL 0.9% NaCl IV to be infused over 1 h prior to IV contrast administration, then decrease IV rate to 250 mL per hour until and during procedure; postprocedure place IV rate at 500 mL per hour for 2 h postcontrast or 250 mL per hour over 4 h depending on MD order on length of stay.

Patient with known diagnosis of congestive heart failure: No bolus fluids. Administer 0.9% NaCl IV at 250 mL per hour preprocedure, during procedure, and postprocedure for length of stay.

The rate of infusion may be different based on new data that emerge in preventing contrast induced nephropathy.

After fluids have been administered, RN to administer medications intravenously if the procedure is being performed under conscious sedation.

RN or medical assistant or radiology technician. Prepare Heparinized Saline

250 mL 0.9% sodium chloride with 0.5cc of heparin (5000 USP units/mL)

500 mL 0.9% sodium chloride with 1cc of heparin (5000 USP units/mL)

1000 mL 0.9% sodium chloride with 2cc of heparin (5000 USP units/mL)

Before first case of the day mix amount needed for daily schedule: 500 mL placed on sterile field per case so if four cases are scheduled for the day then mix up a quantity of two 1000 mL bags of heparinized saline and place stickers on bag to label contents. Spike one bag with bag decanter.

Get lidocaine 1% and sodium bicarb 8.4% out of cupboard and check expiration dates and open dates—place on medication cart. Also get heparin 5000 USP units/1 mL out of drawer of medication cart and check expiration date and open date—place on medication cart for use throughout day.

Radiology technician. Take the current day's schedule and highlight the current day's procedures with a green highlighter for those procedures using the C-ARM and a purple highlighter for those procedures not using the C-ARM. Log onto EMR and pull up the patients scheduled for the day to get their social security number, date of birth, and any other pertinent information needed for placing patient information in the EMR being used in the lab for procedure documentation, inventory control, and structured operative note. Place the daily schedule on the C-ARM for reference. Turn C-ARM on.

RN or radiology technician. Assist scrub technician with arranging the room for the procedure. Place extension on end of bed, bring ultrasound in room, place C-ARM and monitor in correct area around room. Assist scrub technician with placing fluids on the sterile field—using sterile technique pour 500cc of heparinized saline into large bowl. Mark the bowl. Wipe off top of lidocaine and bicarb vials with alcohol swab, hold for scrub technician to withdraw in a sterile manner amount needed for the case. Cover camera on C-ARM and foot pedal of C-ARM with plastic bag.

RN, radiology technician, or scrub technician. Set up power injector for the case. Turn power injector on and follow instructions as to how to set up.

Scrub technician. Scrub with 4% chlorohexidine if this is the first case of the day. Don sterile gloves and open sterile field for procedure.

RN, radiology technician, or scrub technician. Wheel patient on gurney from preop area and take to procedure room. Have family members of patient follow and take them to the waiting room.

RN. Chart amount of normal saline patient received in preop area. Review preoperative procedure record and make sure all necessary information has been filled in and make sure patient received sedation.

During the operative procedure

RN, radiology technician, or scrub technician. In procedure room, assist patient in moving from gurney to procedure room bed, cover patient with warm blanket. Place blood pressure cuff on arm, and place pulse oximetry probe on finger. Place EKG stickers on pt.—white on patient's right upper back, black on patient's left upper back, and red on patient's left side of abdomen. Place the patient on 2 L of oxygen per nasal cannula. Chart or make note of entrance time to procedure room. Turn on monitors.

Scrub technician. Don sterile gown and gloves. Prep the area of patient where the procedure will be conducted with chlorhexidine and drape with sterile drapes.

RN. Call doctor to procedure room when patient is prepped and draped with sterile drapes and equipment is set up.

Scrub technician. When the physician enters the room, assist with gowning and gloving. During the procedure, assist the surgeon throughout the case by retrieving sterile supplies that are handed off, flushing sterile supplies, handling of wires, balloons, watching sterile field to make sure sterility is not broken, making sure amounts of fluids on sterile field are adequate, assist in running power injector. Assist with closing at end of case while using a closure device, a hemostatic patch, or manual pressure. Apply a proper dressing according to the hemostatic method used. For closure devices, use gauze and a transparent dressing. After using a hemostatic patch or handheld pressure place gauze, transparent dressing, and then cover with large kerlix roll and foam tape to apply pressure. Assist in unhooking patient from monitors. Help patient move from procedure bed to the gurney. Take instruments to dirty utility.

Radiology technician. During procedure, operate C-ARM, operate ultrasound machine if needed, assist doctor with getting the supplies needed and opening them using sterile technique and handing them off to the scrub technician. At end of case turn on lights in procedure room, uncover bags from C-ARM and discard. Make hard copies of images doctor has requested. With scrub technician's approval remove the instruments from the sterile field and take them to dirty utility. Remove sharps from back table and put in large red sharps container, discard fluids down the sink, discard rest of back table disposables into appropriate garbage when finished. Assist in getting patient unhooked from monitors and moving the patient from procedure bed to gurney.

RN. During procedure fill out the procedure record including the name of the doctor and staff present, diagnosis, procedure, medications given during procedure, and vital signs including respirations every 5 min. Observe heart rhythm for EKG changes throughout procedure and inform the doctor of any changes. Check on patient every 5 min or sooner if needed. Check pain level for the patient, assist in gathering and opening supplies needed by doctor using sterile technique. Print three EKG strips during the procedure: one preprocedure, next during the procedure, and the last one postprocedure, and label them properly. Write name of patient; date of birth; and pre-, intra-, and postprocedure on bottom of the respective strips. Chart fluoroscopic time (time received from radiology technician) at the end of the case, chart amount of fluids and medications given during the case (information received from scrub technician). Chart closure device used and place sticker for closure device on procedure record. Chart amount of fluid patient received during procedure. Record the time procedure finished and the time doctor left procedure room. Open proper dressing needed that will be placed on the procedure site. Remove blood pressure cuff, pulse oximetry, and EKG lead stickers from the patient. Place bed at lowest level, bring gurney in to procedure room and assist patient in moving from procedure bed to gurney. Wheel patient to pre-/postoperative area and give report to MA or RN.

RN, radiology technician, and scrub technician. Clean procedure room—with appropriate cleaner, clean procedure table, C-Arm, back table and any other surfaces that may need it. Break down power injector unless another aortogram is scheduled for the same day. If another aortogram is scheduled then dispose of single patient line only and clean power injector with appropriate cleaner. If there are no other angiograms needing the power injector for the day then break down all disposables from injector and clean with appropriate cleaner. Follow the instructions given by the manufacturer of the power injector. Clean blood pressure cuff, EKG leads, and pulse oximetry with appropriate cleaner. Mop floor. Replace bed sheet and pillow cases to get room ready for next case. Empty garbage and take to back entrance to be taken out to large trash when there is time later in day. If necessary, rearrange the room to prepare for the next case.

Postoperative procedure

RN or medical assistant. Follow instructions for length of stay in postoperative area. It varies depending on the procedure, closure device used, and the amount of bleeding postprocedure. Check length of stay with physician. Take vital signs including respirations, neuro check, and bilateral posterior tibial and dorsalis pedis pulses every 15 min for the first hour, every ½ hour for the second hour, and then every hour and chart in postprocedure record. Every time vital signs are taken, check access site for drainage, pain, hematoma, or tenderness, check distal pulses with doppler and chart in postprocedure record. If there are any abnormalities, report to MD. If the patient is a diabetic, check and record blood glucose level postprocedure and before discharge. Offer patient something to eat or drink. If patient is stable and dressing is dry after required length of stay, RN should perform last assessment on patient and give permission for discharge. Discontinue IV line, review postop instructions with patient and family, make appointment for 7–10 day follow-up or earlier if necessary. Have patient sign postoperative instruction sheet and give copy to patient. If patient is on Glucophage, metformin, or Glucovance and stopped taking the medicine before the procedure, send a lab slip home with the patient to get BUN and creatinine rechecked 48 h postprocedure. Remind patient to take medication only after the office calls the patient to start the medicine. If the patient was on anticoagulants give appropriate instruction to resume the medication. Discharge the patient and assist the patient to the door or to the car. If the patient was on anticoagulant give specific instructions for starting the medicine.

Radiology technician. Plug C-ARM cable into wall for downloading procedure images to the PAC system and confirm that the transfer occurred.

Scrub technician. After instruments have run through ultrasonic cleaner follow the instructions for sterilization as provided by the autoclave manufacturer.

Medication management

Policy: All medications should be administered to the patient in a safe manner.

Procedures: The nurses, medical assistants, and scheduler should follow these guidelines.

Standing Medication Orders

Dye Allergy Prep: Medications for home use PO: medrol 32 mg PO 12 h before procedure, 32 mg 2 h before procedure, and Benadryl 25 mg 1 h before procedure. Call the prescription to the pharmacy used by the patient. If medication was not taken at home give Benadryl 50 mg IV, Solu-Cortef 100 mg IV, 30 min before the procedure.

Prophylactic Antibiotic: if *not* allergic to penicillin: Preoperatively give cephalexin (Keflex) 500 mg (1 tab) 1 h prior to procedure and send patient home with three tablets of 500 mg each to take one tablet every 8 h. If patient is on dialysis; then the patient should take cephalexin 500 mg PO × 1 tab 1 h prior to procedure followed by 500 mg PO daily for 3 days. On dialysis days, medicine to be taken after dialysis.

If allergic to penicillin: Preoperatively give clindamycin (Cleocin) 300 mg (1 tab) 1 h prior to procedure and send patient home with three tablets—300 mg tabs to take one every 8 h × 3 tabs. No change in dialysis patient dosing.

Preprocedure Sedative: Vicodin 5/500 mg tablet × 1 PO and valium 10 mg (or 5 mg) tablet PO × 1 30–60 min prior to procedure, or:

For patient having fistulogram: Vicodin 5/500 mg tab × 1 PO 30–60 min prior to procedure.

Postprocedure Pain: Try positioning and ice pack first. If no relief: Motrin 200 mg tabs × 3 PO × 1 dose. If no relief after 45 min: Norco 5/500 mg one tab PO × 1 dose. If pain has not improved to tolerable level after 1 h, contact the physician for further instructions.

Mild Allergic Reaction to Medication: Rash, itching, hives, localized swelling (no breathing difficulty, cough, facial swelling, or generalized swelling). Always report reaction to the physician. Order Medrol dose pack × 1 to be called in to local pharmacy. To be taken as directed, no refills.

Vomiting/Nausea: For vomiting or persistent nausea give Zofran (ondansetron) give 2 mL/4 mg (2 mg/1 mL) IV undiluted over >30 s × 1 dose (onset 5–10 min) or Tigan 200 mg IM × 1 dose. Onset: IM 15–20 min.

Sentinel event management

Cardiac arrest/respiratory arrest policy. Purpose: To assure prompt and efficient response to a cardiac/respiratory arrest.

Policy: In the event of a cardiac arrest/respiratory arrest there will be a response by all clinical staff in the building.

Procedure: Personnel who encounter a person in a cardiac/respiratory arrest state should initiate basic guidelines for CPR designated as follows:

1. Doctor: Directs emergency, secure airway if necessary and assist where needed. Follow ACLS protocol.
2. Nurse 1: Call doctor stat. Place O_2 and secure airway until medical assistant (MA) relief, place IV line if patient does not already have one, the draw up emergency medication as directed.
3. Nurse 2: Grab defibrillator and bring into room, take over putting in IV line if not already done.
4. Radiology Technician: Chart notes/scribe for emergency, call 911, and assist in gathering the supplies called for.
5. Scrub Technician: Take care of access site for the procedure.
6. Nurse 3 or MA 1: Take over bag/mask ventilations when entering room if needed.
7. Nurse 4 or MA 2: Start chest compressions if needed (preferably male if available).
8. MA 3: Standby to assist as needed.
9. MA/RN in pre-/postoperative area: Continue care of patients.
10. All cardiac arrest resuscitation attempts should be documented (Fig. 10.3).

Facility management

In addition to the policies and procedures for employees and patient-related issues there should also be policies and procedures developed for the facility. Since the endovascular center is an extension of practice, many issues related to facility management would have been already addressed by the practice. The OEC will be clearly identified on the exterior of the building and will be accessible to the physically disabled and mentally disabled. Exits for evacuation will be properly marked and easily seen. Hours of operation will be posted. All areas of movement will be free of obstruction. All other facility policies of the office will be followed by OEC. However, since medical equipment is being used the equipment needs to be serviced as per manufacturer's recommendation. This would usually entail a service contract with the manufacturer. In case of a procedure-related emergency the facility should have quick access to equipment brought in by an ambulance service responding to a 911 call. There should also be a policy for disposing of biological waste in addition to general waste. Here is an example of autoclave maintenance.

Autoclave maintenance

Policy: The autoclave sterilizer will be maintained in optimum status at all times.

Procedure: To ensure performance of the sterilizer, proactively find and correct system problems and comply with manufacturers' recommended care or warranty purposes.

Equipment: automatic sterilizer, 3M Attest spore incubator, cleaning bucket, stiff bristle brush.

Supplies: Distilled water, soft cleaning cloth, Speed-Clean Sterilizer Cleaner, 3M Attest biological indicators, occasionally a filter or a gasket will need to be changed

1. CARDIOPULMONARY RESUSCITATION RECORD

Patient Name:_________________________________ Date:___________

2.

1. Time of arrest: _______ witnessed by: _________________ 911 called: ______

2. Precipitating event: ____

3. Oxygenation: O2 ______ L/Min via Mask: ____ Cannula: _______ Ambu: ____

Ambu bag with airway: Yes: _______ No: ________

CPR initiated at: ______________ Initiated by:___________________________

5. Medications given: IV line started :_________________________________

MEDICATIONS	Dose	Route	Time/init	Time/init	Time/init	Time/init
Atropine 1 mg						
Amiodarone 300mg/150mg						
Calcium Chloride 5-10ml of 10% sol						
Epinepherine 1 mg						
Flumazenil 0.2mg over 15sec						
Lidocaine 1mg/kg						
Nitroglycerin 0/4mg/SL						

3.
4. 6. Defibrillation AED
5.

TIME	RESPONSE

FIG. 10.3 Cardiac arrest record form.

if unable to clean or if excessive wear is noted per manufacturer's instructions.

Method: See manufacturer's care sheet (attached) for weekly and monthly maintenance steps. All preventative maintenance will be recorded on a log sheet (attached) that states the date, person performing task, and type of maintenance performed. It will also include the biological spore test result from the monthly test of performance.

In this chapter, we have given the salient features of policies and procedures needed for an OEC. The center should develop its own policies and procedure and follow them diligently.

CHAPTER 11

Billing and Coding

SEAN P. RODDY, MD • SUNITA SRIVASTAVA, MD

INTRODUCTION

Patient outcomes and quality of care are essential to every vascular surgeon and group. The existence and growth of a surgical practice is rooted in clinical service and the corresponding reimbursement for care. The elements of this process include billing, coding, and reimbursement from third-party payors. The interaction between patient and physician whether during an office visit or procedure is based on a diagnosis. This describes the disease process for which care is being provided and is linked to either a procedure or office visit. The payment process begins with linking the visit or intervention with the diagnosis code. The procedural code may be appended with modifiers to capture the extent of services provided. This claim is submitted to the insurance carrier electronically and is reviewed for reimbursement. Correct coding and medical appropriateness as well as timely submission produce a clean claim without error and increase the chances of timely review and payment. Claim rejections due to error, delay in submission, and medically questionable services decrease the chances of payment even with subsequent corrections. Accurate, timely, and clinically appropriate claim submissions are necessary for efficient reimbursement and to avoid the potential for fraud. This chapter is only a guideline for the physician since each insurance payer has their own rules and regulations. Please consult your local carriers for specific details on claim submission.

DIAGNOSIS CODING

The International Statistical Classification of Diseases and Related Health Problems (ICD) is an internationally recognized classification system and is the foundation of healthcare delivery throughout the world. In the United States, the National Center for Health Statistics (NCHS) updated the ICD system to include more diagnosis codes and categories (ICD-10). The classification system was then clinically modified (ICD-10-CM) to include ambulatory encounters, enhance the specificity of codes, as well as to group diagnosis/symptom combinations more succinctly to describe a clinical condition. The opportunity to generate higher-quality clinical data from the ICD-10-CM may have an impact on outcomes and improve healthcare delivery in the future.

The first section of the ICD-10-CM coding structure is an alphabetical index of the disease entities with corresponding diagnostic code numbers, and the second section is a numerical list of code numbers in a tabular form, which are more specific to the disease condition. Each ICD-10 code is comprised of a three- to seven-digit number. To increase the specificity, more digits and a decimal point follow the first three characters. The alphabetical list is divided into body system or conditions. Modifications included in ICD-10-CM include the laterality or side of body affected, the expanded use of combination codes (certain conditions and associated common symptoms), the inclusion of injuries grouped by anatomic site rather than type of injury, and increased specificity of the code to reflect current practices and conditions listed in the tabular column.

PROCEDURAL CODING

Procedure codes are listed in the Current Procedural Terminology (CPT) book. This manual is created, maintained, and copyrighted by the American Medical Association (AMA) which updates it annually effective January 1 of each year. It is a systematic listing of all procedures that are currently performed in the United States and is a resource utilized by physicians, healthcare delivery systems, and third-party payors. As new technologies emerge, and others become obsolete, new CPT codes are introduced while obsolete ones are terminated. The structure of the CPT code consists of a five-digit number which can be broken down into standard codes and add-on codes. Standard codes are those that can be submitted by themselves and are stand-alone codes. Add-on codes must be accompanied by other specific code(s) and cannot be reported alone. An example of an add-on code is CPT 35700

Office-Based Endovascular Centers. https://doi.org/10.1016/B978-0-323-67969-5.00011-3
Copyright © 2020 Elsevier Inc. All rights reserved.

(*re-operation, femoral-popliteal or femoral-tibial, more than 1 month after original procedure*). This code provides value for the added difficulty in performing reoperative leg bypass surgery. Therefore, payment for CPT code 35700 would also require one of the nine standard lower extremity revascularization codes to be submitted as well.

CPT codes for physician reimbursement are also designated as either Category I or Category III. Category I codes are the typical five-digit number code describing a standard accepted procedure. Category III codes are four-digit codes followed by a "T" assignment identifying it as a temporary or emerging technology code. This category of codes typically describes the use of a device not approved by the Federal Drug Administration or an investigational procedure. Most Category III codes are not reimbursed by insurers until potentially converted to a Category I code. These T codes are useful designations for data collection by Medicare, private insurers, and other interest groups. Category III codes are limited in duration with a maximum of 5 years. These codes can be converted to Category I when sufficient clinical data resulting in FDA approval or data from clinical trials support mainstream utilization and reimbursement.

More than one procedure on the same date, same session, or within a global period may require use of an appropriate modifier. Modifiers are two-digit numbers that can be added to a claim that describes circumstances allowing for full or partial payment in situations that would otherwise be denied by the insurer. Additionally, the National Correct Coding Initiative (CCI) reviews codes quarterly to decide what can and cannot be billed together based on current practice, billing patterns, and trends. For example, the −59 modifier can be used to notate distinct procedural services or an exception to the CCI. The modifiers are listed both in the front of the CPT manual each year as well in a separate section in the Appendix.

It is also important to understand that when more than one CPT code is billed for the same session, the highest valued code is paid in its entirety. All subsequent nonradiologic codes are paid at 50% of their independent value. This modified payment is termed the "multiple procedure payment reduction" or MPPR and accounts for the overlap in work before, during, and after multiple procedures are done on the same date of service. Imaging codes (i.e., the radiology codes that begin with the number 7) and vascular laboratory codes are not subject to this discount. Additionally, add-on codes are exempt from this fee reduction since they are created solely for utilization with other codes.

Radiologic procedures, while described by a single CPT code, include two distinct portions, a technical component, and a professional component. The professional component is the work provided by the physician and includes the supervision and interpretation of imaging. The CPT code is then appended with modifier −26 to claim this work. The technical component of a service includes the equipment, supplies, personnel, and the costs related to conducting the examination. The TC or technical modifier would be claimed by the facility or hospital responsible for these costs. If the equipment is owned by a practice in an office setting, that practice would bill with no modifier; this is termed "billing global." That includes both the technical component and the professional component for a given examination. If a test is performed in the hospital where the hospital owns the equipment, the physician would typically bill with a −26 modifier. This signifies that the physician is performing and interpreting the test but does not own the equipment, purchase the catheters/stents/balloons/contrast, manage the facility, and employ the staff required to perform the procedure.

All radiologic codes in CPT are further classified into one of the three categories: catheter manipulation, imaging acquisition and interpretation, and endovascular intervention. This original coding scheme for endovascular procedures is called component coding. Component coding is still used in certain clinical scenarios such as diagnostic angiography, peripheral (excluding carotid, renal, and lower extremity) procedures. It has essentially been replaced by a bundled coding system. Bundled CPT codes describe an entire procedure and include all the necessary steps needed to accomplish it including the diagnostic and therapeutic elements. The recognition that certain procedures have necessary elements inherent to them has led to the development of the bundled code set for multiple endovascular therapies.

OFFICE-BASED ENDOVASCULAR CENTER

In the Medicare system, the Relative Value Update Committee (RUC) uses relative value units (RVUs) to standardize all procedures across specialties. Each CPT description has a certain amount of physician work, practice expense, and malpractice liability. The summation of these three components corresponds to the total RVUs assigned for any given procedure. Physician providers are compensated based on fee schedules through each insurance carrier that include CPT codes, which may be valued in both a "facility" and a "nonfacility" location. Interventional procedures done in a hospital are reimbursed at the "facility" rate. Reporting inpatient endovascular therapies to an insurance carrier translates into professional fee reimbursement only. The hospital will submit a separate claim for its expenses. On the other hand, "nonfacility" corresponds to an outpatient setting such as an office-based laboratory (i.e., place of service 11) as described in this chapter. Procedures that are performed in an office location are subject to a "site of service differential" because the overhead incurred by the practice is much higher. Reimbursement for each CPT code reported includes the professional fee as well as additional operating costs which include rent, radiology imaging equipment, catheters and balloons, bare metal stents, nursing, and medications. The costlier overhead is offset by higher practice expense assigned to many CPT codes in the "nonfacility." The physician work and the malpractice expense do not differ based on site of service, but the inherent site costs associated with that procedure does.

LOWER EXTREMITY ARTERIAL ENDOVASCULAR THERAPIES

Lower extremity endovascular intervention is reported using bundled CPT codes based on anatomic location and type of vessel treatment with progressive hierarchies that describe more intensive endovascular services inclusive of lesser therapies. The current introductory wording immediately before CPT code 37220 in the 2019 CPT manual states "these lower extremity endovascular revascularization codes all include the work of accessing and selectively catheterizing the vessel, traversing the lesion, radiological supervision and interpretation directly related to the intervention(s) performed, embolic protection if used, closure of the arteriotomy by any method, and imaging performed to document completion of the intervention in addition to the intervention(s) performed." Essentially all steps necessary after diagnostic angiography required to complete the procedure have been included in a single code. Diagnostic angiography has not been included or valued into the CPT code change proposals. The radiology coding for aortography (CPT code 75625) and lower extremity angiography (CPT codes 75710 and 75716) are still reportable but require use of the −59 modifier when submitted at the time of lower extremity arterial intervention provided the following three criteria are met:

1. No prior catheter-based angiographic study is available
2. A full diagnostic study is performed
3. The decision to intervene is based on this study

This also assumes that the medical record justifies the above stipulations.

The patient's lower extremity arterial tree has been divided into three specific territories: iliac, femoropopliteal, and tibial/peroneal. "Iliac" incorporates intervention on the common, external, or internal iliac arteries. "Femoropopliteal" comprises treatment of the common, superficial, and deep femoral arteries as well as the popliteal artery both above and below the knee. "Tibial/peroneal" accounts for the posterior tibial, anterior tibial, and peroneal arteries. The common tibioperoneal trunk, for coding purposes, is included as an extension of either the posterior tibial or peroneal artery for intervention and is not considered a separate vessel. The four therapeutic groups are listed as:

1. percutaneous transluminal angioplasty (PTA)
2. intravascular stent placement with or without PTA
3. atherectomy with or without PTA
4. both intravascular stent placement and atherectomy with or without PTA

The most comprehensive treatment is reported for each territory. Primary stent placement is coded identical to failure of an angioplasty requiring stent salvage. Covered stents are considered identical to bare metal and drug-eluting implants from a coding perspective in these locations when treating atherosclerotic arterial occlusive disease. Intervention upon the femoropopliteal territory results in only one CPT code submission to the insurance carrier. The anatomic definition for the femoral region includes the deep and superficial femoral artery (SFA) as well as the above- and below-knee popliteal arteries. Therefore, treatment of one vessel such as the SFA is identical from a coding perspective to a case where simultaneous intervention on the deep femoral, common femoral, superficial femoral, and popliteal arteries are all performed. The "highest" level of treatment in this vascular bed is most appropriate to bill. For example, PTA of one region of the SFA and stenting within another area of the SFA should be reported using the "stent" code and not the "PTA" code. "Stent" placement is a more comprehensive procedure which includes use of an angioplasty balloon as needed and has a higher RVU content in both the facility and nonfacility.

Unlike the femoropopliteal region which bundles all vessel therapy into a single description, the other two extremity territories have a base code with an add-on code option. Endovascular intervention within the iliac and the tibial/peroneal locations requires use of a base code for the initial vessel. If an additional artery (as defined above) is treated within that same territory, the add-on code is submitted in addition to the base CPT code. Since there are a total of three vessels in each of these two locations for a given extremity, the add-on code can be reported a maximum of once (when two vessels are treated) or twice (when three vessels are treated) in a given territory. The second submission requires use of the −59 modifier to clarify it as distinct anatomic site and not an inadvertent duplicate code submission. If more than one vessel is treated in a given territory, the more comprehensive treatment is reported using the base code and the lesser intense therapy is billed using the add-on code. Each territory in the ipsilateral extremity subject to intervention requires one base code. If a bilateral procedure is reported in similar territories, the base code for each is reported. For example, "kissing" common iliac stents would require reporting the iliac stent base code twice. If different therapies are performed in same territory of the right and left lower extremity arterial circulation, the lesser intense base code necessitates an appended −59 modifier for reimbursement. A special notation was added to the introductory wording for instruction on reporting therapy when a single intervention crosses/spans two vessels in an area that has add-on coding available. It states, "If a lesion extends across the margins of one vessel vascular territory into another, but can be opened with a single therapy, this intervention should be reported with a single code despite treating more than one vessel and/or vascular territory." In contrast, more extensive lesions with plaque burden in both the common and external iliac arteries do not fall under these guidelines since each vessel is considered distinct and treated separately.

The table below outlines the new lower extremity endovascular arterial intervention coding structure:

	PTA	Atherectomy With/ Without PTA	Stent With/ Without PTA	Stent + Atherectomy With/ Without PTA
Iliac	37220	N/A	37221	N/A
Additional Ipsilateral iliac	+37222	N/A	+37223	N/A
Femoropopliteal	37224	37225	37226	37,227
Tibial/peroneal	37228	37229	37230	37,231
Additional ipsilateral tibial/ peroneal	+37232	+37233	+37234	+2735

Suprainguinal atherectomy is also reported with a bundled code set. Unlike the Category I lower extremity codes described above, the catheterization for suprainguinal atherectomy is separate because all of the other vascular interventions in these anatomic regions follow a similar convention. Their code descriptions are listed as "transluminal peripheral atherectomy, open or percutaneous, including radiological supervision and interpretation" and are numbered as follows:

Renal artery	0234T
Visceral artery (except renal), each vessel	0235T
Abdominal aorta	0236T
Brachiocephalic trunk and branches, each vessel	0237T
Iliac artery, each vessel	0238T

Generic Stenting

Placement of an endovascular stent in vessels outside the lower extremity, cervical carotid, extracranial vertebral or intrathoracic carotid, intracranial, or coronary arteries has a separate and distinct coding scheme. One CPT code is used to designate the first vessel treated by stenting, and a separate CPT code is used for "each additional vessel" stented. When these codes were created, the specialties felt there was a difference in the physician work associated with placement of a stent in the arterial system compared to the venous system, which resulted in separate code description dividing the two vascular regions. As such, these codes are based on the number of blood vessels treated and designated as "initial arterial stent," "subsequent arterial stent," "initial venous stent," and "subsequent venous stent." Despite reporting "per vessel" treated, the intervention should be submitted only once if a lesion extends across the margins of one vessel into another but can be treated with a single therapy.

These four code descriptions were created by bundling the surgical procedure code with the radiologic supervision and interpretation. Included with each procedure are all balloon angioplasty performed in the treated vessel including treatment of a lesion outside the stented segment but in the same vessel, any predilation (whether performed as a primary or secondary angioplasty—i.e., failed angioplasty requiring stent salvage), postdilation following stent deployment, radiological supervision and interpretation directly related to the intervention performed, closure of the arteriotomy by pressure, application of an arterial closure device or standard closure of the puncture by suture, and completion angiography. Excluded and separately reportable are angioplasty in a separate and distinct vessel, nonselective and/or selective catheterization (unlike in the lower extremity where the catheter is bundled), extensive repair or replacement of an artery (e.g., CPT codes 35226, 35286, or 35371), ultrasound guidance (e.g., CPT code 76937) for vascular access, intravascular ultrasound (IVUS) (i.e., CPT codes 37250, 37251), and the initial diagnostic angiogram (as defined under "Vascular Procedures" in the CPT manual Radiology section).

The codes are as follows:

37236 Transcatheter placement of an intravascular stent(s) (except lower extremity, cervical carotid, extracranial vertebral or intrathoracic carotid, intracranial, or coronary), open or percutaneous, including radiological supervision and interpretation and including all angioplasty within the same vessel, when performed; initial artery

37237 Transcatheter placement of an intravascular stent(s) (except lower extremity, cervical carotid, extracranial vertebral or intrathoracic carotid, intracranial, or coronary), open or percutaneous, including radiological supervision and interpretation and including all angioplasty within the same vessel, when performed; each additional artery

37238 Transcatheter placement of an intravascular stent(s), open or percutaneous, including radiological supervision and interpretation and including angioplasty within the same vessel, when performed; initial vein

37239 Transcatheter placement of an intravascular stent(s), open or percutaneous, including radiological supervision and interpretation and including angioplasty within the same vessel, when performed; each additional vein

Covered stents are considered identical to bare metal or drug-eluting implants from a coding perspective in these locations when treating atherosclerotic arterial occlusive disease. Specific descriptors have been added for the treatment of arterial aneurysms by thromboexclusion: when an endovascular stent is deployed as a cage to trap embolization coils, the embolization code is reported and not the stent code. Alternatively, the stent deployment code should be reported and not the embolization code if a covered stent is inserted as the sole treatment of the vascular abnormality.

PTA BUNDLING

PTA in vessels outside lower extremity arteries for occlusive disease, intracranial, coronary, pulmonary, or dialysis circuit also has a separate and distinct coding scheme. Please remember that PTA is included in all stenting codes and is not separately billable when codes 37236-9 are reported. One CPT code is used to designate the first vessel treated by PTA, and a separate CPT code is used for "each additional vessel." A similar difference in the physician work associated with PTA in the arterial system was identified as compared with the venous system. As such, these codes are based on the number of blood vessels treated and designated as "initial arterial PTA," "subsequent arterial PTA," "initial venous PTA," and "subsequent venous PTA." Despite reporting "per vessel" treated, the intervention should be submitted only once if a lesion extends across the margins of one vessel into another but can be treated with a single therapy.

The PTA codes are as follows:

37246 Transluminal balloon angioplasty (except lower extremity artery/arteries for occlusive disease, intracranial, coronary, pulmonary, or dialysis circuit), open or percutaneous, including all imaging and radiological supervision and interpretation necessary to perform the angioplasty within the same artery; initial artery

37247 Transluminal balloon angioplasty (except lower extremity artery/arteries) for occlusive disease, intracranial, coronary, pulmonary, or dialysis circuit), open or percutaneous, including all imaging and radiological supervision and interpretation necessary to perform the angioplasty within the same artery; each additional artery (list separately in addition to code for primary procedure)

37248 Transluminal balloon angioplasty (except dialysis circuit), open or percutaneous, including all imaging and radiological supervision and interpretation necessary to perform the angioplasty within the same vein; initial vein

37249 Transluminal balloon angioplasty (except dialysis circuit), open or percutaneous, including all imaging and radiological supervision and interpretation necessary to perform the angioplasty within the same vein; each additional vein (list separately in addition to code for primary procedure)

These new codes bundle the surgical procedure with the radiologic supervision and interpretation. They include all balloon angioplasty performed in the treated vessel and any predilation, the radiological supervision and interpretation directly related to the intervention performed, closure of the arteriotomy by pressure, application of an arterial closure device or standard closure of the puncture by suture, and completion angiography.

HD INTERVENTIONS

Endovascular hemodialysis access imaging and intervention is described by a bundled code set. Three codes (36901, 36902, 36903) were developed to bundle all work involved in the percutaneous management of a patent dialysis access, and three codes (36904, 36905, 36906) were created to bundle endovascular dialysis access thrombectomy procedures. Both code sets are hierarchical and describe increasing intensity of intervention. In addition, three add-on codes (36907, 36908, 36909) were created to reflect additional work in the central veins and/or branch vessel embolization.

For coding purpose, the hemodialysis circuit is comprised of a "peripheral" segment and a "central" segment. The "peripheral" segment begins at the arterial anastomosis and extends up to and includes the axillary vein and entire cephalic vein, while the "central" segment includes the subclavian and innominate veins through the superior vena cava. In the lower extremity, the "peripheral" segment extends up to and includes the common femoral vein while the "central" segment includes the external iliac and common iliac veins through the inferior vena cava.

Code 36901 describes a traditional diagnostic fistulogram with assessment of the circuit from arterial anastomosis through the vena cava. All needle placements, as well as nonselective catheter manipulations within the circuit, are included in the code and are not separately reportable. If the catheter is advanced to the vena cava, code 36010 is not additionally reported. Additionally, angiography with arm access of the superior vena cava (75827) and with leg access of the inferior vena cava (75825) is bundled. If ultrasound guidance is required for access into the vessel, this is separately reported with code 76937.

Codes 36901–36906 include all catheter placement(s) and manipulation(s) to perform a graft/fistula diagnostic radiological study. However, 36215 (*selective catheter placement, arterial system; each first order thoracic or brachiocephalic branch, within a vascular family*) is not inherent to the work of 36901–36906 and separately reportable. When a catheter is maneuvered from a puncture of the dialysis graft/fistula into the proximal inflow vessel for formal extremity diagnostic arteriography, code 36215 is reported in addition to 36901–36906. Reporting 36215 to position the catheter tip simply near the arterial anastomosis of the AV access is not appropriate. If such an inflow catheterization is performed with extremity arterial angiography as well as AV access imaging, report one of the base codes (36901–36906) in addition to 36215 and the unilateral extremity arterial imaging code 75710.

If the dialysis access requires balloon angioplasty in the "peripheral" segment, use code 36902. In addition to including the work of balloon angioplasty within the "peripheral" segment, code 36902 includes all the diagnostic services and therefore 36901 may not be reported in conjunction with 36902. Code 36902 may only be reported once per session. If two or more lesions are treated within the "peripheral" segment using balloon angioplasty, code 36902 bundles all additional "peripheral" segment angioplasty regardless of the number of inflations or balloons used. There is no difference between treatments at the arterial anastomosis versus the venous outflow in the "peripheral" segment.

Code 36903 describes all work to deploy an intravascular stent within the "peripheral" segment. Code 36903 may only be reported once per session. If more than one stent is deployed within the "peripheral" segment, code 36903 is only reported once regardless of the number of lesions treated. Code 36903 applies to any type of stent deployed and is appropriate for bare metal, covered, or drug-eluting stents. Additionally, any PTA performed in the "peripheral" segment in the same setting is bundled into 36903 even if the angioplasty treats a lesion within the "peripheral" segment but in an area separate and distinct from the stented lesion. For example, if a brachiocephalic fistula is found to have a perianastomotic stenosis as well as a stenosis in the midcephalic vein, treatment with balloon angioplasty at the perianastomotic region followed by a cephalic vein stent would all be reported with 36903.

Three codes describe mechanical thrombectomy of an AV access (36904–36906), and there is no distinction between the "peripheral" and "central" dialysis segments in this setting. If clot extends into the central veins, its removal is included in codes 36904–36906. If PTA (e.g., 36907) or stent placement (e.g., 36908) is required in the central veins after successful thrombectomy, this remains separately reportable as detailed below.

Code 36904 incorporates all components of a mechanical or pharmacological "declot" procedure (e.g., mechanical thrombectomy, thrombolytic infusion, thrombolytic bolus). Thrombectomy of an occluded dialysis access which involves balloon angioplasty would be reported with 36905. Similar to code 36902, code 36905 reflects all angioplasty within the "peripheral" segment regardless of number of inflations or number of balloons used. Inflating a balloon to push clot centrally is not considered "angioplasty." Code 36905 implies that a stenosis is identified before or after thrombectomy requiring a therapeutic dilatation to help maintain longer term patency. Stent placement in the "peripheral" segment would be reported with 36906, which is a comprehensive code involving all stents placed and all balloon angioplasty performed within the "peripheral" segment during the thrombectomy.

Two add-on codes (36907, 36908) were created to describe work performed in the central veins. Catheter placement and angiography are bundled into these codes and are not separately reportable. As with the base codes (36901–36906), codes 36907 and 36908 may be reported only once per session regardless of the number of lesions treated. Code 36908 includes all the work of code 36907, and therefore these two codes may not be reported together. Add-on codes must be reported with a primary procedure, which will typically be 36901–36906. However, if central venous angioplasty or stenting is performed as part of the open surgical creation of an AV access (e.g., 36818–36830) or open surgical revision and/or thrombectomy (e.g., 36831–36833), the central venous intervention may be separately reported with 36907 or 36908.

Code 36909 describes all embolization procedures performed on branch vessel(s) emanating from the hemodialysis circuit. Code 36909 may be reported with any of the base codes (36901–36906); however, code 36909 may also be reported if the embolization is completed from an access other than the dialysis circuit. For example, if a brachiocephalic fistula side branch is cannulated through an ipsilateral radial artery, code 36909 would be reported for the embolization. Selective venous catheterization(s) of branch vessel(s) (e.g., 36011) is bundled and not separately reportable.

VENOUS INSUFFICIENCY

Endovenous ablation therapy in the lower extremity was introduced over a decade ago. Treatment is based on catheter techniques which ultimately occlude the incompetent vein. The initial technologies involved venous access under ultrasound guidance using thermal energy (radiofrequency or laser) to occlude the greater saphenous vein, typically performed under tumescent anesthesia in an office setting. Therefore, there are two sets of code descriptions created to describe these separate technologies.

CPT code 36475 states "endovenous ablation therapy of incompetent vein, extremity, inclusive of all imaging guidance and monitoring, percutaneous, radiofrequency; first vein treated" while CPT code 36478 denotes "endovenous ablation therapy of incompetent vein, extremity, inclusive of all imaging guidance and monitoring, percutaneous, laser; first vein treated." The majority of cases use this technology on the greater saphenous vein. However, the lateral accessory saphenous vein and the lesser saphenous vein are alternatives based on clinical indication.

If two or more veins are ablated in the same setting, add-on codes were created to describe the additional work. CPT code 36476 depicts "endovenous ablation therapy of incompetent vein, extremity, inclusive of all imaging guidance and monitoring, percutaneous, radiofrequency; second and subsequent veins treated in a single extremity, each through separate access sites (List separately in addition to code for primary procedure)," while CPT code 36479 states "endovenous ablation therapy of incompetent vein, extremity, inclusive of all imaging guidance and monitoring, percutaneous, laser; second and subsequent veins treated in a single extremity, each through separate access sites (List separately in addition to code for primary procedure)." In CPT terminology, "second and subsequent" means that the add-on code is reported only once per session regardless of the number of veins treated. For example, if two veins are treated with radiofrequency in the same leg, CPT codes 36475 and 36476 would be submitted to the insurance carrier. If three or more veins are treated in the same leg and in the same setting, the billing is identical to the "two vein scenario" above (CPT code 36476 is not reported more than once or with a unit value greater than one). However, bilateral intervention requires the −50 modifier (bilateral procedure) and is applicable to all four vein ablation codes listed above.

Ultrasound imaging is bundled into these CPT codes. CPT codes 93970 (duplex scan of extremity veins including responses to compression and other maneuvers; complete bilateral study), 93971 (duplex scan of extremity veins including responses to compression and other maneuvers; unilateral or limited study), 76937 (ultrasound guidance for vascular access requiring ultrasound evaluation of potential access sites, documentation of selected vessel patency, concurrent real-time ultrasound visualization of vascular needle entry, with permanent recording and reporting (List separately in addition to code for primary procedure)), and 76942 (ultrasonic guidance for needle placement (e.g., biopsy, aspiration, injection, localization device), imaging supervision and interpretation) are all considered inherent to these CPT codes and therefore not separately billable.

Code descriptions for direct puncture sclerotherapy (36468–36471) were revised in 2018 to distinguish them from two new codes (36465, 36466) that describe injection of a new noncompounded proprietary foam sclerosant into a truncal vein. Code 36468 sclerotherapy for telangiectasia (spider veins) may only be reported once per extremity per session, no matter how many separate injections are performed. Sclerotherapy for a single incompetent vein (36470) or multiple incompetent veins (36471) may be reported only once per extremity, no matter how many veins were treated. Injections performed to treat incompetent lower-extremity nontruncal veins are reported with 36470 or 36471 regardless of whether a standard sclerosant, a compounded foam sclerosant, or a noncompounded foam sclerosant is utilized. If ultrasound guidance is used from these nontruncal sclerotherapy, then code 76942 is also reported. Codes 36465 and 36466 involve noncompounded foam sclerosant (commercially manufactured proprietary chemical) injection into a truncal vein with ultrasound compression of the outflow to prevent dispersion of the foam to unintended anatomy. Therefore, ultrasound guidance is included in 36465 and 36466 and not separately reportable. Codes 36465 and 36466 are reported once per extremity; 36465 for a single vein or 36466 for multiple veins. Sclerotherapy coding is as follows:

36468 Injection(s) of sclerosant for spider veins (telangiectasia), limb, or trunk
36470 Injection of sclerosant; single incompetent vein (other than telangiectasia)
36471 Injection of sclerosant; multiple incompetent veins (other than telangiectasia), same leg
36465 Injection of noncompounded foam sclerosant with ultrasound compression maneuvers to guide dispersion of the injectate, inclusive of all imaging guidance and monitoring; single incompetent extremity truncal vein (e.g., great saphenous vein, accessory saphenous vein)
36466 Multiple incompetent truncal veins (e.g., great saphenous vein, accessory saphenous vein), same leg

Additional technological advances in catheter properties and chemical agents resulted in four new codes in 2017 and 2018 for endovenous ablation therapy of incompetent veins. Mechanochemical (MOCA) and chemical adhesive (glue) ablation modalities are nonthermal and nontumescent and thus require only local anesthesia. However, similar to RFA and EVLT therapies, MOCA and glue ablation includes ultrasound guidance, which when utilized, may not be separately reported. Although the clinical work is similar for many of the procedures that treat incompetent veins, creation of separate and distinct CPT codes was the most appropriate solution to differentiate the practice expense associated with each of the modalities. It is important to note that, when performed in an office setting, all supplies and equipment necessary to perform the procedure (e.g., catheters, injectable medications, ablation "kits," compression dressings/stockings, etc.) are included and may not be reported separately. These additional CPT codes include the following:

36473 Endovenous ablation therapy of incompetent vein, extremity, inclusive of all imaging guidance and monitoring, percutaneous, mechanochemical; first vein treated
36474 Endovenous ablation therapy of incompetent vein, extremity, inclusive of all imaging guidance and monitoring, percutaneous, mechanochemical; subsequent vein(s) treated in a single extremity, each through separate access sites (List separately in addition to code for primary procedure)
36482 Endovenous ablation therapy of incompetent vein, extremity, by transcatheter delivery of a chemical adhesive (e.g., cyanoacrylate) remote from the access site, inclusive of all imaging guidance and monitoring, percutaneous; first vein treated
36483 Endovenous ablation therapy of incompetent vein, extremity, by transcatheter delivery of a chemical adhesive (e.g., cyanoacrylate) remote from the access site, inclusive of all imaging guidance and monitoring, percutaneous; subsequent vein(s) treated in a single extremity, each through separate access sites (List separately in addition to code for primary procedure)

As the technology associated with venous ablative therapies expands, additional codes will likely be created.

INTRAVASCULAR ULTRASOUND

Two new CPT code descriptions were recently created that describe the IVUS transducer placement and manipulation as well as the radiologic supervision and interpretation of the IVUS imaging. CPT code 37252 denotes "Intravascular ultrasound (noncoronary vessel) during diagnostic evaluation and/or therapeutic intervention, includes radiological supervision and interpretation, when performed; initial noncoronary vessel (List separately in addition to code for primary procedure)." Examples of this procedure include intravascular ultrasound evaluation of the lower extremity during revascularization or intravascular ultrasound evaluation of the iliac vein for the treatment of May-Thurner Syndrome. CPT code 37253 denotes "Intravascular ultrasound (noncoronary vessel) during diagnostic evaluation and/or therapeutic intervention, includes radiological supervision and interpretation, when performed; each additional noncoronary vessel (List separately in addition to code for primary procedure)."

CPT codes 37252 and 37253 are both add-on codes, and therefore must be reported as part of a primary procedure. They may be reported with diagnostic angiography (e.g., iliac and inferior vena cava angiography without intervention) and/or therapeutic endovascular therapy (e.g., assessment of an arterial dissection after intravascular stent deployment). Importantly, the multiple procedure payment reduction does not apply for add-on codes. CPT code 37252 is reported for IVUS in the initial vessel and may only be reported once per procedure. CPT code 37252 reflects all IVUS performed in the first vessel for the entire procedure. For example, IVUS may be used to diagnose a dissection in the SFA and then utilized again to assess the adequacy of stent deployment to repair the dissection; CPT code 37252 would be reported once to reflect all IVUS performed regardless of the number of probe introductions. For any additional noncoronary vessels imaged with IVUS, CPT code 37253 may be reported. If more than one additional vessel is evaluated, CPT code 37253 may be reported in multiple units. However, if pathology crosses more than one vessel, a single code would be reported. A deep venous thrombosis imaged with IVUS extending from the femoral vein into the external iliac vein would be reported as a single vessel with CPT code 37252.

Several additional procedures have been adjusted to bundle IVUS into their primary codes. Vena cava filter insertion (37191), vena cava filter repositioning (37192), vena cava filter removal (37193), and intravascular foreign body retrieval (37197) include IVUS in their description of work, and therefore CPT codes 37252 and 37253 may not be separately reported when performed in conjunction with these services.

MODERATE SEDATION

Coding to describe moderate sedation administered by the surgeon became effective in 2017. Timing of this service begins with the administration of the sedating agent and requires face-to-face time by the physician. Additional face-to-face time with the patient after the physician has completed the procedure and left the procedural suite is not added to this intraservice time calculation. For time less than 10 min, no code is reported, and the sedation is assumed inherent to the base procedure. Two codes are important in the OEC setting:

99152 Moderate sedation services provided by the same physician or other qualified healthcare professional performing the diagnostic or therapeutic service that the sedation supports, requiring the presence of an independent trained observer to assist in the monitoring of the patient's level of consciousness and physiological status; initial 15 min of intraservice time, patient age 5 years or older.

99153 Moderate sedation services provided by the same physician or other qualified healthcare professional performing the diagnostic or therapeutic service that the sedation supports, requiring the presence of an independent trained observer to assist in the monitoring of the patient's level of consciousness and physiological status; each additional 15 min intraservice time (List separately in addition to code for primary service) (Table 11.1).

TABLE 11.1
Time Requirement for Moderate Sedation Billing.

Total intraservice time for moderate sedation	CPT Code(s) Reported
Less than 10 min	Not separately reported
10–22 min	99152
23–37 min	99152 + 99153 × 1
38–52 min	99152 + 99153 × 2
53–67 min	99152 + 99153 × 3
68–82 min	99152 + 99153 × 4
83 min or longer	Add 99153

SUMMARY

Open and endovascular coding for vascular surgery can be complex and challenging. Physicians are integral to the billing and reimbursement process. Keeping pace with the temporal changes in the CPT codes, RVU valuations and yearly Medicare Physician Fee Schedule promote physician advocacy and contribution to the optimum delivery of healthcare.

FURTHER READING

1. *2019 Physicians' Professional ICD-10-CM International.* Salt Lake City: The Medical Management Institute; 2018.
2. *Current Procedural Terminology Cpt 2019 Professional Edition.* Chicago: American Medical Association; 2018.
3. National Correct Coding Initiative Edits https://www.cms.gov/Medicare/Coding/NationalCorrectCodInitEd/index.html?redirect=/nationalcorrectcodinited/.
4. Medicare Claims Processing Manual https://www.cms.gov/regulations-and-guidance/guidance/manuals/internet-only-manuals-ioms-items/cms018912.html.

CHAPTER 12

Anesthesia for Office Based Procedures

DEEPAK NAIR, MD, MS, MHA, RVT, FACS

The advances in anesthesia and the increasing management of anesthesia by the vascular specialist have allowed the interventionalist to perform more complex procedures in the office-based endovascular center (OEC). Common office-based vascular procedures are varied and simple to challenging, ranging from visual sclerotherapy to complex endovascular intervention of peripheral aneurysms. The advances in technology and procedural techniques have also been instrumental in increasing the shift of vascular procedures from the hospital to the office environment. It is important to remember that an office-based procedure is one that is done in a doctor's office. These are generally exempt from federal and state regulation, though less so every year. Most states do not even require accreditation of office facilities that perform procedures. Only 22 states have clear specific laws that govern office-based surgery. These offices are not, generally, required to report adverse events. The responsibility for patient safety rests squarely on the physicians providing the care. It is thus crucial that anesthesia be administered in the office carefully and in a safe manner.

The American Society of Anesthesiologists (ASA) Guidelines for Office-Based Anesthesia[1] offer an excellent resource for standards when running an OEC. The ASA recommends offices to have a reliable source of oxygen, suction, resuscitation equipment, and emergency drugs if performing procedures. Table 12.1 offers recommended equipment to have on hand. The ASA Statement on Nonoperating Room Anesthetizing Locations provides specific guidance on the matter. These guidelines strongly recommend that an individual be designated as the medical director and thus responsible for all procedural policies and procedures in the center/office. The ASA guidelines and others have called for anesthetic care in the office to be equivalent to what you would expect for a similar patient having a similar procedure in an ambulatory surgery center or hospital.[2] The ASA describes four levels of sedation (Table 12.2).[1] Levels 0, 1, and 2 are appropriate for in-office settings. Level 3 (deep sedation) and level 4 (general anesthesia) are considered less safe in the office.[3]

LOCAL ANESTHESIA

Local anesthesia is used in nearly all office-based vascular procedures. Lidocaine is the most common medication used for local infiltration. The maximum lidocaine dose for an adult is 4.5 mg/kg. If the lidocaine is mixed with epinephrine (a vasoconstrictor), the dosage can be increased to 7.0 mg/kg. Needle aspiration prior in injection is considered a proper technique, especially when injecting around vascular structures, to avoid intravascular administration. In patients with known lidocaine allergy, an ester family local anesthetic is recommended (i.e., procaine and tetracaine).[4]

The potential for toxicity of local anesthesia must be known, assessed for, and be able to be managed if side

TABLE 12.1
Necessary Equipment for Sedation.

Equipment
Oxygen supply from a portable or permanent source
Airway equipment including nasal cannula, oral airways, nasal trumpet, ambu bag, mask ventilation, and intubation equipment
Continuous functioning suction
Emergency code cart with defibrillator
Physiological monitoring equipment for continuous monitoring including pulse oximeter, respirations, blood pressure, pulse, cardiac monitoring, and capnography
Stethoscope
Reversal agents
IV access equipment
Telephone
Intraosseous access kit for emergent situation

Office-Based Endovascular Centers. https://doi.org/10.1016/B978-0-323-67969-5.00012-5
Copyright © 2020 Elsevier Inc. All rights reserved.

TABLE 12.2
Continuum of Sedation and Anesthesia.

Level of Sedation/ Anesthesia	Description
Level 0	No sedation/local anesthesia only
Level 1	Minimal sedation/anxiolysis
Level 2	Moderate sedation/analgesia (conscious sedation)
Level 3	Deep sedation/analgesia
Level 4	General anesthesia

effects occur. Patients may develop mild symptoms such as tinnitus, circumoral paresthesia, or a metallic taste sensation with increased administration/absorption. Severe signs such as dysarthria, seizures, loss of consciousness, and ultimately respiratory arrest can also occur with higher doses of local anesthesia. Local anesthesia should be administered carefully in patients who have a history of seizures. Careful calculation and administration is vital to avoid overdose that can lead to clinical sequelae. The American Society of Regional Anesthesia and Pain Management recommends that anyone performing local anesthesia maintain a local anesthetic systemic toxicity (LAST) rescue kit. This is to include 1 liter of 20% lipid emulsion, several large syringes and needles for rapid infusion, standard intravenous tubing, and a printed LAST checklist.[5]

SEDATION

Procedural sedation is used for most endovascular procedures. At its core, the sedation provided during vascular in-office procedures is meant to allow the patient to tolerate the unpleasantness of the procedure with decreased anxiety while maintaining full control of their airway and respiration. Level 1 or minimal sedation allows for anxiolysis while the patient has full ability to respond to verbal stimuli without any depression of cardiovascular function or spontaneous ventilation. Level 2 or conscious sedation allows patients a deeper level of sedation and may require tactile, in addition to verbal, stimuli to illicit a response. Nevertheless, spontaneous ventilation is maintained and cardiovascular function is not depressed. Level 3 sedation is deep sedation with analgesia that requires repeat, painful stimuli to elicit a response from the patient. Airway intervention may be required if there is inadequate spontaneous ventilation; however, cardiovascular function is maintained. Level 4 sedation is defined as general anesthesia. This is rare or nonexistent as a sedation strategy in office-based vascular procedures. Proper supplies for airway management and proper personnel with basic life support and advanced cardiovascular life support (ACLS) are essential as an individual patient's response to sedation can be hard to predict.[6]

Interventionalists and the registered nurses should be ACLS certified. The physician should have education in conscious sedation. Many of the interventionalists would already have privilege in providing conscious sedation in the hospital setting. This should suffice for the education and training required for privileging in the office. In case the physician does not have privilege in the hospital for conscious sedation, it is recommended that the physician participate in education and acquire the knowledge to provide conscious sedation in a safe manner.

Sedation is achieved with a very few medications in most vascular cases. Benzodiazepines such as diazepam, lorazepam, or midazolam are often the most common drugs given to achieve amnesia, anxiolysis, and sedation. They do not provide analgesia. Flumazenil should be readily available to treat any overdose of benzodiazepines. Common opioids generally administered in conjunction with benzodiazepines and local anesthesia, for analgesia include fentanyl and morphine. Naloxone should be readily available for acute reversal. If administering or supervising the administration of these medications, the interventionalist must have an understanding of the dosages, pharmacokinetics, and side effects of these drugs.

PATIENT AND PROCEDURE SELECTION

Proper patient selection is key in mitigating adverse events in office-based procedures. It is highly recommended that a statement about why the patient is a candidate for an in-office procedure be included in the preoperative and/or intraoperative record. Procedural sedation needs to be planned, prescribed, selected, ordered, and supervised by the physician who is ACLS certified, a trained anesthesiologist, or a certified registered nurse anesthetist. A set of selection criteria for patients who are deemed to be appropriate candidates for office procedures is ideal. Table 12.3 lists conditions which may have a higher risk of periprocedural adverse events.[1,2,7] These conditions should be specifically evaluated at the preoperative visit. A decision then should be made as to the general fitness of the patient to undergo a surgical procedure. This can be best done by using the ASA Physical Status

TABLE 12.3
Patient Comorbidities That are High Risk for Adverse Events in Office-Based Vascular Procedures.

Comorbidities
Previous problems with anesthesia or sedation
Potential for a difficult airway
High aspiration risk
Abnormal bleeding or thrombotic disorder
Severe anxiety
Morbid obesity (especially involving the neck and facial structure)
Severe obstructive sleep apnea
Anaphylaxis risk
Inability to cooperate
Recent myocardial infarction
Recent stroke
Active seizure disorder

Severe chronic obstructive pulmonary disease.

TABLE 12.4
ASA Physical Status Classification System.

ASA Physical Status Classification	Definition	Examples
ASA I	Healthy patient	Healthy nonsmoker
ASA II	Patient with mild systemic disease	Current smoker, pregnancy, obesity (BMI<40), controlled diabetic or hypertensive
ASA III	Patient with severe systemic disease	Morbid obesity (BMI>40), implanted pacemaker, end stage renal disease, poorly controlled diabetes, poorly controlled hypertension
ASA IV	Patient with severe systemic disease that is a constant threat to life	Stroke or myocardial ischemia <3 months, active cardiac ischemia, severe reduction of ejection fraction, sepsis, end stage renal disease not on dialysis
ASA V	Patient who is not expected to survive without the operation	Ruptured aortic aneurysm, intracranial bleed with mass effect
ASA VI	Brain-dead patient whose organs are to be harvested for donor purposes	

Classification System.[8] Table 12.4 provides a synopsis of the system. ASA I and II patients are suitable for office-based endovascular procedures using moderate sedation or lesser degree of anesthesia. ASA III patients must be chosen more carefully. For example, most end stage renal disease patients undergoing dialysis can have interventions on their access safely and more cost-effectively via percutaneous techniques with Level 1 or lesser anesthesia in the office site-of-service.[9–12] However, most patients with severe cardiac dysfunction are not suitable for procedures in the office. ASA IV and V patients are not candidates for office-based intervention.

Physical examination may identify a patient with facial and neck features that makes airway management more challenging and may put the patient at greater risk. Such features in the head and neck include short neck, limited neck extension, decreased hyoid-mental distance (less than 3 cm in an adult), neck mass, cervical spine immobility, and obvious tracheal deviation. A small opening in the mouth (less than 3 cm in an adult), macroglossia, and a non-visible uvula are features in the mouth that will limit access to a patient's airway. Abnormalities of the jaw such as micrognathia, retrognathia, trismus, and significant malocclusion are pathologies that can make airway management difficult. The presence of these features should trigger a consultation for the patient with an anesthesiologist. These patients may be better suited to have the procedure performed in the hospital.

Procedure selection is as important as patient selection. Procedures with high potential for major complications should be avoided in the office setting. Prolonged procedural time has the greatest correlation for periprocedural adverse events.[8] The American Society of Plastic Surgeons recommends office-based

TABLE 12.5
Modified Aldrete Score.

Activity	Respiration	Circulation	Consciousness	Oxygen Saturation	Score
Moves 4 extremities voluntarily or on command	Able to deep breathe	Blood pressure ±20–30 mm Hg of preprocedural level	Awake and alert	SpO_2 above 92% on room air or equal to preprocedural level	2
Moves 2 extremities voluntarily or on command	Dyspnea, limited breathing, or tachypnea	Blood pressure ±31–49 mm Hg of preprocedural level	Drowsy, arousable to oriented state	SpO_2 greater than 92% with O_2 inhalation	1
No movement of extremities	Apneic or on ventilator	Blood pressure ±50 mm Hg or more of preprocedural level	Responds vaguely, unresponsive	SpO_2 below 92% with oxygen	0

procedures be limited to 6 h duration and be completed by 3 p.m.[13,14] This is a reasonable blueprint to follow for office-based endovascular procedures, though it is the opinion of this author that procedures should be limited to a planned 2 h. Occasionally the planned procedure may last more than 2 h.

POSTPROCEDURE RESPONSIBILITIES

Patient management post office-based intervention needs to be standardized, documented, and safe. The physician should validate and document indicating the total amount of medication administered during the procedure, including local anesthesia used. An immediate postprocedure note should be completed. A discharge order with any specific discharge instructions should be entered in the patient's medical record. The patient's level of pain and their modified Aldrete Score (Table 12.5) need to be determined and documented immediately postprocedure and during the postprocedure period at regular intervals. Patients may be discharged with a physician's order when the discharge criteria are met. Appropriate outpatient discharge criteria include a modified Aldrete score above 8, vital signs stable or back to baseline, mental status that is alert and oriented or a return to baseline, and discontinuation of supplemental oxygen for at least 15 min unless there is an order for it to be continued. If a patient received a reversal agent (Naloxone, Flumazenil), postprocedure monitoring should continue for a minimum of 2 h after the last administration of the reversal agent to guard against the patient becoming resedated after reversal effects have abated. Outpatients should be discharged in the presence of a responsible adult who will drive/accompany them home and be able to report any postprocedure complications. Discharge instructions need to be explained to the patient and their accompanying adult, along with written instructions. Discharge instructions should include information regarding diet, medications, activities (no driving, operating machinery, drinking alcohol, making important or legal decisions for 24 h postprocedure), and a number to call for new or severe symptoms.

PROTOCOLS AND ALGORITHMS FOR EMERGENCIES

All offices should have protocols in place for emergencies regardless of the level of sedation used in procedures (Chapter 2). It is the responsibility of the person administering anesthesia to ensure that the proper personnel and resources are available for the performance of the procedure and monitoring of the patient during sedation and recovery. Emergencies such as allergic reaction, respiratory depression, vasovagal response, and hypoglycemia may occur without much warning. Protocols for such situations and algorithms for their treatment need to be in place. Hospital agreements if applicable for accepting patients from the office and transfer policies must be established before any procedure is done. Many states require such arrangements. It is advisable to have dry runs for an emergency requiring transfer to a hospital. Our practice is to run a "Mock Code Day" annually to practice ACLS protocols and emergency case scenarios with staff and physicians.

SUMMARY

Anesthetic management by interventionalists has allowed for an increasing number of peripheral arterial and venous interventions to be performed in the OEC. This brings with it increased patient satisfaction and improved cost-effectiveness for most procedures. Patient safety in these settings must be assured by proper patient and procedural selection, physician and staff training, adequate supplies and emergency rescue medication, and expedient methods to get patients stabilized and transferred to a higher level of care if needed. Following established guidelines as demonstrated in this chapter is paramount to patient safety. Continuing education should be obtained specifically in local anesthesia and sedation by providers involved in these therapies to maintain a high level of care.

REFERENCES

1. *Guidelines for office-based anesthesia. Schaumburg (IL): American Society of Anesthesiologists Ambulatory Surgery Care Committee*; 2009. Available at: https://www.asahq.org/standards-and-guidelines/guidelines-for-office-based-anesthesia. Accessed May 1, 2019.
2. Shapiro FE, Punwani N, Rosenberg NM, et al. Office-based anesthesia: safety and outcomes. *Anesth Analg*. 2014;119:276–285.
3. Continuum of depth of sedation: definition of general anesthesia and levels of sedation. American Society of Anesthesia. Available at: http://www.asahq.org/quality-and-practice-management/standards-guidelines-and-related-resources/continuum-of-depth-of-sedation-definition-of-general-anesthesia-and-levels-of-sedation-analgesia.
4. Kouba DJ, LoPiccolo MC, Alam M, et al. Guidelines for use of local anesthesia in office-based dermatological surgery. *J Am Acad Dermatol*. 2016;74:1201–1219.
5. Checklist for treatment of local anesthetic systemic toxicity (LAST). American Society of Regional Anesthesia and Pain Medication. Available at: https://www.asra.com/advisory-guidelines/article/3/checklist-for-treatment-of-local-anesthetic-systemic-toxicity. Accessed May 1, 2019.
6. Practice guidelines for moderate procedural sedation and analgesia 2018. : a report by the American society of anesthesiologists task force on moderate procedural sedation and analgesia, the American association of oral and Maxillofacial Surgeons, American college of radiology, American dental association, American society of dentist anesthesiologists, and society of intraventional radiology. *Anesthesiology*. 2018;128:437–480.
7. Standard for office based anesthesia practice. American Association of Nurse Anesthetists. Available at: https://www.aana.com/patients/office-based-anesthesia.
8. *American Society of Anesthesiologists Physical Status Classification System*. American Society of Anesthesiologists House of Delegates/Executive Committee; 2014. Available at: https://www.asahq.org/standards-and-guidelines/asa-physical-status-classification-system.
9. Jain KM, Munn J, Rommel M, et al. Future of vascular surgery is in the office. *J Vasc Surg*. 2010;51:509–513.
10. Jain K, Munn J, Rommel MC, et al. Office-based endovascular suite is safe for most procedures. *J Vasc Surg*. 2014;59:186–191.
11. Dobson A, El-Gamil AM, Shimer MT, et al. Clinical and economic value of performing dialysis vascular access procedures in a freestanding office-based center as compared with the hospital outpatient department among Medicare ESRD beneficiaries. *Semi Dial*. 2013;26:624–632.
12. Kian K, Takesian K, Wyatt C, et al. Efficiency and outcomes of emergent vascular access procedures performed at a dedicated outpatient vascular access center. *Semin Dial*. 2007;20:346–350.
13. Mingus ML, Bodian CA, Bradford CN, et al. Prolonged surgery increases the likelihood of admission of schedule ambulatory surgery patients. *J Clinton Anesth*. 1997;9:446–450.
14. Iverson RE. ASPS task force on patient safety in office-based surgery facilities. Patient safety in office-based surgery facilities: I. Procedures in the office-based surgery setting. *Plast Reconstruct Surg*. 2002;110:1337–1342.

FURTHER READING

1. Statement on nonoperating room Anesthetizing locations. In: *American Society of Anesthesiologists Standards and Practice Parameters Committee*; 2018. Available at: https://www.asahq.org/~/media/Sites/ASAHQ/Files/Public/Resources/standards-guidelines/statement-on-nonoperating-room-anesthetizing-locations.pdf.

CHAPTER 13

Quality and Safety

KRISHNA JAIN, MD, FACS

For an office-based endovascular center (OEC), patients are essential to the success of the practice. Maintaining patient satisfaction and quality of care is of paramount importance. A visit to the physician's office can be a stressful situation for the patient. Culture dictates the assumption that the physician will deliver quality care. However, when the endovascular procedure is being performed in the office, the stress level of patients is likely to increase because patients are used to having the procedure done in a large hospital where there are many services available to ensure the safety of the patient. This is in contrast to the OEC, where emergency services are less obvious. On the other hand, the patient is used to coming to the office and is comfortable with the physical structure and the employees working in the office. Therefore, it behooves the treating physician to provide the highest quality of care in the office, which matches or surpasses the care provided in the hospital, to ensure that the patient continues to come to the practice for their endovascular care. Quality care invariably results in improved patient satisfaction. The patients become ambassadors of the practice. This becomes quite apparent in taking care of patients on dialysis. In a dialysis unit, typically there are several patients getting treatment at the same time. A patient who had a procedure performed in the OEC and was pleased with the care because of the satisfactory outcome and overall quality of the experience at OEC will share their positive experience with the other patients in the unit. In our practice, patients loathe to go to the hospital for a procedure because of the overall quality of care and experience in the OEC.

It is very difficult to measure quality in healthcare, yet every segment of society demands quality. This includes patients, physicians, healthcare workers, payers, and the government. In 2016, more than 80,236 medical publications were published in PubMed discussing quality. There is no question that quality healthcare should be provided to every person. Quality in Webster's dictionary is defined as "peculiar and essential character or nature; degree of excellence," thus quality is an abstract term. In real-life quality healthcare means different things to different people. It may mean a pleasant experience at the physician's office, pleasant surroundings, less hassle with scheduling, decreased number of visits to have the procedure done, avoiding the walk through the labyrinth of a hospital, or having the desired outcome of a procedure. Quality improvement or continuous quality improvement has become the buzzword that executives live by. While quality may be abstract, safety can be measured. It is easy to quantitate the outcome of a procedure. There are complications that can be identified, counted, and compared. Mortality rate, the ultimate measure, is easy to tabulate. Sometimes safety is used to define quality. Safety is an integral part of quality care, but there are other factors that need to be addressed. OECs can be a model for defining quality care and safety for endovascular procedures because the variables are controlled by a solo practitioner or a single group of physicians.

Quality and safety can be improved only by developing a culture of quality and reliability throughout the organization. There are several tools that can be used to improve quality. These include Six Sigma, Lean, change management and others. Most of the safety tools utilized in the healthcare segment are from the manufacturing industry and airlines. These mostly deal with the safety of the product and safe landing of the aircraft. It is important to use tested principles from various industries to improve safety. However, safety is only one part of the quality measurement.[1] A noted heath quality proponent, Dr Donabedian, suggested the following attributes to measure quality in healthcare.[1]

Efficacy: The ability of care, at its best, to improve health

Effectiveness: The degree to which attainable health improvements are realized

Efficiency: The ability to obtain the greatest health improvement at the lowest cost

Office-Based Endovascular Centers. https://doi.org/10.1016/B978-0-323-67969-5.00013-7
Copyright © 2020 Elsevier Inc. All rights reserved.

Optimality: The most advantageous balancing of cost and benefits

Acceptability: Conformity to patient preferences regarding accessibility, the patient-practitioner relationship, the amenities the effect of care, and the cost of care

Legitimacy: Conformity to social preferences concerning all of the above

Equity: Fairness in the distribution of care and its effects on health

In the same article, he further wrote: "The quality of care is judged by its conformity to a set of expectations or standards that derive from three sources: (a) the science of health care that determines efficacy, (b) individual values and expectations that determine acceptability, and (c) social values and expectations that determine legitimacy."[1]

Below we will review the various quality measurement and improvement processes that can help an OEC meet the quality expectations of individuals, society, and the payers. In a quality-driven organization, the quality of the center should meet the expectations of the providers of care because their success depends upon proper alignment of their expectations with societal expectations.

SIX SIGMA

In 1980, a Motorola engineer named Bill Smith introduced set of techniques and tools to improve processes. A Six Sigma process is one in which 99.99966% of all outcomes for a process are statistically expected to be free of defects. The term "Six Sigma process" comes from the notion that if one has six standard deviations between the process mean and the nearest specification limit, practically no items will fail to meet specifications. Processes that operate with "Six Sigma quality" over the short term are assumed to produce long-term defect levels below 3.4 defects per million opportunities. The goal of Six Sigma is to improve all parts of the processes. An OEC needs to determine an appropriate sigma level for each of its processes and strive to achieve that level. To meet this goal, it is incumbent on management to prioritize areas of improvement.

Application of the Six Sigma Doctrine to Medicine

Continuous efforts to achieve stable and predictable process results are of vital importance for business success. The same can be said for the medical practice. This is where a policy and procedure manual in an OEC can be an effective tool (Chapter 10). Utilizing policy and procedures allows the organization to preestablish the standard operating procedures of the practice to systematically preplan the procedures for optimal patient care and outcomes, such that there are no essential components that are lost or forgotten. This ensures each patient will receive the same level of care, creating consistency between patients and reliability for patients in the practice. Once the policies are written, it is incumbent upon the center to follow them. This is the one best method of decreasing variation. For example, if a patient has renal insufficiency and needs a contrast study, there should be a hydration protocol that should be followed each and every time to decrease postprocedure renal failure.

As in business, medical procedures processes have characteristics that can be defined, measured, analyzed, improved, and controlled. This is where a registry can be very helpful (Chapter 19). Using a registry, procedure outcomes can be measured, documented, and compared with others. If the outcomes do not meet local, regional, and national standards, efforts can and should be made to improve outcomes. This may mean complete analysis of the process from proper indication for the procedure to the planning, procedure execution, and ending with follow-up after the procedure in the short and long term.

To achieve sustained quality improvement, commitment from the entire organization is required. Top-level management needs to be committed to the process and lead the way. In an OEC, the top-level management are the physicians leading the practice, thus they have ultimate control of the entire process and can readily control the quality and quality improvement efforts. In a hospital setting, surgeons or interventionalists can only control part of the process in the operating room or catheterization lab environment. All the other aspects of care such as registration process, nursing and ancillary staff care are beyond the physicians' control. This can result in an uneven experience for the patient. In the OEC, all aspects of care being provided are under the leadership of the interventionalist. This includes preprocedure evaluation, completion of the procedure, discharge, and follow-up. All care provided to the patient by the physician and the OEC staff is controlled and managed by the physician. Many variables that are present in the hospital setting are eliminated, resulting in a more satisfying patient experience. Above all, the physician is responsible for providing the highest level of care.

Six Sigma Implementation

The acronym **DMAIC**—*Define, Measure, Analyze, Improve, and Control*—can be used for implementation of the Six Sigma program. DMAIC refers to a data-driven cycle used to improve and sustain the improved results. The DMAIC improvement cycle is the core tool used to drive Six Sigma projects. However, DMAIC can be used as the framework for other improvement applications as well.[2,3]

Define

The purpose of this step is to clearly identify the problem, goal, potential resources, project scope, and timeline. Take the example of excessive bleeding postprocedure. The current incidence rate forms the baseline to improve upon. A clear goal needs to be established within a certain time period with the currently available resources. For the excessive bleeding example, the practice goal may be to meet the national incidence rate of bleeding in the next 6 months.

Measure

This step establishes the current baseline as the basis for improvement. The definition of "excessive bleeding" needs to be agreed upon by all operators. The incidence of bleeding may already be known, and if not known the data need to be collected. This forms the baseline, which the performance metric will be compared with at defined intervals. The whole team involved in the care of the patient needs to be vested in this process.

Analyze

The purpose of this step is to identify, validate, and select a root cause for elimination. The cause may be multifactorial. In the case of bleeding it may be due to excessive anticoagulation, inappropriate site selection, inappropriate sheath size, procedural difficulties, improper use of manual compression, inappropriate use of closure devices, failure of a particular device, or postprocedure early ambulation. If there are multiple operators, it may be operator specific. These variables need to be measured consistently to determine the root cause of excessive bleeding, and again the cause may be multifactorial.

Improve

Once the root cause or causes are identified, the solutions should be implemented and tested. Once the cause of bleeding is identified, steps need to be taken to rectify the problem. Teams should start with the simplest solution first, followed by more difficult processes to implement. The implementation plan needs to be agreed upon by the whole team, carefully documented, and implemented. In the bleeding example, it may be a systemic problem or an operator-specific problem. It is possible that the operator may not be well trained in using the closure device or the OEC may be using a device that is know to have high bleeding complication rate. Appropriate steps can be taken for proper training or changing the devise if indicated.

Control

Control is the final step within the DMAIC improvement method. In this step, procedures should be amended and the benefit of the quality improvement efforts should be quantified and celebrated. Improvements should be tracked over time. In the excessive bleeding example, once the acceptable level of bleeding complication is achieved all the changes needed to reach that level should be documented, agreed upon by the whole team and become part of the processes used by the practice to take care of future patients. Just because a process has been improved once, does not mean it may not be targeted again in future improvement cycles. If other modalities to control bleeding complications become available, they should be utilized. The ultimate goal should be to have zero bleeding complications. This means that the OEC will continuously look at the ways to decrease the incidence of complications.

Six Sigma Team Member Roles

Prior to Six Sigma, quality management was the function of a separate quality department. Various terminologies adapted from a sport like Judo are adopted for various roles played by employees and create a hierarchy. The following key roles are played by various members of the team for its successful implementation.[4]

Executive Leadership: In the context of an OEC, this includes the CEO and President of the group. These leaders are responsible for establishing a vision for Six Sigma implementation and empower the other role holders. They provide the freedom and resources to explore new ideas by breaking natural barriers and overcoming inherent resistance to change.

Champions take responsibility for implementation across the organization. The Executive Leadership may use an office/business manager to fulfill this role. Champions also provide mentorship to Black Belts.

Master Black Belts, identified by Champions, act as in-house coaches, devoting 100% of their time to guide Black and Green Belts. In an OEC, this may not be possible and the role may be carried out by the champion instead.

Black Belts operate under Master Black Belts and spend 100% of their time applying Six Sigma methods to specific projects, providing leadership to specific tasks. In an OEC a nurse manager of the center may take this on as an added responsibility.

Green Belts are the employees who implement the Six Sigma process in addition to other job responsibilities, operating under the guidance of Black Belts. In an OEC, this would mean that all the employees participate.

Six Sigma Certification

While Six Sigma certification is not mandated, a quality-driven organization may want to be certified to bring consistent quality to the center. Various organizations provide Six Sigma certification including professional associations, university certification programs, and for profit training organizations. Motorola, created a certification process early on, subsequently the Lean Six Sigma Society of professionals, American Society of Quality, Institute of Industrial and Systems Engineers, and Chartered Quality Institute created their own certifying processes. Currently there are close to 50 universities offering a certification program.

Six Sigma in Healthcare

Benefits of using Six Sigma have been documented in the literature. The program should be integrated into the business plan for the executives to have total buy-in. If the process is looked upon only as a quality initiative, it tends to be diluted and does not get the necessary commitment from the whole organization. The reason the program works well at Motorola and other companies is because the quality improvement process has become part of the companies' DNA.

Here are some examples of impact of Six sigma in healthcare[5]:

- Mount Carmel Health System: Saved $3.1 million focusing on operational issues and business management and at the same time employee and physician satisfaction rates improved.
- Boston Medical Center: Saved more than $2.2 million while focusing on diagnostic imaging.
- Rapides Regional Medical Center: Saved $950,000.00 annually by decreasing wait time in the emergency room.
- The Women and Infants Hospital of Rhode Island: The hospital standardized its procedures for embryo transfer, thereby increasing the implementation rates by 35%.
- Valley Baptist Health System: Potential increase in income by reducing surgery turn over time. Additional 1100 additional cases per year could be performed.
- Yale-New Haven Medical Center: Potential savings of $1.2 million by reducing bloodstream infection in intensive care unit by 75%.

LEAN

Taiichi Ohno was a Japanese industrial engineer and businessman. He is considered to be the father of the Toyota Production System, which became Lean Manufacturing in the United States. The Lean method is a quality system that reduces or eliminates activities that do not add value. The "value" as defined by the customer is the price a customer is willing to pay for the services provided. The LEAN method helps ensure high quality and customer satisfaction. For an OEC the, patient defines "value." With current changes in payment system, CMS is defining "value." There are three type of activities defined in the LEAN method: (1) activities that do not add value and are total waste, (2) activities that add value, and (3) activities that enable value-added activities and are necessary for the process to continue. The goal is to reduce or eliminate wasteful activities, thereby improving efficiency and providing greater value.

Principles of LEAN

There are five fundamental principles of LEAN process:

1. **Define value:** The customer (patient) defines the value of a service. So the first step is to identify the patient's expectations from the services being provided. Process activities then can be classified into non-value added, value added, and enabling value added.
2. **Map the value stream:** The workflow steps need to be identified and documented for every service being provided. Value stream mapping helps to identify nonvalue activities so that they can be eliminated thereby improving the efficiency of the process. For example, if a patient has to spend time reregistering at every encounter, this may be a non-value-added activity for the patient.
3. **Create flow:** Smooth flow needs to be created so that there are no wasted services or wasted time. Patient coming in for a procedure should not wait in waiting room or wait for lab results.

4. **Establish pull:** The pull approach is used to provide the customer with services on demand. There is no reason patient should have to wait for an intravenous infusion started or experience a delay caused by late arrival of the interventionalist. The time these events take should be accounted for in the appointment process, so that care is provided in a timely, efficient manner.
5. **Seek continuous improvement:** There must be consistent efforts toward continuous quality improvement. If all the waste has been eliminated, future technologies and innovation will continue to offer opportunities for improvement

Removing Waste

In Lean methodology process, waste is identified as Muda, a Japanese term for waste. Using the Lean methodology, there are eight types of waste, defined with the acronym DOWNTIME, which can be eliminated. The eight types of waste are defects, overproduction, waiting, nonutilized talent, transportation, inventory, motion, and extra processing. One example of waste that is very prevalent occurs in the interventional suite where every operator has a preference card that the nurse or the surgical assistant refers to before starting the case. At the start of the case, disposable equipment like sheaths, wires, and balloons are taken out of the sterile sheath and placed on the table before the operator arrives in the room. If the operator decides to use a different piece of equipment because of patient characteristics or the procedure that was planned has changed, then that equipment is disposed of and thus wasted. Instead, catheters, devices, and other disposable equipment should be opened in consultation with the operator for every procedure. Another area of waste deals with inventory control; most products have to be used by a certain date. If the product is not used in a timely manner it is wasted and money is lost. To avoid this waste, the products and their expiration dates should be documented and tracked.

Six Sigma and Lean processes have different strengths in improving quality and providing value. This has resulted in a combination of the two systems, termed Lean Six Sigma.

LEAN SIX SIGMA

According to The American Society for Quality, "Lean Six Sigma is a fact-based, data-driven philosophy of improvement that values defect prevention over defect detection. It drives customer satisfaction and bottom-line results by reducing variation, waste, and cycle time, while promoting the use of work standardization and flow, thereby creating a competitive advantage. It applies anywhere variation and waste exist, and every employee should be involved".[6] The Lean process helps in reducing or eliminating wastes using the "DOWNTIME" methodology. Six Sigma focuses on eliminating variation in process thereby reducing errors. The two quality management systems can work hand in hand complementing each other. This approach can result in increased safety for patients while delivering higher value care. An integrated approach of Lean Six Sigma at OEC helps improve process efficiency, optimizes resource utilization while increasing patient satisfaction. This would also result in increased profits for the OEC.

Seventy-seven hospitals deploying Lean Sigma method reported following results.[7] Greater than 95% of operating rooms and 86% of emergency rooms had improved clinical success after utilizing LEAN techniques. For Six Sigma, the results were similar with 95% clinical success in operating rooms and 95% success in other inpatient areas. Similar results were seen after use of Lean or Six Sigma in ancillary or support services (94% vs. 90% in admissions/discharge, and 87% vs. 88% in radiology). Lean and Six sigma processes have also been shown to be successful in improving processes for information systems, administration, and pharmaceutical services.[7]

CHANGE METHOD

Change is the only constant.

HERACLITUS, GREEK PHILOSOPHER

There is no business that does not change over time. Healthcare is no different. Who knew that we would be utilizing electronic medical records or using virtual reality to teach medical students and residents. Over the last several decades, various change models have been created and used for quality improvement efforts. The plan-do-check-act cycle was created by W. Edwards Deming. The Change Quest Model, created by Dr Britt Andreatta, is based on neuroscience and how humans respond to change. The eight-step process was developed by Dr John Kotter, a Harvard business professor.[8] Kotter suggested that in order to accomplish change, at least 75% of the company's management team needs to buy into the need for change.[9] Successful use of the Kotter model has been shown in the clinic, specifically improving the hand off between nurses in the hospital. Using the Kotter model changes were made to the way nurses communicate at the bedside at shift change, resulting in improved compliance as well as patient and nurse satisfaction with the handoff process. The key feature of the success of this model is incorporation of feedback and ideas from the stakeholders involved, creating a coalition for change.[10]

THE KOTTER MODEL

Step 1. Create urgency: People in the organization need to understand the need for change. The threats and problems need to be identified so that opportunities to address those threats can be found. All members of the organization need to be part of the discussion to understand the urgency for change.

Step 2. Create a coalition: Change requires a group of influential leaders that are invested in the change. Leaders should be found throughout an organization and may bring status, power, expertise, and political importance to the change. The team should work together to develop the plan for change.

Step 3. Create a vision for change: A clear vision and strategy to execute that vision is required for change. The vision must be a value-driven plan that is shared with the participants in a short and succinct manner.

Step 4. Communicate the vision: Most visions fail because of poor communication. Let everyone know your vision and repeat it often with conviction. The vision should be a part of everyone's work life. Vision should drive decision-making and problem-solving. Any concerns or anxieties that crop up as a result of the vision should be addressed promptly without bias. You should lead by example.

Step 5. Remove obstacles: There will always be obstacles that come with any change. These barriers need to be removed as soon as identified. It may be necessary to look at the organizational structure, compensation system, or job descriptions hindering change. People helping the change should be rewarded and the ones hindering change should be convinced to become a part of the process.

Step 6. Create short-term wins: There should be short-term and long-term targets. The short-term targets should be achievable, as early success is a great motivator. This helps neutralize critics and negative thinkers. Each win helps motivate the entire staff. People helping achieve these wins should be rewarded.

Step 7. Build on the change: Declaration of victory too early may result in ultimate defeat. Lots of small victories will amount to the ultimate victory. Each successful change provides an opportunity to learn from mistakes made or the reasons for success. As the goals are achieved the momentum should be kept up and more people should become change agents.

Step 8. Anchor the changes in corporate culture: Changes that have been achieved should become part of the core of the organization. Continuous efforts are needed for change to be a part of the whole organization. Leaders need to continue to support the change. Changes that have been made need to be discussed with the current employees and future hires. People instrumental in change need to be publicly recognized and new change leaders need to be groomed.

QUALITY IMPROVEMENT OPPORTUNITY IN OEC

All aspects of patient care in the OEC should be reviewed, and everyone should follow policies and procedures as mandated by the practice. Certain areas of the OEC can be targeted for data collection to make sure the procedures are being followed. For example, postoperative complications are easily quantifiable. The goal of the center should be to have a 0% incidence of postprocedure bleeding. This is a hard goal to achieve but with attention to detail, effort should be made to eliminate every possible reason for bleeding. The process will start at the time of history taking followed by hematological evaluation, avoidance of drugs that could result in bleeding, ultrasound-guided access of the blood vessel, use of smallest catheters and devices possible, judicious use of anticoagulants during the procedure, appropriate use of closure devices or manual compression, postprocedure care, and after discharge care instructions. If a patient does have a postprocedure bleeding, a root cause analysis should be performed to identify the cause of bleeding, and the practice should apply appropriate safeguards for the next procedure. Other areas that could be targeted are inventory control, patient satisfaction, employee satisfaction, clinical criteria i.e. incidence of infection, appointment timeliness, patient comfort, waiting time, etc.

It is very important for the employees to have a stake in the quality improvement process. Many of the initiatives could and should be driven by employees. They see things from a different perspective and spend much more time with the patient and the family as compared to the physician. Employees who come with ideas and solutions that improve quality should be encouraged and rewarded for their efforts.

SAFETY

Agency for healthcare research and quality working with several other organizations and stakeholders developed a toolkit for improving safety in ambulatory surgery centers.[11] Though the toolkit was not developed for the OEC, the principles apply to OEC as well. The toolkit is divided in three sections: implementation, sustainability, and resources. Each section contains guides, tools, slide sets, videos, and audio files. The toolkit can be tailored to the needs of OEC.

The American College of Surgeons has developed a manual entitled *Optimal Resources for Surgical Quality and Resources* that describes the attributes of high reliability organization.[12] These attributes are preoccupation with failure, sensitivity to operations, reluctance to simplify interpretation, commitment to resilience, and deference to expertise.

Preoccupation with failure. Awareness of all the areas that may result in failure is essential to plan properly. In an OEC, the plan may be to use a certain closing device after the procedure. The physician may ask if the device is available. The answer may be yes without actually checking availability of the device. At the end of the procedure, the closure device is brought to the table but it is the wrong device. The physician and the staff should have checked the availability of the desired device. Check, double check, and triple check!

Sensitivity to operations. Uneventful lapses, near misses, and close calls should be carefully investigated. One of these events may give the opportunity to improve the processes. For example, if a patient in the OEC, who has significant renal insufficiency, is being prepared for an angiogram and the nurse announces that the serum creatinine level is 4, the procedure should not be started. The creatinine level was not available the day before the procedure resulting in this near miss. Appropriate procedures need to be developed so that all events are planned for and this occurrence is not repeated.

Reluctance to simplify interpretation. If a close call or error occurs, a full root cause analysis should be completed, rather than accepting the first obvious reason for the mistake. For example, an OEC patient is having an angiogram and during the procedure the blood sugar is found to be very high despite the fact that the patient received insulin preprocedure. The first thought would be that patient did not receive enough insulin. However, on further analysis, it may be found there was no process in place for identifying patients who may have uncontrolled diabetes or a process to make sure that the blood sugar is appropriately controlled after receiving the insulin before the patient is on the table for angiogram.

Commitment to resilience. This applies to using safeguards like marking the right limb for the procedure, and establishing time-outs before the procedure. Every process step needs to be carefully executed and double checked. There is no room for shortcuts.

Deference to expertise. Traditionally, the surgeon/interventionalist is the captain of the ship and everyone follows the direction. However, if a member of the team recognizes an event that may harm the patient that person needs to speak up. In OEC, if the interventionalist is about to deliver a stent in the superficial femoral artery which could occlude the origin of profundal femoris artery, any member of the team should feel comfortable pointing out this situation to the interventionalist without any fear of repercussion.

CONCLUSION

The quality improvement methods described in this chapter can help improve quality and meet the expectations of the individual, society, and the payers. Some areas where the OEC can focus to improve quality include interactions between patients and employees, employee communication, patient comfort, patient safety, follow-up, ease of use of the facility, inventory control, and meeting the regulatory requirements. To help establish, measure, and meet quality standards, the center can participate in a registry (Chapter 19) and follow guidelines and standards put forth by societies and regulatory bodies. National, regional, and international societies in vascular surgery, interventional cardiology, and interventional radiology have worked in unison or separately to establish guidelines and standards published in peer-reviewed journals. It is important to know these guidelines and follow them. Above all, it is essential that every OEC provides a safe environment for patients. The whole team in the OEC should be dedicated toward providing quality care safely. All employees should be empowered to meet these goals, encouraged to develop ideas to improve quality and rewarded accordingly.

To conclude, let us go back to the seven pillars of health quality article by Avedis Donabedian, "the care being provided should be efficacious, effective, efficient, optimal, acceptable, legitimate and be provided equally to every member of society."[1]

REFERENCES

1. Donabedian A. The seven pillars of quality. In: *Archives of Pathology and Laboratory Medicine*. Vol. 1990.
2. InvisibleC. DMAIC. Invis Consult blog. https://invisibleconsultant.co.uk/dmaic-define-stage/.
3. Webber L, Wallace M. *Quality Control for Dummies*. 2006.
4. Harry M, Schroeder R. *Six Sigma*. Random House Inc; 2000.
5. A Look at Six Sigma's Increasing Role in Improving Healthcare. Villanova Univ.
6. What Is Six Sigma. Am Soc Qual.
7. Hospitals see benefits of lean and six sigma. *Am Soc Qual*; 2009. http://asq.org/qualitynews/qnt/execute/displaySetup?newsID=5843.
8. Kotter J. Kotter's 8-step change model - change management tools from mind tools. *MindtoolsCom*. 1995.
9. Kotter JP. *Leading Change, With a New Preface by the Author*. Harvard Bus Sch Press Books; 2012.
10. Small A, Gist D, Souza D, Dalton J, Magny-Normilus C, David D. Using Kotter's change model for implementing bedside handoff: a quality improvement project. *J Nurs Care Qual*. 2016;31(4):304–309. https://doi.org/10.1097/NCQ.0000000000000212.
11. Toolkit to improve safety in ambulatory surgery centers. *Agency Helathcare Res Qual*. 2014.
12. Hoyt D, Clifford K. *Optimal Resources for Surgical Quality and Safety*. American College of Surgeons; 2017.

CHAPTER 14

Management of Complications

KRISHNA JAIN, MD, FACS

There is no open surgical procedure that does not have inherent complications. The same holds true for endovascular procedures.

Potential complications can occur if the procedure is done in the hospital or carried out in the office-based endovascular center (OEC). The procedures that were done in the hospital are gradually migrating to the OEC. The same interventionalists who were performing the procedures in the inpatient setting are now operating in the OEC. The complications encountered in OEC will be similar to those seen after the procedure is done in the hospital. Various types of procedures are carried out in the OEC. These procedures include arterial procedures, dialysis access–related procedures, venous procedures for superficial and deep venous disease, insertion of ports and indwelling catheters, and embolization procedures. Some potential complications are common to all procedures while others are specific to each procedure type. Ideally speaking, it is best not to have a complication. Risk of complication can be decreased by proper selection of patients, and attention to detail.

PATIENT SELECTION AND PREVENTIVE MEASURES

The resources in the OEC are significantly limited as compared with the hospital. Operating in a hospital gives a sense of security because it is a much larger facility. Physicians have traditionally worked in the hospital and all resources needed to manage a complication are under one roof. However, with appropriate selection of patients the complications in the OEC can be minimized and managed as shown in publications by Jain et al.[1] and Lin et al.[2] In general, following type of patients should not have a procedure done in the OEC: patients above 400 lbs, patient with low pain tolerance if only local anesthesia is used at the center, patient in ASA class 4 unless they are coming for dialysis access management (this should be infrequent and the procedure should be done under local anesthesia), patients with severe dye allergy, patients with low comprehension who may not be able to follow instructions, and patients who cannot lay flat for the procedure because of back pain, respiratory issues.

Other preventive measures that can be taken start with a comprehensive history taking. A checklist before starting the procedure can be very helpful (Table 14.1). If the patient has any allergies to medication, is using anticoagulants or antiplatelet drugs, or is taking medications like Glucophage, the medicines need to be adjusted before and after the procedure is performed. If the patient is diabetic, Hgb A1C should be checked and optimized. Blood sugar should be checked prior to the initiation of the procedure. If conscious sedation is planned, the patient's airway should be checked (Chapter 12). The patients, not on dialysis, with compromised renal function should be appropriately hydrated prior to the use of contrast agent. The appropriate measures to decrease radiation exposure to the patient and the staff should be taken to prevent radiation injury. If the patient is in childbearing age, pregnancy test should be performed prior to the procedure. All the supplies needed for the procedure should be available including the supplies that may be needed to take care of intraoperative complication. This may include disposable items such as covered stents, thrombectomy/aspiration catheters, detachable coils, or nondisposable items, such as intravascular ultrasound, medications, and equipment for airway management and defibrillator as per advanced cardiac life support (ACLS) protocol should be readily available. The interventionalist and the nurses should be ACLS certified. The following drugs should be available: epinephrine, amiodarone, lidocaine, magnesium

Office-Based Endovascular Centers. https://doi.org/10.1016/B978-0-323-67969-5.00014-9
Copyright © 2020 Elsevier Inc. All rights reserved.

TABLE 14.1
Checklist Before Starting the Procedure.

Name, Date of Birth, Sex, Medical Record Number
Consent
Procedure
Type of procedure site of procedure, site marked
Anticoagulants
Blood sugar
Allergies
Glomerular filtration rate (GFR)
Antibiotics
Allergy prevention medicine
Special equipment
Cardio pulmonary status
Radiation precautions

atropine, dopamine, adenosine, diltiazem, beta-blockers, amiodarone, digoxin, and verapamil.

PRECAUTIONS DURING THE PROCEDURE

Appropriate access site should be selected to carry out the intervention. Ultrasound guidance while accessing the vessel is known to decrease the incidence of postoperative bleeding.[3] Smallest sheath possible for the procedure should be used. During the procedure, intravascular guidewires, catheters, etc. should be used carefully. Manufacturers' recommendation should be followed. Use of fluoroscopy and contrast media should be minimized. Hemostasis should be achieved by manual compression or use of a closure device. If CO_2 angiography is used it should be used only for procedures below the diaphragm.

Despite all the precautions that are taken each procedure has inherent potential complications. Let us look at general complications and the complications that are specific to each procedure.

GENERAL COMPLICATIONS

Cardiac
Pulmonary
Renal
Infection
Others

Cardiac: The patient should have been screened before the procedure to avoid intraoperative or postoperative cardiac event. However, despite proper optimization of cardiac status, patient may have a cardiac event. If the patient is having cardiac symptoms during the procedure or changes in cardiac rhythm, these should be addressed and procedure shortened to the extent that it can be done safely. If the patient shows signs of cardiac compromise in the recovery, the patient should be treated. Patient should be transferred to the emergency room after discussing with patient's cardiologist and/or primary care doctor.

Pulmonary: If the patient becomes short of breath it may be due to fluid overload, patient's underlying pulmonary disease, or an allergic reaction to contrast agent or other drugs. Each cause of pulmonary symptoms will need to be treated in a different fashion. Patient may need diuresis or a bronchodilator or treatment of the allergic reaction. If the patient continues to be symptomatic the patient should be sent to the emergency room after discussion with the primary care doctor and/or the pulmonologist.

Renal: Contrast-induced nephropathy[4] is a serious complication caused by the use of contrast media. Patients with poor kidney function could be candidates for CO_2 angiography. Hydration[5] before the procedure and continued after the procedure may minimize the kidney injury. Low-osmolar contrast agent may also help prevent injury to the kidney.

Infection: Every precaution should be taken to prevent postprocedure infection. The site of intervention should be properly prepared and cleaned with chlorhexidine. Antibiotic prophylaxis should be used as indicated. In a study by Jain et al.[1] the incidence of cellulitis and infection was 0.001% in 6458 procedures carried out in the OEC. All patients received one dose of antibiotic orally preprocedure and three doses postprocedure. One has to be especially careful if foreign bodies like stents, filters, indwelling catheters, and ports are inserted in patients for short duration or permanently. The stents can get infected[6] in short term or long term with serious consequences.

Others: The patients being treated in the OEC have multiple other underlying comorbidities like hypertension, diabetes, etc. Patients with end stage renal disease and venous disease may have other underlying medical conditions that could potentially cause complications. The interventionalist should be aware of these conditions and be prepared to manage these conditions on a short-term basis. The patients with epilepsy may have a tendency to get a seizure during the procedure.[7] This can happen even with the use of local anesthesia.

COMPLICATIONS AFTER LOWER EXTREMITY ARTERIAL INTERVENTION AT THE ACCESS SITE

Bleeding

The commonest complication after lower extremity arterial intervention is bleeding in the groin since transfemoral approach is the commonest approach used. This can happen with or without the use of closure devices. This can present as swelling, ecchymosis, pulsatile mass, pain, bleeding, or neuralgia. If there is significant bleeding, patient may be hypotensive. It is rare for a patient to be hypotensive unless patient develops retroperitoneal hematoma. After physical examination, an ultrasound of the femoral artery should be carried out to make sure there is no pseudoaneurysm and the hematoma is confined to the groin. Most of these patients can be treated with manual compression, warm compress, and antiinflammatory drugs. If the patient has significant symptoms like severe pain, necrosis of the skin, or neuralgia, operation may be required to evacuate the hematoma. If transaxillary approach is used a hematoma can cause nerve compression and ensuing symptoms. The hematoma should be evacuated in an urgent manner to avoid long-term sequelae of nerve compression. It is rare to have bleeding after radial or tibial approach. This can be managed by local compression.

PSEUDOANEURYSM

In case the patient develops a pseudoaneurysm (PSA), this can cause pain, rupture and significant bleeding, nerve compression, skin necrosis, or distal embolization. Small PSA, less than 3 cm in size can be observed. The patient can be followed up with serial ultrasound exams, provided the patient is not on anticoagulant and is reliable for follow-up. There was 86% chance of spontaneous closure in one study.[8] Ultrasound-guided compression of the pseudoaneurysm has been found to be successful.[9] However, this can be very painful, time-consuming,[10] may not work if the patient is on anticoagulant, and may result in rupture of the pseudoaneurysm, thrombosis of the vessel or distal embolization. Ultrasound-guided thrombin injection into the pseudoaneurysm has become the first-line therapy. Pseudoaneurysm can be treated with ultrasound-guided thrombin injection[10] and compression and followed for complete thrombosis. The main risk of this approach is thrombosis of the artery caused by thrombin. Use of thrombin in this scenario is off-label. A surgical repair may be required in a patient in case of failure of thrombin injection, patient with large pseudoaneurysm, pseudoaneurysm with large neck or pseudoaneurysm with arteriovenous fistula (AVF). The repair may be an open procedure entailing resection of PSA and repair of the artery[11] or an endovascular approach using covered stent.[12] There is not enough published data to recommend the endovascular approach on a routine basis.

ARTERIOVENOUS FISTULA

AVF is a rare complication of the procedure. These are usually diagnosed during physical examination as a thrill is felt or during auscultation when a bruit is heard. Ultrasound examination of the site confirms the diagnosis. Most AV fistulas are benign and can be left alone. Many of these will spontaneously close. If they become symptomatic then a surgical repair or endovascular repair using a covered stent[13] may be indicated. In a high-risk patient, a covered stent may be the treatment of choice.

THROMBOSIS

Thrombosis can occur at the access site or anywhere in the arterial system where intervention has been carried out. Thrombosis of common femoral artery, axillary artery, or brachial artery will usually manifest immediately. If the access vessel thromboses and patient is symptomatic, surgical exploration and repair of the vessel are the best options. The thrombosis occurs because of the diseased vessel, use of large sheaths, complication of a closure device, or inadequate anticoagulation. Patient will have symptoms of acute arterial ischemia. Patient should not leave the operating table before the distal pulses are checked manually or using a Doppler. When the femoral approach is used and the extremities are under the drapes the pulses should be checked with Doppler before the procedure is started and skin marked. Flat Doppler probe could be taped to the skin where the pulses are found. It should be done for both lower extremities. Radial artery occlusion in the presence of a normal Allan test is usually asymptomatic. Tibial artery occlusion after using the tibial approach is rare and usually asymptomatic.[14]

COMPLICATIONS OF THE PROCEDURE IN TREATED VESSELS

These complications include dissection, perforation, thrombosis of the treated vessel and embolization.

DISSECTION

If the subintimal dissection is used to perform an angioplasty then proper technique for reentry and angioplasty should be followed. However, when the intent is to carry out angioplasty without entering the subintimal plane a flap caused by the dissection can completely close the artery. During angioplasty, if a dissection occurs which is not uncommon, it can be diagnosed using contrast injection or using intravascular ultrasound. Intravascular ultrasound can be an useful adjunct in assessing the significance of the flap. The flap can be treated by using a self-expanding or balloon-mounted stent. The goal should be to have less than 30% stenosis at the end of the procedure. Small flaps in large normal vessels may not need to be treated.

PERFORATION

Perforation of the vessel can be caused by a wire or during balloon angioplasty. If the wire traverses outside the vessel it should be easily seen under fluoroscopy as the wire will be outside the normal course of the vessel and will start to curl in the soft tissue. The wire should be pulled out and a hand injection should be carried out. A crossing device may be needed to cross the lesion. Stiffer wires tend to cause more perforations. Once the wire is pulled back in the artery, usually the procedure can be continued. If the lesion cannot be crossed in an antegrade manner a retrograde tibial approach may be successful in crossing the occluding lesion in the artery in the leg. If the patient becomes uncomfortable, the procedure should be stopped. Patient should be carefully followed in the recovery area for an expanding hematoma or ischemia to the foot.

Perforation during angioplasty or atherectomy can have serious consequences. This is the most dreaded complication in an OEC. These can result is severe hemorrhage in the soft tissue or in the retroperitoneum depending on the site of angioplasty. The patient can suddenly become hemodynamically unstable. In the OEC, it can be treated using a covered stent[15] after tamponading the perforation site with a compliant balloon. If this fails, the patient should be transferred to the hospital immediately for surgical repair.

THROMBOSIS

Thrombosis of the treated vessel can potentially occur any time after treatment. This can present as an acute severe ischemia to the leg in the recovery area or after discharge, or patient may go the baseline symptoms for which the procedure was initially carried out. Depending on the severity of the symptoms it may be appropriate to proceed with repeat endovascular procedure. However, if the acute closure results in limb-threatening ischemia, surgical approach may be more suitable and the patient may need a bypass.

EMBOLIZATION

In the vessels with severe disease, thrombus, or exophytic plaque, the risk of embolization can be significant. The embolization can cause severe ischemia. If the risk of embolization is considered to be high, minimal manipulation should be carried out, patient should be anticoagulated early and use of embolic prevention filters[16] may be warranted. Various atherectomy devices have different rate of embolization. The appropriate device should be used. In case of embolization, patient should be anticoagulated and various techniques can be used to remove the embolus. These techniques include use of aspiration catheters,[16] percutaneous embolectomy, use of penumbra device (Penumbra, Alameda, CA), use of AngioJet (Possis medical, Minneapolis, Minnesota), or use of thrombolytics. If these techniques cannot be carried out in the OEC or fail, an open procedure is warranted. Thromboembolectomy with or without a bypass can restore circulation to the limb. This may need to be performed on an emergent basis. There can also be embolization of wires or catheters being used during the procedures. A segment of wire or the catheter can be accidently sheared off resulting in embolization. These can be retrieved using snares, etc.[17] Rarely an open approach may be needed. Depending on the size of the embolus, there is a risk of severe complications in these patients.

COMPLICATIONS DUE TO VASCULAR CLOSURE DEVICES

The use of vascular closure devices (VCDs) has been quite popular in OEC because of the advantages VCDs provide. The time to hemostasis is decreased so that the patient can be moved out of the procedure room faster as compared to the use of manual compression. Time to ambulation is decreased. This can permit the procedures to be carried out later in the day. The recovery area may need fewer beds because of decreased length of stay in the recovery area. Despite these advantages, the use of the devise remains controversial because overall risk of bleeding after the procedure is the same as after manual compression.[18] There is also risk of embolization with certain devices and fibrosis caused in the long term. There is also the issue of added cost of the device. The VCD should be used as per instructions for use by the manufacturer. If larger sheaths are used, multiple VCD may be required for hemostasis.

VENOUS COMPLICATIONS

Complications can occur after management of superficial venous disease as well as deep venous disease. The complications related to superficial venous disease are addressed in Chapter 29.

Venous complications can occur during a variety of procedures. These procedures include dialysis-related angioplasty of venous stenosis, during iliac vein dilatation and stenting, inferior cava reconstruction, insertion and removal of inferior vena cava filters, and during insertion of catheters and ports. These complications may result in perforation and bleeding, inadvertent cannulation of an artery or migration of stents and filters. During insertion of a catheter, pneumothorax or hemothorax is a known complication of the procedure. Almost all complications of venous procedures occur intraoperatively and are diagnosed immediately and treated according to the complication. Some of the stents in larger veins may migrate at a later time.

VENOUS ANGIOPLASTY

Most commonly, venous angioplasty is carried to maintain the patency of a dialysis fistula or a bridge graft. In the case of fistula, the stenosis can occur anywhere in the outflowing vein. It is commonly seen at the cannulation site, near the anastomosis, in the cephalic vein axillary vein confluence or at the site of a previous ipsilateral catheter. The stenosis may also be central if the patient had a previous indwelling catheter for a long period of time. The area of the stenosis is usually quite fibrotic because of intimal hyperplasia and may need high-pressure balloons to dilate the area of stenosis. It is not uncommon to use pressures exceeding 20 atm. The high-pressure balloon may cause the rupture of the arterialized vein. The flow through the vein is brisk and depending on the site, rupture may cause a large hematoma or bleeding in the mediastinum. The bleeding should be controlled by using a balloon inflated at low pressure and covering of the disrupted area using a covered stent. The stenosis in a bridge graft usually occurs at the graft vein anastomosis. This can be treated by angioplasty, and if there is disruption at the anastomosis a covered stent can be used to cover the area of disruption. In general, use of covered stent at the graft vein anastomosis has been shown to be beneficial in improving the patency of the graft.[19]

During dilation and stenting of an occluded or severely diseased iliac vein a wire may inadvertently be pushed outside the lumen. The venous system is low pressure system and once the wire is pulled back in the vein bleeding usually stops. If the rupture occurs during dilation, the inflated balloon at low pressure should be able to stop the bleeding. During the planned procedure a stent is usually planned, and placement of a bare metal stent should stop the bleeding. Sometimes a covered stent may be needed. However, the covered stent may not be available in large enough sizes. In follow-up, if patient continues to complain of pain or if there is a drop in hemoglobin, a CT scan may be needed to assess the extent of retroperitoneal hematoma. Patients usually complain of some discomfort on the treated site even without a complication.

Migration of the stent is a much larger concern. It can happen during the procedure or soon after if the stent is not appropriately sized. The stents should be appropriately sized since the veins can be in spasm during the procedure and diameter also changes based on respiratory cycle. It is more likely to happen during angioplasty of central veins like brachiocephalic vein or superior vena cava.[20] This can also happen during iliac vein intervention.[21] The migration of the stent can be life threatening as it can migrate to pulmonary artery or damage valves. Most of the time the stent can be retrieved percutaneously from the right atrium using snares and balloons. A cut down may be needed to remove the stent form the entry site. Occasionally, open-heart surgery may be performed to retrieve the stent from the heart or pulmonary artery. If smaller coils or plugs are used during the procedure, they may migrate and end up in the lung and may be innocuous.

INFERIOR VENA CAVA FILTER

Complications can occur while inserting the filter or retrieving it. The filter is inserted via femoral or internal jugular approach. Each site has its own inherent complications. Common femoral approach is more commonly used. Some of the complications of inserting a filter are pneumothorax, carotid artery injury, misplacement of the filter, access site thrombosis, hematoma, air embolism, and, worse of all, migration of the filter. Some of the complications can be avoided by using ultrasound-guided access of the vein. If the filter is released at the wrong spot another filter can be added. If the appropriate size filter is used the chance of migration is small. Inferior cava should be measured prior to deployment of the filter to be able to use the correct size filter. If the filter migrates to the heart it may be possible to retrieve it percutaneously using snares and large sheaths. The filter will have to be crushed into a large sheath and removed using a cutdown. If this approach fails open surgery may be required. Long dwelling filters may cause vena cava thrombosis. Every attempt should be made to retrieve the retrievable filter. Longer the filter stays in place higher the number of complications including fracture of the legs of the filter, tilting of the filter, and perforation of adjoining structures like duodenum and aorta. Retrievable filter can be easily removed in the OEC[22]

DIALYSIS ACCESS–RELATED COMPLICATIONS

The procedures that are carried out to maintain the dialysis access function include balloon angioplasty, balloon angioplasty and stent, coiling of vein tributaries, and thrombectomy of the dialysis access. Many of the complications as a result of these procedures have been described in other sections of this chapter. Complications related to percutaneous thrombectomy of the access are specific to this particular procedure. There can be significant load of thrombus in a large thrombosed AVF. Various techniques are used for thrombectomy.[17] During thrombectomy, the clot can migrate to the lung and cause pulmonary embolus. Usually small amount of clot traveling to the lung is well handled by the patient. In case of a symptomatic pulmonary embolus, appropriate anticoagulation treatment should be initiated. During thrombectomy if lytic enzyme is used the enzyme also helps lyse the clot in the lung due to its systemic effect. In a large series[17] of 2975 dialysis graft thrombectomy performed percutaneously the incidence of arterial embolism was 3.9%. Most of the emboli could be managed using percutaneous balloon embolectomy or aspiration. Surgical embolectomy was rarely required. The circulation to the extremity should be checked before the sheaths are removed. In case of inadvertent embolization, the sheaths can be used for endovascular procedure to retrieve the embolus.

CATHETER- AND PORT-RELATED COMPLICATIONS

Complications related to insertion of indwelling catheters and ports are described earlier in the chapter. The main risk for leaving an indwelling catheter for a long time is venous stenosis, thereby diminishing the chance for a successful dialysis access on ipsilateral side and sometimes on both sides as patient may develop central stenosis. Other risk is catheter infection or systemic sepsis caused by the catheter. In either case, the catheter will need to be removed. In addition to the risks described earlier, the main risk of inserting a port is bleeding in the pocket and infection. Bleeding will have to be stopped surgically and if the port gets infected it usually needs to be removed.[5]

EMBOLIZATION PROCEDURES

Various embolization procedures are being carried out in the OEC. Embolization of the uterine fibroids is becoming increasingly popular in an OEC. The complications of the procedure will mostly be the same as any arterial intervention. In a study reported by de Bruijn et al., there were no complications after uterine fibroid embolization. In any embolization procedure, extreme care should be taken to make sure that the embolization substance does not travel beyond the intended target.

Interventionalists working in the OEC should be prepared to manage the complications that may occur during or after the procedure. If the complication cannot be managed by conservative approach or endovascular techniques, patient should be transferred to an acute care hospital with proper consultation between the interventionalist, emergency room doctor, and preferably the physician who will be treating the patient. Every transfer to the hospital may not automatically need an operation.[23] Some patients are transferred for observation, others for nonsurgical complications like a cardiac or respiratory event.

REFERENCES

1. Jain K, Munn J, Rummel MC, Johnston D, Longton C. Office-based endovascular suite is safe for most procedures. *J Vasc Surg.* 2014. https://doi.org/10.1016/j.jvs.2013.07.008.
2. Lin PH, Yang K-H, Kollmeyer KR, et al. Treatment outcomes and lessons learned from 5134 cases of outpatient office-based endovascular procedures in a vascular surgical practice. *Vascular.* 2017;25(2):115–122. https://doi.org/10.1177/1708538116657506.
3. Kalish J, Eslami M, Gillespie D, et al. Routine use of ultrasound guidance in femoral arterial access for peripheral vascular intervention decreases groin hematoma rates. *J Vasc Surg.* 2015;61(5):1231–1238. https://doi.org/10.1016/j.jvs.2014.12.003.
4. Mohammed NMA, Mahfouz A, Achkar K, Rafie IM, Hajar R. Contrast-induced nephropathy. *Heart Views.*

2013;14(3):106–116. https://doi.org/10.4103/1995-705X.125926.
5. Pinelli F, Cecero E, Degl'Innocenti D, et al. Infection of totally implantable venous access devices: a review of the literature. *J Vasc Access.* 2018;19(3):230–242. https://doi.org/10.1177/1129729818758999.
6. Hogg ME, Peterson BG, Pearce WH, Morasch MD, Kibbe MR. Bare metal stent infections: case report and review of the literature. *J Vasc Surg.* 2007;46(4):813–820. https://doi.org/10.1016/j.jvs.2007.05.043.
7. DeToledo JC, Minagar A, Lowe MR. Lidocaine-induced seizures in patients with history of epilepsy: effect of antiepileptic drugs. *Anesthesiology.* 2002;97(3):737–739. http://www.ncbi.nlm.nih.gov/pubmed/12218544.
8. Toursarkissian B, Allen BT, Petrinec D, et al. Spontaneous closure of selected iatrogenic pseudoaneurysms and arteriovenous fistulae. *J Vasc Surg.* 1997;25(5):803–808. discussion 808-9 http://www.ncbi.nlm.nih.gov/pubmed/9152307.
9. Fellmeth BD, Roberts AC, Bookstein JJ, et al. Postangiographic femoral artery injuries: nonsurgical repair with US-guided compression. *Radiology.* 1991;178(3):671–675. https://doi.org/10.1148/radiology.178.3.1994400.
10. Kuma S, Morisaki K, Kodama A, et al. Ultrasound-guided percutaneous thrombin injection for post-catheterization pseudoaneurysm. *Circ J.* 2015;79(6):1277–1281. https://doi.org/10.1253/circj.CJ-14-1119.
11. Huseyin S, Yuksel V, Sivri N, et al. Surgical management of iatrogenic femoral artery pseudoaneurysms: a 10-year experience. *Hippokratia.* 2013;17(4):332–336. http://www.ncbi.nlm.nih.gov/pubmed/25031512.
12. Calligaro KD, Balraj P, Moudgill N, Rao A, Dougherty MJ, Eisenberg J. Results of polytetrafluoroethylene-covered nitinol stents crossing the inguinal ligament. *J Vasc Surg.* 2013;57(2):421–426. https://doi.org/10.1016/j.jvs.2012.05.112.
13. Thalhammer C, Kirchherr AS, Uhlich F, Waigand J, Gross CM. Postcatheterization pseudoaneurysms and arteriovenous fistulas: repair with Percutaneous implantation of endovascular covered stents. *Radiology.* 2000;214(1):127–131. https://doi.org/10.1148/radiology.214.1.r00ja04127.
14. Lai SH, Fenlon J, Roush BB, et al. Analysis of the retrograde tibial artery approach in lower extremity revascularization in an office endovascular center. *J Vasc Surg.* February 2019. https://doi.org/10.1016/j.jvs.2018.10.114.
15. Sato K, Orihashi K, Hamanaka Y, Hirai S, Mitsui N, Chatani N. Treatment of iliac artery rupture during percutaneous transluminal angioplasty: a report of three cases. *Hiroshima J Med Sci.* 2011;60(4):83–86. http://www.ncbi.nlm.nih.gov/pubmed/22389952.
16. Siablis D, Karnabatidis D, Katsanos K, Ravazoula P, Kraniotis P, Kagadis GC. Outflow protection filters during percutaneous recanalization of lower extremities' arterial occlusions: a pilot study. *Eur J Radiol.* 2005;55(2):243–249. https://doi.org/10.1016/j.ejrad.2004.07.010.
17. Jain K, Munn J, Rummel M, Johnston D, Longton C. VS6. Percutaneous thrombectomy of a dialysis graft in the office setting. *J Vasc Surg.* 2012;55(6):28S. https://doi.org/10.1016/j.jvs.2012.03.092.
18. Starnes BW, O'Donnell SD, Gillespie DL, et al. Percutaneous arterial closure in peripheral vascular disease: a prospective randomized evaluation of the Perclose device. *J Vasc Surg.* 2003;38(2):263–271. http://www.ncbi.nlm.nih.gov/pubmed/12891107.
19. Abreo K, Sequeira A. Role of stents in hemodialysis vascular access. *J Vasc Access.* 2018;19(4):341–345. https://doi.org/10.1177/1129729818761280.
20. Taylor JD, Lehmann ED, Belli A-M, et al. Strategies for the management of SVC stent migration into the right atrium. *Cardiovasc Intervent Radiol.* 2007;30(5):1003–1009. https://doi.org/10.1007/s00270-007-9109-3.
21. Mullens W, De Keyser J, Van Dorpe A, et al. Migration of two venous stents into the right ventricle in a patient with May–Thurner syndrome. *Int J Cardiol.* 2006;110(1):114–115. https://doi.org/10.1016/j.ijcard.2005.05.070.
22. VanderVeen NT, Friedman J, Rummel M, et al. PC190. Improving the retrieval rate of inferior vena cava filters: impact of inferior vena cava filter retrieval in the office endovascular center. *J Vasc Surg.* 2018. https://doi.org/10.1016/j.jvs.2018.03.339.
23. Jain KM, Munn J, Rummel M, Vaddineni S, Longton C. Future of vascular surgery is in the office. *J Vasc Surg.* 2010. https://doi.org/10.1016/j.jvs.2009.09.056.

CHAPTER 15

Radiation Safety and Ultrasound-Guided Procedures

JESSE CHAIT, BS • ALBERT PAVALONIS, DO • ADBELHAMID ELFAHAM, PHD • ENRICO ASCHER, MD, FACS

GENERAL RADIATION SAFETY FOR THE OEC

Introduction

Fluoroscopic-guided interventions have revolutionized the modern management of vascular disease. Regardless of the procedure or target anatomy, imaging is required to safely and effectively perform both simple and complex endovascular interventions. With the inevitable shift of vascular disease management from open surgery to minimally invasive, endovascular procedures, the minimization of harmful radiation exposure has become of paramount concern for both patients and providers[1,2].

To best understand the ways in which operators can reduce radiation exposure, we must first discuss radiation safety in the OEC. As rigorously practiced in the inpatient setting, the paradigm of time, distance, and shielding remain true for office-based labs. Furthermore, the mantra of "as low as reasonable achievable"—or ALARA—should be adhered to in all settings where ionizing radiation is utilized. ALARA can be successfully practiced through a variety of adjunctive techniques, including liberal use of duplex ultrasound guidance, utilization of intravascular ultrasound (IVUS),[3] as well as conservative use of fluoroscopy during endovascular procedures. While designing an OEC and evaluating the purchase of capital equipment, one of the parameters that should be taken into account when acquiring a C-arm is radiation safety. Some C-arms are designed to decrease radiation exposure to the patient and the operating team, and these products should be selected over those without such safety capabilities.

Reduction of Radiation Exposure to Patient and Staff

In our practice, we strive to minimize exposure to ionizing radiation. Although some local health departments do not require it, procedure rooms should be designed with lead-lined walls to protect the rest of the office from scattered radiation. The key to successful adherence to the ALARA principle is efficiency in the procedural area, and we believe the OEC is an ideal environment for this practice, as it is not always possible in the hospital operating room, radiology suite, or catheterization laboratory. Some best practices include:

1. Consistency of the procedural team throughout the day
2. Clear familiarity of roles and responsibilities before each case
3. Accessibility of all necessary equipment within the operating suite
4. Defined procedural goals prior to the start of every case

The relationship of distance to source of ionizing radiation is important for both procedural and nonprocedural staff in an OEC. Considerations that we find important to reduce radiation exposure to the patient and staff are:

1. Use pulse mode instead of continuous fluoroscopy. Our practice is to use 8 pulse per second (8PPS). Dose reduction to the patient using 8PPS is about 50% without compromising image quality. Reduction of patient dose by about 50% will also reduce exposure to staff from scattered radiation.
2. Avoid using fluoroscopic magnification mode because it increases radiation dose to patient and staff. For example, the radiation for the entrance skin dose is 100 μGy/min for normal 30.38 cm (12″) image, the entrance skin dose will increase to 235 μGy/min if mag 1 is used, and it will increase to 440 μGy if mag 2 is used.
3. Keep the image intensifier as close as possible to the patient, which reduces entrance skin exposure to patient and scattered radiation to staff.
4. Keep the X-ray tube as far as possible from patient to avoid skin injury.
5. Collimation of X-ray beam to the area of clinical interest which reduces radiation dose to patient and scatter radiation to staff while improving image quality.

Office-Based Endovascular Centers. https://doi.org/10.1016/B978-0-323-67969-5.00015-0
Copyright © 2020 Elsevier Inc. All rights reserved.

6. Use of catheters with radiopaque tips.
7. Annual testing of the fluoroscopic unit by a consultant medical physicist to insure compliance with health and safety regulations.

Protection of Radiation Workers from Scattered Radiation

1. Monitored egress to the procedural area
2. Clear signage regarding use of ionizing radiation
3. Annual mandatory radiation safety in-service on ionizing radiation safety for all procedural staff provide by a consultant medical physicist
4. Communication with nonprocedural staff conducted though hands-free devices
5. Shielding of the procedural staff is of utmost importance, as we consider our employees to be our best assets. The proceduralist should strive to reduce radiation exposure by all available means. Proper shielding and protection for the staff is achieved through a variety of methods:
   1. All personnel within the lab are required to use the following shielding equipment:
      a. Two-piece wraparound lead apron (0.5 mm lead equivalent)
      b. Thyroid shield
      c. Radiation glasses
      d. Lead-lined hats
      e. Lead-lined gloves for the physician and scrub technician

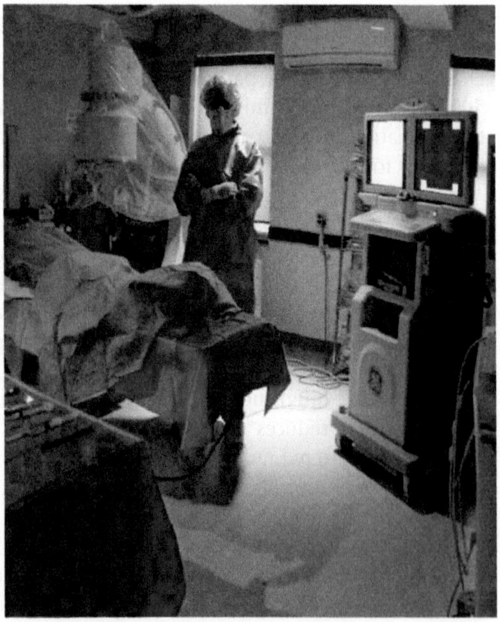

OEC Surgeon with full shielding

   2. Annual inspection of all personnel radiation protective equipment.
   3. Radiation badges for all procedural staff that are monitored and reviewed monthly by the radiation safety officer. The physician may also be doing procedures in the hospital. The dose received by the physician should be calculated by adding the dose from two badges.

The concern with radiation exposure provides a nice transition into the next section where the discussion will focus on several techniques that eliminated the need for radiation and require few procedural modifications.

TRANSCUTANEOUS ULTRASOUND-GUIDED PROCEDURES

Introduction

The OEC offers a great advantage in the delivery of endovascular therapy. Advancements in endovascular technique have given rise to increased utilization of ultrasound guidance to limit or eliminate the use of contrast and ionizing radiation. Our lab routinely uses both transcutaneous and intravascular ultrasonography to perform interventions, especially in patients who suffer from contrast allergy or impaired renal function. To be able to perform these procedures, it is important to have a good ultrasound machine and a well-trained ultrasound technician. While using IVUS, the operator should be familiar with interpretation of intravascular images. Techniques that are commonly performed under ultrasound guidance, with limited or no fluoroscopy, include vascular access, arteriovenous fistula maturation, infrainguinal angioplasty, inferior vena cava filter (IVCF) placement, pseudoaneurysm injection, iliac vein stenting, and endovenous thermal ablation. The aim of this section is to discuss utilization technique in regards to transcutaneous ultrasound guidance.

Ultrasound-Guided Access

Access site complications are especially problematic in the outpatient setting and can result in severe injury or death. As multiple systematic reviews and meta-analyses have confirmed that ultrasound guidance increases initial success rate and reduces the complications associated with both arterial and venous catheterization,[4–7] we believe palpatory or landmark-guided percutaneous vascular access is needlessly dangerous. Our group advocates the utilization of ultrasound-guided venous and arterial access in all

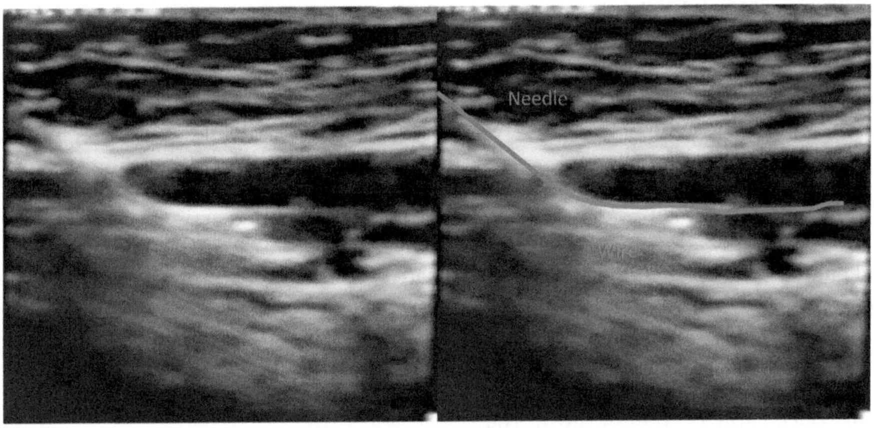

Ultrasound Guided Access

percutaneous access situations. Besides proven superiority in terms of first-attempt success and reduction in complications, further advantages of ultrasound guidance include:

1. Safe and efficacious vessel puncture away from areas of severe calcification or stenosis.
2. Allowance for real-time inspection following sheath removal for early detection of access site complications in the setting of absent external hemorrhage.

Additionally, we have modified this procedure to include periadventitial injection of local anesthetic. In general practice, local anesthetic for percutaneous access involves injection of a small volume into the subcutaneous space. Our periadventitial injection technique involves injection of local anesthetic under ultrasound guidance. A favorable spot, as defined as a noncalcified vessel segment with an adequately sized lumen for initial cannulation, is first identified and then a 50/50

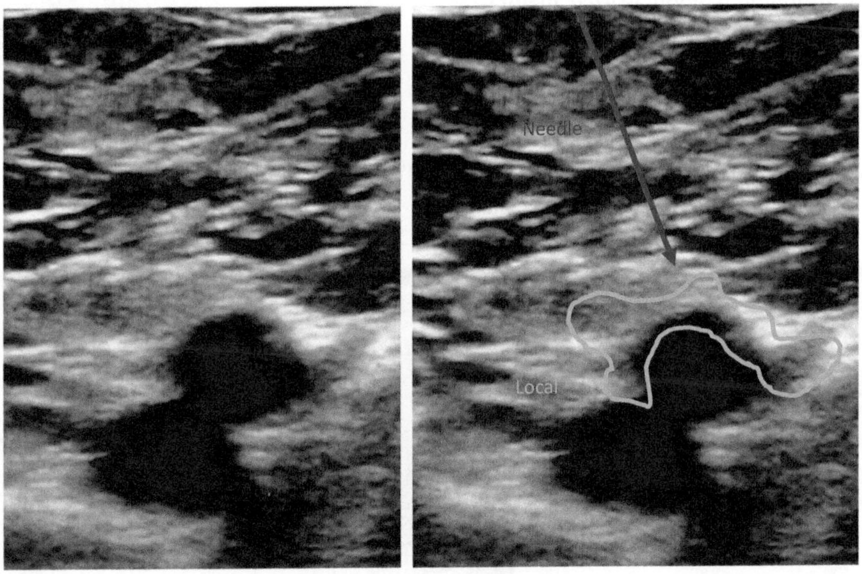

Periadventitial Injection

mixture of 0.25% Marcaine/1% lidocaine is infiltrated in the tissue just above the adventitial layer. In our experience, the addition of this technique significantly reduces discomfort during sheath manipulation and requires less procedural sedation, allowing for faster recovery time and discharge.

Ultrasound-Guided Arteriovenous Fistuloplasty

Use of ultrasound guidance for interventions involving arteriovenous fistulae is advantageous. The benefits are several: no contrast or radiation is required, the stenotic fistula segment can be treated without additional equipment, and the response to treatment can be immediately assessed with calculation of volume flow. The preoperative fistula sonogram provides valuable information regarding the etiology of the underlying culprit lesion. We utilize a linear ultrasound probe to access the fistula in retrograde fashion after determining the location of the most proximal stenosis.[8] Advancement of an access sheath and wire with negotiation of stenotic areas is easily performed under ultrasound guidance. Fistuloplasty is performed with the benefit of direct visualization, and standard or cutting balloons can be used without problem. During the procedure, pre- and post-intervention peak systolic velocities as well as volume flow are measured to monitor treatment response. This technique has been successfully applied by our group in multiple situations involving arteriovenous fistulae and grafts, including balloon-assisted maturation,[8] management of failing access,[9] and treatment of acute occlusive lesions.[10]

Ultrasound-Guided Infrainguinal Arterial Interventions

The treatment of infrainguinal arterial disease is the most common arterial procedure performed in the OEC. Our lab alone has seen arterial patient volume increase by over 200% in the past 3 years. With that volume increase, patients with renal insufficiency and contrast-sensitive patients are more routinely encountered. Almost all patients who receive infrainguinal arterial interventions undergo contrast angiography, but when the use of contrast is contraindicated or can be avoided, ultrasound-assisted arterial intervention is proven to be an excellent alternative. Our group has had success with ultrasound-guided management of both native vessel disease using angioplasty,[11] as well as endovascular treatment of failing bypass grafts.[12]

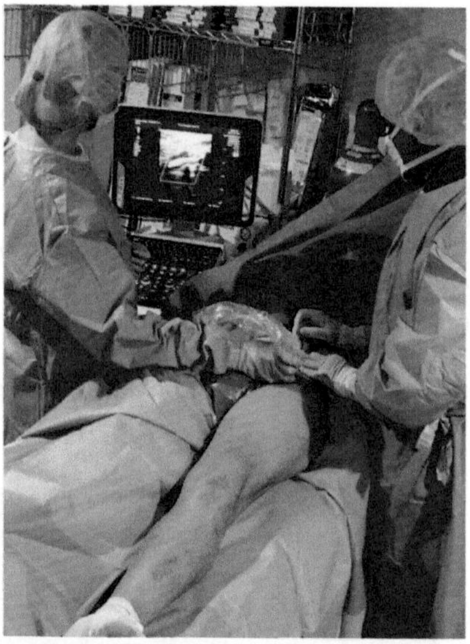

Procedural configuration for US guided infrainguinal intervention

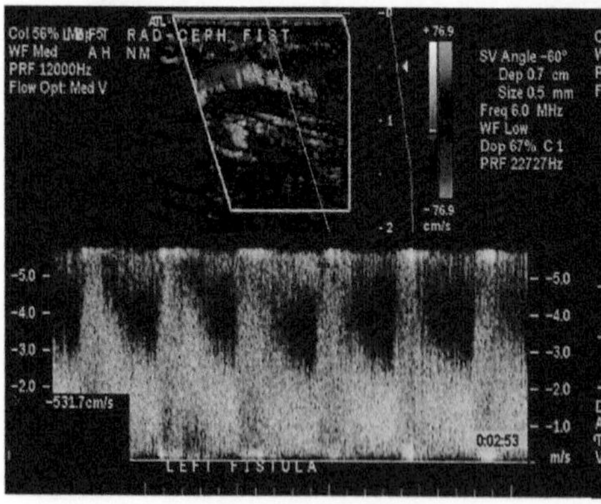

Pre-Balloon Angioplasty

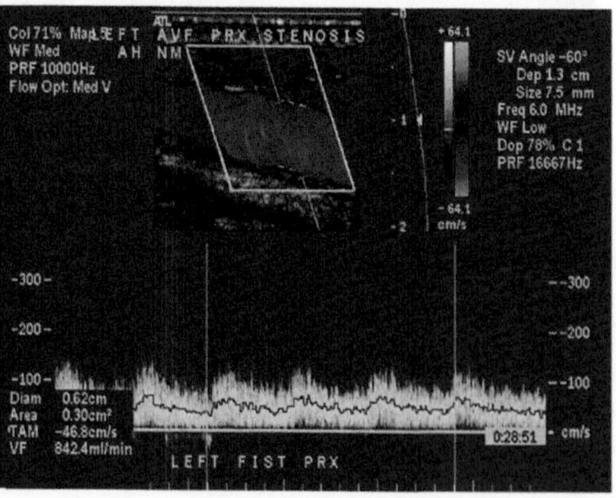

Post-Balloon Angioplasty

The planning for such a case starts with high-quality diagnostic ultrasonography involving aortobiiliac and infrainguinal arterial studies. This diagnostic preplanning is important when determining access site and identifying the location of hemodynamically significant lesions. The entire target extremity should be draped and prepared in sterile fashion to allow for the sonographer to fully participate in the intervention. If contralateral common femoral access is desired, the brief use of fluoroscopic guidance without contrast may be required to negotiate the aortic bifurcation. If an ipsilateral approach is preferred or deemed more clinically appropriate, fluoroscopic guidance can be eliminated completely. A standard 0.035 wire is easily seen and followed with a linear ultrasound probe. If difficulty is encountered with crossing a lesion, standard guiding catheters may be utilized. Again, no special preparation of angioplasty balloon is required, as most balloons are well visualized on ultrasound. With ultrasound guidance, subintimal dissection can be performed with better appreciation of local arterial anatomy as compared to fluoroscopic imaging. When the target lesion is crossed with a wire, balloon angioplasty and stenting can be safely performed under direct ultrasound visualization. Once a lesion has been treated, immediate quantitative and qualitative results can be realized and documented

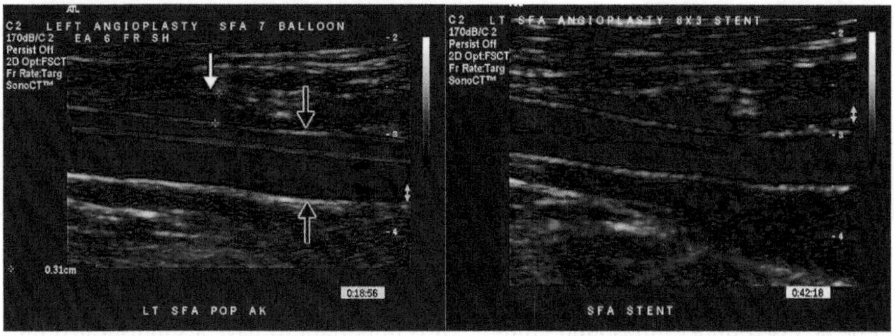

Ultrasound-Guided SFA Balloon Angioplasty

Ultrasound-Guided SFA Stenting

Ultrasound guidance has also been used, with success, in the infrapopliteal arteries. Treating lesions in the tibial vessels via common femoral access is without much added difficulty. Greater than 90% technical success has been achieved with this modality.[13] With the wide acceptance and use of pedal access, sonographic guidance can again be employed in a similar but retrograde fashion and without added cost or equipment.

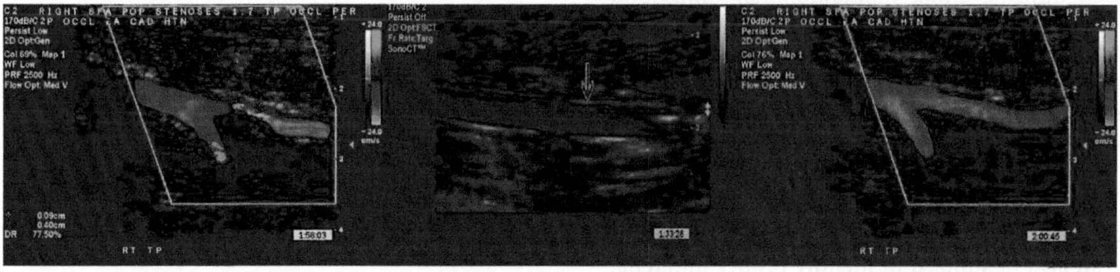

Severe stenosis of the proximal tibioperoneal trunk

Angioplasty under ultrasound guidance

Post-intervention result

In addition to treatment of atherosclerotic lesions, ultrasound-assistance can also be utilized for the treatment of popliteal artery aneurysms. The approach and patient setup is similar to other infrainguinal procedures. The advantage of deploying a stent graft under ultrasound guidance is that the proximal and distal landing zones are visualized in real time. Additionally, after stent graft deployment, the sonographer can detect any early endoleaks (typically IA/B or II), which can be addressed immediately. With type II endoleaks, the

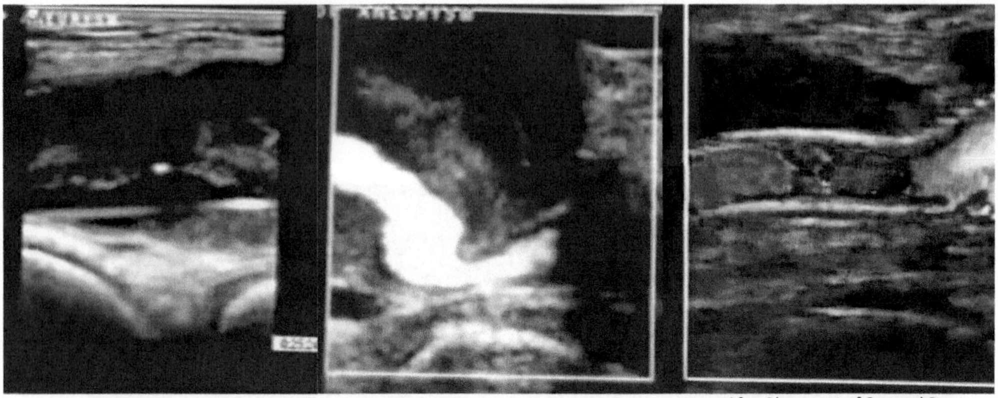

Wire Traversing Aneurysm Extent of Thrombosed Aneurysm Sac After Placement of Covered Stent Without Evidence of Endoleak

aneurysm sac can be accessed under ultrasound guidance and treated using coil embolization.

Ultrasound-Guided Inferior Vena Cava Filter Placement

Office-based considerations, techniques, complications, and retrieval strategies for IVCFs are covered extensively in Chapter 33. This section will briefly focus on ultrasound-guided placement of IVCFs, as patient referral to the OEC for acute deep venous thrombosis is not uncommon in our practice. In patients with contraindication to contrast use, the procedure can be modified utilizing either transabdominal ultrasound (TAUS) or IVUS. Initial ultrasound-guided access can be safely obtained via the jugular or femoral vein. Fluoroscopy is used to monitor guidewire advancement through the IVC to minimize the potential of inadvertent wire perforation. At this point, the sonographer identifies the junction of the inferior vena cava and right renal vein, measures inferior vena cava diameter, allowing for the operator to select a properly sized filter.[14] IVUS can also be utilized to identify proper infrarenal filter placement.[15,16] The delivery sheath can be positioned and the filter deployed below the renal veins. Postdeployment, the sonographer can identify and record the location and potential angulation of the filter.

It should be the goal of OEC operators to minimize radiation exposure to the patient as well as the operating team. All precautions should be taken to minimize radiation exposure. Judicious use of transcutaneous ultrasound and IVUS can minimize the radiation exposure.[3] Patients with compromised renal function and patients with contrast allergy are particularly suited for ultrasound-guided intervention. It is important to have a sophisticated ultrasound machine and highly trained ultrasound technician.

REFERENCES

1. Hegedus F, Mathew LM, Schwartz RA. Radiation dermatitis: an overview. *Int J Dermatol.* 2016;56(9):909–914.
2. Albert JM. Radiation risk from CT: implications for cancer screening. *Am J Roentgenol.* 2013;201(1):W81–W87.
3. Chait J, Davis N, Ostrozhynskyy Y, et al. Radiation exposure during non-thrombotic iliac vein stenting. *Vascular.* 2019 (Epub ahead of print).
4. Brass P, Hellmich M, Kolodziej L, Schick G, Smith AF. Ultrasound guidance versus anatomical landmarks for subclavian or femoral vein catheterization. *Cochrane Database Syst Rev.* 2015.
5. Brass P, Hellmich M, Kolodziej L, Schick G, Smith AF. Ultrasound guidance versus anatomical landmarks for internal jugular vein catheterization. *Cochrane Database Syst Rev.* 2015.
6. Sobolev M, Slovut DP, Lee Chang AL, Shiloh A, Eisen L. Ultrasound-guided catheterization of the femoral artery: a systematic review and meta-analysis of randomized controlled trials. *J Invasive Cardiol.* 2015;27(7):318–323.
7. Bhattacharjee S, Maitra S, Baidya DK. Comparison between ultrasound guided technique and digital palpation technique for radial artery cannulation in adult patients: an updated meta-analysis of randomized controlled trials. *J Clin Anesth.* 2018;47:54–59.
8. Alsheekh A, Hingorani A, Aurshina A, et al. Early results of duplex guided trans-radial artery fistuloplasties. *Ann Vasc Surg.* 2019;60:178–181.
9. Ascher E, Hingorani A, Marks N. Duplex-guided balloon angioplasty of failing or nonmaturing arteriovenous fistulae for hemodialysis: a new office-based procedure. *J Vasc Surg.* 2009;50(3):594–599.

10. Aurshina A, Ascher E, Hingorani A, Marks N. A novel technique for duplex-guided office-based interventions for patients with acute arteriovenous fistula occlusion. *J Vasc Surg*. 2018;67(3):857–859.
11. Ascher E, Hingorani A, Marks N. Duplex-guided balloon angioplasty of lower extremity arteries. *Perspect Vasc Surg Endovasc Ther*. 2007;19(1):23–31.
12. Marks N, Hingorani A, Ascher E. Duplex guided balloon angioplasty of failing infrainguinal bypass grafts. *Eur J Vasc Endovasc Surg*. 2006;32(2):176–181.
13. Ascher E, Marks N, Hingorani A, Schutzer R, Nahata S. Duplex-guided balloon angioplasty and subintimal dissection of infrapopliteal arteries: early results with a new approach to avoid radiation exposure and contrast material. *J Vasc Surg*. 2005;42(6):1114–1121.
14. Qin X, Lu C, Ren P, et al. New method for ultrasound-guided inferior vena cava filter placement. *J Vasc Surg*. 2018;6(4):450–456.
15. Gunn AJ, Iqbal SI, Kalva SP, et al. Intravascular ultrasound-guided inferior vena cava filter placement using a single-puncture technique in 99 patients. *Vasc Endovasc Surg*. 2013;47(2):97–101.
16. Passman MA, Dattilo JB, Guzman RJ, Naslund TC. Bedside placement of inferior vena cava filters by using transabdominal duplex ultrasonography and intravascular ultrasound imaging. *J Vasc Surg*. 2005;42(5):1027–1032.

CHAPTER 16

The Role of IVUS in Arterial and Venous Procedures in the Office-Based Laboratory

PAUL J. GAGNE, MD • JON BOWMAN, MD • TARAS KUCHER, MD

The standard of care for patients with peripheral vascular disease (PVD) is unaffected by the venue where care is provided. We approach the care of our patients with PVD, and especially interventions for advanced PVD, in the same way whether the procedure is performed in the traditional setting of a hospital or in our office endovascular center (OEC). The safety and quality of the procedure is uncompromised. We have found patient satisfaction is typically higher after care in the OEC compared with the hospital. The hospital is an environment that patients, especially older patients, find overwhelming.

High-quality transcutaneous duplex ultrasound imaging has been an essential part of the office-based practice of vascular surgeons and interventionalists for decades. Extending this practice of excellence in vascular imaging in the OEC is logical (Fig. 16.1). As vascular interventionalists, we depend upon quality imaging to consistently achieve successful revascularization with endovascular procedures when treating peripheral artery occlusive disease (PAD), chronic deep venous occlusive disease (CVD), and failing arteriovenous (AV) access in hemodialysis patients. Appropriate imaging is critical to reproducibly achieving good clinical outcomes.

In the last decade, significant interest has grown in the use of intravascular ultrasound (IVUS) to supplement, and in some instances, largely replace the imaging information gained from traditional angiography. The benefits of IVUS in improving the imaging of diseased vessels have been well reported.[1–5] Using IVUS for evaluating limbs for PVD frequently results in the identification of lesions that otherwise would require multiview contrast angiography to identify. IVUS therefore often lowers radiation exposure and intravenous contrast volume[6] for patients. The use of IVUS and the pathology identified is different for treating patients with PAD, CVD, or AV access.

IVUS AND LOWER EXTREMITY PERIPHERAL ARTERY OCCLUSIVE DISEASE

IVUS allows accurate measurement of an artery's diameter to properly size the balloon and stent required for treatment. IVUS, compared with arteriography, is also more exact in identifying the extent and severity of significant arterial occlusive disease requiring treatment. IVUS is able to characterize the composition of an atherosclerotic plaque and more specifically, the extent of calcium in the artery wall. For example, circumferential calcification in the arterial wall would require a different endovascular approach and vessel preparation with atherectomy as compared with an artery with sparse arterial wall calcification. Postintervention, IVUS can identify not only if an arterial dissection is present but also the significance of the dissection (Fig. 16.2A and B) and whether further treatment requiring a stent placement, is necessary.

PAD AND IVUS CLINICAL DATA

The benefits of IVUS for decreasing radiation exposure to a patient and the medical staff during an involved and lengthy lower extremity intervention are obvious (Chapter 15). For retroperitoneal procedures involving the aorta or iliac arteries, where radiation dose increases due to the depth of the arteries, the decrease in radiation exposure through the use of IVUS is compounded. We can complete the procedure by only performing a diagnostic and completion angiogram. Multiple view angiograms to determine the presence or severity of a stenosis

Office-Based Endovascular Centers. https://doi.org/10.1016/B978-0-323-67969-5.00016-2
Copyright © 2020 Elsevier Inc. All rights reserved.

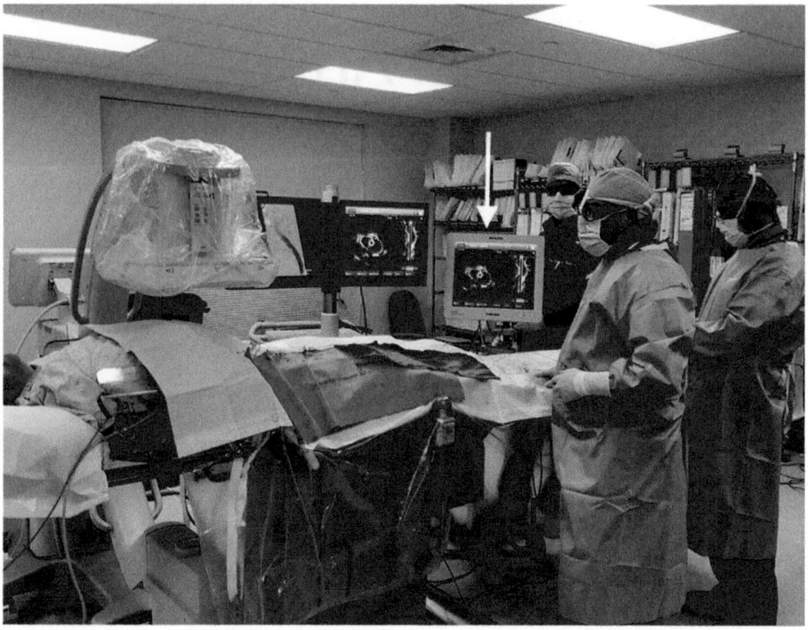

FIG. 16.1 Office-based laboratory setup with intravascular ultrasound.

are unnecessary since IVUS provides a multidimensional view.

What has been less obvious in the past is the improved clinical outcomes that IVUS helps achieve in treating symptomatic PAD. Several studies have shown the importance of accurate artery sizing for successful long-term endovascular revascularization and clinical improvement. The VIPER trial, a multicenter US trial, showed that oversizing a superficial femoral artery (SFA) stent greater than 20% compared with the artery diameter decreased stent primary patency from 88% at 1 year to 70% ($P < .05$). This study observed that oversizing was largely attributed to the interventionalist overestimating the diameter of the artery. Quantitative imaging techniques such as IVUS allow accurate artery sizing that enables proper stent sizing and improved patency.[7] In the Superb Trial, PTA was compared with PTA plus stenting with the

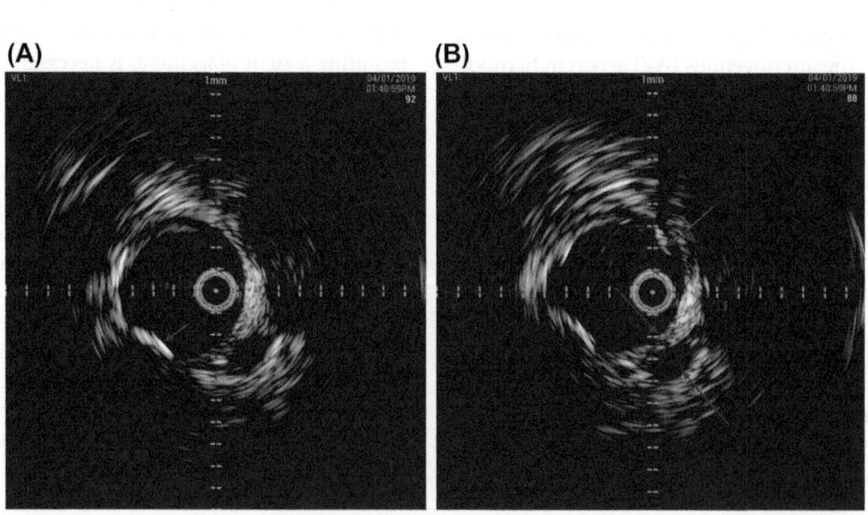

FIG. 16.2 **(A)** Mildly stenosed artery with peripheral artery disease; **(B)** Post-PTA dissection.

Supera stent (Abbott, North Chicago, IL) for PAD in the SFA and proximal popliteal artery. The Supera stent is designed to match the artery size. It is not to be oversized more than 1 mm compared with the artery. In this study, primary patency was 90.5% when the stent was sized appropriate to the vessel. Primary patency dropped to 57.7% ($P < .026$) when the stent was oversized leading to elongation. Quantitative IVUS imaging provides precise arterial diameter measurement for proper stent sizing.[8] Lida et al.[9] reviewed their experience with endovascular interventions in 1198 limbs with TASC IIA-C femoral popliteal lesions. IVUS was used in 22% (n = 268) of the procedures. IVUS was used in cases with more severe TASC II class, longer lesion length, and smaller reference vessel diameter. They analyzed 234 propensity score-matched pairs at a mean follow-up of 1.9 + 1.5 years for IVUS versus no IVUS use. Primary patency ($P < .001$), assisted primary patency ($P < .001$), and freedom from reintervention ($P < .001$), all were significantly improved in the group where quantitative imaging with IVUS was used. At 1 year, primary patency improved by 18%. Though this is a retrospective study, the findings suggest a favorable impact from the use of IVUS in infrainguinal PAD endovascular procedures.

IVUS PROTOCOL FOR DIAGNOSING PERIPHERAL ARTERY OCCLUSIVE DISEASE

When performing endovascular interventions for lower extremity PAD, the access vessel and procedure are as per standard technique for these procedures, using contralateral or ipsilateral common femoral artery approach. We also use pedal access and radial access. The initial imaging is performed using arteriography to identify overall disease distribution and visualize the runoff vessels.

Based on the clinical indication (i.e., claudication, rest pain, nonhealing ischemic wound), we proceed with intervention as per standard technique. In the OEC, we perform all appropriate interventions available for treating PAD. This includes atherectomy, percutaneous transluminal angioplasty (PTA), and stenting. Paclitaxel drug-coated technologies, both paclitaxel-coated stents (DCS) and balloons (DCB) are used as appropriate. We use IVUS before and after atherectomy and usually prior to other interventions. The use of IVUS to help guide the type of atherectomy device and monitor the amount of plaque debulking appears to improve clinical outcomes.[10] IVUS is used to properly size a balloon or stent based on the artery diameter rather than the lumen diameter. Several authors have reported that angiography underestimates artery size in as many as 40% of cases compared with IVUS.[11,12]

Additionally, we use IVUS to evaluate the artery post-PTA or atherectomy to assess both for a significant dissection (Fig. 16.2A and B) and the length of disease to be treated with a stent or DCB when necessary. Stenting should be performed from normal artery to normal artery completely covering the diseased segment. Whether adequate lumen gain has been achieved is also assessed using IVUS after interventions, since lumen size can impact patency and clinical outcome.[13]

Use of IVUS has also been reported to aid in "true lumen" reentry when crossing chronic total arterial occlusions. In a study, the addition of IVUS was associated with both expedited crossing of the chronic total occlusion and higher technical success for revascularization. No IVUS-related complications were reported.[13]

The IVUS catheter we use is either a Visions PV 0.018p, 0.014P, or 0.014P RX (Royal Phillips, Netherlands) catheter depending upon the working wire being used for the intervention. We use the 0.014 IVUS catheters most frequently. This can be used through a 5 or 6 Fr sheath.

In patients with chronic renal insufficiency, we use IVUS to limit the amount of contrast we use during endovascular interventions for treating lower extremity PAD. We also use IVUS in conjunction with CO_2 angiography for some of these procedures. In these instances, the CO_2 angiogram is the "road map" for proper wire and device placement and location, and IVUS is used before any intervention to diagnose and characterize the degree of stenosis and character of the plaque.

IVUS AND LOWER EXTREMITY CHRONIC DEEP VEIN OCCLUSIVE DISEASE

For decades, venography has been the gold standard for imaging the pelvic veins and diagnosing iliac and common femoral vein occlusive disease (IFVOD). There was not any other dynamic imaging technique available for the deep venous system that was suitable for use during interventions. However, prior work has questioned whether venography is adequately sensitive for diagnosing different types of venous lesions.[14] Patients with severely symptomatic chronic lower extremity venous insufficiency (CVI) CEAP (clinical, etiology, anatomy, pathophysiology) 4 to 6 clinical classification of venous disease[15] often suffer from nonthrombotic compression of the iliac veins. These lesions are often misdiagnosed with multiplanar venography; however, when these lesions are identified using IVUS and treated with stents, the treatment commonly results in clinical improvement. This clinical response in patients emphasizes the flow limiting significance of these lesions.

In 2002, Raju and Neglen[16] published their experience combining single plane venography and IVUS to diagnose IFVOD. They noted that IVUS visualized significant iliac vein and common femoral vein (CFV) stenosis due to extrinsic compression not detected with venography. They also noted that many patients had postthrombotic scar and damage from prior acute DVT that was not diagnosed with venography but was identified using IVUS. They concluded that IVUS imaging was necessary for both diagnosing and guiding endovascular interventions for IFVOD in patients with clinically advanced chronic venous hypertension. Gagne et al.[17] have reported on the results of the VIDIO (venography vs. IVUS for diagnosing iliofemoral vein occlusive disease) study for patients with CEAP 4–6 chronic venous disease. This prospective, multicenter study showed that IVUS was more sensitive in identifying significant IFVOD than multiplanar venogram ($P < .05$) and in 57% of the CEAP 4–6 patients examined, IVUS changed the treatment recommendation. Furthermore, when IVUS identified "significant" IFVOD and patients were treated with stents, their chronic venous disease (i.e., CEAP 4–6) improved. This same cohort of patients with significant stenosis identified by multiplanar venograms, when treated with stents, did not reliably improve in any statistically significant way. The conclusion from this post hoc analysis of the VIDIO data is that IVUS diagnosed IFVOD in CEAP 4–6 patients, when treated with stenting, better predicts subsequent clinical improvement than IFVOD diagnosed with multiplanar venogram.[18] This published clinical data have resulted in expanding interest in using IVUS for both identifying symptomatic CVI patients and guiding treatment of patients with severe symptomatic chronic IFVOD.

We use IVUS to evaluate patients for IFVOD only when they present with severe (i.e., clinical CEAP 3–6) lower extremity chronic venous hypertension. We have found that the details of the history, physical exam, and infrainguinal venous duplex exam identify patients who may benefit from IVUS evaluation for IFVOD. When the physical findings of chronic venous hypertension seen while examining the leg are not explained by the degree of deep and superficial reflux or deep vein occlusive disease identified on infrainguinal duplex ultrasound (DUS), we suspect IFVOD and proceed accordingly.

Patients who have limb edema alone (clinical CEAP 3), without symptoms of heaviness or venous claudication, may have IVUS-identified IFVOD due to compression. Unfortunately, treatment of these stenoses with stents will result in clinical improvement in only half the patients treated. Our clinical experience has led us to limit our evaluation and intervention in these CEAP 3 patients. We follow them, and if their symptoms persist or worsen then we consider IVUS evaluation for IFVOD. We have found that these patients often do not exhibit a clinical picture of progressive deterioration from venous hypertension. When there is a combination of physical finding of edema, with recurrent symptoms of limb heaviness, pain, venous claudication, or skin damage such as hyperpigmentation or hyperemia, evaluation with IVUS and appropriate intervention of IFVOD can lead to satisfying clinical improvement.

IVUS PROTOCOL FOR DIAGNOSING CHRONIC DEEP VEIN OCCLUSIVE DISEASE

The popliteal vein is our preferred access site when evaluating and treating IFVOD. Ultrasound-guided cannulation is simplified in most patients, given the superficial course of the popliteal vein compared to the femoral vein in the midthigh. This access is also excellent for executing diagnostic imaging and any intervention in the iliac and CFV segments. Some patients are not suitable for the prone position required for popliteal vein access, especially when using intravenous conscious sedation. Our experience has shown that patients with obesity, back problems, COPD, and sleep apnea are often not candidates for this approach. These patients are then imaged and treated in the supine position, either through the midthigh femoral vein or the internal jugular vein.

The midthigh femoral vein access can present several challenges. When cannulating the femoral vein, a "window" around the superficial femoral artery to introduce the needle and sheath into the adjacent vein must be identified to avoid arterial trauma. This often requires changing the angle of transcutaneous insonation, to guide the entry point and course of the needle from simple medial thigh imaging. Patients with "large" thighs present equipment and technical challenges. Echogenic access needles and micropuncture sheaths for DUS-guided venous access can be "short" due to the depth of the femoral vein from the skin. To minimize the distance from the skin to the vessel and compensate for the finite length of the access needle and sheath a more perpendicular cannulation angle to the vein in "large" thighs might be utilized to gain vascular access. This acute angle can then lead to subsequent "kinking" of the working sheath if the sheath is "soft," interfering with the planned endovascular procedure. Also, we often access the femoral vein more cranially in the "large" thigh because of the limited visibility and needle length for more distal thigh access. Since we wish to maintain sheath access to the entire CFV in case stenting is indicated, the length of the FV visible and accessible for cannulation is often limited. If the access site is cranial to the lesser trochanter of the femur, it is likely that you will be unable to fully image and treat any CFV occlusive disease identified through that access. Finally, our protocol for access site management at the end of our deep vein interventions is to compress our access site for 15 min after sheath removal and then place a compression bandage for 2 h. We do not reverse anticoagulation which is therapeutic during the procedure. Femoral vein access in large thighs has been associated with more ecchymoses and hematomas than popliteal vein or internal jugular vein access. We believe the superficial thigh muscles interfere with effective compression when the femoral vein is "deep."

The internal jugular vein (IJV) is an effective access site for bilateral IVUS imaging of the iliac and CFVs. Postprocedure access site compression is almost unnecessary in most patients once the patient assumes the sitting position. We have found that intervening on the iliofemoral veins with IJV access is sometimes difficult. Crossing occluded or severely scarred iliac veins can be challenging from the IJV. The maneuverability and "pushability" of wires and catheters is diminished in the relatively large IVC due to bowing. Even with long working sheaths this loss of technical advantage is not fully recovered. However, crossing from the IJV is sometimes the only way to successfully cannulate and treat long segment IFVOD. One advantage of the IJV access is the ability to cannulate both the femoral and the deep femoral veins (DFVs) with the IVUS catheter and determine if there is significant, flow limiting occlusive disease in these critical inflow vessels. This can be valuable information in determining if post-stenting there will be adequate flow into iliac and CFV segments previously occluded by postthrombotic scar or acute DVT.

We routinely use the Philips-Volcano PV .035 IVUS catheter (Royal Phillips, Netherlands), placed through an 8 Fr sheath, and image from the renal veins to the DFV, which is usually found at the level of the lesser trochanter of the femur. This IVUS system has a 60 mm field of view necessary to image the large diameter deep veins of the pelvis and groin. The smaller fields of view (<24 mm) associated with Volcano's 6 or 5 Fr catheter systems (i.e., PV 0.014 or PV 0.018) are inadequate for visualizing the entire diameter of the iliac veins due to wire bias as the catheter tracks through the pelvis.

Following cannulation, wire access is gained from the FV to the IVC, using a relatively soft wire, like a 0.35 Bentson wire, to perform IVUS imaging. This limits distortion of the venous structures during the IVUS "pull-back" that can occur with stiff wires (e.g., Amplatz wires). Sometimes, the wire is pulled out of the IVUS catheter tip before imaging the veins to better center the catheter in the lumen if the field of view is limited or if it appears that the wire/catheter bias in the tortuous veins of the pelvis is causing distortion and an artifactual stenosis. This is a helpful technique in some patients.

A comprehensive IVUS study for IFVOD in symptomatic CVI patients should evaluate the pararenal IVC, the infrarenal IVC, the CIV, the EIV, and the CFV. Arterial landmarks identified with IVUS help to confirm the corresponding vein segments, especially when the vein pathology is severe and diffuse due to postthrombotic scar. Such arterial landmarks include the left renal artery crossing the IVC, the bifurcation of the aorta, the bifurcation of the common iliac artery, and the bifurcation of the common femoral artery. During the pullback of the IVUS catheter through the various vein segments, the orientation of the arteries to the corresponding vein segments can be variable in the image. The physician must be familiar with the relation of the veins and arteries even when not anatomically oriented.

During IVUS imaging of the IVC, we evaluate the vein for phasic changes with deep breathes. When the IVC is distended and phasic changes are absent, a diagnosis of congestive heart failure or other systemic condition resulting in general fluid overload is evident. The aorta bifurcates at or sometimes cranial to the CIV confluence. The aortic bifurcation can help to locate the CIV confluence when severe bilateral postthrombotic scar is present. We also measure the most inferior IVC for diameter when needing to extend a stent from the CIV into the IVC. The IVC can be very variable in size at the confluence of the CIVs and sometimes is the same size as a dilated CIV. If the CIV stent diameter is as big or bigger than the IVC lumen, then a stent extending into the IVC can "jail" the contralateral CIV causing a contralateral leg deep vein thrombosis. Kissing CIV stents to rebuild the CIV confluence in order to protect the contralateral CIV may be necessary in occasional patients depending on the type of venous stent used.

The CIV, EIV, and the CFV are routinely assessed with IVUS for nonthrombotic extrinsic compression

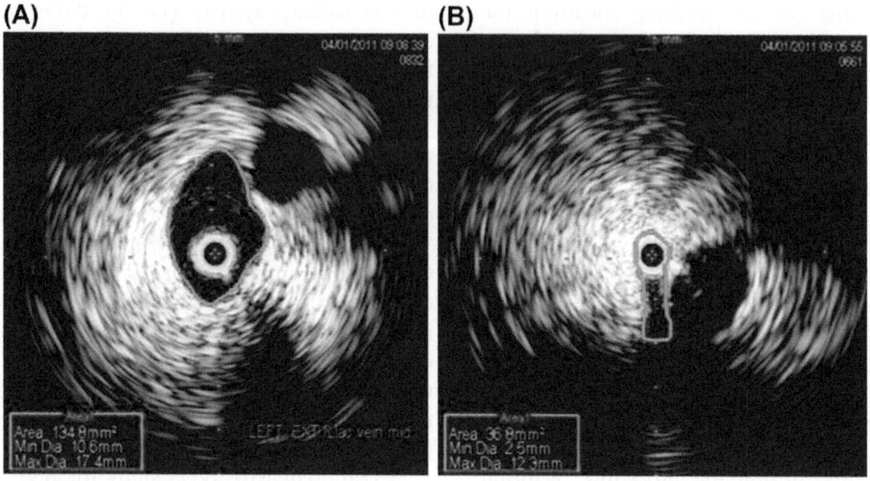

FIG. 16.3 **(A)** Normal external iliac vein; **(B)** Compression stenosis of external iliac vein.

(Fig. 16.3A and B) as well as intramural and intraluminal postthrombotic scar (Fig. 16.4A–C). Compression by the adjacent common iliac artery can be identified with IVUS anywhere along the length of the left or right CIV. Compression of the EIV is commonly at or adjacent to the CIA bifurcation into the external (EIA) and internal iliac (IIA) arteries. This bifurcation is usually easily evident with IVUS. Though the most cranial portions of the CIV and EIV are the segments most commonly compressed, compression is not always limited to these segments. Compression can occur anywhere along the length of these veins. The CFV can be compressed at the inguinal ligament, though postthrombotic scar is the most common cause of narrowing in the vein. We have seen a number of patients with peri- and intraluminal scar in CFV, and stenosis following total hip arthroplasty.

It is important to identify the bifurcation of the CFA during evaluation of the CFV with IVUS. The DFV is generally observed traversing between the superficial femoral artery (SFA) and the profundal femoris artery (PFA). The DFV is also often duplicated which can be easily identified with IVUS. The DFV is usually the most caudal extent of the IVUS study and is an important vessel to identify when placing a CFV stent. The DFV is an important inflow vessel to any CFV stent and should not be covered. Radiographically, the lesser trochanter of the femur marks the approximate junction of the FV and DFV, and this confluence is easily confirmed with IVUS. Routine identification of these

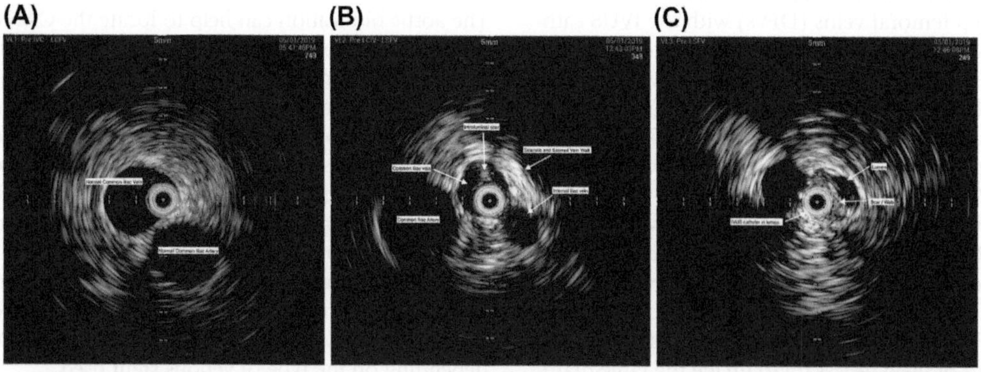

FIG. 16.4 **(A)** Normal iliac vein; **(B)** Stenosed iliac vein and intraluminal scar; **(C)** Sclerotic and contracted vein with Intraluminal web.

landmarks is particularly important when stents are necessary in postthrombotic patients with disease extending into and caudal to the CFV. Insuring that DFV flow into the stent is preserved is important for securing stent patency and avoiding thrombosis.

IVUS AND MAINTENANCE THERAPY FOR FAILING ARTERIOVENOUS DIALYSIS ACCESS

Patients on chronic hemodialysis require a well-functioning arteriovenous fistula (AVF) or graft (AVG) for therapy, on average three times weekly. There are multiple factors that affect the patency of AVF and AVG. Having a reliable AV access is an important component of maintaining a good quality of life for chronic dialysis patients. We have found that the care of these patients and their AVFs and AVGs is enhanced because of ready availability of a surgeon and staff in the OEC. The ability to provide same day treatment for a failing or nonfunctioning AV access can only be achieved by having access to an OEC (Chapter 32).

Our standard protocol is to study these patients' failing AVF or AVG, with a limited fistulogram to identify the vascular anatomy and then use IVUS to evaluate for stenosis within the access or obstruction in the venous outflow tract. We regularly observe that IVUS simplifies and expedites selecting proper balloon and stent size. IVUS is a time and cost-saving maneuver in that, once added to the workflow regimen, it is quick and informative. You also save time and money by choosing the proper balloon and stent size the first time for optimal outcomes. In fact, the addition of IVUS imaging to traditional digital subtraction angiography leads to improved outcomes that prolongs AV access function as compared with DSA-guided interventions without the use of IVUS.[6] IVUS use decreases the number of fistulograms required and thus also decreases the amount of contrast and radiation needed to identify a stenosis threatening patency.[6] The need for multiplanar views to identify a lesion is avoided. Furthermore, in patients with significant thoracic outlet compression of the subclavian vein in the AV access outflow tract, IVUS is especially valuable. Not only is the degree of stenosis easily assessed with IVUS, but the size of balloon or stent necessary to treat the stenosis following thoracic outlet decompression is best assessed with IVUS. The large size of these central veins leads to large stents and significant morbidity should they embolize to the heart or pulmonary arteries. Accurate sizing of the subclavian and central veins is critical to avoid this complication. Like the large veins stented in the pelvis for chronic venous hypertension, IVUS is the gold standard for sizing the central veins prior to stent placement. Depending on the age and size of the AV access, we use various IVUS catheters depending on the field of view needed and the suitable access sheath. The Philips 0.14, 0.18, and 0.35 IVUS catheters all have a role, though the 0.18 catheter is the workhorse catheter for these cases. Following diagnosis, we also use IVUS to ensure that a PTA or stent has achieved adequate lumen gain to insure the technical success of the procedure.

In patients with failed AVFs or AVGs who require thrombolysis and endovascular reconstruction, we find IVUS identifies the cause of the thrombosis (Fig. 16.5) and the presence of unresolved intraluminal thrombus better than angiography. The presence of persistent thrombus has been found to predict early rethrombosis of AV access after intervention.[19] This capability of IVUS may not only provide a clinical benefit to the dialysis patient but may also be cost-effective for promoting long-term function of a salvaged AVF or AVG.

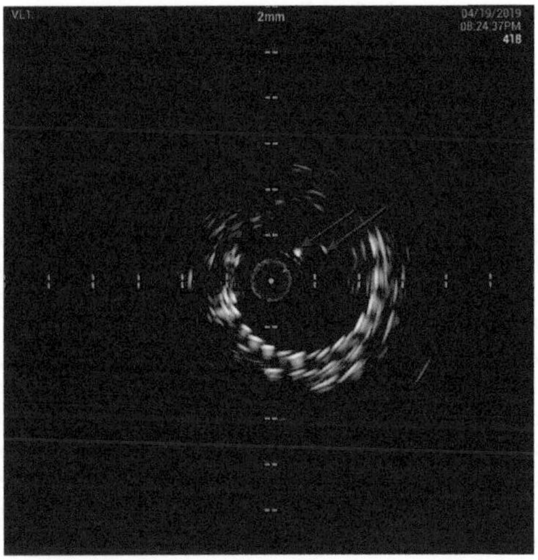

FIG. 16.5 Fractured stent in axillary vein of arteriovenous fistula as cause of in-stent thrombosis; not evident on fluoroscopy due to overlapping stents.

An additional consideration emphasizing the value of IVUS in these patients is the ability to decrease recurrent exposure to radiation to the patients and the staff since patients with vascular access for hemodialysis require recurrent intervention. The emerging data on long-term risks of radiation exposure in other patient populations, though inadequately studied and measured in this patient cohort, shows the deleterious effect of radiation on patients and treating physicians. IVUS is an invaluable tool for decreasing radiation exposure to a minimum for our dialysis patients. Finally, in patients with contrast allergies, IVUS is a reliable way to diagnose and treat stenosis in an AV access without the need for premedication or the risk of the life-threatening side effects from iodinated contrast.[20] Quality patient care is preserved and simplified.

IVUS has been available in the hospitals for several years. Only recently, CMS approved reimbursement for the use of IVUS in OEC. Since the endovascular procedures are gradually moving from the hospital to OEC, there will be greater use of this technology in providing improved health care by decreasing radiation exposure, appropriate sizing of balloons and stents, and visualization of lesions missed by traditional angiography. It has really revolutionized the management of patients with chronic venous occlusive disease.

REFERENCES

1. Tabbara M, White R, Cavaye D, Kopchok G. In vivo human comparison of intravascular ultrasonography and angiography. *J Vasc Surg*. 1991;14:496–502.
2. Arthurs ZM, Bishop PD, Feiten LE, et al. Evaluation of peripheral atherosclerosis: a comparative analysis of angiography and intravascular ultrasound imaging. *J Vasc Surg*. 2010;51:933–938.
3. Cooper BZ, Kirwin JD, Panetta TF, et al. Accuracy of intravascular ultrasound for diameter measurement of phantom arteries. *J Surg Res*. 2001;100:99–105.
4. Schwarzenberg H, Müller-Hülsbeck S, Gluer CC, et al. Restenosis of peripheral stents and stent grafts as revealed by intravascular sonography: in vivo comparison with angiography. *AJR Am J Roentgenol*. 1998;170:1181–1185.
5. van Sambeek MR, Qureshi A, van Lankeren W, et al. Discrepancy between stent deployment and balloon size used assessed by intravascular ultrasound. *Eur J Vasc Endovasc Surg*. 1998;15:57–61.
6. Ross JR, Franga DL, Gallichio M, et al. *J Vasc Surg*. 2017; 65(5):1383–1389.
7. Saxon R, et al. Heparin-bonded, expanded polytetrafluoroethylene- lined stent graph in the treatment of femoropopliteal artery disease: 1-year results of the VIPER (viabahn endoprosthesis with heparin BioacMve surface in the treatment of superficial femoral artery obstructive disease. *Trial J Vasc Interv Radiol*. 2013;24:165–173.
8. FDA PMA P120020: SUPERA Perpipheral Stent System, Summary of Safety and Effectiveness Data.
9. Iida O, et al. Efficacy of intravascular ultrasound in femoropopliteal StenMng for peripheral artery disease with TASC II class A to C lesions. *J Endovasc Ther*. August 2014;21(4):485–492.
10. Scoccianti M, Verbin CS, Kopchok GE, et al. Intravascular ultrasound guidance for peripheral vascular interventions. *J Endovasc Surg*. 1994;1:71–80.
11. Arko F, Meettauer M, McCollough R, et al. Use of intravascular ultrasound improves long-term clinical outcome in the endovascular management of atherosclerotic aortoiliac occlusive disease. *J Vasc Surg*. 1998;27(4):614–622.
12. Kashyap VS, et al. Angiography underestimates peripheral atherosclerosis: lumenography revisited. *J Endovasc Ther*. 2008;15(1):117–125.
13. Makris GC, Chrysafi P, Little M, et al. The role of intravascular ultrasound in lower limb revascularization in patients with peripheral arterial disease. *Int Angiol*. 2017; 36(6):505–516.
14. Negus D, Fletcher EW, Cockett FB, Thomas ML. Compression and band formation at the mouth of the left common iliac vein. *Br J Surg*. 1968;55:369–374.
15. Eklöf B, et al. Revision of the CEAP classification for chronic venous disorders: consensus statement American venous forum international ad hoc committee for revision of the CEAP classification. *J Vasc Surg*. 2004;40(6): 1248–1252.
16. Raju S, Neglén P. High prevalence of nonthrombotic iliac vein lesions in chronic venous disease: a permissive role in pathogenicity. *J Vasc Surg*. 2006;44:136–143.
17. Gagne PJ, et al. Venography versus intravascular ultrasound for diagnosing and treating iliofemoral vein obstruction. *J Vasc Surg*. 2017;5:678–687.
18. Gagne PJ, et al. Analysis of threshold stenosis by multiplanar venogram and intravascular ultrasound examination for predicting clinical improvement after iliofemoral vein stenting in the VIDIO trial. *J Vasc Surg*. 2018;6:48–56.
19. Arbab-Zadeh A, et al. Hemodialysis access assessment with intravascular ultrasound. *Am J Kidney Dis*. 2002;39(4): 813–823.
20. Oakley M, Amankwah KS. *J Vasc Ultrasound*. 2014;38(4): 214–217.

CHAPTER 17

Management of Periprocedural Anticoagulation

SHIKHA JAIN, MD

INTRODUCTION

The management of periprocedural anticoagulation in the age of novel oral anticoagulant (NOAC) therapy requires a multidisciplinary approach for the best overall outcomes. It is essential that all members of the healthcare team are informed regarding the anticoagulation plan and educated on appropriate guidelines for perioperative anticoagulation, as well as strategies to prevent both bleeding and thromboembolic complications. From 1964 to 2010, warfarin was the only oral anticoagulant approved by the US Food and Drug Administration (FDA). The approval of dabigatran in 2010 and rivaroxaban and other factor Xa inhibitors in 2011 changed the landscape of anticoagulation care plans[1]. With the increasing utilization of NOACs, the decision of which anticoagulant to use has become more complicated. The management of these drugs in the perioperative period can be complex, and a comprehensive plan must be put in place.

The most common reasons patients are placed on anticoagulants include a history of venous thromboembolism (VTE), stroke prevention due to arrhythmias such as atrial fibrillation or atrial flutter, and after the placement of a coronary stent or replacement of a heart valve. The management of these medications in the perioperative setting can be complicated by the fact that while anticoagulation is on hold, the risk of thromboembolism transiently increases. However remaining on anticoagulation in the operative setting can increase the risk of bleeding complications. The amount of time each drug takes to achieve peak and trough level and leave the system varies, and these facts must be taken into account when determining management in these patients. Finding a balance and weighing the risk benefit ratio for those on anticoagulation are essential for appropriate perioperative management.

The recommendations presented here will incorporate best practice utilizing the current best available data; however, it is important to acknowledge that this evidence is not always supported by large trials and may be based simply on small observational studies, or expert opinion.

In order to utilize these agents in a safe and effective manner in the periprocedural period, it is important to understand the differences in anticoagulation therapeutic options that currently exist.

Antiplatelet Agents

This category of drugs irreversibly inhibits ADP receptors on platelets by binding the P2Y12 receptors which then prevent the aggregation of platelets.[2] These drugs are most often given to patients who have a history of cardiac stent placements, peripheral vascular disease, or cerebral vascular accidents. The most commonly utilized antiplatelet agents are aspirin and clopidogrel. Prasugrel and ticagrelor are other new agents that also fall into this category and are more potent.

Vitamin K Antagonists

Warfarin

Warfarin remains the gold standard by which all new thrombotic therapeutic agents are measured against. It has proven to be efficacious in decreasing the risk for recurrent thrombotic events and fatal pulmonary embolisms (PEs) as well as has a known safety profile.[3] Warfarin is a vitamin K inhibitor that inhibits the activity of vitamin K–dependent factors II, VII, XI, and X. Warfarin also decreases the anticoagulant activity of protein C and S.[4,5] For patients on vitamin K antagonist (VKA) therapy for VTE indications who optimally require a minimum of 3 months of anticoagulation, the estimated risk of recurrence in the first month after clot diagnosis if therapy is discontinued is 40% and during the subsequent 2 months the risk is 10%. The overall recurrence risk after 3 months of VKA therapy is estimated at 15% for the first year.[6] This does not

Office-Based Endovascular Centers. https://doi.org/10.1016/B978-0-323-67969-5.00017-4
Copyright © 2020 Elsevier Inc. All rights reserved.

TABLE 17.1
CHA_2DS_2-VASc Score.[20]

CHA_2DS_2-VASc	Score
Congestive heart failure/LV dysfunction	1
Hypertension	1
Age >75 years	2
Diabetes mellitus	1
Stroke/TIA/TE	2
Vascular disease (prior MI, PAD, aortic plaque)	1
Age 65–74 years	1
Sex category (i.e., female)	1
Maximum Score	9
Score	**Annual stroke risk (%)**
1	1.3
2	2.2
3	3.2
4	4
5	6.7
6	9.8
7	9.6
8	6.7
9	15.2

take into account patients with acquired hypercoagulable states such as hereditary thrombophilia, active malignancy, or antiphospholipid syndrome, which are all independent risk factors for recurrence of VTE and may require indefinite anticoagulation therapy. For patients who require 3 months of anticoagulation for treatment of a VTE, if elective surgery can be delayed by at least 1 month, and ideally 3 months, this will allow for the safest perioperative anticoagulation plan. If anticoagulation is held in the initial 3 month period, this transient interruption in therapy will increase their risk of clot propagation or the development of new clots.

Patients on VKA therapy for arterial indications, those with mechanical heart valves, and those with nonvalvular atrial fibrillation (NVAF) are at increased stroke risk when anticoagulation is subtherapeutic, or held.[7] In those with NVAF, the validated clinical prediction score (CHA_2DS_2-VASc) uses congestive heart failure, hypertension, age, diabetes, and history of stroke or transient ischemic attack, vascular disease, and female sex to estimate the stroke rate per 100 patient years in a nonsurgical setting. The 2016 European Society of Cardiology (ESC) guidelines recommend using this score to estimate the risk of stroke in AF patients and to start oral anticoagulation in men with a score of 1 or higher and women with a score of 2 or higher[8] (Table 17.1). Thus patients with a high score will be at higher risk for developing a thrombotic episode while transiently off therapy.

Novel Oral Anticoagulant

The group of drugs known as NOACs has become increasingly more utilized over the last decade. There are two subsets of NOACs, factor Xa inhibitors and direct thrombin inhibitors. Currently, there are four NOACs approved for the treatment of the following diagnoses: deep vein thrombosis (DVT); PEs; stroke prevention in NVAF, and DVT prophylaxis for certain surgical procedures. They are also known by the term direct oral anticoagulants or target-specific oral anticoagulants. These drugs include apixaban, dabigatran, betrixaban, edoxaban, and rivaroxaban. Contrary to warfarin, NOACs reach therapeutic levels quickly and do not require frequent monitoring, do not come with dietary restrictions, and have a significantly decreased chance of a drug interaction with other medications.[9] However, the NOAC class of medication does not have the robust collection of randomized control trials demonstrating their safety in surgical procedures. Until 2018, there were no specific reversal agents for the NOACs, but with the approval of idarucizumab in the spring of 2018, one previous hurdle for those on dabigatran requiring urgent or emergent surgery was seemingly overcome. The accelerated approval of andexanet alfa in the spring of 2018 for the reversal of low molecular weight heparin (LMWH) and factor Xa inhibitors provided a similar solution for patients on those agents.[10,11]

Factor Xa inhibitors

The factor Xa inhibitors that are currently commercially available include rivaroxaban, apixaban, betrixaban, and edoxaban. These drugs bind to factor Xa and prevent the formation of thrombin by interrupting the extrinsic and intrinsic coagulation cascades.[2]

The first Xa inhibitor available on the market was rivaroxaban. It is most often utilized for the treatment of VTE, prevention of VTE after orthopedic surgery, stroke and VTE prophylaxis in patients with NVAF, and for VTE prophylaxis in patients with malignancy.[2]

Rivaroxaban has a rapid onset of action with concentrations reaching peak within 2.5–4 h of administration. In patients who are overall in good health, maximum effects are achieved around 3 h and last for approximately 12 h.[12] Its terminal half-life ranges from 5.7 to 9.2 h. This may be longer in the elderly patient population due to the increase in renal dysfunction.[12] It is contraindicated in those with severe liver dysfunction and also in those with creatinine clearance below 30 mL/min as it is renally excreted. There is no standard mechanism for monitoring, and it can be reversed with 4-factor prothrombin complex, or with active charcoal if administered within 8 hours of ingestion.[13] The agent andexanet alfa was also recently approved as a factor Xa reversal agent. It is important to remember activated partial thromboplastin time (aPTT) and international normalized ratio (INR) are not reliable methods to monitor the effects of factor Xa inhibitors such as rivaroxaban. However, antifactor Xa activity can be utilized for monitoring if necessary.

Apixaban is approved for stroke prophylaxis in atrial fibrillation patients with nonvalvular disease, stroke prophylaxis, and treatment of pulmonary emboli as well as for VTE prophylaxis in cancer patients. Peak concentrations are achieved in about 3 to 4 h, thus it also has a rapid onset of action. Its half-life is approximately 12 h and is prolonged in those with renal dysfunction. Apixaban is metabolized through the liver, and 25% is estimated to be excreted renally, 75% by the biliary system.[2] Apixaban does prolong aPTT and PT/INR in a direct dose-dependent relationship, but there is no consistency in the lab values thus it is not utilized for the purposes of monitoring.[14,15] Antifactor Xa activity can be used for monitoring if necessary.

The two remaining Xa inhibitors, edoxaban and betrixaban, are not as commonly utilized. Edoxaban is used to treat and prevent VTEs and for stroke prevention in patients with atrial fibrillation as well as for VTE prophylaxis in oncologic patients. Neither should be used in patients with prosthetic heart valves. Betrixaban is occasionally used in the prevention of VTE in hospitalized adult patients.

Direct thrombin inhibitor

The only current oral direct thrombin inhibitor available is dabigatran etexilate. Dabigatran etexilate is approved for the prevention of VTE after joint surgery, the treatment of VTE, and for prevention of stroke in NVAF. It inhibits thrombin by binding reversibly. In doing so, it prevents the activation of factors V, VIII, and X, thus preventing fibrinogen to fibrin conversion. Peak plasma concentrations are achieved at 2 h. It can be reversed with activated charcoal or hemodialysis. Idarucizumab, a humanized monoclonal antibody fragment, is a specific reversal agent currently available as well.[16]

NOAC REVERSAL

With the approval of idarucizumab and andexanet alfa, the landscape of perioperative anticoagulation in the case of urgent/emergent surgical scenarios has shifted. Idarucizumab was approved in October 2015 as the first NOAC reversal agent based on the results of the RE-VERSE AD phase 3 trial. This trial looked at 503 patients at 173 sites across the world. Patients were split into Group A (n = 301) and Group B (n = 202). In Group A, 60% of patients presented with uncontrolled or life-threatening bleeding, and in Group B, 40% required an invasive procedure or an emergency surgery or intervention. The final results showed that in the 90 patients that received idarucizumab (51 people in Group A and 39 in Group B) the median maximum percentage reversal was 100% (95%CI 100 to 100). In Group A, mean hemostasis was restored at a mean of 11.4 h in the 35 patients that could be assessed. In Group B, 33 of the 36 patients who underwent a procedure reported intraoperative hemostasis. Only one thrombotic event occurred within 72 h after idarucizumab was administered to a patient who was not reinitiated on anticoagulants.[17] Idarucizumab is a dabigatran-specific Fab fragment and has no activity against direct factor Xa inhibitors or other anticoagulants.

Andexanet alfa is a reversal agent for factor Xa inhibitors. It was approved in May 2018 for the reversal of rivaroxaban and apixaban; however, its availability is limited. If available, it should be utilized for patients with life-threatening bleeding associated with active, direct factor Xa-associated anticoagulation that cannot be managed with more conservative interventions.

Periprocedural Management

Before the decision is made as to whether interruption of anticoagulation is required for a procedure, it is important to understand the risk of bleeding with that particular procedure, the effect of a perioperative bleed if it were to occur, and whether the patient has other comorbidities that would increase bleeding risk.

There are several important factors that must be taken into consideration when developing a plan for perioperative anticoagulation:

1. The history of bleeding diathesis.
2. The length of time in which hemostasis is anticipated to be achieved.

3. The risk of complication from not being on the anticoagulant (e.g., stroke, VTE).
4. The patient's renal and hepatic functions which could impact drug clearance.
5. The pharmacokinetics of the drug (vitamin K antagonists such as warfarin have a longer half-life compared with NOACs).
6. Some procedures such as implanting a pacemaker or cardioverter-defibrillator have been found to have a lower bleeding risk when VKA therapy is continued rather than bridging with a heparin drip.

Typically, it takes the body five half-lives to clear any drug. NOACs have a significantly shorter half-life when compared with warfarin (5–17 h vs. 40 h), and due to this short half-life, NOACs do not need to be held for as long a period preoperatively as warfarin (only 24–48 h for NOACs compared with 4–5 days for warfarin). However, as described above, there are other factors that must also be taken into account. Many NOACs are cleared through the renal system (e.g., apixaban, rivaroxaban, dabigatran, edoxaban), and thus renal function must be taken into account when determining the amount of time an agent must be held. Among them, apixaban is the only agent that has lower clearance through the kidney (25%). Therefore in some cases of mild kidney injury, this would be the drug of choice.

TABLE 17.2
HAS-BLED Score to Assess Bleeding Risk.[11]

HAS-BLED	Score
Hypertension (uncontrolled BP) systolic >160 mmHg	1
Abnormal renal function (chronic dialysis, renal transplant, serum Cr ≥ 200 μmol/L	1
Abnormal liver function (chronic hepatic disease, biochemical evidence of significant hepatic derangement bili >2 × ULN, AST or Alt>3×ULN	1
Bleeding tendency or predisposition	1
Labile INR on VKA (time in therapeutic range <60%)	1
Age >65 years	1
Drugs (e.g., concomitant aspirin or NSAID) or ETOH	1 or 2
History of a stroke	1
Alcohol or drug use history (≥8 drinks/ week)	9

Assessing risk of bleeding due to the planned procedure

The risk of procedural bleeding is typically extrapolated from small, observational studies and/or case series involving specific procedures. Due to this, most recommendations and guidance on periprocedural anticoagulation is based on expert consensus.[18] It should also be considered while performing procedures with low rates of bleeding, but significant morbidity or mortality associated with a potential bleed such as spinal or intraocular surgery.

The consensus from multiple professional societies deems four main levels of bleeding risk: (1) No clinically important bleeding risk; (2) Overall low risk of procedural bleed; (3) Uncertain risk of procedural bleed; (4) Intermediate/high risk of procedural bleed. It is important to remember that it is up to the proceduralists discretion as to what the anticipated risk of bleeding would be as the degree of difficulty and complexity of any given procedure will vary, e.g., all surgeries of the hip do not carry with them the same risk of bleeding.

There are several consensus documents that have been published dividing the most commonly performed procedure by risk of bleeding (high or low risk). However, there are many procedures where disagreements exist on how bleed risk is categorized.

Assess patient-related risk of bleeding

The HAS-BLED score is the score recommended by the European Society of Cardiology and Canadian guidelines to assess the bleeding risk in patients on anticoagulation (Table 17.2). A history of prior bleeding event (highest risk if in the preceding 3 months), history of a bleeding event with a similar procedure or bleeding with prior bridging, an abnormality of platelet function (either qualitative or quantitative), concomitant use of medications that can be associated with platelet dysfunction such as aspirin would all increase the potential risk of periprocedural bleeding. A HAS-BLED score of >3 is indicative of the necessity for close monitoring and has been shown to be highly predictive of a bleeding event, however, is not an absolute in requiring the interruption of anticoagulant therapy. Because some of these same risk factors also increase the risk for thrombosis, the score should be used to identify modifiable risk factors to decrease the risk of bleeding. It is predictive of major bleeding in patients both with and without AF, and it also forces clinicians to assess the patient's reversible risk factors that may impact bleeding risk.[11,19]

Periprocedural Management: Recommendations

Antiplatelet therapy

Many patients with cardiovascular (CV) disease or significant CV risk factors require long-term aspirin therapy for risk reduction and when making the determination of holding this agent prior to the procedure there should be discussion with the patient's cardiologist.

The large randomized POISE-2 trial found that administering aspirin (acetylsalicylic acid or ASA) during the perioperative period in patients undergoing noncardiac surgery does not change the risk of having a CV event, and may result in an increased risk of bleeding. A substudy of this trial also found that there was no benefit at reducing the risk of acute kidney injury or prevention of VTE.[21,22]

ASA should not be given to patients undergoing surgery unless there is a definitive evidence-based indication for primary or secondary prevention. Patients without definitive guideline based need for ASA should have the agent held in the preoperative period, and it should not be reinitiated with the purpose of thrombosis prevention postoperatively. There are other agents that are more effective and indicated for postoperative thrombosis prevention if needed. In moderate- and high-risk patients on lifelong ASA for an evidence-based primary or secondary preventative purpose, indication may warrant continuing the agent throughout the perioperative period. Patients undergoing a procedure where the complications from a potential bleed may be catastrophic, such as an intramedullary spine surgery or other closed-space procedures should have their ASA held in the perioperative period with multidisciplinary consultation.[23]

In a moderate- to high-risk patients receiving ASA and undergoing a noncardiac surgery, ASA can be continued in the perioperative setting. If a patient has a coronary stent and requires a nonemergent surgery, the procedure should be delayed for at least 6 weeks after bare metal stent is placed and at least 6 months after a drug-eluting stent is placed. If patients require surgery within that time frame, continuing the antiplatelet medication perioperatively would be recommended.

In patients who are on other forms of antiplatelet therapy for cardiac indications, it is important to discuss the risks and benefits of holding therapy depending on the clinical scenario. In patients who are on clopidogrel, prasugrel, or ticagrelor, after a percutaneous coronary intervention (PCI) the drug should be held for 7 days prior to the procedure, only if cardiologist approves of this disruption in therapy. In most cases, patients who have had a bare metal stent should wait 30 days before disruption in dual antiplatelet therapy, and in patients with drug-eluting stents, it is preferred the patient delay nonurgent procedures for 6 months prior to disruption in dual antiplatelet therapy.[24]

In patients receiving antiplatelet therapy for secondary prevention such as in patients with a history of stroke, coronary artery disease or myocardial infarction, peripheral arterial disease or a history of venous, or arterial thrombosis, antiplatelet therapy should be held for 7 days prior to the procedure. The patients ordering service (cardiology, vascular, or neurology) should be conferred with to discuss this disruption in therapy prior to scheduling the procedure. The timing of resuming antiplatelet therapy would be based on the assessment of postprocedural hemostasis.[24]

Vitamin K antagonists

There is no need to interrupt VKA therapy in patients with no clinically significant risk or low risk of bleeding, and no patient-related factors that could increase risk of bleeding (Fig. 17.1).

If the patient's VKA is held, in certain scenarios the use of parenteral heparin for bridging purposes may be necessary. This would be recommended if the patient is on VKA and has a high risk of stroke or systemic embolism (>10% per year). This would include patients with a history of an ischemic stroke within the last 3 months, those with a CHA_2DS_2-VASc (Table 17.1) score of 7–9, or those patients with a previous stroke or systemic embolism more than 3 months previously who do not have a significant periprocedural bleeding risk.[25]

The CHEST guidelines suggest patients with mechanical heart valve, AF, or VTE at high risk of thromboembolism should undergo bridging during the interruption in therapy.

Prior to restarting VKA, it is important to ensure complete hemostasis. Typically, VKA therapy can be restarted within 24 h postoperatively. If the patient requires bridging with heparin, this can be initiated within 24–72 h prior to the procedure depending on the bleeding risk postprocedure.

It is important to check the INR level 5–7 days prior to procedure for several reasons. If the patient's medication is not planned to be held, it would be important to note if the INR is greater than 3. If bridging is intended, the INR level will be helpful in determining how many days prior to the procedure the VKA should be held.

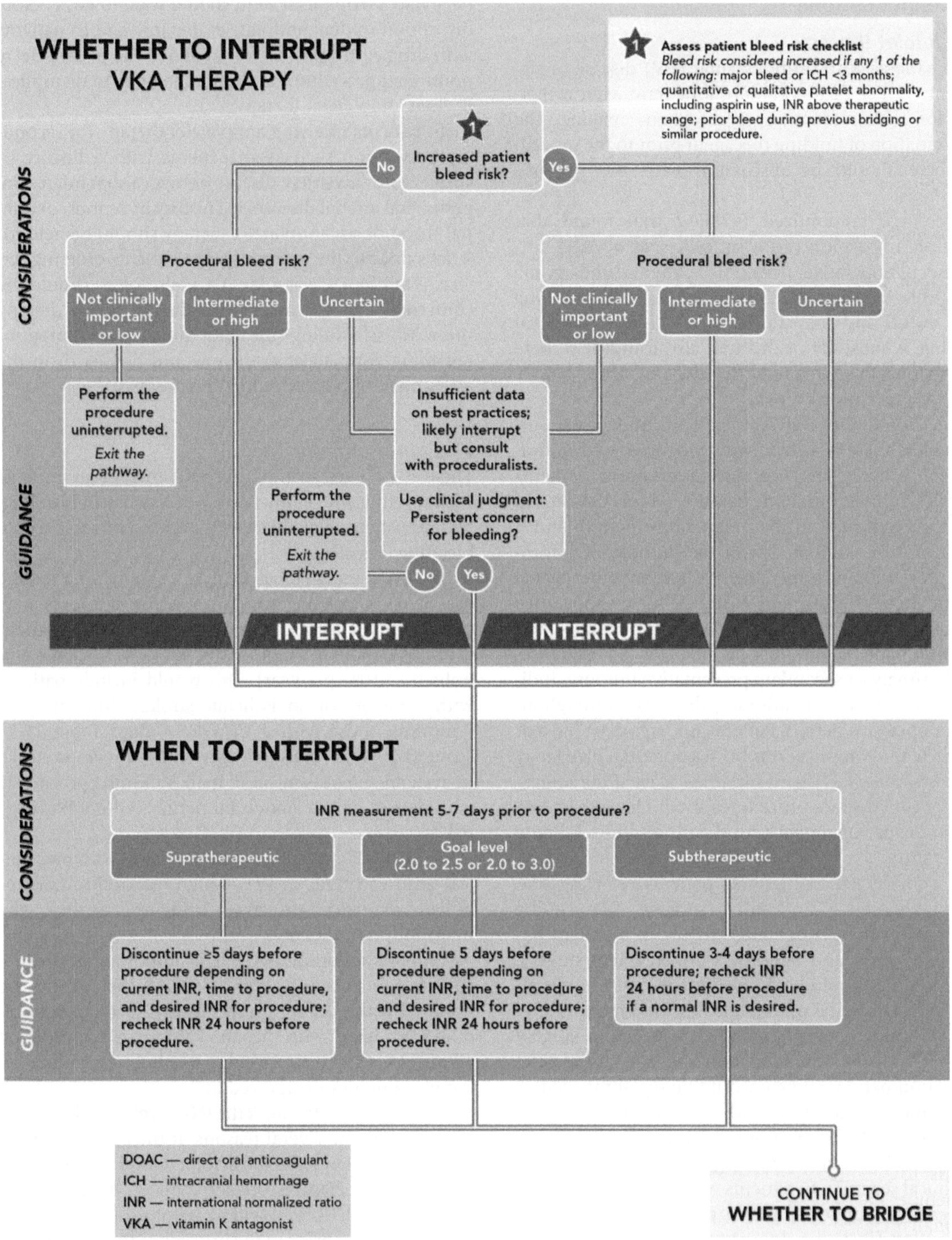

FIG. 17.1 How to determine if vitamin K antagonist (VKA) therapy should be held, and when to interrupt therapy. (Reproduced with permission from JACC Services UMA. No Title.)

Recommendations for Periprocedural interruption of VKA[25]:

- Hold therapy with a VKA
  - Patients having a procedure that has an intermediate or high bleeding risk
  - Patient having a procedure with an unclear bleeding risk, and presence of factors intrinsic to the patient that may increase the risk of bleeding
- Continue VKA therapy
  - In patients with low bleeding risk
  - No patient-related factors that increase bleeding risk
- Consider holding VKA therapy if:
  - Procedure has no clinically significant or low bleeding risk and the patient has medical problems/patient-related factors that increase the risk of bleeding
  - Patient's planned procedure has an unknown bleeding risk and no patient-related factors that would increase the risk of bleeding

Recommendations for periprocedural VKA hold based on INR[25]:

In the majority of patients, when the INR reaches 1.5, it is safe to perform surgery. After resuming warfarin postprocedure, the INR should reach therapeutic values after approximately 3 days.[6]

Recheck INR within 24 h of procedures. If INR remains persistently elevated, delay any elective procedure until INR is in a safe range.

- INR 1.5–1.9: Hold the VKA 3–4 days prior to surgery if normal INR needed for procedure. If low risk of periprocedural bleeding and subtherapeutic INR would not result in added risk, a VKA can be held for less time.
- INR 2.0–3.0: VKA should be held 5 days prior to procedure.
- INR >3: VKA should be held for at least 5 days prior to the procedure. The INR would need to be rechecked 24 h prior to procedure to determine if it will need to be held longer.
- In some patients, the INR is known to normalize in a shorter amount of time. For those patients, a shorter period of time for discontinuation is possible.

NOAC

When making the determination if the patient's NOAC needs to be held periprocedure, it is important to remember the bleeding risk of the procedure, the drugs estimated clearance from the system, and the patient-related factors that would increase the risk of periprocedural bleed. For elective procedures, the procedure should be delayed until reversible patient-related factors can be corrected.

The short half-lives of these agents allow for a bit more flexibility in perioperative management. It is important to remember that these drugs are administered either once or twice a day resulting in some variations in peak/trough drug levels. In patients undergoing a low-risk procedure with a low risk of bleeding, it may only be necessary to hold the patients NOAC for one dose if the drug is given once a day. It may also be possible to schedule the surgery at a time when the NOAC is at a nadir during its trough (Fig. 17.2).

Renal function must be closely monitored to determine the amount of time the drug's anticoagulant properties will remain in the patient's system. This can be analyzed using the Cockcroft-Gault equation to estimate creatinine clearance (CrCl).[25] It is recommended that the drug be held for a certain amount of time depending on bleeding risk of the procedure, and half-life of the drug. For a procedure with a low risk of bleeding, the goal should be completion of two to three half-lives. For high or intermediate risk, or in procedures where the level of risk is unknown, 4–5 half-lives should suffice.[12,14,26–30] There is limited data on best practices for patients with end stage renal disease or on dialysis, thus in those situations, laboratory testing such as dilute thrombin time (dtt) for patients on dabigatran and agent-specific antifactor Xa activity testing for apixaban, edoxaban, and rivaroxaban should be utilized.

The number of doses these patients will require to be held preoperatively would depend on the estimated creatinine clearance and the level of risk of bleeding associated with the procedure. There is no use for parenteral heparin bridging in patients on NOAC agents (Table 17.3). Those at very high thrombotic risk should limit the period that anticoagulation is held (Fig. 17.2).

Special Scenarios

In neuraxial procedures, the risk of spinal or epidural hematoma could be devastating. The NOACs carry a black box warning for these scenarios, and the American Society of Regional Anesthesia and Pain Management have developed specific guidelines for these procedures. They recommend holding dabigatran for 4–5 days and factors Xa inhibitors 3–5 days prior to a neuraxial procedure. They recommend restarting the drug 24 h post-procedure.[31] If the patient is at an elevated thrombotic risk, a drug-free interval of 2–3 half-lives or bridging with LMWH may be reasonable in order to lower the risk of spinal hematoma (Fig. 17.3).

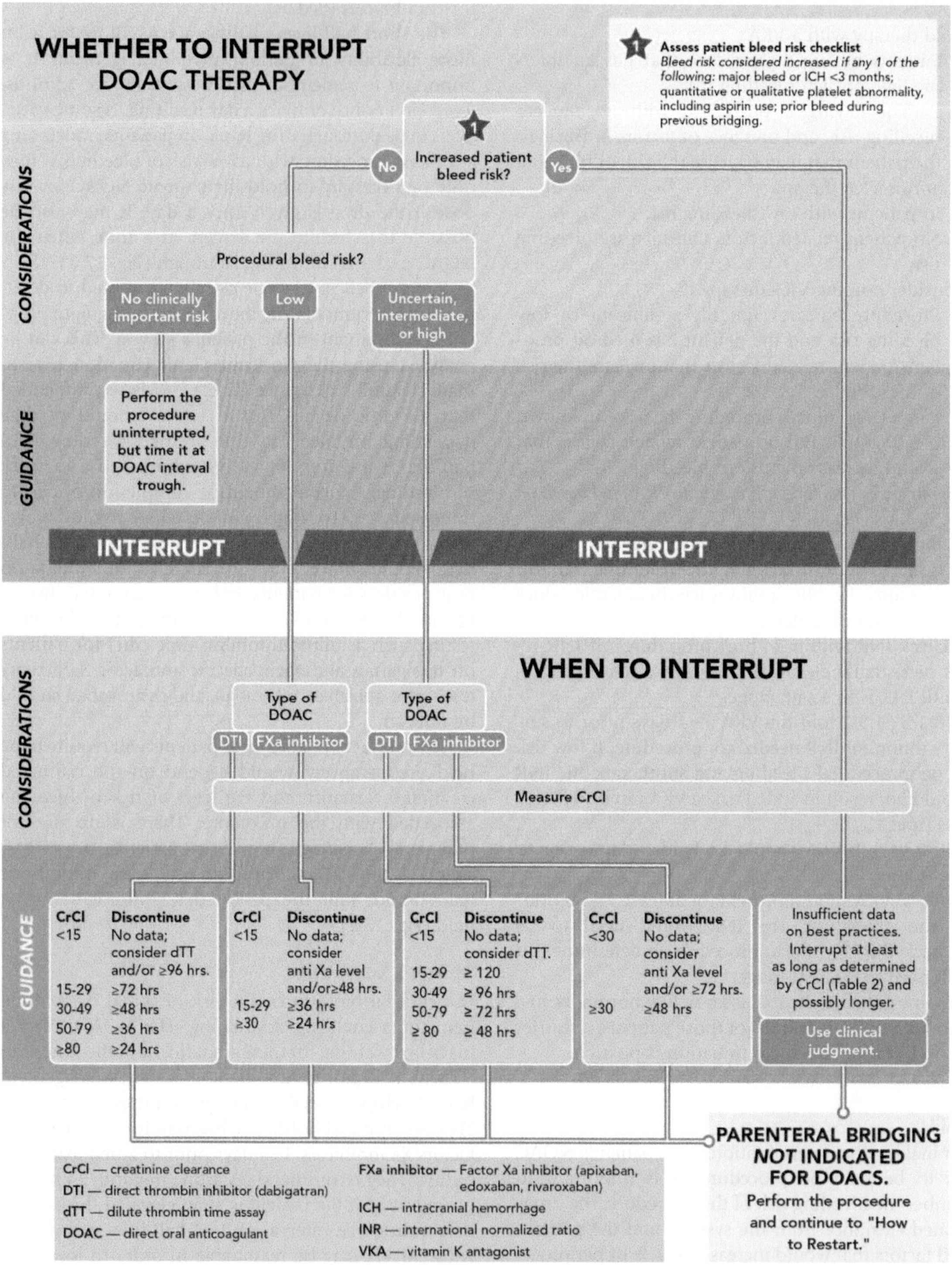

FIG. 17.2 Interruption of novel oral anticoagulant therapy: Indications and timing. *DOAC*, Direct oral anticoagulant. (Reproduced with Permission from JACC Services UMA. No Title.)

TABLE 17.3
Summary of American College of Cardiology Guidelines for Recommended Duration of Withholding NOAC Periprocedurally and Restarting Postprocedure.[25]

	DABIGATRAN					APIXABAN, EDOXABAN, RIVAROXABAN		
Cr Cl (ml/Min)	>80	50–79	30–49	15–29	<15 (off dialysis)	≥30	15–29	<15 (off dialysis)
Estimated drug half-life (hours)	13	15	18	27	30	6–15	A: 17 E: 17 R: 9	A: 17 E: 10–17 R: 13
Procedural bleeding risk								
Low	≥24 h	≥36 h	≥48 h	≥72 h	No data Consider measure dTT and/or hold >96 h	≥24 h	≥36 h	No data Consider measuring agent-specific anti-XA and/or hold ≥48 h
Uncertain Intermediate High	≥48 h	≥72 h	≥96 h	≥120 h	No data Consider measuring dTT	≥48 h E: 72 h	No data Consider measuring agent-specific anti Xa level and/or withholding ≥72 h	
Resume after procedure	**Dabigatran**					**Apixaban, edoxaban, rivaroxaban**		
Low bleed risk	Resume at reduced dose 75 mg on night of procedure (≥4 h postneuraxial anesthesia). Resume full dose next morning. OR resume 24 h postprocedure					R: As soon as hemostasis achieved		
Uncertain Intermediate High bleed risk	Resume 48–72 h after procedure.					48–72 h postprocedure		

dtt, dilute thrombin time.
Studies summarized: RE-LY and ROCKET-AF. ARISTOTLE.

Bridging and Resuming VKA Therapy Postprocedure

For patients on VKA, bridging therapy may be necessary if the patient is at high risk of developing a thrombotic event. Unfractionated heparin (UFH) or low LMWH are the most commonly utilized agents. For patients with a history of heparin-induced thrombocytopenia, a non-heparin agent would need to be utilized.

- The parenteral anticoagulant should be initiated when the INR is no longer therapeutic.
- UFH should be discontinued at least 4 h prior to the procedure. Residual effect can be monitored using the aPTT.
- LMWH that is being given at therapeutic doses should be held at least 24 h prior to surgery. The residual effects of the drug can be monitored using an LMWH-specific antifactor Xa assay. However, prophylactic doses can be held for 12 h prior to procedure.

VKA therapy can be reinitiated when hemostasis is achieved; however, it will be important to discuss with the proceduralists and team the estimated bleeding risk. The dose can be restarted at the previous dose. VKAs typically takes 24–72 h for the anticoagulant to be effective, thus early resumption does not increase the risk of bleeding. If the INR is normal at time of reinitiation, full therapeutic effect typically occurs between 5 and 7 days. Bridging is often not necessary and can lead to increased risk of postprocedural bleeding complications. Thus it is important to balance the risk of bleeding with the risk of thrombosis and may be necessary in certain patients at high risk of developing thrombosis. For those with moderate to high risk for stroke or systemic thromboembolism, bridging therapy with parenteral agents may be necessary. If parenteral anticoagulation is required, this can be initiated within 24 h postprocedure if hemostasis has been received. If the procedure has a high bleeding risk, initiating at 48–72 h may be safer.[18,32]

There are procedures where continuing VKA therapy results in a lower risk of bleeding than bridging

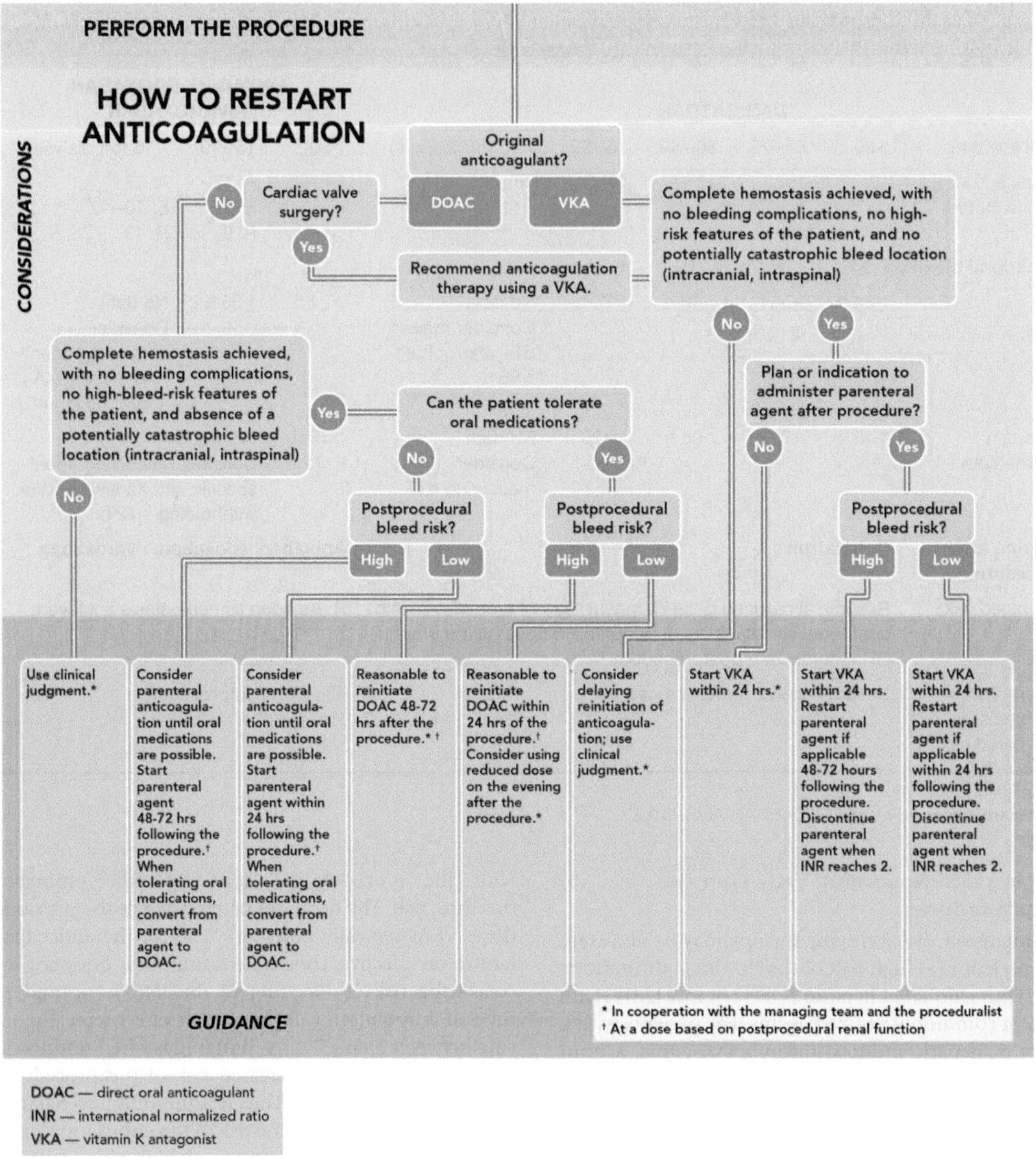

PERFORM THE PROCEDURE
HOW TO RESTART ANTICOAGULATION
CONSIDERATIONS
Original anticoagulant?
DOAC
VKA
Cardiac valve surgery?
No
Yes
Recommend anticoagulation therapy using a VKA.
Complete hemostasis achieved, with no bleeding complications, no high-risk features of the patient, and no potentially catastrophic bleed location (intracranial, intraspinal)
No
Yes
Plan or indication to administer parenteral agent after procedure?
Complete hemostasis achieved, with no bleeding complications, no high-bleed-risk features of the patient, and absence of a potentially catastrophic bleed location (intracranial, intraspinal)
Yes
Can the patient tolerate oral medications?
No
Yes
Postprocedural bleed risk?
High
Low
Use clinical judgment.*
Consider parenteral anticoagulation until oral medications are possible. Start parenteral agent 48-72 hrs following the procedure.† When tolerating oral medications, convert from parenteral agent to DOAC.
Consider parenteral anticoagulation until oral medications are possible. Start parenteral agent within 24 hrs following the procedure.† When tolerating oral medications, convert from parenteral agent to DOAC.
Reasonable to reinitiate DOAC 48-72 hrs after the procedure.*†
Reasonable to reinitiate DOAC within 24 hrs of the procedure.† Consider using reduced dose on the evening after the procedure.*
Consider delaying reinitiation of anticoagulation; use clinical judgment.*
Start VKA within 24 hrs.*
Start VKA within 24 hrs. Restart parenteral agent if applicable 48-72 hours following the procedure. Discontinue parenteral agent when INR reaches 2.
Start VKA within 24 hrs. Restart parenteral agent if applicable within 24 hrs following the procedure. Discontinue parenteral agent when INR reaches 2.
GUIDANCE
* In cooperation with the managing team and the proceduralist
† At a dose based on postprocedural renal function
DOAC — direct oral anticoagulant
INR — international normalized ratio
VKA — vitamin K antagonist

FIG. 17.3 How to restart anticoagulation.[24]

therapy. The BRUISE CONTROL (Bridge or Continue Coumadin for Device Surgery Randomized Controlled) trial looked at patients having implantation of a defibrillator or pacemaker. They found that maintenance of therapeutic anticoagulation with a VKA resulted in significantly less bleeding than bridging with heparin.[33] There is less prospective data on the safety and efficacy of uninterrupted anticoagulation for the NOACs.

Resuming NOAC Therapy Postprocedure

Prior to resuming therapy, local hemostasis is necessary. When this has been achieved, resuming anticoagulation requires consideration of the potential risk of bleeding at the procedural site, and patient-related factors that may increase that risk. This must be balanced with the patients risk of thrombosis while anticoagulation remains on hold.

The RE-LY (Randomized Evaluation of Long-Term Anticoagulation Therapy) trial found similar rates of major bleeding in patients receiving dabigatran at the standard dose of 150 mg twice a day and VKA therapy (3.8 vs. 3.3%, respectively). Dabigatran therapy was interrupted for a shorter period of time.[34] ROCKET-AF (Rivaroxaban Once Daily Oral Factor Xa Inhibition Compared with Vitamin K Antagonism for Prevention of Stroke and Embolism Trial in Atrial Fibrillation) looked at periprocedural outcomes in patients on warfarin and rivaroxaban. The rate of thromboembolism was comparable, and there was no difference in major bleeding events. Rivaroxaban, apixaban, and edoxaban can safely be restarted postprocedure as soon as adequate hemostasis is established.[35]

Due to NOAC short half-lives, bridging is rarely needed prior to procedures. Postprocedure reinitiation of therapy may be delayed secondary to the risk of postprocedural bleeding, the need for further procedures, or patient's inability to take oral medications. In situations where anticoagulation is needed but the patient is unable to take pills, or further procedures are planned, a short acting agent such as UFH may be required if the patient remains at high risk for thrombosis. If the patient is not at high risk and prophylactic medications are needed, this can also be managed with UFH or LMWH. These types of decisions would need to be made on a case by case basis.

Angiography Periprocedural Management

Angiography, or arterial intervention with up to a size 6 French catheter, would be considered a low bleeding risk procedure. The length of time of interruption of the drug is dependent on several factors, including renal function and risk of thrombosis. If the patient is at high thrombotic risk, dabigatran should be held for 2 days in a patient with normal renal function, 3 days with a CrCl 50–79, 4 days for CrCl 30–49, and 5 days for a CrCl less than 30. Rivaroxaban should be held for 2 days if the CrCl is 50 or greater and held for 3 days if the CrCl is less than 50. Apixaban and edoxaban should be held for 2 days if CrCl is greater than 80, 3 days if Cr Clr is 30–79, and 4 days if CrCl is less than 30.

If the patient is on warfarin and at high risk for thrombosis, a bridging protocol should be implemented. If bridging is initiated with heparin, enoxaparin, or dalteparin, warfarin should be held 5 days prior to procedure. Heparin can be initiated the same day warfarin is held, and dosed as a continuous infusion until 4–5 h prior to procedure. If the patient is being bridged with enoxaparin, after the warfarin is held, 4 days prior to the procedure no anticoagulant should be given. On day three and two prior to the procedure, a weight-based dose of enoxaparin should be given. On the day prior to the procedure, the patient should receive half of the dose of enoxaparin in the morning. On the day of the procedure, neither enoxaparin nor warfarin should be given. The patient's INR should be monitored during the perioperative period as well. The patient's renal function should also be considered when determining anticoagulation plan. If the patient is in low thrombotic risk and on warfarin, bridging is not required. Postprocedure, the risk of bleeding should be assessed by the interventionalist, and anticoagulation should be resumed when deemed safe from a bleeding standpoint. For patients at high risk of thrombosis, a bridging protocol can be initiated until the patient's INR is therapeutic.[25]

Almost all procedures can be carried out safely in patients on anticoagulation. However, it is important to know patient's risk factors, indication for anticoagulation, renal, and hepatic function. If the periprocedural anticoagulation is difficult to manage because of various factors, the procedure may need to be performed in the hospital.

REFERENCES

1. How CH. Novel oral anticoagulants for atrial fibrillation. *Singapore Med J*. 2015. https://doi.org/10.11622/smedj.2015184.
2. Lemay A, Kaye AD, Urman RD. Novel anticoagulant agents in the perioperative setting. *Anesthesiol Clin*. 2017. https://doi.org/10.1016/j.anclin.2017.01.016.
3. Smith M, Wakam G, Wakefield T, Obi A. New trends in anticoagulation therapy. *Surg Clin North Am*. 2018. https://doi.org/10.1016/j.suc.2017.11.003.
4. Mega JL, Simon T. Pharmacology of antithrombotic drugs: an assessment of oral antiplatelet and anticoagulant treatments. *Lancet*. 2015. https://doi.org/10.1016/S0140-6736(15)60243-4.
5. Yorkgitis BK, Ruggia-Check C, Dujon JE. Antiplatelet and anticoagulation medications and the surgical patient. *Am J Surg*. 2014. https://doi.org/10.1016/j.amjsurg.2013.04.004.
6. Kearon C, Hirsh J. Management of anticoagulation before and after elective surgery. *N Engl J Med*. 2002. https://doi.org/10.1056/nejm199705223362107.
7. Dentali F, Pignatelli P, Malato A, et al. Incidence of thromboembolic complications in patients with atrial fibrillation or mechanical heart valves with a subtherapeutic international normalized ratio: a prospective multicenter cohort study. *Am J Hematol*. 2012. https://doi.org/10.1002/ajh.23119.

8. Kirchhof P, Benussi S, Zamorano JL, et al. 2016 ESC guidelines for the management of atrial fibrillation developed in collaboration with EACTS. *Russ J Cardiol.* 2017. https://doi.org/10.15829/1560-4071-2017-7-7-86.
9. Tate A, Taranu R, Williams P, et al. Use of anticoagulants remains a significant threat to timely hip fracture surgery. *Geriatr Orthop Surg Rehabil.* 2018. https://doi.org/10.1177/2151459318764150.
10. Ansell JE. Universal, class-specific and drug-specific reversal agents for the new oral anticoagulants. *J Thromb Thrombolysis.* 2016. https://doi.org/10.1007/s11239-015-1288-1.
11. Omran H, Bauersachs R, Rübenacker S, Goss F, Hammerstingl C. The HAS-BLED score predicts bleedings during bridging of chronic oral anticoagulation: results from the national multicentre BNK online bridging registry (BORDER). *Thromb Haemost.* 2012. https://doi.org/10.1160/TH11-12-0827.
12. Kubitza D, Becka M, Mueck W, et al. Effects of renal impairment on the pharmacokinetics, pharmacodynamics and safety of rivaroxaban, an oral, direct Factor Xa inhibitor. *Br J Clin Pharmacol.* 2010. https://doi.org/10.1111/j.1365-2125.2010.03753.x.
13. Miyares MA, Davis K. Newer oral anticoagulants: a review of laboratory monitoring options and reversal agents in the hemorrhagic patient. *Am J Heal Pharm.* 2012. https://doi.org/10.2146/ajhp110725.
14. Chang M, Yu Z, Shenker A, et al. Effect of renal impairment on the pharmacokinetics, pharmacodynamics, and safety of apixaban. *J Clin Pharmacol.* 2016. https://doi.org/10.1002/jcph.633.
15. Frost C, Wang J, Nepal S, et al. Apixaban, an oral, direct factor Xa inhibitor: single dose safety, pharmacokinetics, pharmacodynamics and food effect in healthy subjects. *Br J Clin Pharmacol.* 2013. https://doi.org/10.1111/j.1365-2125.2012.04369.x.
16. Stangier J, Rathgen K, Stähle H, Gansser D, Roth W. The pharmacokinetics, pharmacodynamics and tolerability of dabigatran etexilate, a new oral direct thrombin inhibitor, in healthy male subjects. *Br J Clin Pharmacol.* 2007. https://doi.org/10.1111/j.1365-2125.2007.02899.x.
17. Reardon DP, Owusu K. Idarucizumab for dabigatran reversal guideline. *Crit Pathw Cardiol.* 2016. https://doi.org/10.1097/hpc.0000000000000074.
18. Douketis JD, Spyropoulos AC, Spencer FA, et al. Perioperative management of antithrombotic therapy. Antithrombotic therapy and prevention of thrombosis, 9th ed: American College of Chest Physicians evidence-based clinical practice guidelines. *Chest.* 2012. https://doi.org/10.1378/chest.11-2298.
19. Lip GYH, Zarifis J, Watson RDS, Beevers DG. Physician variation in the management of patients with atrial fibrillation. *Heart.* 1996. https://doi.org/10.1136/hrt.75.2.200.
20. Hedna VS, Favilla CG, Guerrero WR, et al. Trends in the management of atrial fibrillation: a neurologist's perspective. *J Cardiovasc Dis Res.* 2012. https://doi.org/10.4103/0975-3583.102690.
21. Kumar PA, Mrkobrada M, Lurati Buse G, et al. Aspirin in patients undergoing noncardiac surgery. *N Engl J Med.* 2014. https://doi.org/10.1056/nejmoa1401105.
22. Garg AX, Kurz A, Sessler DI, et al. Aspirin and clonidine in non-cardiac surgery: acute kidney injury substudy protocol of the Perioperative Ischaemic Evaluation (POISE) 2 randomised controlled trial. *BMJ Open.* 2014. https://doi.org/10.1136/bmjopen-2014-004886.
23. Gerstein NS, Carey MC, Cigarroa JE, Schulman PM. Perioperative aspirin management after POISE-2: some answers, but questions remain. *Anesth Analg.* 2015. https://doi.org/10.1213/ANE.0000000000000589.
24. Services UMA. No Title.
25. Doherty JU, Gluckman TJ, Hucker WJ, et al. 2017 ACC expert consensus decision pathway for periprocedural management of anticoagulation in patients with nonvalvular atrial fibrillation: a report of the American College of cardiology clinical expert consensus document task force. *J Am Coll Cardiol.* 2017. https://doi.org/10.1016/j.jacc.2016.11.024.
26. Nutescu EA. Oral anticoagulant therapies: balancing the risks. *Am J Heal Pharm.* 2013. https://doi.org/10.2146/ajhp130040.
27. AG B. Xarelto (Rivaroxaban). Prescription Information.
28. Boehringer Ingelheim Pharmaceuticals I. Pradaxa (dabigatran) prescribing information. *Interactions.* 2015.
29. Dias C, Moore KT, Murphy J, et al. Pharmacokinetics, pharmacodynamics, and safety of single-dose rivaroxaban in chronic hemodialysis. *Am J Nephrol.* 2016. https://doi.org/10.1159/000445328.
30. Parasrampuria DA, Marbury T, Matsushima N, et al. Pharmacokinetics, safety, and tolerability of edoxaban in end-stage renal disease subjects undergoing haemodialysis. *Thromb Haemost.* 2015. https://doi.org/10.1160/TH14-06-0547.
31. Narouze S, Benzon HT, Provenzano D, et al. Interventional spine and Pain procedures in patients on antiplatelet and anticoagulant medications (second edition): guidelines from the American society of regional Anesthesia and Pain medicine, the European society of regional anaesthesia and pain thera. *Reg Anesth Pain Med.* 2018. https://doi.org/10.1097/AAP.0000000000000700.
32. Malato A, Saccullo G, Lo Coco L, et al. Patients requiring interruption of long-term oral anticoagulant therapy: the use of fixed sub-therapeutic doses of low-molecular-weight heparin. *J Thromb Haemost.* 2010. https://doi.org/10.1111/j.1538-7836.2009.03649.x.
33. Verma A, Leiria TLL, Wells GA, et al. Pacemaker or defibrillator surgery without interruption of anticoagulation. *N Engl J Med.* 2013. https://doi.org/10.1056/nejmoa1302946.
34. Healey JS, Eikelboom J, Douketis J, et al. Periprocedural bleeding and thromboembolic events with dabigatran compared with warfarin: results from the randomized evaluation of long-term anticoagulation therapy (RE-LY) randomized trial. *Circulation.* 2012. https://doi.org/10.1161/CIRCULATIONAHA.111.090464.

35. Acosta RD, Abraham NS, Chandrasekhara V, et al. The management of antithrombotic agents for patients undergoing GI endoscopy. *Gastrointest Endosc*. 2016. https://doi.org/10.1016/j.gie.2015.09.035.

FURTHER READING

1. Kubitza D, Becka M, Voith B, Zuehlsdorf M, Wensing G. Safety, pharmacodynamics, and pharmacokinetics of single doses of BAY 59-7939, an oral, direct factor Xa inhibitor. *Clin Pharmacol Ther*. 2005. https://doi.org/10.1016/j.clpt.2005.06.011.
2. Castillo J, Wiens BL, Crowther MA, et al. Andexanet alfa for the reversal of factor Xa inhibitor activity. *N Engl J Med*. 2015. https://doi.org/10.1056/nejmoa1510991.
3. Ageno W, Mantovani LG, Hass S, et al. Safety and effectiveness of oral rivaroxaban versus standard anticoagulation for the treatment of symptomatic deep-vein thrombosis (XALIA): an international, prospective, non-interventional study. *Lancet Haematol*. 2016. https://doi.org/10.1016/S2352-3026(15)00257-4.
4. Eikelboom JW, Connolly SJ, Brueckmann M, et al. RE-ALIGN (Dabigatran vs warfarin mechanical heart valves). *N Engl J Med*. 2013. https://doi.org/10.1056/NEJMoa1300615.
5. Parasrampuria DA, Truitt KE. Pharmacokinetics and pharmacodynamics of edoxaban, a non-vitamin K antagonist oral anticoagulant that inhibits clotting factor Xa. *Clin Pharmacokinet*. 2016. https://doi.org/10.1007/s40262-015-0342-7.

CHAPTER 18

Patient Satisfaction

KRISHNA JAIN, MD, FACS

We are witnessing rapid changes in healthcare. The healthcare expenditure continues to outpace general inflation. The Centers for Medicare and Medicaid Services (CMS) predicts annual healthcare costs will be $4.64 trillion by 2020, which represents nearly 20% of the US gross domestic product. The nation is looking toward a more fiscally responsible healthcare system. The patient has become a client, customer, or a consumer. The patient expects success after every intervention, while rest of the parameters that go into determining patient satisfaction are maintained at an optimal level. There is a high correlation between meeting the patient expectation and patient satisfaction.[1] CMS is tying payment to physicians based on quality matrix, and patient satisfaction is a part of it.

There was a time when all that mattered was that the patient had a satisfactory outcome after a surgical procedure. The landscape has changed dramatically. There were excellent surgeons with pristine reputation for their surgical skills but not necessarily for their bedside manners. In today's environment they will not do well. There are surgeons with a beautiful office, excellent staff, great communication skills but marginal surgical skills. Their overall patient satisfaction scores are likely to be great, and they will do well with the regulatory agencies and payers alike. It is not given that a satisfied patient receives the best medical care. One of the risk factors for vascular disease is obesity. Discussions with the patient about weight loss are not always perceived by the patient to be of a friendly nature and may result in lower patient satisfaction. In general, the office-based endovascular center (OEC) should strive to have patients who are satisfied with the care provided to them in the OEC. Happy patients are the best ambassadors of the practice.

There are two terms used to describe patient interaction with a healthcare system: patient satisfaction and patient experience. These two terms have different meaning. They are not interchangeable. It is difficult to define patient satisfaction. In general, a satisfied patient has a feeling that the patient was respected, had a good outcome, and overall the doctor and staff showed empathy and the patient expectation were met or exceeded. In comparison, patient experience is defined differently. The Agency for Research and Quality defines patient experience as follows: "Patient experience encompasses the range of interactions that patients have with the healthcare system, including their care from health plans, and from doctors, nurses, and staff in hospitals, physician practices, and other healthcare facilities. As an integral component of healthcare quality, patient experience includes several aspects of healthcare delivery that patients value highly when they seek and receive care, such as getting timely appointments, easy access to information, and good communication with healthcare providers." Most of the published patient experience data comes from the hospital system. In an OEC, patient satisfaction is paramount to its success. High patient satisfaction results in patient retention as well as increased referrals from the patients and referring physicians. This also prevents medical malpractice lawsuits.

Healthcare delivery system is changing. With the corporatization of medicine, the individual touch patient expects and aspires for is rapidly disappearing. The delivery of care is becoming much more impersonal. The care provided by physicians is measured in relative value units and to some degree by patient satisfaction surveys compiled by outside consulting firms. OEC provides an opportunity for the healthcare team to deliver the highest quality of care without losing the personal touch. In 2001, Institute of Medicine (IOM) published a report titled,[2] "Crossing the Quality Chasm." In this report, IOM set forth six goals for a quality healthcare system. The care provided to the patient should be (1) safe; (2) equitable; (3) evidence based; (4) timely; (5) efficient; and (6) patient centered.

If these six aims along with three others described later in the chapter are met, it is very likely that patient satisfaction will approach 100%. In reality, in the OEC,

Office-Based Endovascular Centers. https://doi.org/10.1016/B978-0-323-67969-5.00018-6
Copyright © 2020 Elsevier Inc. All rights reserved.

patient satisfaction did reach 99%.[3] Let us look at the process of applying these six goals in an OEC.

SAFETY

The care provided in the OEC is as safe as in any hospital setting. Jain et al., in 6458 cases performed in the OEC, reported overall complication rate of 0.8%. Arterial procedures with intervention had the highest complication rate (10 of 368 [2.7%]), followed by venous ablation procedures (22 of 1019 [2.2%]). In 5134 consecutive cases, Lin[4] et al. published progressive decrease in complication rates from 3% to 0.7% in the latest period. Once precautions are taken to avoid complications (Chapter 14) and the selection of patients is appropriate, the complication rate should be the same or better than the hospital. The risk of nosocomial infection is eliminated. In the OEC, the same team works in the preoperative area, procedure room, and the postoperative area on a daily basis. This helps decrease lack of communication and inherent risk of complication caused by miscommunication.

EQUITABLE

Based on the geographical area and the socioeconomic status of the community where the practice is located the practice would be serving the community at large. Majority of patients seen in a practice dealing with vascular disease come from referrals from the local physicians. If the physicians in the area are serving the community well, it will be reflected in the practice, and since OEC is an extension of the practice the OEC will be serving the patients in an equitable manner. Medicaid in general plays less than Medicare for any given procedure. The reimbursement varies from state to state. In our experience we did not loose money for any procedure performed in the OEC while taking care of patients on Medicaid. Though, the profit margin was minuscule to nonexistent.

EVIDENCE BASED

Medicine continues to be an art as well as science. There are guidelines for management of most of the diseases being treated in the OEC. However, the guidelines written by different societies for the same disease process may differ from each other. There are intersocietal guidelines that are usually more comprehensive and should be followed as much as possible. Since the medicine is still an art to some extent, there may be an occasional patient that falls outside the guidelines. The interventionalist should follow the guidelines as much as possible. There is no peer review process in place for the OEC. This makes it even more crucial that the care being provided in the OEC is evidence based. Every interventionalist should take the "Mirror test," When looking in the mirror in the morning one should think of the patient as their immediate family and ask the question, "Will I operate on this patient if the person was my mother?"

TIMELY

One thing that is very evident is the timeliness of care in the OEC as compared with the hospital. Think of a patient admitted through the emergency room by a hospitalist with a gangrenous toe. Usually it will take a couple of days for medical workup. At some point, vascular consult will be requested. Depending on the hospital, the procedure for endovascular revascularization may be scheduled in the hybrid operating room, cardiac Cath lab, or an interventional radiology suite. Depending on the procedure, room schedule, and the interventionalist's schedule, a procedure may be performed anywhere from 1 to 3 days after the call is made to schedule the procedure. Depending on the time of the day when the procedure is performed, patient may have to wait another day to be discharged. If the same patient comes to the office, patient can be examined, assessed, have the noninvasive vascular imaging of the lower extremity arterial system and blood work to check the kidney function on the same day. On the next day patient can have total revascularization of the extremity with critical limb ischemia and go home. In follow-up, patient may have debridement in the office or minor amputation in the hospital on an outpatient basis. Since the interventionalist controls the schedule in the OEC, it is a lot easier to provide care for the patients in a timely manner.

For patients on hemodialysis, OEC is the ideal place to maintain their dialysis access. Number of missed dialysis can be minimized and patient can have more catheter-free days. Failing access can be easily managed using endovascular techniques on nondialysis days. In case of thrombosis of the dialysis access percutaneous thrombectomy can be carried out on the same day and patient dialyzed. If the hemodialysis catheter is not needed any more, the catheter can be removed on the same day. In a study by El-Gamil et al.,[5] patients being treated in an OEC had lower annual mortality, lower access-related infections, fewer hospitalizations, and lower total per member per month payments as compared with hospital outpatient department.

Patients with retrievable inferior cava filters need to have the filters removed in a timely manner. This can easily be done in the OEC. In one study,[6] it seems to improve the retrievable rate of these filters. Patients needing ports can have the port inserted on the same day as they are seen in consultation in the office so long as they are not on anticoagulants and white count and platelet count is normal.

EFFICIENT

Timeliness and efficiency go hand in hand. The OEC usually opens before the main office and closes at the same time as the office. This would be a 10-hour day. There is no provision for overnight stay in the OEC. That means all the work needs to be done during these hours. Since the physician owners have a vested financial interest in the center, every effort is made by the team to eliminate wasted time. The techniques will include, a) doing cases in the morning that will require longer time in the recovery room, b) turnover time between cases being 6–15 min, c) working through the lunch break with appropriately trained people, d) availability of all procedure-related data before the patient arrives in the OEC etc. During the course of the day of the procedure, patient does not have to go through more than 30 touches by different people, quite common in the hospital even for outpatient procedures.

PATIENT CENTERED

Patient comes for the procedure at the same place, where the patient has received nonoperative clinical care. The culture of the office should be patient centric. The only reason the practice exists is because it cares for the patients. If there are no patients there is no practice. It behooves the owners of the practice to make the patient comfortable and be treated with respect during every encounter with staff as well as the medical personnel. This culture permeates into the OEC. Patient's privacy and confidentiality should be maintained at all times.

In addition to the goals set by IOM there are other factors that impact patient satisfaction in an OEC.

FINANCIAL

In today's healthcare environment, patients carry insurance policies with very large deductibles. The patients on Medicare may be barely managing their lives on social security checks. The office should work with the patient and the family if necessary to make sure that there is a financial plan in place before the procedure is done. There are strict rules laid out by CMS that need to be followed in billing and collection for patients on Medicare and Medicaid. As per the rules the patient balance can only be written off if proper procedure is followed. A payment plan can also be agreed upon before the procedure is performed on patients with any kind of insurance or self-paying patients.

COMMUNICATION

The thought of having an invasive procedure is scary for everyone. Timely communication plays a great role in alleviating anxiety in the patient. Since OEC is an extension of the practice, the practice should have the policy of open communication with the patient. Every employee should be able to communicate with the patient and share information pertinent to their level in the organization. Physicians should be able and willing to discuss all aspects of care with the patients and family members designated by the patient.

EMPATHY

In Merriam-Webster Dictionary, empathy is defined as "(also the capacity for) the action of understanding, being aware of, being sensitive to, and vicariously experiencing the feelings, thoughts, and experience of another of either the past or present without having the feelings, thoughts, and experience fully communicated in an objectively explicit manner." Any invasive procedure causes anxiety in the patient and the family. To have a good doctor-patient relationship, it is crucial that the doctor and the whole team has empathy toward the patient. It lays the foundation for high patient satisfaction.

In the functioning of the OEC, patient satisfaction is driven by three factors contributing to their care.

Doctor
Organization
Office environment

DOCTOR

For patient to be fully satisfied the patient must feel that the patient got undivided attention of the doctor. Usually, it is the same doctor who has been managing the patient in the office who will carry out the procedure in OEC. Sometimes, another doctor in the practice may carry out the procedure because of scheduling reasons, or different skill sets possessed by doctors in the practice. In case another doctor is going to do the procedure, the operating physician should meet the patient in advance and build a relationship. There should be frank and exhaustive discussion about the pros and cons of planned procedure. Alternatives to the invasive procedure should be discussed. The appearance of the doctor is important. A chronically tired looking doctor in shabby clothes does not build confidence in the patient. Without violating the HIPAA rules, it is important to have good relationship with the patient's family or the caretaker. They are concerned about the care the patient will get as well as they will be responsible for the care after the procedure, and many times will be bringing patient to the follow-up appointments. Doctor is the leader of the organization and needs to lead by example.

ORGANIZATION

The whole organization needs to be quality driven. In today's environment, the office is exposed to the world even before the patient comes to the office. Majority of patients or the relatives of the patient are looking up information about the OEC on the Internet. They are doing independent research about the doctor and the practice. They are looking for a practice website, researching on social media and other Internet sites. The OEC website should be pleasing, informative, and updated as necessary. The patient should feel welcome starting from the time a call is made to make an appointment and throughout all encounters. Well-informed patient is a happier patient. There should be clear-cut delineation of duties. Since the OEC is an extension of the office practice, if the patients are unhappy in the office it is most likely that they will be unhappy in the OEC. Beyond the usual office staff, the patient will interact with the OEC staff which will include the scheduler, recovery room staff, and procedure room staff. All these staff members need to be courteous, respect patient privacy, and answer questions appropriate for their level. Organization should make sure that the staff members are happy doing their job. Happy staff members make the patients happy. There should be clear-cut chain of responsibility.

There should be a mechanism to answer patient concerns and complaints in a timely manner. According to the joint commission a mechanism must exist for receiving complaints, and patients should be informed of this mechanism and their right to complain. The organization should respond to the complaint, take appropriate action and share the outcome with the patient.

OFFICE

The physical structure of the office should be pleasing and patient friendly. The reception area is usually shared by the patients coming to the office for office visits as well as the patients coming to OEC for a procedure. The OEC facility should not be cramped and be designed in a way to have comfortable space for patients and their families. The procedure rooms should be designed for patient comfort and safety. There should be space for family members while waiting for the procedure to be completed. Since there is no cafeteria in the office, the waiting family should be offered light snacks. The reception and waiting area should have appropriate current reading material.

MEASURING PATIENT SATISFACTION

Satisfaction is part subjective and part based on reality. The surveys are created in an attempt to translate subjective feelings into meaningful, quantifiable data that can be acted upon. The survey can be done via mail, telephone call, or face to face with the patient at the post-procedure office visit. The survey should be short and ask pertinent questions about the care provided in the OEC. Patient interacts with different people in the OEC. Survey can be designed to ask questions about each point of contact and the operative experience.

The hospitals have used Hospital Consumer Assessment of Healthcare Providers and systems (HCAHPS) for quite some time. This was the first national, standardized survey of patients that was publicly reported regarding the patient's perspective of hospital care. The survey is also known as CAHPS. This survey compares the hospital locally, regionally, and nationally. The survey has three goals: (1) provide objective data about patient's perspective of care at the hospital, (2) public reporting of the results that may help hospital improve quality of care, (3) public reporting increases accountability and transparency of quality of care provided by the hospital. This results in a better accounting of public investment in healthcare. The survey consists of 27 questions and is sent to discharged patients from the hospital. Eighteen questions out of 27 are directly related to patient's experience at the hospital. Nine questions are asked related to other items. The survey is sent to random patients every month between 48 h and 6 weeks postdischarge. The survey can be conducted by mail, telephone, mail followed by telephone call, or interactive voice recognition.

In addition to authorizing payment for certain procedures in the OEC by CMS, the Deficit Reduction Act of 2005 created an additional incentive for acute care hospitals to participate in HCAHPS. More incentives were created in the Patient Protection and Affordable Care Act of 2010.

ONLINE REVIEWS

Online reviews have taken a life of their own. There are countless reviews online. These reviews are on non–healthcare websites like Google or Yelp and on healthcare websites like Healthgrades, RateMDs, Zocdoc, etc. In addition, many healthcare organizations have their own websites. A significant number of patients look at online reviews in making healthcare decisions. The negative reviews cause stress among physicians. In a study published by Holliday et al.,[7] 53% of physicians and 39% of patients reported visiting a physician rating website at least once. The physicians trusted data on health system patient experience surveys more often than the data on independent websites while the opposite was true for the patients. Widmer et al.[8] compared Press Ganey–conducted patient satisfaction survey with the online review by patients of physicians who had a negative review and the ones who did not. In Press Ganey survey, there was no difference in patient satisfaction score in the two groups. However, when comparing non–physician-specific factors in those with negative online reviews versus the ones without negative online reviews there was a significant difference. This has implications in the OEC. Despite the patient being satisfied with the services provided by the physician there may be other factors in the OEC that can result in a negative online review. The online reviews are here to stay and the OEC should make an active effort to address any issues that may result in negative reviews. There is a debate as to how to handle a negative online review. Some experts recommend addressing the negative review while others do not. If there is merit in the negative review the issue should be addressed. For example, if the review says the staff is rude, staff may need further training. I would recommend a strategy that is proactive. If any member of the practice sees a negative comment about the practice or the OEC, the patient should be contacted observing HIPAA rules. Do not post comments on the website. Once the problem is resolved, the patient is very likely to take down the negative post. Comments on social media stay forever and it is in the best interest of the OEC not to have any negative comments on social media.

MIPS and MACRA

The Medicare Access and Chip Reauthorization Act was passed in 2015. In the act, Merit-Based Incentive payment (MIPS) system was created. As per CMS website, in MIPS, "Performance is measured through the data clinicians' report in four areas—Quality, Improvement Activities, Promoting Interoperability (formerly Advancing Care Information), and Cost. We designed MIPS to update and consolidate previous programs, including Medicare Electronic Health Records (EHR), Incentive Program for Eligible Clinicians, Physician Quality Reporting System (PQRS), and the Value-Based Payment Modifier (VBM)." In addition, an advanced alternative payment system (APM) was also created. As per CMS website, "An APM is a payment approach that gives added incentive payments to provide high-quality and cost-effective care. APM can apply to a special clinical condition, a care episode, or a population." Physicians working in the OEC are ideally suited to participate and take advantage of these programs. When the physician is in charge of the total care being provided to the patient in the OEC, variables can be controlled and improvements made to deliver quality care at the highest level. If the practice wants to participate in an APM, it may be possible to create a model to take care of patients on hemodialysis and patients with critical limb ischemia. OEC is ideally suited to take care of these patients. Participation in a quality clinical data registry can help meet some of the requirements of MIPS.

Survey Tool

The OEC may contract with an outside agency to carry out a survey. This kind of survey may be acceptable to payer, but is expensive. If the goal is to assess the quality of care being delivered for internal use the survey can be developed by the practice (Table 18.1).

Patient satisfaction is important to the patient, patient's family, and the physician alike. Every doctor wants the patients to be happy with the care they receive. When the physician provides care in the hospital there are many factors that are not in the control of the physician. However, when the care is provided in the office and OEC, almost all foreseeable aspects of care are controlled by the doctor and the staff. In this setting if patients are unsatisfied by the care they are receiving, the doctor and the team needs to analyze the cause of this dissatisfaction and correct the deficiency. There will be an occasional patient who will

TABLE 18.1
Sample Survey Questionnaire (on the Scale, 1 is Poor and 10 is Excellent).

Question	Scale
Was the staff courteous	1 2 3 4 5 6 7 8 9 10
Communication with staff	1 2 3 4 5 6 7 8 9 10
All questions about procedure answered	1 2 3 4 5 6 7 8 9 10
Satisfied with results	1 2 3 4 5 6 7 8 9 10
Will you come back for a procedure if needed	Yes/No
Will you recommend the center	Yes/No
Comment	

be dissatisfied despite the best efforts on part of the practice. Even that patient needs to be treated with respect and compassion. OEC is the site of service which lends itself to strive for 100% patient satisfaction.

REFERENCES

1. Hamilton DF, Lane JV, Gaston P, et al. What determines patient satisfaction with surgery? A prospective cohort study of 4709 patients following total joint replacement. *BMJ Open*. 2013;3(4). https://doi.org/10.1136/bmjopen-2012-002525.
2. *Crossing the Quality Chasm*. Washington, D.C.: National Academies Press; 2001. https://doi.org/10.17226/10027.
3. Jain KM, Munn J, Rummel M, Vaddineni S, Longton C. Future of vascular surgery is in the office. *J Vasc Surg*. 2010. https://doi.org/10.1016/j.jvs.2009.09.056.
4. Lin PH, Yang K-H, Kollmeyer KR, et al. Treatment outcomes and lessons learned from 5134 cases of outpatient office-based endovascular procedures in a vascular surgical practice. *Vascular*. 2017;25(2):115–122. https://doi.org/10.1177/1708538116657506.
5. El-Gamil AM, Dobson A, Manolov N, et al. What is the best setting for receiving dialysis vascular access repair and maintenance services? *J Vasc Access*. 2017;18(6):473–481. https://doi.org/10.5301/jva.5000790.
6. VanderVeen NT, Friedman J, Rummel M, et al. PC190. Improving the retrieval rate of inferior vena cava filters: impact of inferior vena cava filter retrieval in the office endovascular center. *J Vasc Surg*. 2018. https://doi.org/10.1016/j.jvs.2018.03.339.
7. Holliday AM, Kachalia A, Meyer GS, Sequist TD. Physician and patient views on public physician rating websites: a cross-sectional study. *J Gen Intern Med*. 2017;32(6):626–631. https://doi.org/10.1007/s11606-017-3982-5.
8. Widmer RJ, Maurer MJ, Nayar VR, et al. Online physician reviews do not reflect patient satisfaction survey responses. *Mayo Clin Proc*. 2018;93(4):453–457. https://doi.org/10.1016/j.mayocp.2018.01.021.

CHAPTER 19

Registry

BOB TAHARA, MD, FSVS, FACS, RVT, RPVI • JEFFREY G. CARR, MD, FACC, FSCAI

INTRODUCTION

Office-based endovascular centers (OECs) also known as outpatient interventional suites (OISs) or office-based labs (OBLs) have continued to grow throughout the United States with an accompanying shift from inpatient and hospital-based care to outpatient and office-based interventions.[1,2] This has included marked increase in the number of outpatient peripheral interventional procedures, cardiac diagnostic/interventional procedures, dialysis interventions, interventional oncology-related procedures and a wide array of both superficial and deep venous procedures. As this shift has become more pronounced, there has been a corresponding increase in concern and focus on quality of care provided in the outpatient sites of service. This focus has included questions on appropriateness, patient selection, procedural conduct and safety, and ultimately outcome measures.[2,3] While there have been multiple peer-reviewed publications documenting the safety and efficacy of office-based interventions, the majority of these papers report results from a single center or data from relatively small series.[4,5] A broad-based multicenter documentation of interventional experience in an office or freestanding facility has been elusive and challenging but is desirable.

Participation in a Quality Clinical Data Registry (QCDR) is one option that can be utilized to address some of these questions and concerns on a broader basis. Generally speaking, a clinical data registry enables the collection of clinically relevant data about a specific disease state, condition, or procedure(s) with the goal of documenting and understanding basic patient characteristics and demography, disease morphology and expression, risks and exacerbating factors, procedural characteristics, and outcomes. Specific registries may also concentrate on tracking data such as safety and efficacy, complications, cost data, and any other cogent variables and factors. The data can then be analyzed to allow the assessment and provide useful information regarding real-world practice patterns, clinical pathways or guidelines, risk stratification, cost-benefit ratios, optimal use of new or existing treatments or devices, and potential contraindications.

In addition to the analytics and pure scientific utility of clinical registries, there are a growing number of federal regulations which require data reporting through a QCDR. Registry participation may also be used to satisfy some or all of the requirements attendant to the Merit-Based Incentive Payment System (MIPS) as mandated by the Medicare Access and CHIPs Reauthorization Act (MACRA) which was signed into law in 2015.[6]

Desired Features and Value of Clinical Data Registries

Ideally a clinical data registry should have several desirable characteristics:

1) Reasonably easy data entry
2) Collection of the clinically relevant variable information in a manner that makes sense to the participating clinician
3) Scalable architecture which allows or already incorporates implementation of different modules or modalities to accommodate changing care patterns
4) Adequate and timely reporting and analytics
5) Reasonable cost basis
6) Data that support a site's quality improvement functions and the ability to satisfy statutory and/or regulatory reporting requirements

We will broadly examine some of these characteristics and then describe specific currently available clinical data registries which are in use and applicable to the OEC/OIS.

REGISTRY CHARACTERISTICS

Data Entry

For a clinical data registry to have any utility at all, one must first enter relevant data into the registry! Data entry is fundamentally impacted by the design and

Office-Based Endovascular Centers. https://doi.org/10.1016/B978-0-323-67969-5.00019-8
Copyright © 2020 Elsevier Inc. All rights reserved.

architecture of a particular database. Initially, many databases or tracking programs were individually hosted on hardware resident in a particular hospital, facility, or office leading to implementations that were potentially "one off" and limited by both the systems utilized as well as the technical support personnel and programmers available to that site. Additionally, these databases were proprietary to the group or institution and inherently were limited in scope. Modern "big data" paradigms have fundamentally shifted this architecture to a virtual, cloud-based hosting environment that now encompasses a wide array of SQL and NoSQL database architectures allowing accumulation and rapid processing of a staggering number of variables and data points.

The majority of currently available clinical data registries utilize a web-based electronic data collection (EDC) format. The advantage of this approach is wide accessibility of data from any device capable of running a compatible web browser, near instant upload of the entered information into the database, and the ability to edit entries if appropriate. Typically, current registries incorporate fairly robust security provisions with granular role-based permissions that allow both clinicians and their ancillary staff to enter and review patient data during and after entry into the EDC.

Disadvantages include the need for reasonably robust Internet access, the need for accurately typing in free text if required or making appropriate menu or drop-down selections, difficulties with passwords and usernames, and any or all of the attendant technical difficulties websites may experience.

Web-based EDCs frequently incorporate multiple entry mechanisms including free text, numerical data, multiple choice selections, and/or menu-based options. Free entry options for both textual strings and numerical data allow a basically unlimited and a long range of data entry. Disadvantages of free entry include the interjection of variability in format and values that could potentially render the data difficult or impossible to analyze, transcriptional errors, and a greater time/typing requirement. Menu-based or multiple-choice options allow for standardization of values, formats, and speedy entry but decrease the possible data entry range as compared with free entry.

Even more efficient and idealized mechanism for data entry potentially is either by direct transfer or some type of export/import facility of structured data transfer from an electronic medical record (EMR) into the registry database. Advantages of this approach would include an elimination of transcriptional or selection errors, elimination of hand entry and the attendant savings in both personnel time and costs. Disadvantages include direct transfer of data which was erroneously entered into the EMR, a host of potential technical hurdles to implementation, and the cost of implementation on a widespread basis. At the current time, despite data transfer standards such as HLA7, there is substantial variation between different EMR products' capability to store their own data, database architecture support, and implementation of data transfers and/or exports. This functionally leads to a situation where each individual product requires individual programming or mapping to enable a direct transfer or export/import functionality, which in turn substantially increases the cost of implementation. Smaller organizations, offices, or physician practices rarely have the resources to implement these types of transfers at the local level and larger organizations may have a host of competing technical demands. Both scenarios often preclude development of transfer and/or export/import facilities to a clinical registry. Despite these technical hurdles, there will likely be automatic electronic transfer of data from EMRs into clinical registries in the future to improve efficiencies and reduce the burden of data entry duplication.

REGISTRY ARCHITECTURE

While a complete discussion of back-end database architecture is beyond the scope of this chapter, we will briefly explore characteristics the authors believe are desirable in a clinical data registry.

Both SQL and NoSQL database engines provide advantages and disadvantages in the architecture of the database. Both types are broadly incorporated into several clinical data registries, allow appropriate queries and data analysis, and have mature enterprise level support for clinical registry vendors. Regardless of the basic database engine used, it is absolutely essential that the database structure incorporates appropriate relationships between the variables and between different table and file structures so that proper analytics can be performed. This basic structure generally needs to be established very early in the database design phase and essentially requires some understanding of desired and required analysis of data as the end product. Data should be collected based on the questions that are being asked and need an answer.

Development of various database modules for different disease states and procedures is a basic requirement to meet the evolving needs of the OEC/OIS/OBL. Considering the range of cardiovascular procedures that are currently performed in outpatient environment, there is a need for either (1) individual clinical registry for specific category of disease/interventions or (2) more comprehensive registries that have multiple disease-specific/intervention-specific modules. Using multiple individual registries for each specific type of disease or intervention rapidly complicates the logistics, data entry complexity, staff time, and cost of participation for practices or sites that perform multiple types of interventions that include peripheral arterial, venous, cardiac, dialysis access, and other interventions. A possibly easier and more cost-effective option would be to utilize a clinical data registry that has a common entry and cost structure but incorporates multiple modules to report on different disease processes or interventions. Potential required modules include peripheral arterial interventions, diagnostic coronary angiography and coronary interventions, cardiac rhythm interventions/management, dialysis access formation and interventions, and superficial/deep venous interventions. Unfortunately, as detailed further in this chapter, no single clinical registry currently fulfills and supports all of these module requirements.

REPORTING AND ANALYTICS

The ability to analyze the raw data entered into a clinical data registry is another basic required function. Ideally this reporting would update either in real-time or on a regular and frequently scheduled basis, be available for viewing online and provide the ability to download reports and results, provide participating clinicians with information that is meaningful and answers cogent clinical questions. The ability to benchmark individual physicians, groups or virtual groups against the aggregated data may provide valuable insights into care patterns, utilization rates, and allows the reporting of data for quality assurance/improvement activities.

Basic reporting should allow analysis of patient demographics, risk factors, disease severity, identification of complications and complication rates, and intervention-specific outcome measures. More sophisticated analytics may provide subgroup analysis which allows drilling down to an individual risk or morphology in an effort to find optimal treatment modalities and minimize complication potential. For example, basic reporting could give a range and average of patient ages, incidence of diabetes and/or hypertension etc., and the overall complication rate for a particular intervention such as angioplasty. More detailed analysis might provide a more granular report. It may be possible to study patient outcomes using a specific device or modality for a specific subset of patients, i.e., vessel patency at various intervals while using a particular atherectomy device or stent in patients over the age of 70 with elevated LDL levels.

Reports may take a multitude of forms ranging from simple tabular results to very sophisticated visualizations using a variety of line graphs, bar graphs, or pie charts (Fig. 19.1). Interactive reporting where queries or graphs can be clicked on to drill down to more granular details is often desired by clinicians. Well-designed clinical reporting dashboards help consolidate reporting in an accessible manner and simplify viewing of both site-specific and aggregated results. Leveraging cloud-based computing resources so that all of the CPU-intensive computation is performed on the hosting server is faster and more scalable than downloading raw data and performing the analysis on a local machine or device. Additionally, mobile-optimized websites can potentially offer this type of reporting accessible via handheld devices allowing the data to be viewed at the bedside and across different locations.

REGULATORY/STATUTORY REQUIREMENTS

Clinical data registries can be used to meet certain federal requirements. QCDRs are a subset of all existing clinical data registries and can be used to report data satisfying a portion of the MIPS requirements that were established under MACRA. A clinical data registry may nominate itself to the Center for Medicare Services (CMS) in order to be considered for QCDR status. If the registry meets CMS-defined requirements, it may be granted QCDR status which allows the registry to be used by eligible clinicians/groups for MIPS reporting. These requirements are posted on the CMS website. Reporting requirements have changed significantly since originally approved in 2015. There are additional ongoing requirements to maintain QCDR status including meeting and conference participation, documentation review and revision, auditing functions, and quality measure reviews that must be conducted in accordance with the current CMS regulations and guidance. The authors anticipate that there will continue to be quite a bit of fluidity in the QCDR/MIPS/MACRA reporting and qualification requirements in the future and that the one constant we can count on is that, there will be changes in reporting requirements. Notwithstanding these challenges, possessing a designated QCDR status is a highly desirable quality for registries.

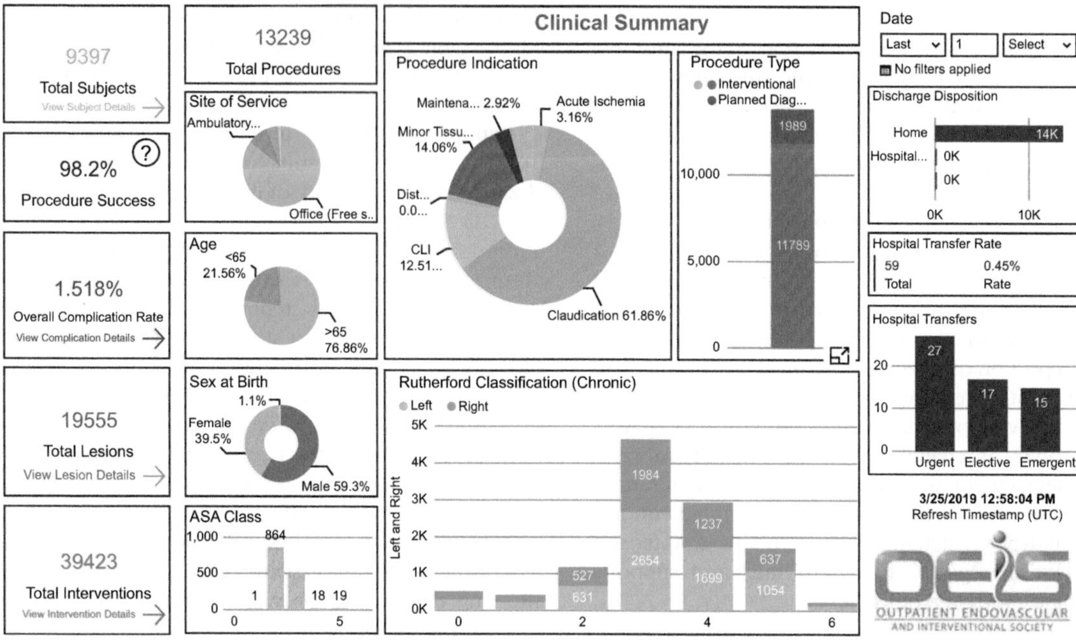

FIG. 19.1 Screenshots of Outpatient Endovascular and Interventional Society (OEIS) National Registry Dashboard.

Currently Available and Applicable Clinical Data Registries

There are several clinical data registries that are currently in operation and support in whole or part many of the interventions being performed in outpatient settings. Some of these are outpatient focused, i.e., Outpatient Endovascular and Interventional Society (OEIS) National Registry, while others really began and are primarily focused on hospital-based care but allow for outpatient case data entry, i.e., VQI. Some are split between the inpatient and outpatient intervention, i.e., National Cardiovascular Data Registry (NCDR). Some registries are very specific to single disease entities, i.e., American Vein and Lymphatic Society (AVLS formerly ACP) Venous Registry and NCDR peripheral vascular intervention (PVI) Registry. Some have started with a particular facet of care and have plans to add modules, i.e., OEIS National Registry currently enrolls only peripheral arterial interventions but has plans to add coronary and rhythm management, venous, and dialysis modules. Unfortunately, no single registry that is currently available meets the requirements of all the procedures carried out in OEC. We briefly summarize the key attributes of the currently available registries.[7]

OEIS National Registry

The OEIS was founded in 2013 for the express purpose of promoting high-quality patient-centric care in the outpatient interventional suite. Membership in this organization is deliberately multidisciplinary and primarily composed of vascular surgeons, interventional cardiologists, and interventional radiologists performing cases in an outpatient or office environment. To advance the goal of reporting outcomes and serve as a platform for research, the OEIS National Registry was conceived and became operational in January 2017. The first module to come online was the Peripheral Arterial Interventions module. This collects and analyzes data related to lower extremity arterial intervention in the outpatient and office sites of service. The registry is structured around a NoSQL back end (MongoDB, MongoDB Inc.) with a proprietary web-based EDC (Syncrony-Syntactx Corporation) which is utilized by participating sites for data entry and accessing reports. The registry allows for exporting of raw data and completed analytics. Aggregated and site-specific data/analytic dashboards are available online to participating sites, and some summary data are available publicly. Direct export/import from EMRs is not currently available but is under development at the time of this publication. Reporting is currently in the form of a set of fairly sophisticated dashboards which allow the participating sites/clinicians to view the results of a defined set of CMS-approved quality measures, patient demographic and comorbidity data, procedural and interventional data, complications, and long-term outcomes such as patency and amputation rates. Interactive dashboards allow subgroup analysis.

At the time of this writing, the registry has 62 sites and has enrolled nearly 17,000 peripheral arterial intervention cases in its first 2 years of existence. The OEIS NR is an approved QCDR and supports reporting of CMS-approved Quality Measures and Improvement Activities as part of MIPS. This provides a vehicle for registry subscribers to submit their performance on certified quality measures to receive an adjustment for reimbursement for their Medicare cases. Costs to subscribe to the OEIS registry are modest with a defined monthly fee, a discount for active OEIS members, and zero setup fees. At the time of writing, the monthly OEIS member rate is $175.00/month per site. Further information can be found by accessing the OEIS NR webpages at https://oeisociety.com/oeis-national-registry/.

The Vascular Quality Initiative[8,9]

The Vascular Quality Initiative (VQI) was originally created in 1982 as a regional effort by the Vascular Study Group of New England (VSGNE) to track, standardize, and improve vascular care and outcomes. The VQI underwent further development in content, scope, and platform and was subsequently adopted by the Society of Vascular Surgery (SVS) in 2011. The VQI is now more than a registry and is a formally recognized Patient Safety Organization (PSO). It currently offers 12 modules including AAA, TEVAR, carotid interventions (both CEA and CAS), venous interventions, hemodialysis access, peripheral vascular interventions (PVIs), infrainguinal and suprainguinal bypass, and others. Additional modules being actively developed include a noninvasive vascular ultrasound module and vascular medicine management module. VQI has robust support from the SVS. PSO is an LLC owned and administered by SVS with a formal governance and administrative structure for the PSO itself. A formal VQI Research Committee exists and is active in directing and facilitating data harvest and publications documenting results from enrolled cases. The PSO also has established specific Arterial and Venous Quality Councils and has a number of ongoing Quality Initiatives that are actively managed.

The database structure is SQL based for transactions and NoSQL for the actual analytics. The EDC is web-based and currently developed and administered by M2S (West Lebanon, NH). Collected data fields are both comprehensive and detailed which requires a significant investment in staff time for data entry and typically requires institutional support. VQI has recently developed a "basic" input version which reportedly markedly decreases the collected data points in response to user concerns about the time required for data entry in the office/outpatient venue. Direct EMR imports/exports are not yet fully enabled. The registry does allow for exporting of data and completed analytics in various formats. Aggregated and site-specific data/analytic dashboards are available online to participating sites, and some summary data are publicly available. The dashboard reports are comprehensive, and subgroup analysis is available. At the time of this writing, the VQI has 557 participating centers, 18 regional groups, and over 576,000 entered cases including about 183,000 peripheral interventions. The overwhelming majority of these enrolled cases were performed in inpatient hospital setting in North America and none of the modules is outpatient specific. VQI is an approved QCDR and supports reporting of CMS-approved Quality Measures and Improvement Activities as part of MIPS. Costs, however, are substantial with an initial setup fee of $5000.00 and a subscription fee of $2500.00 per module utilized. Some variable discounts are available dependent on institution and number of participating centers subscribed via a particular site. VQI is the most comprehensive and expensive registry for PVI. Further information can be found by accessing the VQI website at https://www.vqi.org/about/.

National Cardiovascular Data Registry[10]

The National Cardiovascular Data Registry (NCDR) was originally developed in 1997 by the American College of Cardiology (ACC). The original focus was on cardiology-specific intervention and has been expanded to currently offer eight hospital-based registries including acute STEMI/NSTEMI interventions, elective percutaneous coronary intervention, implantable cardioverter-defibrillator, congenital heart disease, and PVIs. There is also a module for atrial fibrillation ablation and a module jointly managed with the Society for Thoracic Surgery (STS) analyzing transcatheter valve therapies. There are two outpatient-specific registries which track (1) outpatient medical management of coronary artery disease, hypertension, heart failure, atrial fibrillation, and diabetes, and (2) a diabetes-specific registry which is used to track diabetes care across a wider spectrum of providers, not simply cardiology. Currently, there is no outpatient-specific procedural module or registry.

The database structure and back end are not disclosed. Data entry is enabled via a web-based EDC or hospitals may choose from several software/service vendors to enable transfer from hospital EMR and internal data collection methods into the applicable NCDR registry. Collected data fields are extensive and detailed but there has been significant development allowing EMR import/exports particularly from the outpatient registry modules and thus often minimizing staff data entry time. Basic analytics and dashboard functions are available for each applicable registry within the NCDR portfolio and more extensive reporting is available. Public reporting of aggregate data is not available. Site-specific reporting has been made voluntary but reporting without explicit hospital permission is not allowed. Custom analytics with relatively sophisticated drill down capabilities are available but require both time and additional costs to develop and generate. At the time of this writing, NCDR has more than 2400 participating hospitals. The two outpatient-specific registry modules, PINNACLE Registry and the Diabetes Collaborative Registry, are designated QCDRs and support reporting for MIPS requirements. The web address for NCDR is https://cvquality.acc.org/NCDR-Home. The cost for NCDR is $5920 per annum for the PVI Registry with a one time implementation fee of $1000. Additional information may be found at https://www.ncdr.com.https://www.ncdr.com

XL-PAD Registry[11,12]

The XL-PAD Registry was launched with the support of an NIH grant and seeks to publish clinical data related to PVI from participating sites. The registry was designed to close enrollment after 14,000 patients were entered and was designed to describe three main clinical outcomes (1) to compare stent versus nonstent outcomes as a composite of repeat revascularization and ipsilateral target limb amputation at 12 months postintervention, (2) to compare stent versus nonstent composite outcomes including death, myocardial infarction, and the outcomes listed in (1), and finally (3) to compare functional outcomes including walking distance and Rutherford classification for stent versus nonstent interventions. The registry utilizes approximately 60 sites for enrolling the 14,000 patients. The database structure appears to be an SQL-type database and the web-based EDC is based on data entry utilizing the University of Texas Southwestern REDCap program. The XL-PAD requires mandatory submission to a core lab to adjudicate angiographic findings and degree of stenosis for interventions. The registry is limited to infrainguinal peripheral arterial interventions and specifically excludes failed attempts at revascularization, surgical bypass procedures, or when only the iliac artery is treated. Dashboards and site-specific analytics are not available nor does it appear that there is the ability to export either raw data or analytics. As of the writing of this document, this registry is not a CMS-certified QCDR. More information can be found at the XL-PAD website https://www.xlpad.org/studies-and-research.

The PRO Registry[13]

The PRO Registry is AVLS registry that is used for superficial venous disease interventions and therapies. The AVLS was originally founded in 1985 as the North American Society of Phlebology and subsequently in 1997 changed its name to the American College of Phlebology. In 2018, the name was changed to AVLS. The PRO Registry was initiated in 2014 and as of this writing has over 24,000 superficial venous procedures entered including over 18,000 endovenous thermal ablations and 6000 chemical ablations. The registry also incorporates reporting of noninterventional therapy such as compression and noninterventional treatment modalities for venous ulcers. The registry database structure is an SQL at the back end. There is a web-based EDC that allows manual entry of data, but the AVLS encourages usage of import/export directly from a limited number of EMRs that have been certified to work with the registry system. The overwhelming majority of data currently entered into the registry has been inputted via EMR import/export. A current listing of those EMR products is posted on the AVLS PRO Registry webpage at www.veinandlymph.org. Aggregated and physician-specific dashboards and analytics are available, and these data are incorporated into the AVLS quality initiatives and research programs. The PRO Registry is not currently a QCDR and consequently, there is no provision for MIPS reporting incorporated into the registry product. Costs are $4000 for non-AVLS members and $2000 per annum per participating physician for an AVLS member. There is no setup fee and discounts on subscription costs are available for physicians that contribute to the Foundation for Venous and Lymphatic Disorders. More information can be found at the AVLS website https://www.veinandlymph.org.

Summary and Conclusions

Clinical data registries are a growing and vital part of the value-based healthcare era. The available clinical data registries have grown and evolved to support specific

TABLE 19.1
Summary Table Comparing Registries.

Registry	Outpatient Specific?	Peripheral Arterial Module?	Venous Module?	Cardiac Module?	Dialysis Module?	Additional Modules?	Direct EMR Import	QCDR	Setup Fees
OEIS NR	Yes	Yes	Planned	Planned	Planned	No	No	Yes	No
SVS VQI	No	Yes	Yes	No	Yes	Multiple, 12 total	No	Yes	Yes
NCDR	No	Yes	No	Yes	No	STS, medical Rx, etc.	No	No	Yes
XL-PAD	No	Yes	No	No	No	No	No	No	No
AVLS PRO	No	No	Yes	No	No	No	Yes	No	No

procedure-based interventions in hospital and outpatient settings. It is essential to ensure that increasing volume of high-quality data that is generated is captured in a registry in a way that accurately portrays the real-world conduct and outcomes of cardiovascular and PVIs in the office and outpatient environment. As the number of outpatient procedures continues to increase, there is mounting interest by patients, physicians, and healthcare organizations to optimize care in this setting. The aim of the participants and the registries is to be able to perform procedures in any setting for the right indications, resulting in optimal outcomes, be cost-effective, and provide data for future innovation. Additionally, clinical data registries are useful tools in continuous quality improvement in any organization. There is also mounting pressure on the physicians brought about by payers and regulatory agencies to furnish clinical data points so that reasonable decisions regarding insurance coverage, appropriateness, and quality assurance can be made. Registries have been developed in part to help answer these and many other questions.

As described in this chapter, currently available registries vary in their complexity, cost, and comprehensiveness, and span a wide range of structures and formats (Table 19.1). It is incumbent on physicians and organizations offering procedures in the outpatient setting to participate and actively enter data into the registry most appropriate or germane to the cases being performed. Challenges remain in creating uniform reporting standards, enhancing the electronic transfer of desired data points from EMRs directly into the various databases, and in translating the analytic results to quality care metrics and healthcare policy decisions that benefit the patients and make sense to the clinicians. Ultimately, registry supported analytics and lessons learned can provide the platforms and roadmaps for providing optimum care in a cost-effective manner to this very complex group of patients with cardiovascular disease.

REFERENCES

1. National trends in lower extremity bypass surgery, endovascular interventions, and major amputations Goodney, P.P. et al. J Vasc Surg, Volume 50, Issue 1, 54–60.
2. Jones WS, et al. Trends in settings for peripheral vascular intervention and the effect of changes in the outpatient prospective payment system. *J Am Coll Cardiol.* 2015;65: 920–927.
3. The disproportionate growth of office-based atherectomy Mukherjee, Dipankar et al. J Vasc Surg, Volume 65, Issue 2, 495–500.
4. Office-based endovascular suite is safe for most procedures Jain, Krishna et al J Vasc Surg, Volume 59, Issue 1, 186 – 191.
5. Treatment outcomes and lessons learned from 5134 cases of outpatient office-based endovascular procedures in a vascular surgical practice. L., Peter et al. Vascular Volume 25, Issue 2, 115–122.
6. https://www.cms.gov/Medicare/Quality-Initiatives-Patient-Assessment-Instruments/Value-Based-Programs/MACRA-MIPS-and-APMs/MACRA-MIPS-and-APMs.html. Accessed May 2019.
7. https://oeisociety.com/oeis-national-registry/. Accessed May 2019.
8. https://www.vqi.org/wp-content/uploads/VQI-Summary-Sides-March-2019.pdf. Accessed May 2019.
9. https://www.vqi.org/wp-content/uploads/YearinReview-2017-18-Digital.pdf. Accessed May 2019.

10. https://cvquality.acc.org/NCDR-Home/Registries. Accessed May 2019.
11. https://clinicaltrials.gov/ct2/show/NCT01904851 XL-PAD clinical trial listing. Accessed May 2019.
12. https://www.xlpad.org/s/XLPAD-Manual.pdf. XL-PAD user manual Accessed May 2019.
13. http://www.phlebology.org/member-resources/acp-pro-venous-registry. Accessed May 20129.

CHAPTER 20

Marketing

ELIAS H. KASSAB, MD, FACC, FSCAI, FACP, FASA, RPVI, FAHA, FSVM • ANNA LEYSON-FIEL, BSN, RN, CCRC

Patients have more options than ever before. With so much information available online, they no longer feel the need to visit the hospital or practice closest to their location. That is why it is crucial to have a planned marketing strategy to reach out to new and returning patients to your practice and endovascular center. To be successful in your healthcare business, it must have a strong identity. Branding is the process which builds this identity and differentiates your practice from others.[1]

Branding and marketing are the same thing—this is untrue!

Marketing is the act of promoting a product to earn revenue. Marketers push out a message, usually telling the consumer why their product is better than a competitor's product. Branding is completely different. Branding should occur before a marketing strategy ever begins. Branding is not the act of pushing out a message. On the contrary, it is the pulling in of a message. It is listening to the consumer and using that information to build a brand strategy.[2]

According to the *Harvard Business Review*, the benefit of consciously shaping a leading brand is that it allows the physician to focus. When the physician knows with the utmost clarity what he/she wants to be known for, it is easier to let go of the tasks and projects that do not focus on delivering on the brand, and on concentrating on activities that do.[13]

Decide what you wish to be known for, develop a list of characteristics to help define identity and your brand. Characteristics should include putting patients first, unsurpassed service, superior patient outcomes, patient-friendly environment, accepts widest range of insurance, compassionate, advanced technology and research, knowledgeable and friendly staff, easy to schedule appointments etc.[3]

Combine the list of characteristics to form the desired identity:

- "Putting patients first by combining leading technology with superior outcomes."
- "Patient-friendly environment accepting all types of insurance with easy to schedule appointment."
- "Compassionate, knowledgeable, and friendly staff focused on superior patient outcomes based on science."

Branding is a service based on trust, time, deliverability, and relationships. It takes 12 positive experiences to make up one unresolved negative experience.[4] According to Warren Buffett, "It takes 20 years to build a reputation and 5 min to ruin it." It is easier to deliver this service in an office-based endovascular center (OEC) than in a hospital setting. Your brand is more than your logo, name, or slogan—it is the entire experience your prospects and customers have with your company, product, or service. Your brand strategy defines what you stand for, a promise you make, and the personality you convey.[5]

Successful healthcare marketing is complicated and sometimes confusing. These six fundamental elements, (1) Professional Referral Marketing, (2) Internet Marketing, (3) Branding, (4) Internal Marketing, (5) External Marketing, (6) Public Relations and the SCALE method (Satisfaction, Collaboration, Adaptation, Location, Education), demystify the healthcare market.

PROFESSIONAL REFERRAL MARKETING

A reliable and continuing stream of patient referrals from other medical or other professional sources is the lifeblood of many specialty providers, including your endovascular practice.

Doctor referrals do not happen by magic or simply because you are a good doctor.

Success requires a written plan and an unfailing system to preserve and grow the flow of professional referrals.[5]

These are the essential elements for success in Professional Referral Marketing:[6]

Office-Based Endovascular Centers. https://doi.org/10.1016/B978-0-323-67969-5.00020-4
Copyright © 2020 Elsevier Inc. All rights reserved.

Confidence

Other professionals will refer patients to you if they like and trust you. "Like" is vital, but "trust" is paramount. It is a matter of *confidence* in you that the referral will be appropriate and beneficial to the patient's care. "Confidence" never happens without a stable *relationship*. Of course, there is an assumption of professional competence, but that alone is not sufficient to distinguish and differentiate between physicians. Professionals will refer with confidence when there is a reliable and robust relationship in place.

Credibility

First of all, proper credentials are a must—your education, training, experience form a foundation for *credibility*. Credentials and a professional CV are essential, but a deep sense of credibility is about the experience. Delivering what the referral sources value most in caring for their patients and making their life more comfortable. Credibility grows when a referral source truly appreciates you as a valuable resource or extension of their work. (It is that *relationship* thing again.)[3]

Consistent Communications

"Failure to communicate" regularly with the sources of referrals can cause lasting damage.

Consumer satisfaction translates into current business, repeat business, and referral business. People enjoy doing business with people they like. Conversely, dissatisfied customers head over to the competition.[7]

Constant communication with the source of referrals results in satisfaction. The referral source is also your customer and needs to be satisfied.

Positive patient satisfaction helps retain existing customers. Marketing pros understand the value of current customers, as well as the added expense related to replacing a dissatisfied customer.[7]

Negative patient experience results in a direct deposit to the competition. The loss of a patient typically results in the growth of your competitor's practice. To make things worse, it is likely that the departing patient was instrumental in the defection of one or more friends or family members.[7]

Facts about customer experience

- 96% of unhappy customers do not complain; however, 91% of those will leave and never come back—1st Financial Training Services
- A dissatisfied customer will tell 9–15 people about their experience. Around 13% of dissatisfied customers tells more than 20 people.—White House Office of Consumer Affairs
- 70% of buying experiences are based on how the customer feels they are being treated—McKinsey
- 55% of customers would pay extra to guarantee a better service—Defaqto research
- Price is not the main reason for customer churn. It is actually due to the overall poor quality of customer service—Accenture Global Customer Satisfaction Report, 2008
- 94% of customers do not want to be transferred to another representative more than once—Mobius Poll 2002
- 80% of customers prefer to speak with a representative on weekends—Mobius Poll 2002
- 84% of customers are frustrated when a representative does not have immediate access to account information—Mobius Poll 2002
- It takes 12 positive experiences to make up for one unresolved negative experience—"Understanding Customers" by Ruby Newell

INTERNET MARKETING

From websites and social media tools to patient portals and mobile apps, online marketing is a mainstream channel for marketing, advertising, and public relations. Exactly how you use the muscle of the digital freeway can be highly effective and profitable, or a huge waste of time and money.[8]

US Internet users conduct 5 billion searches every month directly on major search sites. Furthermore, a recent Harris Interactive Poll reported that more than 80% of consumers now research health information online.[9] Imagine how many of those Internet users are prospective patients in your area looking for the services you offer. It is crucial to have a website for the practice and OEC that is pleasant, informative, easy to navigate, and current. There are websites created by practices that were created a few years ago and never updated. In addition to giving the basic information about the practices like location, parking, office hours, etc., the site can be a great source of patient education. The procedures done in the office can be described. Preprocedure and postprocedure instructions can be included. The links can be created to take patients to a reputable source of information. You have an opportunity to educate the patients in the right way. The website is an extension of you and the practice and should be developed and maintained in that spirit.

Use of social media depends on the type of practice and competition. It is essential to market a venous practice in this manner but may not be equally important in marketing a limb preservation practice. There are experts in the social media marketing space and should be utilized if the practice wants to spend money in this market. Social media is continually evolving, make sure there is no HIPAA violation.

BRANDING

It is all about standing out from the crowd in a positive way, and it includes virtually everything you do. A powerful, differentiating brand for your healthcare business is part of your reputation. Meaningful and effective branding does not occur without a deliberate effort to shape and express the right message at the right time.[8]

Seven reasons why you should brand your healthcare organization[10]:

1. People prefer to buy brands because they reduce perceived risk.
2. People buy brands for status.
3. People refer more often and more passionately to a brand they like and trust.
4. You can build and accelerate your reputation through branding.
5. You can attract more of the cases you want through branding.
6. Branding will give you a competitive advantage.
7. A branded healthcare organization will be worth more than a nonbranded business.

Strong brands are more profitable and increase company value.[11]

INTERNAL MARKETING

The patients who know you are happy will market your practice to their family members and friends at no cost to you. Loyal patients are a great source of internal marketing. They can be a precious resource of referrals, testimonials, and word of mouth advertising. Usually forgotten, the source of internal marketing is your employees. Employees have friends and family members who may need your services. Happy employees become your brand ambassadors. The hospital employees where you practice have the potential of referring a significant number of patients to you. So, be kind to them.

Keep your name in front of patients and referrals.

It takes five or more encounters with your practice's name for it to be recognized. Your name should appear anywhere potential patients would possibly look.[12] These would include the local phone book (not yellow pages), physician directories, physician-listing services, digital media, etc. Free-standing office signs are one of the most effective marketing investments if the location allows it. Twice a year, mailings to patients and residents can also be useful.

Every patient should leave your office with a piece of literature at every visit. Do not let them leave empty handed! Quality pamphlets, like those offered by the many vendors, are an inexpensive way of spreading awareness about your unique practice services. Consider your own, practice-specific, brochure with a relevant appointment and procedure/educational information.

EXTERNAL MARKETING

External marketing uses the media that reach prospective patients who do not know you. Advertising in newspapers, radio, television, billboards, etc. target an audience that needs to know the services you provide to take care of their healthcare need. The margin for error is minimal in an external media budget that is expected to produce a measurable return on investment.

Audiovisual Marketing

Advertisements on radio and television are expensive and should be used with a specific purpose in mind. Television ads are more expensive than radio ads. Direct to consumer marketing needs to be focused and needs to be a part of the overall marketing strategy.

Print Media

Gradually, more and more consumers are getting their information from the Internet. It may not be advisable to spend money on advertisements in newspapers. The telephone books are almost dead. Spending money on yellow pages advertising is not desirable.

PUBLIC RELATIONS

Among other things, planning and generating healthcare publicity, "free press" exposure and public relations activities start with the physician. The physician is the best marketer and instrumental in developing positive public relations. Physicians should dress appropriately at all times and be pleasant in interaction with the referring physicians, coworkers, and patients. The physician should have an aura of authority while being compassionate, knowledgeable, accessible, honest, and trustworthy. The office staff should be cooperative, friendly, and easily approachable. It is all "about the patient." The practice exists because of the patients, and the practice should reflect this in its attitude. The office environment should be patient-friendly. A dirty, unkempt office does not build confidence. The magazines and brochures in the reception area should be updated promptly.

Local media outlets are always looking for reliable medical information to take to their consumers. The practice can make itself available for radio and television interviews, and the physician can write articles for the newspapers. The practice can participate in local, regional, and national health events, like health fare, PAD screening programs, etc.

Satisfaction

Patient satisfaction is the key to the success of an OEC. Your brand grows one patient/family at a time. The OEC can accomplish this by providing a patient-friendly environment, consistent/familiar staff, timely service, and same-day patient discharge. The data are clear; OEC makes life safe and convenient for patients. There are fewer complications and hassles. Patients go home the same day, and there is a significant cost reduction. Plenty of patient satisfaction data are now available, showing patients are delighted with their experience at outpatient centers.

The Harvard Business Review suggests asking patients two questions: (1) Were you satisfied with the quality of your experience and (2) would you come to us again. This strategy comes from the work of Andy Taylor, CEO at Enterprise Rent-A-Car. He discovered these two simple questions that helped the company gain its industry-wide advantage among stiff competition, all without elaborate questionnaires and cumbersome survey.

Collaboration

Working together provides an advantage to all, and in the process makes everyone better. Working with the industry, government, and service partners in healthcare will pay dividends later. The CMS Medicare Physician Fee Schedule Proposed Rule, released on July 8, 2013, articulated CMS's intention to reduce the "nonfacility" reimbursement by up to 50%. This proposed methodology spanned over the gamut of all outpatient services. These were very alarming to the OEC owners and their constituents and sparked the need for physicians to come together (Chapter 37) and educate the CMS. This was marketing at the national payer level. Afterall as an individual organization CMS is the biggest payer of health services.

The Outpatient Endovascular and Interventional Society (OEIS) was developed after the landmark meeting in Dallas, Texas, by the 15 founding fathers: five vascular surgeons, five interventional cardiologists, five interventional radiologists. The OEIS rapidly evolved into the voice of OEC owners. Because of the collaborative efforts of outpatient vascular center leadership, other organizations and the OEIS efforts the final CMS ruling published in November 2013 did not include the proposed changes to the methodology for determining payments for procedures performed in the OEC. The potentially cataclysmic proposed 50% reduction in reimbursement was marginally decreased.

Adaptation

ASCs/OEC can adjust to the fluid healthcare climate without compromising quality and excellent clinical outcomes. It is easier to streamline services and manage costs in an OEC as compared with a broader hospital environment. The physician owners of the OEC must remain current with the regulations affecting their business. The business can be only adept if it stays current with the changes affecting the OEC. As the technological advances come and patients demand the "latest and the greatest" the OEC should be able to adapt to follow the best clinical practice guidelines. AS the practice adapts to changing clinical indications and introduces new procedures, the OEC should continue to educate the referring physicians about the new services being provided through the OEC.

Location

The physical location of the ASC/OEC is essential. It should be near the target patient population, near public transportation and easy access to a highway and close to a hospital. While determining the location, the location of competitors should also be taken into account. If the practice is going to serve a large number of dialysis dependent patients it is prudent to have an OEC close to the dialysis unit. For limb preservation proximity to a wound center is extremely desirable.

Educate

The OEC must maintain the competitive edge in providing healthcare in the local market by staying current with the advances in endovascular therapy offered and by learning from one another. Ben Franklin wrote, "An investment in knowledge pays the best interest." Physicians are not trained in branding or marketing but must know when to get the advice of the branding and marketing experts. As novelist and scholar Ralph Ellison wrote: "Education is all a matter of building bridges." We must continue to build bridges with our colleagues, with the public, with insurance companies, and with the government.

The success of your practice depends on your marketing efforts. In today's competitive landscape, you cannot increase the return on investment simply by employing a tailored marketing strategy. There is no "one size fits all" formula to market your medical practice.

Create a unique selling proposition, a strategy that may work for one practice may not work for others. Focus your marketing efforts based on your skills and specialty. Brand your practice using the right marketing tools. The brand will outlast your practicing years and will benefit your current and future partners. Knowing your niche and marketing your medical practice is critical to your success.[14]

REFERENCES

1. Gandolf S. 15 Healthcare Marketing Strategies That Bring More Patients. Healthcare Success. https://www.healthcaresuccess.com/blog/healthcare-marketing/healthcare-marketing-strategy.html. Accessed August 6, 2019.
2. The Difference Between Marketing and Branding Strategies. Universal Class. https://www.universalclass.com/articles/business/the-difference-between-marketing-and-branding-strategies.htm. Accessed August 6, 2019.
3. Kassab EH. Business 101: Marketing Your Practice. http://media.oeisociety.org/multimedia/files/2018/pdf_fri/0945_Elias_Kassab.pdf. Accessed August 6, 2019.
4. Shaw C. *15 Statistics that Should Change the Business World – but Haven't.* Beyond Philosophy; June 10, 2013. https://beyondphilosophy.com/15-statistics-that-should-change-the-business-world-but-havent/.
5. Brand S.. Marketing MO. http://www.marketingmo.com/strategic-planning/brand-strategy/. Accessed August 6, 2019.
6. Hirsch L, Gandolf S. *The 3 C's for Winning Professional-To-Professional Referrals.* Dentistry IQ; October 5, 2010. https://www.dentistryiq.com/practice-management/article/16365058/the-3-cs-for-winning-professionaltoprofessional-referrals.
7. Gaughran KR, Gandolf S. Why patient satisfaction is key to physician marketing. Healthcare Success. https://www.healthcaresuccess.com/blog/physician-marketing/patient-satisfaction.html. Accessed August 6, 2019.
8. Gandolf S. 6 Proven ways to market any healthcare organization. Healthcare Success. https://www.healthcaresuccess.com/blog/healthcare-marketing/there-are-six-and-only-six-ways-to-market-any-healthcare-organization.html. Accessed August 6, 2019.
9. Gandolf S.How to start getting patients from your healthcare website tomorrow. Healthcare Success. https://www.healthcaresuccess.com/blog/healthcare-marketing/how-to-start-getting-patients-from-your-healthcare-website-tomorrow.html. Accessed August 6, 2019.
10. Gandolf s. Creating a powerful, differentiating brand. Healthcare Success. https://www.healthcaresuccess.com/blog/healthcare-marketing/branding.html. Accessed August 6, 2019.
11. Need to give your brand a health check? get brand audit. Persona Design. https://www.personadesign.ie/brand-audit/. Accessed August 6, 2019.
12. Borglum KC. *Top 10 Marketing Tips for Your Practice.* American Academy of Ophthalmology; March 1, 2008. https://www.aao.org/young-ophthalmologists/yo-info/article/top-10-marketing-tips-your-practice.
13. Smallwood N. Define your personal leadership brand in five steps. *Harv Bus Rev.* March 29, 2010. https://hbr.org/2010/03/define-your-personal-leadershi. Accessed August 6, 2019.

CHAPTER 21

Interventional Cardiologist's Perspective on Ambulatory Surgical Center / Office Based Labs

ELIAS H. KASSAB, MD, FACC, FSCAI, FACP, FASA, RPVI, FAHA, FSVM • ANNA LEYSON-FIEL, BSN, RN, CCRC

HISTORY OF INTERVENTIONAL CARDIOLOGY

The first insight into the usefulness of interventional cardiology techniques was shown by Stephen Hales in 1727, who performed the first cardiac catheterization in a horse using brass pipes to reach the ventricles. The term catheterization was coined in 1844 when French physiologist Claude Bernard recorded the first intracardiac pressure via a catheter. Around 50 years later, in the mid-1890s, German scientist Wilhelm Röntgen discovered X-rays, a discovery hailed as a medical miracle and one that made current day interventional cardiology practice possible.[1]

Throughout the 1900s, many advances were made in this evolving field. In 1929, Werner Theodor Otto Forsmann inserted a urinary catheter in the antecubital vein and threaded it to the right ventricle for which he received the Nobel Prize with two other physicians in 1956.

Andreas Grüntzig in 1977 performed the first human percutaneous transluminal coronary angioplasty procedure. Building on the work by Charles Dotter, Grüntzig's perseverance was extraordinary and resulted in the successful treatment of a patient, whose original lesion remained open at 37-year follow-up. He then continued his work by organizing the first demonstration course in 1978 and publishing his first results in 1979.

As the discipline of interventional cardiology entered the 21st century, dual antiplatelet therapy, primary balloon angioplasty, and selective stenting have become the mainstay of treating coronary artery disease (CAD). The first percutaneous transluminal angioplasty also marked a new era in the treatment of peripheral atherosclerotic lesions.

The early techniques used in peripheral and coronary percutaneous transluminal angioplasty are largely due to the contribution of Charles Dotter. Dotter was the first to describe flow-directed balloon catheterization, the double-lumen balloon catheter, the safety guidewire, percutaneous arterial stenting, and more. This practical genius dedicated his considerable energy to the belief that there is always a better way to treat a disease. His contributions to clinical medicine, research, and teaching have saved millions of limbs and lives all over the world.[2]

Ambulatory Surgery Center (ASC), Office-Based Lab (OBL)

The scope of practice of interventional cardiology is no longer limited to coronary intervention but also includes structural and peripheral vascular interventions.[3] Currently, these procedures are not limited to the inpatient hospital setting. In this chapter, I am going to address the broader issues that have impacted me as a cardiologist and other interventionalist as well.

Approximately in the last 30 years, a shift in having medical procedures done in an outpatient setting started with the formation of ambulatory surgical centers (ASCs) and renal dialysis centers. The first ASC was opened in Phoenix, Arizona, in 1970 by two physicians who saw an opportunity to establish a high-quality, cost-effective alternative to inpatient hospital care for surgical services.[4] As patient care continues to

Office-Based Endovascular Centers. https://doi.org/10.1016/B978-0-323-67969-5.00021-6
Copyright © 2020 Elsevier Inc. All rights reserved.

transition to the outpatient setting, the number and type of services, including cardiology, offered in the ASC have significantly expanded.

Improvements in medical technology continues to support this trend. New technologies offer high-quality imaging equipment with smaller footprints and efficient device delivery systems, making it easier and cost-effective to treat increasingly complex diseases on an outpatient basis. For the patient, it provides convenience—shorter wait for procedure time, customer focus and familiar staff, safety, and excellent patient outcomes. For the physicians, it offers them control over the entire medical process from the official greeting, treatment choice, to discharge. Healthcare savings come from reduced overhead, and no overnight stays.[5]

There are three possible models for outpatient delivery of care: (1) hospital outpatient department, (2) freestanding ASC, and (3) office-based endovascular center (OEC), also known as office-based lab (OBL), or office-based interventional suite (OIS), a term preferred by Jeffrey G. Carr, a contributor to this book, as it conveys the totality of cardiovascular, endovascular, venous, and nonvascular services performed in the office environment.

Safety

As interventional cardiologists have become more experienced and comfortable with outpatient endovascular procedures, significant cost savings are achieved without sacrificing patient safety. Patient satisfaction and security are the keys to the success of outpatient centers.

Samuel Ahn et al. analyzed the safety and efficacy of endovascular procedures in 3174 endovascular cases completed in their office-based suites between 2006 and 2011. Their data indicated that the OEC setting is a safe and productive environment for a patient undergoing an endovascular procedure. (Ahn S, et al. Outpatient office-based endovascular procedures are safe and effective: a 5-year experience in over 3000 cases).

In his landmark article in 2014 published in the *Journal of Vascular Surgery*, Krishna Jain et al. evaluated the safety and patient satisfaction in 2822 patients who underwent 6458 procedures in an OEC suite between 2007 and 2012. They concluded that with appropriate screening, almost all peripheral interventions (arterial, endovenous, and dialysis access) could be performed in an OEC with a low rate of complications. For dialysis patients, outpatient interventions have very low complication rates and are the mainstay of treatment to keep the dialysis access patent. Venous insufficiency, when managed in the office setting, also has a low complication rate. They opined that office-based procedural settings should be seriously considered for percutaneous interventions for arterial, venous, and dialysis-related procedures.

Reimbursement

The **Centers for Medicare and Medicaid Services (CMS)**, previously known as the **Health Care Financing Administration (HCFA)**, is a federal agency within the US Department of Health and Human Services (HHS) that administers the Medicare program and works in partnership with state governments to administer Medicaid, the Children's Health Insurance Program (CHIP), and health insurance portability standards. In addition to these programs, CMS has other responsibilities, including the administrative simplification of the Health Insurance Portability and Accountability Act of 1996 (HIPAA), manage quality standards in long-term care facilities (more commonly referred to as nursing homes) through its survey and certification process, oversee clinical laboratory quality standards under the Clinical Laboratory Improvement Amendments, and oversight of HealthCare.gov.[6]

CMS has the most significant influence of any single agency on medical billing, coding, and reimbursement. CMS has an enormous effect on determining the payment for medical services, and as such, also has a significant influence on private insurance companies since these insurance companies base their fees on Medicare reimbursement for physician services.

Dialysis vascular access services, performed in vascular access centers (VACs), experienced a dramatic overall reduction in reimbursement in 2017, due to a CMS policy requiring services that are billed together more than 75% of the time to be bundled. As a result, new interventional Common Procedural Terminology (CPT) code bundles were developed and resulted in a marked difference in reimbursement for certain interventional dialysis vascular access services performed in a VAC as compared with the same services performed in an ASC setting. These cuts have led many nephrology practices to consider the financial, operational, and legal viability of converting their VAC into hybrid ASC/VAC.[7]

Procedure	2017 Bundled Common Procedural Terminology Code	Office- Based 2917 Final FFS	Approximate ambulatory surgical center Rate	Approximate $ Variance	Percent Change
Angiogram of access	36901	$580.70	$369.36	$211.34	−36%
Angiogram with angioplasty	36902	$1234.97	$3119.32	$1884.35	153%
Angiogram with stent	36903	$5663.44	$6025.55	$362.11	6%
Thrombectomy	36904	$1800.60	$3119.32	$1318.72	73%
Thrombectomy with angioplasty	36905	$2304.14	$6025.55	$3721.41	162%
Thrombectomy with stent	36906	$6867.55	$9341.79	$2474.24	36%

MEDICARE COST SAVINGS TIED TO ASCS[8]

A study on the Medicare Cost Savings Tied to ASC was reported by Dr Brent Fulton and Dr Sue Kim from the Nicholas C. Petris Center on Health Care Markets and Consumer Welfare, School of Public Health, University of California–Berkeley. Their study showed the savings generated by the ASC industry and, the savings were sure to continue for the Medicare program and its beneficiaries over the next decade. The magnitude of these savings, however, will hinge on whether, and how much, the ASC share of surgeries grows within the Medicare program. That growth rate will, in turn, depend on market trends, demographic factors, and how policymakers to act—or decline to act—to encourage the use of ASCs within the Medicare program.

Even the most "optimistic" scenario assumes that ASC share growth for the various procedures will grow modestly as compared with the historical averages and that ASCs have the potential to save the Medicare program and its beneficiaries up to $57.6 billion more over the next decade. The study examined only data from the Medicare program, ASCs typically also serve patients who have private insurance, including the Medicare Advantage program. ASC gets paid less than the HOPD (Hospital Outpatient Department) for the same procedures. Thus, similar cost savings also exist in the commercial health insurance market and the Medicare Advantage program.

POLICY IMPLICATIONS AND CONSIDERATIONS

An aging population, along with inflation in healthcare costs, means that the federal government's Medicare program's disbursements are projected to increase substantially in the coming years. Policymakers in Washington, DC, are exploring potential ways to reduce projected Medicare outlays and extend the program's solvency. The study offers two specific policy concerns:

1. Avoiding ASC to HOPD conversions

Our first and most important observation is that, while the future savings offered by ASCs are easily attainable, they are not inevitable. Because they provide identical services to HOPDs but do so at an average of 58% of the reimbursement rate that the Medicare program pays HOPDs for the same services, ASCs represent a source of value to the program and the taxpayers who fund it. A discrepancy in the way Medicare reimbursement rates are updated, however, threatens to marginalize ASCs' role within the program.

CMS currently applies different measures of inflation to determine the adjustments it provides to its payment systems for ASCs and HOPDs each year. For ASCs, that measure is the CPI-U, which is tied to consumer prices. The index for HOPD reimbursements, on the other hand, remains tied to the hospital market basket, which measures inflation in actual medical costs. Since consumer prices have inflated more slowly than medical costs, the gap in ASC and HOPD reimbursement rates has widened over time. As the reimbursement rate for ASCs continues to fall relative to their HOPD counterparts, ASC owners and physicians will face increasing pressure to leave the Medicare system and allow their facilities to be acquired by hospitals.

When an ASC is acquired by a hospital, in what is known as "an ASC to HOPD conversion," the Medicare reimbursement rate jumps roughly 75% and all savings to the Medicare program, and its beneficiaries, are promptly lost. The continuing reduction in reimbursement led more than 60 ASCs to terminate their participation in Medicare over the last 3 years. If policymakers allow this gap in reimbursements to continue to widen, the cost-saving advantage that ASCs offer could morph into a perverse market incentive that drives ASCs away from the Medicare program.

Some in Congress have introduced legislation, which is titled the "Ambulatory Surgical Center Quality and Access Act," that aims to fix this problem. This bill would correct the imbalance in reimbursement indices and ensure that ASC reimbursements do not continue to fall relative to their HOPD counterparts. Additionally, it would establish an ASC value-based purchasing program designed to foster collaboration between ASCs and the government and create additional savings for the Medicare system in the process.

2. ASCs as part of broader cost-saving efforts

Many of the policy options aimed at reducing Medicare costs that are being considered in Congress today involve important "trade-offs," where reduced outlays come at the expense of retirees' benefits. Often-discussed options such as raising the Medicare retirement age or increasing cost-sharing, for example, generate savings as a direct result of reducing the number of benefits delivered by the Medicare program.

The savings offered by ASCs, however, do not involve such trade-offs; they make it possible for the Medicare program, and its beneficiaries, to realize significant savings without any corresponding reduction in benefits.

There are more than 5300 Medicare-certified ASCs throughout the country, all of which represent an essential source of efficiency for the Medicare program and the taxpayers who fund it. The study recommends that policymakers explore all potential options for encouraging further growth of ASC share within the Medicare system.

The CMS Newsroom reported on November 2, 2018, that the CMS finalized the changes that removed unnecessary and inefficient payment differences between certain provider and supplier types so that patients can have more affordable choices and options. The final rule with comment period updates and revises policies under the Medicare Hospital Outpatient Prospective Payment System (OPPS) and ASC payment system. These changes will further advance the agency's priority of creating a patient-centered healthcare system by achieving greater price transparency and significant burden reduction so that hospitals and ASCs can operate with better flexibility and patients have access to the tools they need to become active healthcare consumers.[9]

The final rule with comment period contains several policies that reduce payment differences between hospitals and ASCs so that patients may benefit from high-quality care at lower costs while receiving care that is provided safely and is clinically appropriate.[9]

For Calendar Year (CY) 2019, CMS finalized the proposal to include additional CPT codes outside of the surgical code range that directly crosswalk or are clinically similar to procedures within the CPT surgical code range on the CPL (Covered Procedures List). As a result, CMS its proposal to add 12 cardiovascular codes to the ASC CPL and adding five additional codes as a result of stakeholder comments the agency received.[9]

Common Procedural Terminology	Procedure
93451	Right heart catheterization
93452	Left heart catheterization w/ventriculography
93453	Righ and left heart cath w/ventriculography
93454	Coronary artery angiogram S&I
93455	Coronary art/graft angiogram S&I
93456	Right heart coronary artery angiogram
93457	Right heart art/graft angiogram
93458	Left heart artery/ventricle angiogram
93459	Left heart art/graft angiogram
93460	Right and left heart art/ventricle angiogram
93461	Right and left heart art/ventricle angiogram
93462	Left heart cath transeptal puncture
93566	Inject right ventricle/atrial angiogram
93567	Inject suprvlv aortography
93568	Inject pulm art heart cath
93571	Heart flow reserve measure
93572	Heart flow reserve measure

As of January 2019, physicians can begin to perform these procedures in the ASC setting. However, this is subject to individual state laws and regulations. This is a critical step for the addition of percutaneous coronary intervention procedures to be covered by CMS in the ASC setting.[10]

Certificate of Need State Laws

OECs are increasing in number because of less licensing and paperwork required as compared with the ASC. It is a requirement by Medicare that the ASC be certified as an ASC to be able to receive reimbursement form CMS. There is no such requirement for an OEC.

A Certificate of Need (CON) is an approval that numerous states require before approving the construction of a new healthcare facility. The central idea of a CON is the assertion that overbuilding and redundancy in healthcare facilities lead to higher healthcare costs.

CON is defined as a declaration from a government planning agency indicating that the construction or alteration of an existing health facility is justified. Designed initially in the 1970s to prevent the creation of duplicate healthcare facilities in local or regional markets, some analysts have suggested that CONs have instead defended existing hospitals from the unwanted competition.[11]

The number of Medicare-certified ASCs varies throughout the United States. States with ***CON laws have 1.6 ASCs per 100,000 people*** on average, slightly less than states ***without a CON law—1.8 ASCs per 100,000***, according to the VMG Health 2017 Intellimarker: Multi-Specialty ASC Study.

The table refers to the number of Medicare-licensed ASCs per 100,000 people as of December 31, 2016.[12]

CON states	Non-CON states
Alabama: 0.7	Arizona: 2.5
Alaska: 2	Arkansas: 2
Connecticut: 1.3	California: 2
Delaware: 2.4	Colorado: 2.2
Georgia: 3.2	Florida: 2
Hawaii: 1.5	Idaho: 3.1
Illinois: 1	Indiana: 1.9
Iowa: 0.8	Kansas: 2.2
Kentucky: 0.7	Louisiana: 1.7
Maine: 1.2	Minnesota: 1.2
Maryland: 5.8	Missouri: 1.6
Massachusetts: 0.8	Nebraska: 2.4
Michigan: 0.9	New Hampshire: 2.1
Mississippi: 2.3	New Mexico: 0.8
Montana: 1.6	North Dakota: 1.5
Nevada: 2.3	Ohio: 1.6
New Jersey: 3	Oklahoma: 1.1
New York: 0.7	Oregon: 1
North Carolina: 1	Pennsylvania: 1.8
Rhode Island: 0.9	South Dakota: 2.2
South Carolina: 1.4	Texas: 1.3
Tennessee: 2.1	Utah: 1.3
Vermont: 0.2	Wisconsin: 1.3
Virginia: 0.7	Wyoming: 3.1
Washington: 2.7	
Washington, D.C.: 0.4	
West Virginia: 0.5	

On December 2018, the US Department of Health and Human Services (DHS) recommended states repeal or scale back their certificate of need laws. The report highlights, "States initially adopted CON laws to further laudable policy goals, including cost control and access to care. The evidence to date, however, suggests that CON laws are frequently costly barriers to entry for health care providers rather than successful tools for controlling costs or improving health care quality."[13]

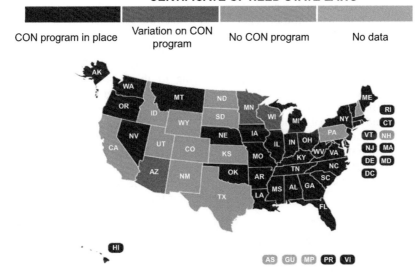

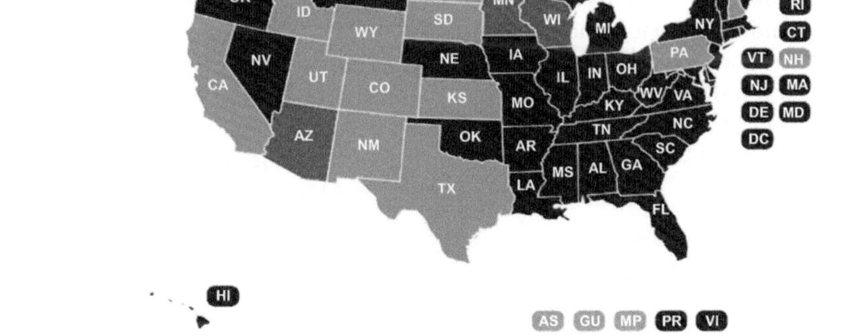

According to George Mason University's Mercatus Center, CON laws lead to higher healthcare spending, fewer hospitals, and a lower quality of care. The research concluded about $200 per capita of healthcare spending would be saved if we repeal the CON laws. Additionally, the same study shows that the presence of a CON program is associated with fewer hospitals in rural, suburban, and urban areas alike.[13]

ARGUMENTS IN FAVOR AND AGAINST CON LAWS[14]

Arguments in Favor of CON Laws

- Healthcare cannot be considered as a "typical" economic product.
- Most health services (like X-ray) are "ordered" for patients by physicians; patients do not "shop" for these services the way they do for other commodities.
- The American Health Planning Association (AHPA) argues that CON programs limit healthcare spending. CON programs can distribute care to areas that could be ignored by new medical centers.

CON requirements do not block change; they mainly provide for evaluation and often include public or stakeholder input.

Arguments Against CON Laws

- By restricting new construction, CON programs may reduce price competition between facilities and keep prices high.
- Some changes in the Medicare payment system (such as paying hospitals according to Diagnostic Related Groups) may make external regulatory controls unnecessary by sensitizing healthcare organizations to market pressures.
- CON programs are not consistently administered.
- Health facility development should be left to the economics of each institution rather than being subject to political influence.
- Some evidence suggest that lack of competition encourages construction and additional spending.
- Potential for CONs to be granted based on political influence, institutional prestige, or other factors apart from the interests of the community.
- It is not always clear what the best interests of the community entail.

The Ambulatory Cardiovascular Center

Several specialties practice in the OEC setting, but the most common are interventional cardiology, vascular surgery, radiology, and interventional nephrology. Significant technological advances have made performing minimally invasive vascular procedures safely and efficiently in the OEC setting. Most peripheral diagnostic and interventional procedures, from peripheral atherectomy to stenting, fistulogram, thrombectomy, and angioplasty are performed in the OEC.[7]

The ambulatory cardiovascular center can be set up as a brand-new surgery center in the same building as the OEC or contiguous with the office, depending on regulations and the configuration of the current facility. It is a Medicare requirement to get certified, licensed, and accredited as an ASC to be able to receive payment from CMS, and some states CON is required to open an ASC. Cases can be scheduled to best maximize reimbursement by operating as an OBL on certain days of the week and an ASC on other days.[7]

With strategic assessments and planning, the OECs and ASC s will be a great model in delivering high-quality, cost-efficient care for the evolving healthcare industry.

Benefits of Physician Ownership[15]

For a cardiologist, the decision to open an OEC/ASC has been driven by the following:

(1) The need to improve work efficiency by removing the unknown variables affecting the hospital schedule and case turnover; procedures are scheduled conveniently for patients and promote more patient-doctor interaction.
(2) The desire to enhance patient satisfaction by being involved in the decisions that impact care, equipment, supplies, and quality outcomes.
(3) Increased productivity by eliminating travel time to hospitals to see other patients in between cases.
(4) Offers the physician the opportunity to increase their revenue by capturing the technical and professional components of reimbursement.
(5) Opportunity to avoid succumbing and surrendering to the hospital PSA (Professional Services Agreement) programs and total loss of autonomy.

BETTER ACCOUNTABILITY

Physician ownership allows for maximum professional control over the clinical environment and the quality of care delivered to patients. This advanced model of service enhances the delivery of care by enabling physician operators to:

- focus exclusively on a small number of procedures in a single setting;
- intensify quality control processes since ASCs rely on a lesser amount of space and fewer operating rooms than most hospitals; and

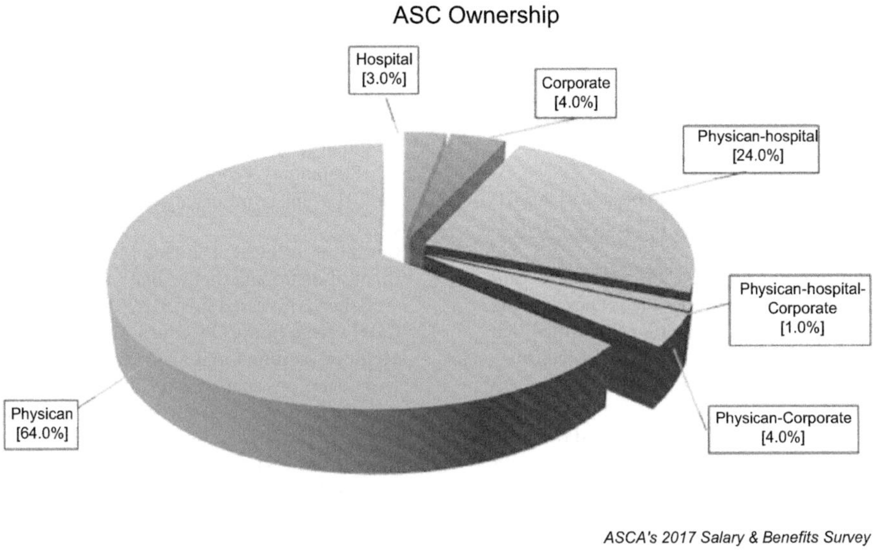

- afford patients the ability to bring any concerns directly to the physician operator who has direct knowledge about each patient's case, rather than deal with hospital administrators who often lack detailed knowledge about individual patients and their experiences.

Unlike large-scale institutions, ASCs:

- serve fewer patients than hospitals and are highly specialized in what they do, allowing them to be more responsive to individual patient needs;
- exercise better control over scheduling, so virtually no procedures are delayed or rescheduled due to the unforeseen emergencies that often take precedent in hospitals; and
- allow physicians to personally guide innovative strategies for governance, leadership, and quality initiatives.

SUMMARY

With the rising pressure from CMS and private payers to hold down prices for procedures while maintaining quality of care, the past 30 years have seen a shift of surgeries from the inpatient to the outpatient setting. The paradigm shift was based on the experience gained from ASCs.

Improvements in medical technology, from open surgical procedures to minimally invasive endovascular treatments, have opened the cath lab to treat beyond the coronaries. Peripheral artery disease (PAD) has been mostly treated by vascular surgeons, but the shift to transcatheter endovascular treatment has led interventional cardiologist to transition from solely treating CAD to PAD. While vessel patency is the goal of addressing the coronaries, in PAD, the goal is limb salvage, to prevent amputation and improve the patient's quality of life.

The main objective of outpatient procedures is to provide a better outpatient experience coupled with a better outcome at a lower cost. The importance of case selection and safety considerations are important factors to consider. Data from ASCs and OECs demonstrate a considerable increase in patient satisfaction and positive outcomes when having their procedures performed in this setting.

Physicians have embraced and adapted to the new health care delivery model. Despite the push back from the hospitals the past 10 years have seen a significant rise in the number of ASCs and OBLs. Amid the increasing prevalence and awareness in cardiac and vascular diseases, bundling of healthcare services, and the steadily decreasing physician reimbursement, doctors are seeking better alternatives to efficiently provide high-quality care for patients.

REFERENCES

1. History of interventional cardiology. *EMJ Int Cardiol.* 2018; 6(1):68–70. https://emj.europeanmedical-group.com/wp-content/uploads/sites/2/2018/07/Interventional-Cardiology-6.1-History.pdf. Published July 2018.
2. Payne MM. Charles theodore dotter. The father of intervention. *Tex Heart Inst J.* 2001;28(1):28–38. PubMed PMID: 11330737; PubMed Central PMCID: PMC101126.

3. Carreras ET, Williams DO. Interventional cardiology: the in and the out. *Circ Cardiovasc Interv*. April 2018;11(4): e006709. PubMed PMID: 29654120.
4. ASCs: A Positive Trend in Health Care – Advancing Surgical. https://www.ascassociation.org/advancingsurgicalcare/aboutascs/industryoverview/apositivetrendinhealthcare. Accessed July 31, 2019.
5. Cross DS, Gonzalez A, Wright KJ. Office-based lab models: getting started. Endovascular Today, Published March 16 (3), 2017. Accessed July 31, 2019.
6. Wikipedia contributors. Centers for Medicare and Medicaid Services. Wikipedia, The Free Encyclopedia. Updated December 19, 2018, 23:36 UTC. https://en.wikipedia.org/w/index.php?title=Centers_for_Medicare_and_Medicaid_Services&oldid=874547407. Accessed July 31, 2019.
7. Toth M, Zasa R. Introducing the ambulatory cardiovascular center. https://www.beckersasc.com/asc-transactions-and-valuation-issues/introducing-the-ambulatory-cardiovascular-center.html. Published May 22, 2017. Accessed July 31, 2019.
8. Study: Medicare cost savings tied to ASCs. Ambulatory Surgery Center Association.https://www.ascassociation.org/advancingsurgicalcare/reducinghealthcarecosts/costsavings/medicarecostsavingstiedtoascs Accessed July 31, 2019.
9. *CMS Finalizes Medicare Hospital Outpatient Prospective Payment System and Ambulatory Surgical Center Payment System Changes for 2019*. CMS-1695-FC; November 02, 2018. Retrieved August 5, 2019, from https://www.cms.gov/newsroom/fact-sheets/cms-finalizes-medicare-hospital-outpatient-prospective-payment-system-and-ambulatory-surgical-center.
10. Lafata T, Toth M, Turmell J. CMS reimbursement and your ambulatory strategy. *Card Interventions Today*. 2019;13(1): 67–70. January/February 2019 https://citoday.com/2019/02/2019-cms-reimbursement-and-your-ambulatory-strategy/.
11. Certificate of need. The Free Medical Dictionary. https://medical-dictionary.thefreedictionary.com/certificate+of+need. Accessed July 31, 2019.
12. CON versus non-CON states: Which regions boast more Medicare certified ASCs? Beckers ASC Review. https://www.beckersasc.com/asc-coding-billing-and-collections/con-versus-non-con-states-which-regions-boast-more-medicare-certified-ascs.html Published June 15, 2017. Accessed July 31, 2019.
13. Mace N. Health Care Needs Market Competition, not Government Restriction. https://www.fitsnews.com/2019/02/02/nancy-mace-health-care-needs-market-competition-not-government-restriction/. Published February 2, 2019. Accessed July 31, 2019.
14. Certificate of need state laws. National Conference of State Legislatures. http://www.ncsl.org/research/health/con-certificate-of-need-state-laws.aspx. Accessed July 31, 2019.
15. Benefits of Physician Ownership. Advancing Surgical Care. https://www.ascassociation.org/advancingsurgicalcare/asc/benefitsofphysicianownership.

CHAPTER 22

Interventional Radiologist's Perspective

DAVID C. SPERLING, MD, FSIR

Interventional Radiology is a subspecialty that one could argue, lends itself to the outpatient endovascular center as well or better than any other specialty. The range and volume of Interventional Radiology procedures that can be accommodated in the outpatient lab is long and varied. To understand this best, a little background is required.

In 1973, the Society of Cardiovascular Radiology was founded by a group of radiologists who wanted to further explore the interventional aspects of radiology. In 1983, the name of the society was changed to the Society of Cardiovascular and Interventional Radiology (SCVIR). Around 2001, a survey had been sent out to patients and physicians to see what kind of name recognition was present regarding the society and its subspecialists. It turns out, the overwhelming majority of patients, and a surprisingly high percentage of physicians, had no idea what we were or what we did. This spurred an intrasocietal debate about changing the society's name yet again in order to gain more patient and physician recognition. Many suggestions for a new name came from this debate. Some of them that I can remember included terms like "Image-Guided Surgery," "Minimally Invasive Surgeons," "Minimally Invasive Specialists," "Vascular and Interventional Radiology," and others. The general sense was that the specialty focused on both image guidance and the minimally invasive nature of the procedures that defined the physicians' practices. In 2002, the Society finally settled on the name that is currently used, the Society of Interventional Radiology. While that name may not be as descriptive as it could be, the thought process in the debate of the name change was what resonated with me. The image guidance and the minimally invasive nature and thought process not only encompass what we do, but also perfectly encapsulate why the outpatient office is ideally suited to Interventional Radiology.

The evolution of Interventional Radiology and its migration to the performance of procedures in the outpatient centers began with hospital-based practices. Interventional radiologists have been pioneers in converting complex, open surgical procedures, into less invasive, percutaneous options. Percutaneous dilation of peripheral arterial stenosis as an option compared with surgical vascular bypass was developed by Dr Charles Dotter in 1963. Further contributions by cardiologists Dr Andreas Gruntzig and Dr Melvin Judkins brought percutaneous intravascular devices and procedures into the modern age. Since that time, many innovators, inventors, and outside-the-box thinkers have contributed to minimally invasive medicine, both vascular and nonvascular, that allow all of us to practice medicine the way we do today.

With that history in mind, we recognize that there was a significant and progressive conversion of open surgical procedures to less invasive percutaneous procedures. Over the decades, many of the less invasive, percutaneous procedures have proven to be safe and effective. Aside from the vascular procedures, biopsies of solid organs and masses also underwent an evolution. Surgical, open, or incisional biopsies have been converted over the years into ultrasound- or CT scan–guided small bore core biopsies or fine needle aspirations. Ultimately, it did not require a big leap to move these safe, minimally invasive procedures from the inpatient radiology suite to the hospital-based outpatient procedure rooms. The patients were discharged on the same day after the procedure. In fact, for several decades, percutaneous image-guided biopsies have been performed in diagnostic radiology offices, as well as by other specialists (kidney biopsies in nephrologists offices, liver biopsies in gastrointestinal physician offices) as outpatient office–based procedures. Taken all together, there seems to be a plethora of options for procedures to be performed in an outpatient, office-based facility, especially if the procedures are performed by interventional radiologists. Realizing the fact that the number of varied procedures could be performed in the office contributed heavily to the decision we made to create our first outpatient office and lab.

When I completed my Interventional Radiology fellowship at Thomas Jefferson University Hospital in

Office-Based Endovascular Centers. https://doi.org/10.1016/B978-0-323-67969-5.00022-8
Copyright © 2020 Elsevier Inc. All rights reserved.

Philadelphia, Pennsylvania, in 1999, I took my first job in a private practice in The Bronx, New York. We were eight radiologists in the practice and practiced out of a 500-bed hospital with an osteopathic radiology residency. We also had an outpatient diagnostic radiology office approximately two miles away from the hospital where we had a CT scanner, an MRI machine, and equipment for mammography, and plain X-ray films. The hospital had not had an interventional radiologist for several years, and I was charged with developing the practice, essentially from the ground up. I welcomed everything, from complex PAD cases to PICC lines. I performed procedures that had never been performed there, like TIPS and thrombolysis, and common procedures like simple biopsies of the liver and thyroid. The mammographer in the group struggled with ultrasound-guided breast biopsies. I was happy to take them off her hands. This was a simple conversion, and I was very comfortable with them, and it made the mammography service much better and responsive to patient's needs, which was ultimately better for the practice. When I first got to the practice, the interventional radiology volume was approximately 1–2 PICC lines a week. By the end of 18 months, we were up to 1500 procedures a year.

As with all practices, academic or private, everyone, including us, was looking to increase revenue in the practice. The outpatient diagnostic office that we owned was busy. There was a 10 x 10-foot room in the back that was not being used. It was essentially a closet with old, useless equipment. I proposed turning the room into a working space to treat patients with varicose veins. It took a bit of convincing, but I was able to persuade my partners to convert this useless space into revenue producing space. Even in the early part of this century, management of varicose veins, diagnosis and treatment, in the office setting was not a new concept. It had already been done successfully by many. There was no reason to perform these procedures in the hospital or in the hospital outpatient department. The reimbursements were not favorable in the hospital, and the hospital environment was stark and unpleasant for a set of procedures that, while meant for symptomatic varicose veins, crossed over to the esthetic side very quickly. The diagnosis and treatment of these patients required a quieter and pleasant space that could be created in our already welcoming and quiet outpatient facility. We began with a small business loan, beautified the room, bought a table and a laser machine, and used one of our older model ultrasounds that, while old and bulky, was still functional. We were able to convert the wasted space into a vein office. We started using the room one afternoon a week and gradually increased the hours as the demand increased. This experiment was successful and profitable to the practice.

At approximately the same time as the development of our office-based vein office, we were so busy in the hospital-based side of our Interventional Radiology practice, that we expanded the facilities in the hospital to two angiography suites and hired a second interventional radiologist. As part of the evaluation process to get the hospital to agree to make the space available as well as to pay for the construction and capital equipment for a second angiography suite, we did a full financial analysis of our financial contribution, resulting from patient care, to the hospital revenue stream. We ran the numbers regarding volume, admissions, downstream revenue, and other benefits to the hospital to "justify" the expansion of the hospital-based practice. One of the most interesting finding that emerged from the data was the fact that we were providing interventional radiology services to a large number of outpatients.

The evaluation had two important findings. First, it showed that 50% of the cases performed by interventional radiologists in our practice were outpatients. This was especially important because as we were streamlining workflow and patient flow in our practice, all outpatients came through the hospital's Ambulatory Surgery unit. This resulted in us identifying the second important finding. Due to this patient flow, Interventional Radiology was the second highest utilizer of Ambulatory Surgery in the entire hospital. This helped justify the expansion of the hospital-based practice. However, based on these data, we posed a question to ourselves; if 50% of our patients are outpatients, why are they being done in the hospital at all?

The procedures that were being performed in the hospital as outpatients through the Ambulatory Surgery unit were varied. Complex procedures such as lower extremity arteriograms with angioplasty or stent placements, uterine fibroid embolization, chemoembolization, percutaneous thermal ablations of liver and kidney tumors were all being performed on outpatient basis, and the patients were sent home the same day after the procedure, usually after a 4- or 6-h recovery period. These procedures, while complex, were typically performed with intravenous moderate sedation, a closure device was used for the access site, and all patients were discharged using the appropriate discharge protocol.

Less complex procedures that also required intravenous moderate sedation were also performed in Ambulatory Surgery and discharged home the same day after 1 to 2 h of observation. Venous port placement for chemotherapy, dialysis access evaluations including percutaneous thrombectomy of access, angioplasty and stent placements, tunneled dialysis catheters, varicocele embolization, liver biopsies, lung biopsies, kidney biopsies, transjugular liver biopsies, biliary drainages, biliary stricture dilations, nephrostomy tubes, nephroureteral catheters, double J nephroureteral stents, suprapubic catheters, IVC filter retrievals, TIPS checks and revisions, and more were all performed in this outpatient manner. Since the workflow was easy and established, even the simpler procedures that did not require sedation or recovery were performed this way. PICC lines, routine nephrostomy, suprapubic catheter and biliary catheter changes, abscess catheter checks and removals, thyroid and lymph node biopsies and fine needle aspirations, and others were performed and the patients were sent home immediately following the procedures.

Only very few patients would come in as an outpatient through the Ambulatory Surgery unit, have their procedure, and be admitted after the procedure for prolonged observation and pain control. These included fresh TIPS procedures, renal artery stents, and some arterial venous malformation embolization. These were low-volume procedures, leaving us to realize that 50% of our case volume was, in fact, outpatient, and the majority of our patients could go home the same day after the procedure.

As we continued to build our practice, we continued to search for alternate revenue streams. We were getting busy enough that our volume was beginning to overwhelm both Ambulatory Surgery center and the inpatient Interventional Radiology suite. The hospital had no space to add another angiography suite or expand Ambulatory Surgery. Both of these projects would be expensive as well. Our practice began to explore the possibility of creating space in our outpatient practice to do these procedures to deal with overflow at the hospital. Unfortunately, we never got a chance to move ahead with the evaluation. The hospital had major economic problems and the Radiology group experienced a major political debacle, and the entire group was forced to move out. Most of the radiologists in our group went their separate ways.

I continued to evaluate the idea of converting most of these hospital-based outpatient procedures into outpatient procedures performed at an office. The billing and reimbursement is done in a global fashion in an outpatient office. The embolizations, angioplasties, stents and ablation of varicose veins are high dollar value procedures. The PICCs, ports, and catheter changes are lower reimbursement procedures, but these procedures also take less time per procedure, and are much more commonly performed than the more complex and time-consuming procedures. Surely, these procedures could be used to fill in the gap between the larger and longer procedures, in a way that would utilize the equipment and personnel for the entire day instead of just being used for one or two big procedures and wasted time between them. We had done this evaluation for our own vein practice. It made sense that it would work well with the rest of the procedures as well. While I thought it was viable to have an office-based endovascular center, I could not do it on my own. The financial outlay and the managerial experience needed can be daunting.

In life, timing is everything. Opportunity is also what you make of it. I was looking for my next job and knew I needed deeper pockets to realize my vision. I met with the leaders of a large tertiary care medical center that was recruiting an interventional radiologist, but was also struggling financially. They needed a way to generate more volume and increase revenue. Working with the financial experts on the institutional side I created a business plan and a proforma, especially paying attention to the expense side and detailing the procedures that could be safely done in the office. Typically, large academic university-based institutions do not overextend themselves, take undue risk, or do things that had not been done before. Luckily, we came to a situation where the correct, open-minded people listened to a sound financial plan, and, for lack of a better term, went for it.

So, in 2008, I signed on to create this outpatient procedural office within the confines of a major academic university practice. We asked the hospital administration if they were interested in partnering with us, and they graciously said "no thank you." Interestingly, they added that they hoped we were successful! Hospitals and academic radiology practices realize that interventional radiologists working in a hospital-based practice cannot realistically show a profit since they only receive the professional component of the procedure. The reimbursement for the technical component, which is much higher than the professional component, is reimbursed to the hospital. The procedures cannot be done without the services of an interventional radiologist, and the hospital cannot collect the technical revenue unless the procedure is done. Since only the professional component is assigned to the radiologist the radiologist is told that hospital is losing money because the radiologist's salary is greater than the total professional reimbursement received by the doctor. Under this scenario, the physicians and their practices traditionally hope to "break even" when comparing their salary to their reimbursements. Unfortunately, this usually does not happen, and there is a deficit that needs to be covered solely based on the professional component reimbursement to the doctor. Most of the time, this deficit is covered by the hospital, as a supplement or a "pass through" payment. The hospital, in our situation, while stating that they hoped we were successful, did have a specific reason. They wanted us to succeed so that our outpatient practice could support our salaries paid by the hospital for the inpatient care provided by us. Other advantages of the office-based interventional practice became clear to the hospital as well. For instance, the outpatient Interventional Radiology office became a way to unclutter the hospital-based practice from the (relatively) healthier outpatients, allowing the procedures on the sicker inpatients to be performed in a timely manner. Additionally, despite increasing procedural volume, the hospital did not have to find more space to add more angiography suites, nor spend the money on construction, capital equipment, more recovery room space, nurses and technologists to staff those spaces and bear all of the other fixed and variable expenses associated with an Interventional Radiology practice. In time, the hospital administration changed its mind and became very willing and active partners in our outpatient procedural suites because of the success of the programs and the advantages to all sides. It became a win-win situation.

Today, we have two outpatient offices, one with two angiography suites and one with one angiography suite. A typical day for each of the rooms encompasses our original thought process about a typical office Interventional Radiology day. At 8:00 a.m. we start with a procedure that does not require an intravenous line for fluids or sedation medications, for procedures such as a thyroid, lymph node, or breast biopsies. At 9:00 a.m., we perform one of the procedures that require extended recovery such as one of the embolization procedures. These include fibroid embolization, chemoembolization, varicocele embolization, or embolization for pelvic congestion syndrome. Over time, we have also added procedures that can now be performed in this time slot. These include Y90 radioembolizations, angiomyolipoma embolizations, portal vein embolizations, as well as TIPS revisions and PAD cases. The 10:00 a.m. and 11:00 a.m. time slots can be filled with any of the less complex procedures, such as dialysis access–related procedures, insertion of venous ports for chemotherapy, PICC, and catheter procedures. The afternoons are reserved for consultations and follow-ups, varicose vein evaluations and procedures, as well as for procedures that do not require any recovery time.

The wide variety of procedures that are available to the interventional radiologist provide an inherent advantage and should be kept in mind while designing the office and the workflow in the office interventional suite. Every Interventional Radiology practice is different from the other. The type and volume of cases is dependent upon referral base, parent institution, local competition, geography, and the other services provided in the community. Regardless, I think that any Interventional Radiology practice can fit into the office model. An additional advantage enjoyed by the interventional radiologist is the fact that should there be a shift in reimbursement of different procedures, changes in local competition, addition of new procedures, etc., the radiologist can easily adapt to new environment because of the radiologist's ability to perform diverse interventional procedures. This provides financial security to the individual and the practice. Ultimately, the interventional radiologist is quite familiar with the minimally invasive procedures performed in a typical Interventional Radiology practice and that makes a transition to performing these procedures in an office-based endovascular center a viable and successful endeavor.

CHAPTER 23

Models for Structuring Office-Based Endovascular Labs

NICHOLAS D. JURKOWITZ, BA, JD • ALEXANDRA DE RIVERA, JD • KRISHNA JAIN, MD, FACS

OVERVIEW OF THE CORPORATE PRACTICE OF MEDICINE DOCTRINE

It is becoming common, and even a major source of venture capital investments, for lay entities to seek investment opportunities in the medical ventures. Before a medical group or physician seeks to associate with a lay entity, it is vital that the potential legal implications are carefully considered. Failing to follow regulations carefully can lead to civil liability, exclusion from private insurance companies/Medicare, and even criminal liability.

What Is the Corporate Practice of Medicine Doctrine?

The Corporate Practice of Medicine ("CPOM") Doctrine ("CPOM Doctrine" or "Doctrine") prohibits any unlicensed person or entity from practicing medicine or interfering with the clinical judgment of a healthcare professional. Developed by the American Medical Association, the Doctrine was designed to protect both the public and healthcare professionals from the commercial exploitation of the practice of medicine. It accomplishes this by prohibiting corporate bodies not subject to professional oversight and ethical restraints from interfering with medical decision-making and preserving a professional's ability to freely exercise autonomy in clinical judgment.

The Doctrine regulates three aspects of the medical industry. First, it restricts who can practice medicine. State licensure requirements provide an absolute barrier to the provision of medical services by unlicensed persons. Moreover, these requirements limit those who can practice medicine to natural persons who, for example, obtain a degree from an accredited school, pass certain testing requirements, and demonstrate both physical and medical soundness. Second, it restricts ownership. All or a majority of equity interests in medical practices, including professional corporations, limited liability companies, partnerships, and nonprofit corporations, must be held by individuals licensed to practice medicine. Third, physicians or other licensed professionals are prohibited from dividing or sharing their professional fees with nonlicensed persons or entities. This conduct is referred to as fee splitting. Fee-splitting arrangements are strongly discouraged because they may be used as a means to influence a medical professional's clinical judgment.

Public policy views profit as inimical to the physician-patient relationship. Whereas a corporation or business partnership's interests are motivated by profit, a physician's interests are governed by the patient's needs and conformity with prevailing medical and ethical guidelines. Accordingly, because the interests of the corporation and the medical professional are asymmetrical, the CPOM Doctrine was put in place to ensure that these competing loyalties should not threaten the public good.

The CPOM doctrine bears directly on the corporate formation and structuring of Office-based endovascular center (OEC). Because physicians looking to establish an OEC will likely seek to engage lay entities to provide practice management services, great care must be taken to develop a structure that avoids any argument that violates the Doctrine.

The Doctrine's Application in Various States

Many states have state statutes and regulations that prohibit lay corporations from engaging in the practice of medicine and, subsequently, have many laws designed to regulate various aspects to medical practice business

Office-Based Endovascular Centers. https://doi.org/10.1016/B978-0-323-67969-5.00023-X
Copyright © 2020 Elsevier Inc. All rights reserved.

operations. Examples of these states are California, New Jersey, and New York. The states that do regulate the corporate practice of medicine can restrict all or some of the basic aspects of a medical practice, including:

- Allowing only licensed physicians or other licensed practitioners to be shareholders and/or directors of a corporation
- Not allowing lay corporations or hospitals from employing physicians
- Restricting medical practices from splitting fees with lay entities or people
- Requirements that all clinical decisions be made by licensees

On the other side of the spectrum, some states have no corporate restrictions on medical practices. In those states, lay entities or individuals can be owners of medical practices and can share in the profits of the business and make vital management and business-related decisions that might be impermissible in states that have stricter regulations. Examples of these states are Utah, Delaware, and New Hampshire.

Several states also prohibit fee splitting arrangements. Fee splitting occurs where the physician is compensated for professional services and proceeds to share his or her compensation with an unlicensed professional. Like the CPOM Doctrine, these laws are designed to prohibit laypersons from deriving profit from the practice of medicine. In establishing payment arrangements between physicians and nonlicensed persons or entities, it is important that such payment be structured in a way that avoids characterization as profit sharing. While some states permit payments based on flat fees commensurate with the value of services performed, others strictly outlaw flat fee arrangements.

The following is a summary of how the CPOM Doctrine functions in California and Michigan.

California

Restrictions on ownership. California law authorizes licensed professionals to establish professional corporations for the delivery of medical care.[1] By law, at least 51% of the shareholders must be licensed in the same category of services as those provided by the professional corporation.[2] Individuals licensed in other professional disciplines can own up to 49% of the total number of shares.[3] The number of licensed individuals owning the majority of shares must exceed the number of shareholders licensed in fields outside of the professional corporation's practice area.[4] Nonlicensed individuals are prohibited from owning any shares in a professional corporation.

Fee splitting prohibitions. California Business and Professions Code § 650(a) prohibits licensed professionals from offering, receiving, or accepting any rebates, refunds, commissions, or any other consideration, as compensation or inducement for patient referral. While the statue expressly permits payments or consideration for services based on gross revenue, it must be "commensurate with the value of the services furnished or with the fair rental value of any premises or equipment leased or provided by the recipient to the payer."[5] When structuring these types of arrangements, it is critical that gross and net revenue are clearly distinguished.

In order to avoid violation of California's fee-splitting prohibition, some management companies will simply charge flat fees. These arrangements ensure compliance with both Business and Professions Code § 650(a) and any federal regulations that prohibit fee-splitting arrangements where the physician renders services to federally funded beneficiaries.

Michigan

Restrictions on ownership. In Michigan, because physicians, dentists, osteopathic physicians, and surgeons render "services in a learned profession,"[6] the CPOM Doctrine is sometimes referred to as the "learned profession doctrine." The Doctrine evolved over the course of several Michigan Attorney General Opinions, and it holds that only a natural person, not a corporation, qualifies to practice a learned profession, and those who belong to a learned profession may organize as either a professional corporation or a professional limited liability company.[7]

Nonprofit corporations formed under the Nonprofit Corporation Act are exempt. In 1993, the Michigan attorney general noted that the Doctrine was intended to prevent the commercial exploitation of the practice of medicine.[8] However, because the risk of commercialization and the limited liability of corporations are neutralized by formation as a nonprofit corporation, the attorney general found that the Doctrine need not be applied to nonprofit corporations.[9] This was later codified in Michigan Compiled Laws § 450.2661(6),

[1]Licensed professionals are prohibited from incorporating as limited liability companies. 4 Op. Cal. Att'y. Gen. 103 (2004).
[2]Cal. Corp. Code § 13401.5.
[3]*Id.*
[4]*Id.*
[5]Cal. Bus. & Prof. Code § 650(b).
[6]Mich. Comp. Laws §§ 450.1109(1), 450.4102(2) (t).
[7]Mich. Comp. Laws § 450.1282.
[8]Op. Mich. Att'y. Gen. No. 6770 at 3 (September 17, 1993).
[9]Op. Mich. Att'y. Gen. No. 6770 at 3–4 (September 17, 1993).

which provides that a nonprofit corporation may provide services in a learned profession.

Fee splitting prohibitions. The Michigan Public Health Code defines as an unethical business practice the "[d]ividing fees for referral of patients or accepting kickbacks on medical or surgical services, appliances, or medications purchased by or in behalf of patients."[10] Moreover, under the Michigan Healthcare False Claim Act and the Michigan Penal Code, fee-splitting arrangements may subject a physician to administrative penalties and criminal liability.[11]

Penalties for Violating the CPOM Doctrine

The CPOM Doctrine should be of significant concern to medical professionals given the hefty penalties that are associated with failure to comply. In general, a violation can result in (1) licensure restriction or revocation; (2) civil and even criminal liability for business partners who are laypersons; (3) voiding the business agreement; and recoupment by both private and governmental insurers.

INVESTMENT STRATEGIES

Management Services Arrangements

While the CPOM doctrine generally forbids a nonlicensed individual or entity from interfering with the affairs of a medical practice, a management services organization ("MSO") owned by a layperson is one way a nonlicensed person can invest in a medical practice without running afoul of a state's CPOM laws. A healthcare MSO, also known as a management company, partners or contracts with a practice to provide administrative services support such as accounting, human resources, advertising, marketing, and billing. The functions performed by the MSO must, in no way, interfere with the professional's ability to exercise independent medical judgment. One of the goals of an MSO is to relieve medical practices of administrative burdens in order to ensure that it can focus primarily on the delivery of quality patient care.

MSOs have become an increasingly popular means for laypersons or entities to invest in medical practices. However, because state guidelines regarding CPOM are sometimes unclear, management services contracts must be carefully structured to ensure that the MSO does not exert undue control over the professional entity.

[10]Mich. Comp. Laws § 333.16221(d) (ii).

[11]Mich. Comp. Laws §§ 750.428, 752-752.1011.

The following is an overview of how MSOs operate in New York and California.

New York

A recent decision issued by the Appellate Division of the New York Supreme Court outlines several factors that courts may consider in determining whether a professional corporation is unlawfully controlled by unlicensed individuals. In *Andrew Carothers, M.D., P.C. v. Progressive Ins. Co.*, 51 N.Y.S.3d 551, 556 (App. Div. 2017), the court upheld a verdict by the lower court, which found that a professional corporation was not entitled to payment under no-fault insurance policies because it was illegally formed. The decision made the following key findings: (1) the physician owner was not engaged in practice and (2) the de facto owners were unlicensed laypersons who exercised substantial control over the practice.

The court's decision also upheld a jury instruction that outlined 13 factors that should be considered when determining whether unlicensed individuals were de facto owners of the professional corporation and exercised substantial control over the professional corporation, including:

(a) Whether the unlicensed individual's dealings with the professional corporation were arm's length or were they designed to give the MSO substantial control over the PC and to channel profits to unlicensed persons;
(b) Whether the owners of the MSO exercised dominion and control over the professional corporation's assets, including its bank accounts;
(c) Whether the funds of the PC were used by the owners of the MSO for personal rather than corporate purposes;
(d) Whether the MSO owners were responsible for hiring, firing, and making salary payments to employees of the professional corporation;
(e) Whether the day-to-day formalities of the corporate existence were followed such as issuing stock, electing directors, holding corporate meetings, keeping contemporaneous corporate books and records, and filing of tax returns;
(f) Whether the professional corporation and the MSO shared a common office space; and
(g) Whether the physician owner of the professional corporation played a substantial role in its overall operation and management.

In reaching its holding, the court also noted that the professional corporation's equipment was leased from an affiliate of the MSO at grossly inflated rates and that checks written from the professional corporation's operating account were signed by an employee of the MSO.

While the court made clear that no factor standing alone could support a finding of fraudulent incorporation, taken together, the factors were relevant for purposes of determining de facto ownership and undue control.

California

The Medical Board of California has published guidelines that may also be instructive for unlicensed MSOs that seek to provide management services to California professional corporations.[12] Its guidance is based on the existing statutory framework, case law, and attorney general opinions that have opined on this subject.

For instance, when confronted with the question of what decisions fall within the provenance of the professional corporation, the California Medical Board provides the following examples:

(a) Determining what diagnostic testing is appropriate.
(b) Deciding what referrals or consultations are necessary.
(c) Responsibility for the ultimate overall patient care.
(d) Determining how many patients a physician must see in a given timeframe or how many hours a physician must work.
(e) Ownership of patient medical records.
(f) Selecting, hiring, and firing (as it relates to clinical competency or proficiency) of physicians, allied health staff, and medical assistants.
(g) Setting the parameters for contractual relationships between third-party payers and physicians.
(h) Decisions regarding coding and billing for care and treatment services.
(i) Approving of the selection of medical equipment and medical supplies for the medical practice.

The California Medical Board notes that examples (e) through (i) may appear to be business or management decisions that fall within the purview of the MSO. However, because these decisions carry implications resulting in the MSO exercising control over the practice of medicine, only a physician licensed to practice in California may make such decisions.

Strategies for structuring management services agreements

Provisions of a management services agreement to protect the manager. Management entities often seek to incorporate into management agreements provisions to protect them from being excluded from continuing to manage the practice in the future. One strategy that can be employed to protect a management entity in this regard is the establishing of onerous terms on termination of the management agreement. For example, the MSA can require that only the manager can terminate the agreement. Or the MSA may permit the medical entity to terminate the MSA or in the limited circumstance of specified breaches. Oftentimes, the MSA, on the other hand, may have the ability to more easily terminate the arrangement, and may even be able to do for no reason at all, which is generally referred to as termination without cause. Prohibiting, or severely limiting, a PC from terminating the MSA protects the MSO because it ensures that the PC cannot replace the MSO with a new manager and thereby exclude the manager from continuing to manage the practice.

Another way in which a management entity can seek to protect itself from being easily replaced is by making the MSA contain a very long term. In some circumstances, the MSO may seek a term of the MSA that lasts 10, 15, or even 20 + years. The long duration, coupled with the above restrictions on early termination, gives protection to the MSO that the PC will not unfairly terminate the relationship.

Whether or not a PC and an MSO should include these provisions in MSAs, or other strategies, is something that should be carefully considered with a healthcare attorney in order to not only make sure that these provisions are advantageous for the entities but also ensure that such provisions do not run afoul of federal and state regulations.

Physician shareholder ownership of the MSO. Another means by which an MSO can protect itself from unfair termination or PC destruction of the practice is to make the physician shareholders of the PC also shareholders of the MSO. Under this strategy, the MSO, in addition to being owned by the lay shareholders, is also at least partially owned by the physician shareholders of the PC. The basic concept under this strategy is that since the PC and MSO have the same shareholders, no one will act in a way that is contrary to the interests of both entities since doing so would be detrimental to all shareholders.

While this may be an effective strategy to employ in order to ensure an efficient and fair operation of the business venture, it still comes with potential complications. First, it requires diluting the shareholder interests of the lay shareholders of the MSO, which can serve as a deterrent for nonphysician investment in the management company.

More importantly, making physicians shareholders of the MSO adds heightened risk of violating state and federal self-referral and anti-kickback laws.

---

[12] Corporate Practice of Medicine, http://www.mbc.ca.gov/Licensees/Corporate_Practice.aspx.

Friendly or Captive Professional Corporations

In the states in which it either completely prohibits for a lay entity to engage in the practice of medicine or in those states in which there are enough restrictions to require a management services organization arrangement, corporations often seek additional protections with respect to the relationship with the PC. One such strategy that a management entity may consider is the captive PC model utilizing a stock restriction agreement.

Stock restriction agreements are not very complicated and are easy to establish. However, while they are a regular tool utilized in general corporate legal structure, the use of a stock restriction agreement in a medical practice setting can be complicated and needs to be carefully considered before implementing. The reason for this is that the states that do restrict the corporate practice of medicine may view the restriction of a PC's stock as demonstrating control of the PC by the lay entity and could be considered practicing medicine or asserting improper control of the PC.

Stock restriction agreements protect an MSO by restricting the ability, or in some cases removing the ability, of a PC's shareholders to transfer their shares. Generally, stock restriction agreements consist of two basic components: (1) a restriction on the ability of the PC's shareholders to sell or transfer the stock of the PC and (2) establishing provisions for the automatic transfer of the PC's shares to a designated individual upon certain specified occurrences. A less aggressive stock restriction agreement can require that prior to any conveyance of stock, the MSO must provide approval for the conveyance in order for it to be effective.

By restricting the ability of the PC shareholders to transfer or sell stock in any way, a lay entity can ensure that the PC does not convey the stock to licensed shareholders and as a result alter the individuals involved in the medical practice.

Hybrid model consisting of an ambulatory surgical center and an office-based endovascular center

In some instances, it may be beneficial for a number of reasons, both practically and financially, to not have a practice be entirely either an ambulatory surgical center ("ASC") or OEC, but rather operate, to the extent permissible under the law, as both. There are many legal implications from this model that need to be considered prior to establishing this model.

Multiple licenses at one location. The first thing that needs to be reviewed and ensured is that there are no state prohibitions on having these two separate entities at one location. Some states may have prohibitions on having two separate entities at one location, each requiring a license. In addition, whether the entities themselves require state licensure to operate is also an issue that needs to be analyzed on a state by state basis.

Medicare Opting In v. Opting Out

Another issue that needs to be addressed is whether the OEC and the ASC will both be enrolled in Medicare or whether it is desired that only one entity will be a Medicare-enrolled provider. Any physician who will bill Medicare is required to enroll as a Medicare provider.[13] In order to enroll, a physician will need to enter into the Medicare Participating Provider Agreement. If enrolled in Medicare, a physician must accept payment on an assignment-related basis for all claims for services provided to Medicare beneficiaries.[14] This means that physicians or groups enrolled are generally prohibited from billing Medicare beneficiaries for any amounts in excess of the Medicare reimbursement rates for covered services and the violation of this can lead to civil monetary penalties, and even Medicare exclusion.[15]

Opting out of Medicare means that a physician or group is choosing to not be enrolled in Medicare and as a result can seek direct payment from the patient and not from Medicare. There are four requirements that are necessary to enter into a private contract with a Medicare beneficiary: (1) no claim for payment may be submitted to Medicare; (2) physician cannot receive any payment from Medicare for the service; (3) the contract with the beneficiary must meet all the requirements under the law; and (4) a valid affidavit has been filed with the Department of Health and Human Services.[16] If a private contract with a Medicare beneficiary lacks these requirements, then it is null and void.[17]

Once opted out, a physician or group cannot submit any claims to Medicare and cannot receive any payment from the Medicare program.[18] This is true even if the physician assigns his billing rights to another entity that is enrolled.[19] Physicians cannot be both simultaneously opted in for some patients and opted out for other. The same is true with a group. If a physician has opted out of Medicare, the group may not submit that physicians' claims to Medicare for reimbursement,

[13] 42 C.F.R. §424.505.
[14] 42 U.S.C. § 1395u(h) (1).
[15] 42 U.S.C. §1320a-7a(a).
[16] 42 U.S.C. § 1395a.
[17] 42 C.F.R. § 405.405.
[18] 42 C.F.R. §405.425.
[19] Id.

even if the group itself has remained opted into the Medicare program.[20]

Thus, one consideration that groups considering this hybrid model must take into account is whether both entities will be Medicare providers or both will opt out. If one will be a Medicare provider and one will opt out, it could be problematic for physicians who will overlap at both entities and provide services. Since, physicians cannot be simultaneously opted in and opted out, services that an opted-out physician provides at one entity will be nonreimbursable to Medicare beneficiaries. This model will likely only make sense when both the OEC and the ASC will either be enrolled or both be not enrolled as Medicare providers.

ASC anti-kickback issues. The OIG has issued opinions that look unfavorably on ASCs that have investors who do not perform procedures at the ASC. In one opinion, the OIG found that optometrists who referred patients to an ASC in which they had an ownership interest in the ASC, that performed ophthalmology procedures would violate the applicable federal kickback statutes since the optometrists would be in a position to refer patients for procedures that they did not perform. Under such an arrangement, the OIG found that there were no safeguards to ensure that the optometrists were not being paid a referral fee as a share of the profits.[21]

Any consideration of establishing an ASC must take into account the need for the physician owners to perform procedures at the ASC. Generally, the physician owners will be required to meet the "one-third" test in order to fall into the ASC safe harbor under the anti-kickback statute.[22] In surgeon-owned and single specialty–owned ASCs, at least one-third of each owner's practice income must come from procedures performed at the ASC over the last 12-month period. As to a multispecialty surgery center, over the past 12 months, one-third of the procedures performed by each physician investor must be performed at the ASC.

Based upon this, it can raise suspicions, and even potentially be a violation of the anti-kickback statute, to have physician owners of an ASC who will not use the ASC. Thus, physicians and groups seeking to form ASCs need to take that fact into consideration. With respect to an OEC, the same is not true. If a group seeks to establish both an ASC and an OEC, it should consider not having physician owners who will not perform procedures as owners of the ASC. Rather, they can be owners of an OEC.

ASC and OEC at same location. One issue that arises in this model is what to do in situations where it is not entirely in the practice's best interest to completely form into an ASC or an OEC. In those circumstances, the practice seeks to be both an ASC and an OEC. There may be several reasons why it is desired, such as economic motives or logistic issues, but there are likely to be scenarios where a location and a group seek to be both simultaneously an ASC and an OEC. Here are some important factors to consider when seeking this model.

Accreditation requirements. ASCs almost always require accreditation from the various accreditation entities, such as the Joint Commission, formerly the Joint Commission on Accreditation of Healthcare Organizations or American Association for Accreditation of Ambulatory Surgery Facilities, Inc. Each of these accreditation entities has specific requirements necessary to receive and maintain accreditation (Chapter 36). Among these are having completely separate medication storage units. Generally, if you will utilize a facility to practice as both an ASC and an OEC, you will have to operate each as separate distinct entities who happen to share space. This can get complicated, especially considering that the same personnel and owners may be present in both entities. Nonetheless, in order to effectively maintain this kind of balance, and to maintain necessary accreditation, an ASC and OEC that share space should establish as many safeguards as possible to operate separate businesses.

Medicare requirements. Federal law defines an ASC as "any distinct entity that operates exclusively for the purpose of providing surgical services to patients not requiring hospitalization and in which the expected duration of services would not exceed 24 h following an admission."[23] ASCs that participate in the federal Medicare and Medicaid programs must satisfy minimum conditions in order to receive reimbursement for patient care and treatment. Those conditions are set forth under 42 C.F.R. §§ 416.20–416.54. In order to ensure compliance with these conditions, the Centers for Medicaid and Medicare ("CMS") contracts with state

[20]Centers for Medicare & Medicaid Services, Medicare Benefits Policy Manual, CH. 15 §40.23 (Oct 1, 2003).

[21]OIG Advisory Opinion 07–13, issued on October 12, 2007.

[22]Not falling into a safe harbor does not automatically mean the conduct violates the statute. Instead, the safe harbors provide assurance to physicians that they are not in violation of the statute. Conduct not contained in the list of safe harbors may still not violate the anti-kickback statute, but there are no assurances of that.

[23]42 C.F.R. § 416.2.

survey agencies to conduct unannounced compliance surveys.

When seeking to operate an ASC and OEC out of the same location, the parties must ensure that the ASC remains a distinct entity within the meaning of federal and state law. The services performed by the entities must not be commingled, and each must ensure that its medical and administrative records are kept physically separate. Non-ASC personnel must not be able to access records ASC record. Records thus should be stored separately, and they should remain locked when the entity is not in operation.

Although the ASC must be distinct, it does not preclude an ASC and OEC from sharing a facility. The State Operations Manual ("SOM") offers additional guidance on this point.

An ASC does not have to be completely separate and distinct physically from another entity, if, and only if, it is temporally distinct. In other words, the same physical premises may be used by the ASC and other entities, so long as they are separated in their usage by time.[24]

In other words, the hours of operation for the ASC and the OEC must never overlap. An ASC should not seek to avoid this requirement be entering into an arrangement whereby the OEC rents out or makes clinical space available to the OEC during the ASC's hours of operation.

To demonstrate that the entities are temporally distinct, each entity should display its hours of operation on signage that is clearly visible to the public. We further suggest that the hours of operation be set forth in any written agreements between the ASC and the OEC. It should also be included in the commercial lease agreement between the entities and the property owner.

Federal law also permits ASCs to share common administrative space with an OEC; however, the use of the common space may not overlap in time. In order to demonstrate the state surveyors that use of common space is not concurrent, signs and schedules should be posted in the space.

States may impose more stringent requirements on ASC sharing space with other entities. The SOM sets forth explicitly that state law controls where it imposes more stringent requirements as compared with federal law.

Maintaining regulatory and corporate formalities between the two entities. As discussed above, it is important to observe necessary corporate and regulatory formalities, which can be easy to overlook. Since the OEC and the ASC will be separate legal entities, they need to be appropriately treated as such. This means separate and distinct corporate documents and avoiding combining patient records. Since the two entities will share the same location, the separate of the two entities needs to be carefully monitored.

Since they will be separate and distinct legal entities, both entities will need to have their own employees and leases at the location. The space lease is an important issue to consider. There are several different ways to set up the two entities. One way to organize the structure is to have separate days of the week for each entity. For example, the ASC can operate on Mondays, Wednesdays, and Fridays, and the OEC can operate on Tuesdays and Thursdays.[25] Another option is to have the OEC occupy a specific portion of the physical space and the ASC to operate another portion of the physical space. No matter the structure, a separate lease or sublease will be necessary for each entity. Generally, one entity will lease the space from the landlord and then will sublease the space to the additional entity. It is important to review the original lease to ensure that subleasing is allowed before proceeding.

Because they are separate entities, both entities will need to have their own employees. If an employee is only employed by the ASC, for example, then there would be no justification for that same employee to provide services for the OEC. It is easy to see how this can cause complications in the structure. It is also a hardship for each entity to have to hire separate and distinct employees. Therefore, the entities should consider a leasing or sharing of the employees. Under this scenario, one entity would be the actual employer. That entity could then enter into an agreement with the other entity to lease the employees on a part-time basis. Both entities would pay for their prorate use of the employees, including taxes and benefits.

CONCLUSIONS

In closing, there are several models that are available to laypersons who wish to invest in medical professional practices. Such arrangements must be carefully structured to avoid running afoul of the laws that govern these types of ventures, but in general, it is important to ensure that these arrangements preserve the professional's ability to exercise independent medical

[24]*CMS Publication 100-07, State Operations Manual*, Appendix L, Part II, § Q-0002 [hereinafter SOM] *available at* https://www.cms.gov/Regulations-and-Guidance/Guidance/Manuals/downloads/som107ap_l_ambulatory.pdf.

[25]Another possible scenario, but generally more difficult to implement properly, is dividing half days, or even on an hourly basis within each day. A careful analysis of these structures should be considered carefully.

judgment. Because state laws governing these investment models vary significantly, one should seek the advice of an attorney to obtain a more complete rendering of a state's laws.

DISCLAIMER

The following information does not constitute legal advice, and readers should not rely on this overview as a complete interpretation of state and federal law on these matters.

CHAPTER 24

Opening an Endovascular Center in an Academic Environment

JOHN BLEBEA, MD, MBA • MAXIM E. SHAYDAKOV, MD, PHD

INTRODUCTION

Historically, both before and after the development of vascular surgery as a recognized specialty, vascular surgical procedures have characteristically been open cases associated with substantial morbidity and mortality. Most of the arterial revascularizations were subsequently performed by board-certified vascular surgeons and the patients were kept in the hospital for days. The more complex cases, such as distal bypasses or aneurysms, were initially done in university hospitals and tertiary referral centers. Although some inpatient postoperative care is still required in certain circumstances, such as carotid endarterectomy, aortic aneurysm repair, or distal bypasses, most hospital care is now reflective of patient comorbidities rather than the procedures themselves. In addition, the significant advancements in endovascular technology, intravenous anesthesia with conscious sedation, and widespread multidisciplinary vascular education have enabled many previously advanced interventional procedures to be performed outside of academic medical centers and carried out on an outpatient basis. Indeed, similar to the dissemination of laparoscopic cholecystectomy, the innovators of surgical outpatient-based endovascular interventions were those in private practice rather than the university surgeons. Even today, academic surgeons and medical centers lag far behind their private practice counterparts in embracing and implementing office-based vascular centers.

The first reports of outpatient transfemoral diagnostic angiography published in the early 1960s were followed by publication of results with outpatient peripheral angioplasty procedures in the 1990s.[1,2] Practice patterns have subsequently evolved such that the majority of percutaneous arterial interventions are no longer performed in the hospital but safely in an office setting with few complications.[3–5] A similar process is now being seen for coronary angiography and same-day cardiac interventions.[6] On the venous side, since the introduction of endovascular laser ablation of the saphenous vein two decades ago, the treatment of patients with venous disease has become almost the exclusive prerogative of the office or outpatient vein centers.[7,8] Outpatient dialysis access centers have become the principal setting for catheter insertion and access maintenance for hemodialysis. Interventionalists from multiple specialties have become involved in outpatient vascular interventions. These have principally included physicians trained as vascular and cardiovascular surgeons, interventional radiologists, interventional cardiologists, as well as interventional nephrologists, dermatologists, primary care physicians, and others.

The major potential benefits of outpatient vascular procedures, such as expedited patient care, lower costs, and higher patient satisfaction, all contribute to an improving quality of care to patients with vascular disease.[9] Excellent reported outcomes with same-day vascular procedures have encouraged the growth of office-based centers specializing in minimally invasive interventions.[10] In association with this, physician compensation (professional component) for hospital-based vascular procedures has been declining. On the other hand, the physician receives a global fee, that includes technical component in addition to the professional component, when the procedure is done in the office. This has attracted physicians to perform more such cases in outpatient facilities.[11,12] The Centers for Medicare and Medicaid Services (CMS) is also trying to reduce inpatient hospital care. Physicians also appreciate the greater control over scheduling and much more efficient procedural performance compared with the hospital environment.

While there are definite benefits to surgical procedures being done in an office setting, questions have been raised about the possible higher risk of morbidity

Office-Based Endovascular Centers. https://doi.org/10.1016/B978-0-323-67969-5.00024-1
Copyright © 2020 Elsevier Inc. All rights reserved.

and mortality.[13] Additionally, the higher reimbursement for office-based procedures may lead to financial conflicts of interests and clinically unjustified interventions.[14] A recent study demonstrated a disproportionate growth of atherectomy compared with other office-based vascular procedures despite the lack of evidence for improved long-term benefits compared with the less costly balloon angioplasty and stenting alternatives.[15] The rapid and substantial growth in the number of these centers has raised concerns on the lack of external oversight, certification of physicians or accreditation of the center, and limited data on outcomes for office-based endovascular interventions.[16–18] These concerns underline the need for careful selection of patients for these procedures, clinical protocols, and experienced physicians and office staff in order to provide high-quality clinical care in the office setting.

While the general benefits and concerns relating to office-based endovascular center (OEC) apply to both private practice and the academic environment, the university setting has its own unique characteristics that provide it with both relative advantages and specific challenges. This chapter will review those characteristics and provide insights into the successful establishment of an OEC by university-employed vascular specialists.

RATIONALE FOR OFFICE-BASED ENDOVASCULAR PROCEDURES IN AN ACADEMIC ENVIRONMENT

An academic endovascular center provides vascular surgeons and other interventionalists with a supportive environment to care for even some of the most challenging patients with vascular pathology. The hospital infrastructure, unavoidable bureaucracy, and challenging logistics are not an ideal setting for many patients. Trying to manage urgent or emergent procedures superimposed on an elective schedule in a large university hospital, where several busy services may be competing for the same operative or interventional block time and human resources, is always a difficult task and leads to repeated unpredictable delays and cancellations. For the vascular surgeon, the ideal setting in the hospital for the majority of vascular interventions is a hybrid operating room which provides them with optimal fixed imaging equipment and a broad assortment of ancillary catheters and guidewires to deal with multiple eventualities, both planned and unexpected. However, although the hybrid operating room was initially envisioned as the protected and sole enclave of the vascular surgeon, its high costs and superior interventional capabilities have attracted other specialists to demand access for its use. These have included interventional cardiologists for the placement of transcatheter aortic valve replacement (TAVR) and difficult pacemaker/defibrillator extractions, cardiothoracic surgeons beginning to do their own endovascular aortic procedures, and trauma surgeons who may also require vascular imaging or interventions. The hybrid room, and even more often its trained nursing personnel, may also be utilized for other elective and emergent procedures when endovascular cases are not scheduled in the room. In such circumstances, when an urgent vascular patient requires intervention, the room or needed personnel may not be readily available. This is particularly problematic at the end of the day or after hours. This may even occur during the scheduled hours during the day because of demand from other specialties thereby delaying elective cases.

Several studies have demonstrated that at least half of all elective surgeries in a hospital may be delayed, significantly affecting patient flow and resources utilization.[19,20] Since complex and life-threatening procedures appropriately have first priority for hospital resources, elective patients or those with less acute interventions are the ones most likely to be delayed or canceled. This reflects the inevitable fact that hospitals have to take care of emergency procedures while at the same time trying to maintain a busy elective schedule. Unfortunately, this inherent conflict translates to elective and outpatient procedures being the ones suffering forced delays and cancellations. This leads to both patient dissatisfaction and ineffective utilization of a physician's time. In an OEC, there are infrequent emergent cases to disrupt the planned elective schedule. This can be especially beneficial for patients with dialysis assess failure to avoid delays in renal replacement therapy or insertion of tunneled catheters. Better control of the schedule in the OEC results in much more efficient care for patients and greatly improved time utilization for the doctor. This provides the academic physician with a more efficient clinical environment in which to deliver excellent patient care while preserving needed time for expected scholarly activities.

An original concern for performing interventional procedures outside the hospital environment was the potential lack of multiple options of specialty catheters and guidewires as well as more specialized and expensive atherectomy or closure devices. However, as hospitals have implemented cost-cutting measures and reduced both the numbers and diversity of endovascular devices, the office-based centers now generally have more of such preferred devices than the hospital. In addition, these devices are generally selected based on their superior utility by the physician using them and not a cost-based decision by a hospital administrator or value-added committee whose primary concern is financial and purchasing agreement requirements. An additional original worry was the fear of hiring inexperienced or untrained nursing staff and assistants for the office. Quite the opposite has occurred. The most experienced and best interventional staff have been recruited to the office setting. They are attracted by the much friendlier work environment, focus on patient care, greater efficiency, and predictable schedules without call or weekend/holiday work. The best nursing and technical staff are now found in the office, not the hospital. The latter is now where the most recent graduates and inexperienced personnel are to be found until they get the needed work experience and then they look for a more desirable position in an office setting.

Vascular interventions performed in the office are significantly less expensive compared with the same procedures performed in the hospital or the hospital outpatient facility.[11,21] An important contributing factor is the more controllable and efficient utilization of human and material resources. Improved efficiency and faster throughput allow for a much higher number of cases to be performed within the same time frame and decreases the procedural costs in the OEC. There are other factors that also improve the cost-effectiveness of procedures performed at the OEC. In both the hospital inpatient and outpatient settings, anesthesiologists are almost always involved in the procedure. There is a greater tendency for patients to undergo general anesthesia in such circumstances. At a minimum, monitored anesthesia care (MAC) is employed by the anesthesiologist with an associated and significant professional fee component. In the office setting, anesthesiologists are rarely employed. Local anesthesia is generally preferred, but physician-supervised intravenous conscious sedation provides very good comfort levels for the patient even for prolonged procedures and at a fraction of the cost of MAC. Extended periods of observation, or overnight in-hospital stays after late interventions, substantially increases treatment costs but are rare after a procedure in the office. There is no provision for the patient to stay overnight in the office. Finally, interventionalists are intimately involved with purchasing, hiring, and staffing decisions. Therefore, they are very cost-conscious and effective managers because, unlike in the hospital, they have both the information and decision-making authority to effect change. Hence, creation of OECs is associated with large savings to patients, insurers, and taxpayers. Unlike previous times, academic physicians are now also held accountable for costs within their divisions or departments. Therefore, having a profitable OEC provides academic interventionalists with a cost center that can support faculty both in terms of research budgets and to provide protected time for scholarly activity.

Recent trends in expectations for greater clinical productivity in association with decreasing physician compensation relative to private practice may force many academic vascular surgeons, especially those at the beginning of their careers, to abandon academia for the more lucrative (both in time and money) private practice opportunities.[22] Reimbursement for office-based procedures are higher because it compensates not only the professional but also the technical services related to vascular interventions. One large retrospective study reported a fivefold increase in revenue for vascular procedures done in the office compared with the hospital.[23] Thus, OECs may serve as a significant source of revenue for underpaid academic physicians. Most importantly, the best argument in favor of outpatient office-based facilities is the significant positive impact on the quality of healthcare. One retrospective review demonstrated that performing vascular access procedures at an outpatient center was associated with a reduction of almost one hospital day per patient year and a decreased rate of missed dialysis treatments.[24]

A multitude of procedures have been safely performed in the OEC setting. These include diagnostic angiography, interventions for peripheral arterial disease (angioplasty, stenting, atherectomy), venous procedures (obliteration of saphenous veins, phlebectomy, sclerotherapy), interventions to maintain hemodialysis access, central venous access, and inferior vena caval filter implantation and removal. Randomized controlled clinical research trials to directly compare the clinical results of vascular interventions performed at a university hospital and an affiliated OEC setting do not exist. However, it is reasonable to expect at least similar outcomes because regardless of the location of an interventional suite the procedures would be performed by the same physicians with the same fund of knowledge and manual skills. Indeed, clinical outcomes would be expected to be better as office-based interventionalists are generally more experienced and in most cases would themselves be doing the procedures instead of supervising less-experienced trainees. On the other hand, published retrospective studies have already shown that percutaneous vascular procedures performed at an OEC are quite safe. One analysis of 6,458 procedures demonstrated zero mortality, a 0.8% overall complication rate, 0.4% hospital transfer rate, and 0.2% rate of open surgical intervention because of complications.[23] Overall patient satisfaction reached 99%. Other authors reported 0.7%–3.0% incidence of complications which is comparable with outpatient hospital-based outcomes.[25,26] These results compare very favorably with a 4.9% complication rate after interventional outpatient procedures performed in a tertiary academic hospital.[27]

PRINCIPLES OF ORGANIZATION OF AN ACADEMIC OEC

Office-based private practice is a well-established and traditional setting for many physicians of different specialties. In modern times, the office has expanded to include ever-more complex procedures. This trend has been especially prevalent in the otolaryngology and plastic surgery specialties.[28] Office-based interventional endovascular centers have more recently joined this trend following the model developed by other specialties with defined processes for creation and development and expected high clinical and financial success rates. However, the establishment of such endovascular centers within academic institutions has been far less common and there is scarce information on how to establish and manage such a center. An academic vascular OEC represents a very different environment with specific advantages and limitations that need to be considered both during the planning stages and implementation.

Establishing an academic OEC is a serious and challenging undertaking which is much more difficult than in the private practice setting. It is particularly demanding because of the multiple individuals that need to support the project within the department, medical school, university, and hospital. Although almost all leaders within the respective institutions must agree, just one alone can prevent it from coming to fruition. Most proposals for an OEC will come from, or will need to be fully championed by, the chief of the respective academic division, most commonly vascular surgery, interventional cardiology, or interventional radiology. This is the individual who will need to invest the large amount of time needed to fully develop the proposal, sell it to all subsequent levels of leadership, explain and respond to the inevitable questions and attempts to derail the project, and ultimately to do the legwork for successful implementation. Although the academic leader can assign partial responsibilities to others, and operation of the OEC once it is successfully running, the sectional or division chief almost always needs to be the one to take on this task. An individual with less administrative status will usually not have the clinical and political experience nor the academic and political authority to successfully carry out such an initiative. If the departmental chair is a vascular specialist, they will be in a stronger position to carry this out although it will be a more difficult task for them because they will have less time for this project due to their other responsibilities which they cannot easily delegate to others.

If the chair is of a different subspecialty, he/she will pose the first challenge to overcome to get the OEC proposal off the ground. The chair is the first supervisor to consider the project. His/her strong and unequivocal support, while not in and of itself sufficient to approve the plan, is absolutely required for it to go anywhere. They cannot make it happen, but they can stop the proposal in its tracks with a simple "no." Important steps in obtaining the chair's support include preparing a convincing financial plan, defining the center as critical to the financial and clinical future of the division, reemphasizing the importance of endovascular interventions for patient care, and potential of strong collaboration with other specialties involved in these procedures. A well-prepared presentation, reflecting much homework already completed, should gain the chair's support. However, even if the chair is sympathetic to the idea, and wants to back it, there may not be enough money in the departmental budget to get the OEC started. In addition, there may be other priorities or commitments already promised by the department which require more immediate attention and financial support. More frequently, there may be strong political challenges from competing departments or specialties which would view an OEC as direct competition for patients and procedures which they are doing or want to do more of in the future. Such antagonism from other specialties need to be considered and, if possible, the divisional or departmental opponent converted to a supporter before an OEC proposal is submitted to higher authority for consideration. Ideally, a collegial relationship between the respective chairs will allow for a constructive meeting in which the OEC can be privately explained to them and support attained. More frequently, other departments will see this as a financial or professional practice threat to them and then the strategy should be to make this into a win-win scenario. The most direct way to achieve this goal would be to allow other specialties to participate in the OEC by granting them practice privileges at the center. As long as the involved individuals get along well with others, this will truly be a winning combination for all. The key in this circumstance is to clearly elucidate right at the beginning that not every physician can be successful in an outpatient environment and they must have the personality, confidence, and interpersonal skills to work well with others.

Once cross-specialty or interdepartmental agreement has been reached, or further attempts felt to be futile in building cooperation, the next step is to obtain approval from the dean of the college of medicine. As the overall leader of all academic faculty, and ultimately responsible for the budget of both the school and faculty practice plan, he is the most important individual to be convinced and potentially the most difficult. His support, however, is the *sine qua non* of this bureaucratic process. Gaining the dean's agreement, however, can be quite problematic as he is not likely to understand details of an OEC proposal, does not have the time to learn, and may not be sufficiently interested. If the university does not own its own medical center, the dean has the biggest potential political risk in dealing with hospital leadership who will see the OEC as a direct financial threat to them. In addition, a divisional chief will have only limited access to and limited influence with the dean. Therefore, they should be completely prepared before meeting with the dean, accompanied by an enthusiastically supportive chair.

An important person to meet prior to the encounter with the dean is the chief financial officer (CFO) of the faculty practice plan. One should have met with the CFO early in the process. The CFO should have been an active participant in developing the business plan and be fully convinced of the financial viability of the proposed OEC. No matter how convinced the dean may be of your plans, he/she will not approve unless the CFO gives financial approval. The discussions with the CFO need to lead to a detailed 5-year financial plan listing expenses with as many details as possible and with justifiable and realistic revenue estimates. A departmental administrator or certified public accountant can be very helpful in this process. The plan should include an estimated number of procedures per year. For an OEC in an academic setting, an estimated annual growth in the number of the procedures would be conservatively projected at 10% for the second year and 20% for each of the third, fourth, and fifth years. Estimated operating expenses should include salaries for surgeons, surgical/radiology technicians, nurses, manager, and front desk clerks. Total human resource costs may vary broadly depending on the patients to be treated and projected number of procedures performed daily. Needless to say, if the champion for the OEC has an MBA and prior demonstrated administrative success as a division chief, their credibility will be much enhanced. Successful examples of established OECs at other academic centers with several years of experience and real objective data, including number of cases, expenditures, and net income, will also be helpful. The most critical part of planning is to make up a detailed and convincing 5-year financial plan.

A proposal to the dean should include providing them with arguments in preparation for pushback from the hospital. If the dean is also vice president of health affairs and chief hospital executive, these will be the final points needed to convince him for approval. The OEC proponent must explain how present hospital facilities are not conducive for optimal patient care, how attempts at improving the process and clinical protocols have proved futile, and how the division has no choice but to pursue an OEC. The hospital chief operating officer (CEO) and administrators will frequently be the biggest obstacles to an OEC initiative because they will see in this effort (erroneously) that they have everything to lose and nothing to gain. Convincing them of this fallacy, however, will not be easy because of multiple reasons: you will most often have had little contact with the CEO, he/she does not have time for you, is not likely to respect you as an equal, and will see you as a competitor who will be taking patients and lucrative procedures away from the hospital. In preparation for this CEO challenge, one should recognize the problem early, document and define lack of adequate access to endovascular suites, insufficient procedure block times, inadequate equipment, and very inefficient patient care. One should keep plans for an independent OEC confidential from hospital administrators but not deny such plans when discovered. Importantly, repeated experience has shown that office-based centers have not been associated with decreased hospital procedure numbers. As the OEC becomes busier, more patients are referred to the hospital for inpatient-based procedures so that the overall financial effect on the hospital is either positive or neutral. Finally, however, unlike the need for concurrence from the other individuals described so far, most CEOs will never be convinced to support the OEC proposal. The objective in these discussions, however, is to provide the dean with the substantive arguments to defend the school's decision to proceed with an OEC.

As has been implied in this discussion, the biggest challenge in an academic environment as compared with private practice is the multiple levels of leadership from which approvals are needed before embarking on an OEC. In a group practice, such a decision can be made relatively quickly by a small group of one to three individuals who own the practice or are in the leadership of a group practice. On the other hand, the biggest problem for a private practice, money, is almost a nonissue for a university. Whereas private groups have to borrow or use mortgage to come up with significant amount of capital upfront, the university does not have to borrow any money. The initial expenses for buying/renovating/building an outpatient center can easily be floated from operating revenues by a faculty practice. The $500,000 to 2 million dollars in initial investment would rarely be a problem for a medical school. In addition, beautiful facilities are occasionally already available from other practices within the medical school or shell space reserved for future needs is available (Figs. 24.1 and 24.2). The building should be large enough to readily accommodate the estimated number of patients per day and provide for expansion with the expectation of future growth. A preoperative holding area, interventional rooms (s), recovery area, physician and manager offices, exam rooms, storage room, space for hazardous waste, and medicine cabinets are the minimum space requirements. Ideally, the OEC building should not be more than 15–30 min from either the hospital or physician academic offices in order to insure minimal time loss for physicians moving between facilities. For patients, being close to the university medical center provides the benefit of rapid transfer should any significant complication occur at the OEC.

In addition to the physical plant, equipment, and supply stock, operating costs of the facility and staffing will need to be covered for the first 3–6 months before a new OEC starts bringing significant income.[29] Having all necessary endovascular devices readily available is critical for procedural safety and success, and to enable

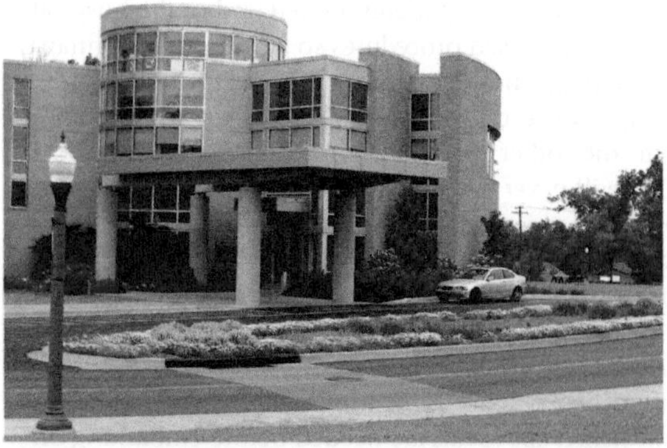

FIG. 24.1 External appearance and entry to a university endovascular center repurposed from an infusion center.

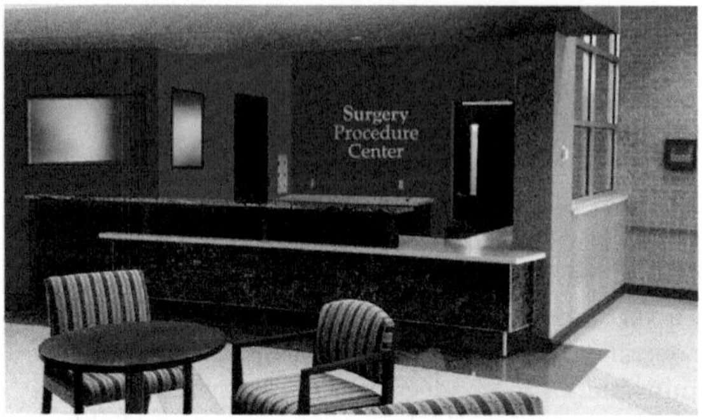

FIG. 24.2 Registration desk and family waiting area.

smooth patient flow. Stock of the most commonly used catheters, guidewires, balloons, stents, sheaths, vessel puncture kits and closure devices are a necessity. Ultrasound-guided access should be the standard of care in the office. Other supplies in required inventory will depend on the number and mix of expected cases. Fortunately, all of these costs are also more easily covered by the deep pockets of a medical school practice plan. In addition, in this scenario, individual physicians are not personally responsible for the legal and financial burdens of the OEC, particularly if it should fail as a business venture.

The bureaucratic challenges of the university environment do not disappear once the plan has been approved by the dean. On the contrary, they now increase almost exponentially in number as the multiple details of facility construction/remodeling begin, permits and contracts are obtained, personnel hiring is begun, and selection/purchasing/stocking of devices is initiated. There are a multitude of previously unidentified offices and individuals who must be involved in this process, few of whom see any urgency in your requests. Be prepared for numerous and ineffectual meetings and a generous amount of paperwork. These cannot be avoided and must be endured. However, going through the process with a positive attitude will help to establish personal rapport with needed individuals, you will discover who can get things done and you will identify talented individuals who will help immeasurably in getting the OEC off the ground and in making it successful. It is at this stage that recruitment should be done for the nurse manager. This person will be one of the most important people in the center, and it is vitally important that the person be a skilled clinician, wise manager, and a mature and positive individual. At this point, it may be worthwhile to seek the assistance of a consultant who may have experience in putting it all together. The medical directorship of the OEC can be transferred from the founding champion and division chief, but only after at least 1 year has passed and the center is running smoothly with stable and experienced personnel. Once opened, there are still multiple issues that will be identified and best resolved by the one who has the knowledge of all of the details and decisions that were required to start. One year also allows sufficient time to identify those interventionalists who thrive and enjoy the outpatient environment that cannot necessarily be predicted beforehand.

A final consideration for an academic-based OEC is the educational aspects which may not be present in the private setting. An important objective of office-based centers is to create an efficient high-flow outpatient setting for ambulatory procedures with low complication rates and high patient satisfaction. However, medical students, residents, and fellows constitute an integral part of patient care in any academic environment and should also be integrated into the activities of the OEC. In this context, we have integrated them into this practice setting. However, in order to fulfill our other objectives, students are in a more observational role then in the hospital, and we prefer to have senior residents or fellows participate in the procedures as there is less time for procedure completion and basic instruction in technique. This has worked out well in our experience.

CONCLUSIONS

Academic institutions will benefit from establishing an OEC through increased patient care efficiency and satisfaction. The majority of patients with peripheral arterial disease, primary chronic venous insufficiency, and dialysis access can receive a more convenient, prompt, and affordable care at the OEC compared with the hospital. These procedures will be done by experienced academic vascular interventionalists who ensure high quality of care. Physicians will benefit from a more predictable schedule and better productivity. Establishing an OEC in an academic environment has significant and unique challenges requiring collaboration and approval among leaders from the department, medical school, and hospital. This will require the time, commitment, and maturity of an experienced and mature individual with a high level of administrative and interpersonal skills. A major advantage is the financial resources that are available to the university which is not seen in private practice and the lack of personal financial responsibility incurred by the academic physician. The benefits to both the patient and physician accrued through practice in an OEC are shared by both those inside and outside the university setting. Opening an endovascular center in an academic environment is possible, good for the patients and the academic physician and should be encouraged.

REFERENCES

1. Straube D. Vertebral angiography. Percutaneous transfemoral technic suitable for outpatient application. *N Z Med J*. 1961;60:697–700.
2. Struk DW, Rankin RN, Eliasziw M, Vellet AD. Safety of outpatient peripheral angioplasty. *Radiology*. 1993; 189(1):193–196.
3. Akopian G, Katz SG. Peripheral angioplasty with same-day discharge in patients with intermittent claudication. *J Vasc Surg*. 2006;44(1):115–118.
4. Zayed HA, Fassiadis N, Jones KG, et al. Day-case angioplasty in diabetic patients with critical ischemia. *Int Angiol*. 2008;27(3):232–238.
5. Kruse JR, Cragg AH. Safety of short stay observation after peripheral vascular intervention. *J Vasc Interv Radiol*. 2000;11(1):45–49.
6. Goss F, Brachmann I, Hamm CW, Haerer W, Reifart N, Levenson B. High adherence to therapy and low cardiac mortality and morbidity in patients after acute coronary syndrome systematically managed by office-based cardiologists in Germany. *Vasc Health Risk Manag*. 2017;13:127–137.
7. Min RJ, Zimmet SE, Isaacs MN, et al. Endovenous laser treatment of the incompetent greater saphenous vein. *J Vasc Interv Radiol*. 2001;12:1167–1171.
8. Aziz F, Diaz J, Blebea J, Lurie F. Practice patterns of endovenous ablation therapy for the treatment of venous reflux disease. *J Vasc Surg*. 2017;5(1):75–81.
9. Kutscher B. Outpatient care takes the inside track. *Mod Healthcare*. 2012;42(32):24–26.
10. Jain K, Munn J, Rummel MC, et al. Office-based endovascular suite is safe for most procedures. *J Vasc Surg*. 2014; 59(1):186–191.
11. Jones WS, Mi X, Qualls LG, et al. Trends in settings for peripheral vascular intervention and the effect of changes in the outpatient prospective payment system. *J Am Coll Cardiol*. 2015;65(9):920–927.
12. Smith ME, Sutzko DC, Beck AW, Osborne NH. Provider trends in atherectomy volume between office-based laboratories and traditional facilities. *Ann Vasc Surg*. 2019. https://doi.org/10.1016/j.avsg.2018.12.059 (in press).
13. Vila Jr H, Soto R, Cantor AB, Mackey D. Comparative outcomes analysis of procedures performed in physician offices and ambulatory surgery centers. *Arch Surg*. 2003; 138(9):991–995.
14. Creswell J., Abelson R. Medicare payments surge for stents to unblock blood vessels in limbs. The New York Times, New York. Available at: https://www.nytimes.com/2015/01/30/business/medicare-payments-surge-for-stents-to-unblock-blood-vessels-in-limbs.html. Accessed April 14, 2019.

15. Mukherjee D, Hashemi H, Contos B. The disproportionate growth of office-based atherectomy. *J Vasc Surg*. 2017;65: 495–500.
16. Blebea J. Accreditation of venous centers: a pathway to improved quality of care. *Endovasc Today*. 2015;14(9): 50–57.
17. Kabnick LS, Passman M, Zimmet SE, Blebea J, Khilnani N, Dietzek A. Exploring the value of vein center accreditation to the venous specialist. *J Vasc Surg*. 2016;4(1):119–124.
18. Lin PH, Chandra FA, Shapiro FE, et al. The need for accreditation of office-based interventional vascular centers. *Ann Vasc Surg*. 2017;38:332–338.
19. Wong J, Khu KJ, Kaderali Z, Bernstein M. Delays in the operating room: signs of an imperfect system. *Can J Surg*. 2010;53(3):189–195.
20. Cox Bauer CM, Greer DM, Vander Wyst KB, et al. First-case operating room delays: patterns across urban hospitals within a single health care system. *J Patient Cent Res Rev*. 2016;3:125–135.
21. Carey K, Burgess JF, Young GJ. Hospital competition and financial performance: the effects of ambulatory surgery centers. *Health Econ*. 2011;20(5):571–581.
22. Khan SM, Nazzal M, Zelenock G, et al. Dissatisfaction with compensation and academic careers may force assistant professor vascular surgeons to abandon academic practice. *J Vasc Surg*. 2015;62(3):832.
23. Jain KM, Munn J, Rummel M, et al. Future of vascular surgery is in the office. *J Vasc Surg*. 2010;51(2):509–513.
24. Mishler R, Sands JJ, Ofsthun NJ, et al. Dedicated outpatient vascular access center decreases hospitalization and missed outpatient dialysis treatments. *Kidney Int*. 2006;69(2): 393–398.
25. Mesbah Oskui P, Kloner RA, Burstein S, et al. The safety and efficacy of peripheral vascular procedures performed in the outpatient setting. *J Invasive Cardiol*. 2015;27:243e9.
26. Lin PH, Yang KH, Kollmever KR, et al. Treatment outcomes and lessons learned from 5134 cases of outpatient office-based endovascular procedures in a vascular surgical practice. *Vascular*. 2017;25(2):115–122.
27. Gradinscak DJ, Young N, Jones Y, et al. Risks of outpatient angiography and interventional procedures: a prospective study. *Am J Roentgen*. 2004;183(2):377–381.
28. Bitar G, Mullis W, Jacobs W, Matthews D, et al. Safety and efficacy of office-based surgery with monitored anesthesia care/sedation in 4,778 consecutive plastic surgery procedures. *Plastic Reconstructive Surg*. 2003;111(1): 150–156.
29. Kho H, Ahn S. Financial considerations for office-based intervention labs. *Endovascular Today*. 2014;Jan:55–58.

CHAPTER 25

Opening a Center in a Private Practice

DANIEL R. GORIN, MD, FACS

In many ways, the most straightforward scenario in which to develop an office-based interventional practice is in the setting of an established private practice. Much of the needed infrastructure is already present. There is staff and processes in place for managing patients, scheduling, billing and coding, payroll, and human resources. The practice is already credentialed with CMS and private payers. There are established relationships with vendors for needed supplies: clerical equipment, bandage and dressing supplies, linen service, waste disposal etc. There is an established referral base and patient flow. All that is needed is to develop, staff, and equip an office-based endovascular center (OEC) that is simply an adjunct to the practice.

In this chapter, I will provide an overview of the various areas that need to be considered when adding an OEC to an established private practice. Many of these subjects are addressed in more depth in other chapters, so I will focus on how to incorporate them in the private practice environment.

- Clinical
- Regulatory
- Financial
- Facility
- Staff and logistics
- Equipment and supplies

CLINICAL

First and foremost, it is vital to ensure that you have the clinical skills and the patient base necessary to perform interventional procedures in the office setting. An OEC is not the place to develop these skills. The physician planning to perform the procedures should have the skills to carry out the endovascular procedures in a safe manner. The best way to achieve the required skills to perform procedures is to use your current hospital-based practice as a "virtual office interventional center." Treat every patient and every procedure as if it was being done in an OEC.

Take the time to develop and refine your method of patient selection. What patients will you opt not to treat in the office? Obese patients? Patients with renal insufficiency and creatinine clearance below a certain level? Patients who will require longer, more complex procedures? Once you gain comfort and experience, you will get more and more comfortable treating complex patients in your OEC, but initially it is wise to be overly conservative. By practicing this triage process ahead of time, you and your staff will be ready when you start.

What procedures will you offer? It is fine to start with a more limited scope, and expand as you and your staff gain comfort and experience. Lower extremity arterial interventions, dialysis access, central venous procedures, embolization procedures, stent grafts for peripheral aneurysms, renal and mesenteric intervention, tunneled catheters and port insertion are appropriate for office-based care. These procedures will constitute the majority of your case volume in the OEC. Start with the procedures in which you have the largest experience, and expand over time.

Access vessel management is a vital part of office-based care. If you are going to use a closure device, use it regularly so that you are facile with it. Be sure that you are expert at ultrasound-guided access of the vessel. Most hospital-based interventional centers have fairly conservative pathways for post procedure mobilization and discharge, and the nursing staff often have a very low threshold for pushing for admission of the patient to the hospital. Develop a sound pathway for early ambulation and discharge, and use it routinely. You may have to gently work to change the culture at your hospital, but it will pay dividends both in getting you ready for office-based care and in increasing the efficiency of your hospital center.

Make sure that you are using the equipment and supplies that you will be using in your OEC. Good office-based care is all about efficient decision-making. Think twice before picking a balloon size, or a guidewire to cross a chronic total occlusion in a vessel. Be sure that when you decide to use expensive technology,

Office-Based Endovascular Centers. https://doi.org/10.1016/B978-0-323-67969-5.00025-3
Copyright © 2020 Elsevier Inc. All rights reserved.

such as covered stents, reentry devices, and drug-eluting balloons and stents, you do so in settings where they are clinically indicated. Successful office-based care, both clinically and financially is thoughtful and orderly. A haphazard approach is bad for patient and the physician alike.

Have a plan to manage complications. Think about what you will treat in the office, and what will require a transfer to the hospital for care. Make lists of equipment that you will need to take care of a complication: covered stents, coils, embolectomy devices, snares, etc. Have a process in place to transfer a patient emergently to the hospital. Contact your local ambulance provider, and have a discussion with your emergency room physicians. Complications will occur. They can easily and safely be managed with planning and foresight.

Careful preprocedure preparation is vital to successful office-based care. Noninvasive imaging is invaluable in planning and performing interventional procedures. ultrasound can not only Ultrasound not only helps define anatomy; it is a great tool for planning safe access. It can help answer the following questions: Is the contralateral femoral artery a good site for access? Is the ipsilateral superficial femoral artery (SFA) a good site for antegrade access? Are the tibial vessels patent for pedal access? Ultrasound, Magnetic resonance angiography (MRA), and computed tomography angiography (CTA) are all good tools to define anatomy and plan treatment as well. Use of these modalities can answer the following questions: Is there unrecognized iliac disease that would change your initial access? Is there an SFA occlusion that would be better managed with a pedal access? Will you use a particular device, or technique to treat the patient? Walking into the room with a plan in place, so that your staff is prepared and ready, will make you much more efficient and result in safer, better care.

What kind of sedation or anesthesia will you use? If you are accustomed to working with an anesthesiologist, do not plan on doing your own sedation in your OEC. If you work with a nurse and manage sedation yourself, think about how you will do this in the office. Preprocedure oral sedation, ultrasound-guided local anesthesia, and nonpharmacologic techniques at stress reduction (music, talking with the patient, patient positioning) are all very helpful in limiting the need for IV sedation. Incorporate them into your hospital practice.

Regulatory

There are a variety of state and local regulations that come into play when developing an office-based interventional center. These often vary significantly from place to place. One of the first steps in planning your center should be to engage an attorney who specializes in healthcare and practices in your state and region. Many states require accreditation of office-based surgery centers that will be using conscious sedation during procedures. Some states have licensing requirements. If you are planning to be an ambulatory surgery center (ASC), there may be a requirement for a certificate of need. States often have radiation safety requirements for locations that are using fluoroscopy. In addition, there are usually local zoning rules and regulations that will need to be complied with. It is important to identify all of these requirements well in advance, so that you can design and equip your center accordingly. In addition, be sure to contact your malpractice provider to ensure that no changes in your coverage are required to perform office-based procedures.

Financial

One of the biggest concerns voiced by physicians thinking about developing an OEC is the expense. At first glance, the prospect of building, equipping, and staffing an office-based center seems daunting. In the setting of an established private practice a careful analysis will usually reveal that it is quite achievable.

Most of the major expenses incurred in setting up an office-based interventional center do not have to be paid up front. Expanding your facility, or moving to a new location, can be financed, often with minimal or no down payment. Office space can be leased as well. In a busy private practice, the cost of office space usually winds up being a small percentage of total overhead. Build-out for the OEC should be properly planned. Too small a procedure room or inadequate recovery area can be problematic in providing safe care and comfort to the patient.

Essentially all of the major equipment can be leased. This includes fluoroscopy equipment, imaging table, pressure injector, ultrasound machine, and patient monitors. This can either be structured as a fair market lease over a defined period of time, after which the equipment is returned, or as a "lease to own" arrangement in which you own the equipment at the end of the lease. The monthly payment will be higher under lease to own arrangement. Fluoroscopy equipment may become obsolete after some period of time, so a fair market lease might be appropriate, while pressure injectors and tables may be better handled under a lease to own arrangement.

Most imaging companies have in-house financing available. In addition, they usually have arrangements with other companies so that they can provide a complete set of equipment for your lab. This can be combined into a single lease, usually at favorable terms and with no up-front expense. Do not scrimp on your equipment. You will be using it every day. Good monitors, a well-built and ergonomically designed procedure table, and high-quality imaging equipment increase the expense only by a small amount per month. The equipment will be invaluable to you as you treat more complex patients in your center.

Most disposable endovascular supplies can be consigned. This provides a number of advantages. It eliminates a large up-front expense to stock your center. Payments are made based on consumption. Consignment allows you to liberally stock your lab and ensure that you always have the equipment that you need. Also, your industry partners will provide indispensable help with inventory management. Overtime, you may find that you can realize cost savings by buying some equipment, but you will have to pay for the supplies between 30 and 90 days depending on the contract. You will have to manage the inventory with your own staff, and will lose money on any product that expires. As you start out, it is most important that you have the equipment that you need at a predictable cost, and that it gets restocked and maintained in a timely manner. Many companies offer volume-based discounts and you should avail them if you like using that particular product. You can also negotiate good payment terms. Inventory control is crucial to your success.

There will be some equipment that has to be paid for up front. Basic nursing supplies, IV equipment, medications, stretchers, clerical supplies all will have to be purchased before you begin caring for patients. In general, these expenses are quite manageable, usually with the cash flow from your current practice, or with a line of credit that can be rapidly repaid.

In the setting of an established private practice, it is fairly easy to predict the income from your lab. This is covered in more detail elsewhere in the book. Briefly, the CPT codes for all of the procedures done in an OEC are valued at a certain RVU level. Each procedure code has a "facility" and a "nonfacility" payment rate. If the physician performs the case in a facility (usually a hospital), the hospital gets paid the technical component and physician bills and gets the professional component. The procedure also has a "nonfacility" payment rate. This rate is paid when the physician performs the procedure in an office. The nonfacility fee reimbursement is a combination of technical component and the professional component. The office gets paid the global fee. This fee is greater than the professional component because it also covers the expense of the procedure. Every OEC procedure has a nonfacility payment associated with it. It is a fairly simple matter to look at an interventional procedure that you currently perform, and see what you would be reimbursed with a nonfacility payment.

You can then look at your practice billing over a recent period of time, say 6 months, and calculate what you would have collected if the procedures had been reimbursed at nonfacility reimbursement rate, rather than the professional component that you have been receiving. Then set a conservative goal of moving a portion of your current procedure volume to the office. Be realistic. Based on these numbers, make a business proforma. Base your calculations on your current volume. You never want to place yourself in the position of feeling pressured to treat a patient in the office in order to make ends meet. You should not look at your OEC as a way to attract new patients; first and foremost, it is simply a better way to care for the patients you are already treating. An initial goal of treating 50% of your current case load in the OEC is a good place to start. Realistically, this number is quite low, but it will give you plenty of room in which to grow slowly and comfortably. In the long run, you will attract new patients because of the quality of care provided in the OEC and extremely high patient satisfaction.

Facility

One of the great aspects of providing interventional in an office-based setting is that it puts the most valuable resource, the physician, in the middle of an environment in which they can provide patient care efficiently in a patient friendly place. In that light, an OEC should be developed as an integral part of your office. As previously noted, much of the infrastructure that you need, noninvasive vascular testing, clerical support, staff and space for consultations, etc., is already present. The first step will be to identify a contractor to help you build out your center. Ideally, this should be a firm that is focused on commercial building, with experience in medical facilities, such as physician offices and ASC and works locally, so that they are familiar with local rules and regulations, and know the town officials who implement them. Early on, some basic decisions have to be made. Do you have enough room in your current office to develop an OEC, or do you need to move? How much extra space do you need? Do you need to meet physical space requirements for accreditation? Will you be required to be within a certain distance of a hospital?

The physical plant requirements are covered in more detail elsewhere in the book (Chapter 5). As a basic tenet, always plan to have more space than you think you require. You will need a good-sized procedure room, with plenty of room for imaging equipment, supply carts, monitoring and sedation equipment, and space for staff to efficiently move around and operate. You will need a good-sized recovery area, with bays for patients, a nursing work area, and a handicap bathroom. You will need plenty of additional storage for nursing equipment, cleaning supplies, drugs and IV supplies, and clerical supplies. Accreditation organizations usually require that the unit be self-contained (that there are doors that can be shut separating the unit from the rest of the office) and have a separate waiting room. Most accreditation organizations will review and approve a floor plan for a nominal fee, this is well worth the time and effort.

You and your patients will be spending a great deal of time in your center. It does not have to be the Taj Mahal, but be sure that you spend the time and effort to build a center that is well laid out, comfortable, and friendly to you, staff, patients, and their families. Spend time visiting other centers to get a feel as to what will work best for you. No one complains that their OEC is too spacious. Almost everyone wishes that they had more room in which to grow.

Staff and Logistics

Your staff is the lifeblood of your facility. Nothing will have a bigger impact on the quality of the care you provide, your patients' experience, and your day-to-day satisfaction. Pick good people, and empower them to create and refine the systems and improve the environment that will allow them and you to be successful. This will create a great facility and will result in a long waiting list of nurses and techs waiting to work in your center.

As noted previously, an established private practice already has a lot of the staff and infrastructure necessary for a successful OEC. You will need to add staff with specific skills that are needed to care for patients undergoing procedures in your center. If you have an active private practice, you likely already know the staff that you would like to hire. Some quiet networking usually results in finding and hiring qualified candidates for the center.

It is ideal if you can identify and hire managers in a couple of key clinical areas. They can help get you organized and can take a leadership role in recruiting, training, and organizing your staff. They may be able to carry out managerial as well as clinical duties. They will also need to be hired several months before your center opens, so they can get your center organized, deal with the vendors, and get it equipped to provide care for patients.

Nursing staff: They will be responsible for all of your pre-, post-, and periprocedural care. It is vital to have well-trained, experienced nurses, with critical care level training. They also need experience in managing arterial access. If you are going to be doing your own conscious sedation, they need experience with that as well. Cardiovascular intensive care unit nurses are ideal. Nurses with Cath lab experience can also be very helpful, but will need to be open to a change in culture from the hospital to the office-based environment. Hire a head nurse. They will help recruit staff and manage the schedule. The nurse manager can help develop protocols and paperwork for patient care, organize staff training and education, and manage preprocedure testing and scheduling. It is a good idea to have at least two registered nurses available at all times, so that there will always be plenty of help in case of an emergency. While one nurse is helping with conscious sedation, the second nurse should be available to monitor patients in recovery area.

Radiation technologist (RT): In most states, only a licensed RT or physician can operate fluoroscopy equipment. Hire an RT with managerial experience as well. As with nursing, they can help recruit staff, manage the RT schedule, and train new staff on protocols and procedures. Your head RT can also be your coordinator with your industry partners. They will handle service and upkeep of your imaging equipment, and work with industry representatives in managing inventory. RT can also be in charge of compliance with radiation safety requirements.

Based on the particulars of your available staff and practice patterns, you may have additional staff. If you plan on using anesthesia personnel for your conscious sedation, you may be able to have a smaller nursing staff. If you have an operating room tech who is facile with catheters and guidewires, you may need only one RT to run the C-arm. You may choose to have nurse practitioners or physicians assistants work with you on particular types of cases. Most importantly, never let your center be short staffed. Patient safety, and a good patient experience, depends on having an adequate number of medical personnel, who are well trained and committed to quality patient care. It will cost your practice much less to have an extra staff person on a light day, as compared with canceling cases because staff is not available. On light days the staff members can be used for other tasks in the office since there is no barrier between the office and the OEC.

Equipment

Interventional procedures require several pieces of complex, expensive equipment. You will need high-quality imaging equipment, the full spectrum of disposable endovascular supplies, and a wide array of ancillary equipment: packs and drapes, patient monitors, stretches, IV equipment, drugs, contras, etc. The list is quite extensive and included in Chapter 7.

This is where industry partners play an important role. They are able to work with your staff to get you the equipment that you need, and organize and maintain it. If you are performing interventional procedures, you already have relationships with industry, and know what companies provide high-quality equipment and support in your area. Imaging companies can help you design and set up your procedure room. They usually can supply, or have relationships with companies that can supply, the additional durable equipment that you need: procedure table, pressure injectors, patient monitors, etc. Similarly, the major device companies are well versed in how to set up and stock a new lab. A good industry partner will know the supplies you need and they cannot provide. No devise company has all the tools you need. They can advise you as to the needs of the lab and how to source the required items. Established medical practices always have a relationship with a vendor for basic medical supplies for their office. These vendors can supply the basic patient care equipment that you need and can guide you on putting together supply lists for your center. Most importantly, properly hired staff, using their experience, will be able to plan and equip the lab adequately. ICU nurses know what they like in their IV kits and other patient-related items. RTs who have worked in a Cath lab know the syringes, basins, and drapes they want in an angiogram pack. Your new staff members, under the direction of a manager along with your industry partners, should be able to get you equipped, organized, and ready to begin treating patients.

CONCLUSION

Adding an OEC to your private practice is a significant undertaking. Take the time to travel and observe care in other office-based centers. Most physicians doing quality office-based interventional care are happy to host you and are generous with their time and knowledge. Your industry partners can often suggest good practices to visit. Join national societies, such as the Outpatient Endovascular and Interventional Society, that are committed to safe, effective, and appropriate office-based care. Hire great staff, and empower them. Pick industry partners who are committed to excellence and supportive of office-based care. As you go through the process of planning, equipping, staffing, and ultimately opening an office-based center, you will likely find it to be one of the most rewarding and fulfilling endeavors in your career. When done well, it will be a wonderful place for you, your staff, and your patients.

CHAPTER 26

Joint Ventures in Office-Based Endovascular Centers

NICOLAS J. MOUAWAD, MD, MPH, MBA, FSVS, FRCS, FACS •
JESSICA L. BAILEY-WHEATON, ESQ •
TODD A. ZIGRANG, MBA, MHA, FACHE, CVA, ASA •
BHAGWAN SATIANI, MD, MBA, DFSVS, FACHE, FACS

While the hospital and physician healthcare sectors are massive ($1 trillion and $600 billion, respectively), they may be considered financially separate.[1] Despite this, they are not only bound in a tight business relationship but have become increasingly more dependent on each other clinically. And while the power equation seems to be shifting to increasingly large health systems, hospitals cannot function efficiently without actively aligned physician groups. In this regard, outpatient joint ventures have been explored for several years to benefit both entities. Patient safety remains the overarching goal in healthcare delivery, including outpatient surgery centers. Compared with their inhospital counterparts, these outpatient surgery centers may include more efficient clinical operations and cost savings to the patient, surgeon, and payers. Furthermore, patients benefit from shorter wait times, easier scheduling, more convenient locations, and consistent on-time appointments, as well as more intimate surroundings and a more satisfying patient experience.[2]

The shift to outpatient care led to the establishment of ambulatory surgical centers (ASCs), renal dialysis centers, cardiac catheterization facilities, and now office-based endovascular centers (OEC). With decreasing reimbursement, physicians have resorted to forming larger single or multispecialty groups to better negotiate insurance contracts, as well as building hospital relationships while concurrently reducing overhead. Groups have also invested in ancillary services in order to receive global fees instead of just declining professional fees. Surgeons invested in ASCs for surgical procedures now increasingly work in the outpatient setting, offering convenience, efficiency, and cost-effective services compared with hospitals for payers interested in further savings.

Ownership and referral to an ASC does not necessarily implicate the Stark Law but does involve the Anti-Kickback Statute (AKBS) and state law. Whereas the federal Stark Law has "exceptions" to allow for legal activities, the AKBS have "safe harbors" (41 C F R. Section 1001.952(r)), which provide that any return on physician investment will not be deemed as remuneration that may have violated the AKBS if the arrangement falls within the safe harbor's criteria. There are also "advisory opinions" issued by the Office of Inspector General (OIG); although these are not legal precedents, they offer guidance for forming or scrutinizing ASC investments.

Specialties like vascular surgery then took this shift to outpatient care a step further by performing venous and arterial procedures such as angiography and endovascular procedures in OEC. Health systems had already started partnering with physicians in managing ASCs, but now are faced with increasing competition for endovascular procedures performed by independent vascular surgeons in their own OECs. Due largely to technologic advances, the shift to outpatient vascular procedures in the last decade has been striking.[3]

OEC LEGAL CONSIDERATIONS

Please note that the information provided in this chapter does not, and is not intended to, constitute legal advice, instead, all information and content are for general informational purposes only.

Stark Law

The Stark Law governs physicians (or their immediate family members) who have a financial relationship (i.e., an ownership investment interest or a compensation arrangement) with an entity and prohibits those

Office-Based Endovascular Centers. https://doi.org/10.1016/B978-0-323-67969-5.00026-5
Copyright © 2020 Elsevier Inc. All rights reserved.

individuals from making Medicare referrals to those entities for the furnishing of *designated health services* (DHS).[4] DHS encompasses the following items and services:

(1) Clinical laboratory services;
(2) Physical therapy services;
(3) Occupational therapy services;
(4) Radiology services, including magnetic resonance imaging, computerized axial tomography scans, and ultrasound services;
(5) Radiation therapy services and supplies;
(6) Durable medical equipment and supplies;
(7) Parenteral and enteral nutrients, equipment, and supplies;
(8) Prosthetics, orthotics, and prosthetic devices and supplies;
(9) Home health services;
(10) Outpatient prescription drugs;
(11) Inpatient and outpatient hospital services; and
(12) Outpatient speech-language pathology services.[5]

OECs are generally not subject to Stark Law restrictions because they typically do not furnish DHS. However, in the event that the OEC is performing DHS (e.g., radiology services), *and* that DHS is not reimbursed by Medicare as part of a composite rate,[6] then the financial relationship between the physicians and the hospital, and their connection to the OEC, may be subject to Stark, the application of which regulations (and any appropriate exceptions) will be determined by the structure of the financial relationship between the parties (e.g., direct/indirect, compensation/ownership investment).

Anti-Kickback Statute (AKBS)

The AKBS makes it a felony for any person (not just a physician) to "knowingly and willfully" solicit or receive, or to offer or pay, any "remuneration," directly or indirectly, in exchange for the referral of a patient for a healthcare service paid for by a federal healthcare program.[7] Of note, interpretation and application of the AKBS under case law has created precedent for a regulatory hurdle known as the *one purpose* test, under which test healthcare providers violate the AKBS if even *one purpose* of the arrangement in question is to offer remuneration deemed illegal under the AKBS.[8]

Due to the broad nature of the AKBS, legitimate business arrangements may appear to be prohibited.[9] In response to these concerns, Congress created a number of statutory exceptions and delegated authority to the HHS to protect certain business arrangements by means of promulgating several *safe harbors*,[9] which set forth regulatory criteria that, if met, shield an arrangement from regulatory liability, and are meant to protect transactional arrangements unlikely to result in fraud or abuse.[10] In contrast to the Stark Law, failure to meet all the requirements of a *safe harbor* does not necessarily render an arrangement illegal.[11]

Under the AKBS, ASCs and OECs are treated differently. Specifically, ASCs meet AKBS *safe harbor* provisions, which state that "'remuneration' does not include any payment that is a return on an investment interest, such as a dividend or interest income, made to an investor," under certain circumstances. For example, the operating and recovery room space must be exclusively dedicated to the ASC, all patients referred to the entity by an investor must be fully informed of the investor's ownership interest, and all of the following applicable standards are met within one of the categories set forth in Table 26.1.[12]

Additionally, the above safe harbors are only available to those ASCs that meet the following statutory definition:

> any distinct entity that operates exclusively for the purpose of providing surgical services to patients not requiring hospitalization and in which the expected duration of services would not exceed 24 hours following an admission. The entity must have an agreement with CMS to participate in Medicare as an ASC...
>
> **"DEFINITIONS" 42 U.S.C. § 416.2**[13]

Because no federal licensing is required to operate an OEC,[14] they would not be considered an ASC under the AKBS. Consequently, the specific facts and circumstances related to the transaction, such as the structure of the hospital-physician joint venture and the various financial relationships included (e.g., OEC space rental, information technology) will guide the applicability of AKBS, and its associated safe harbors.

PARTNERSHIP MODELS

Several functional models for OEC partnership do exist and are based primarily on the relationship among the stakeholders.[15] Multiple combinations are feasible.

1. **Physician-owned.** This is the most basic of all models, where sole ownership of the endovascular center is held by the physicians, and they may or may not retain an outside management group to assist in business operations. In this model, the physicians gain all the returns from the venture. However, they also incur all the risk. Although the physician owners are educated clinically, physician leaders may not be well versed in making strategic business decisions, and therefore lack access to capital, management support, and managed care

TABLE 26.1
Ambulatory surgical center (ASC) Exceptions to the Anti-Kickback Statute.

	A	B	C	D	E
	Category	**Surgeon-Owned ASC**	**Single-Specialty ASC**	**Multispecialty ASC**	**Hospital/Physician ASC**
1	Investor	General surgeons or surgeons engaged in the same surgical specialty, who can refer patients directly to the ASC and perform surgery on such referred patients	Physicians engaged in the same medical practice specialty who can refer patients directly to the entity and perform procedures on such referred patients	Physicians who can refer patients directly to the entity and perform procedures on such referred patients	A hospital
2		Surgical group practices comprised exclusively of such surgeons	Group medical practices composed exclusively of such physicians	Group medical practices composed exclusively of such physicians	General surgeons or surgeons engaged in the same surgical specialty, who are able to refer patients directly the ASC and perform surgery on such referred patients
3		Individuals not employed by the ASC or any other investor, not in a position to provide items or services to the entity or any other investors, and not in a position to make or influence referrals directly or indirectly to the ASC or any other investors	Individuals not employed by the ASC or any other investor, not in a position to provide items or services to the entity or any other investors, and not in a position to make or influence referrals directly or indirectly to the ASC or any other investors	Individuals not employed by the ASC or any other investor, not in a position to provide items or services to the entity or any other investors, and not in a position to make or influence referrals directly or indirectly to the ASC or any other investors	Physicians engaged in the same medical practice specialty who can refer patients directly to the entity and perform procedures on such referred patients
4					Physicians who can refer patients directly to the entity and perform procedures on such referred patients
5					Surgical group practices comprised exclusively of such surgeons
6					Group medical practices composed exclusively of such physicians
7					Individuals not employed by the ASC or any other investor, not in a position to provide items or services to the entity or any other investors, and not in a position to make or influence

Continued

TABLE 26.1
Ambulatory surgical center (ASC) Exceptions to the Anti-Kickback Statute.—cont'd

	A	B	C	D	E
	Category	Surgeon-Owned ASC	Single-Specialty ASC	Multispecialty ASC	Hospital/Physician ASC
					referrals directly or indirectly to the ASC or any other investors
8	Standards	The investment terms offered to an investor may not be tied to the previous or expected number of referrals, services furnished, or the amount of business for the entity otherwise generated by the investor	The investment terms offered to an investor may not be tied to the previous or expected number of referrals, services furnished, or the amount of business for the entity otherwise generated by the investor	The investment terms offered to an investor may not be tied to the previous or expected number of referrals, services furnished, or the amount of business for the entity otherwise generated by the investor	The investment terms offered to an investor may not be tied to the previous or expected number of referrals, services furnished, or the amount of business for the entity otherwise generated by the investor
9		At least one-third of the surgeon investor's practice income for the prior fiscal year or the prior 12-month period must come from the surgeon's performance of procedures	At least one-third of the surgeon investor's practice income for the prior fiscal year or the prior 12-month period must come from the surgeon's performance of procedures	At least one-third of the surgeon investor's practice income for the prior fiscal year or the prior 12-month period must come from the surgeon's performance of procedures	Neither the entity nor any investor can loan funds or guarantee a loan for an investor, if the investor uses any portion of the loan to acquire the investment interest
10		Neither the entity nor any investor can loan funds or guarantee a loan for an investor, if the investor uses any portion of the loan to acquire the investment interest	Neither the entity nor any investor can loan funds or guarantee a loan for an investor, if the investor uses any portion of the loan to acquire the investment interest	At least one-third of the procedures performed by each physician investor must be performed at the investment entity;	An investor's payment in return for their investment must be directly proportional to the amount of capital they invested
11		An investor's payment in return for their investment must be directly proportional to the amount of capital they invested	An investor's payment in return for their investment must be directly proportional to the amount of capital they invested	Neither the entity nor any investor can loan funds or guarantee a loan for an investor, if the investor uses any portion of the loan to acquire the investment interest	The ASC, the hospital. and any physician investors must treat patients receiving medical benefits or assistance under any healthcare program in a nondiscriminatory manner
12		Ancillary services performed for beneficiaries of federal healthcare programs must be related to the primary procedures performed at the ASC and may not be billed separately to Medicare or other federal healthcare programs	Ancillary services performed for beneficiaries of federal healthcare programs must be related to the primary procedures performed at the ASC and may not be billed separately to Medicare or other federal healthcare programs	An investor's payment in return for their investment must be directly proportional to the amount of capital they invested	The ASC may not use (1) space, including operating and recovery room space located in or owned by any hospital investor, unless the space lease complies with the space rental safe harbor; (2) equipment provided by any

TABLE 26.1
Ambulatory surgical center (ASC) Exceptions to the Anti-Kickback Statute.—cont'd

	A	B	C	D	E
	Category	Surgeon-Owned ASC	Single-Specialty ASC	Multispecialty ASC	Hospital/Physician ASC
					hospital investor, unless the equipment lease complies with the equipment rental safe harbor; nor (3) services provided by any hospital investor, unless the services contract complies with the personal services and management contracts safe harbor
13	Standards	The ASC and any investors must treat patients receiving medical benefits or assistance under any healthcare program in a nondiscriminatory manner	The ASC and any investors must treat patients receiving medical benefits or assistance under any healthcare program in a nondiscriminatory manner	Ancillary services performed for beneficiaries of federal healthcare programs must be related to the primary procedures performed at the ASC and may not be billed separately to Medicare or other federal healthcare programs	Ancillary services performed for beneficiaries of federal healthcare programs must be related to the primary procedures performed at the entity and may not be billed separately to Medicare or other federal healthcare programs
14				The ASC and any investors must treat patients receiving medical benefits or assistance under any healthcare program in a nondiscriminatory manner	The hospital's report, or any other claim for payment from a federal healthcare program, may not include any costs associated with the ASC unless the federal healthcare program requires their inclusion
15					The hospital cannot directly or indirectly make or influence referrals to any investor or entity.

contracting that may be available in the joint venture models described below.

Physician-ownership of outpatient endovascular centers has resulted in an increase in outpatient surgical volumes.[16] Many physicians confronting declining reimbursement from insurers have moved their work to such centers where they can exert control over the entirety of the care provided during an interventional procedure. Since the physicians own a stake in the success of the center, this creates a potential conflict of interest between the physicians' financial incentives and the patients' clinical needs. Furthermore, hospital-physician integration trends continue to increase—from July 2012 to July 2018, hospital-employed physicians increased by 55%.[17] In fact, from July 2016 to January 2018, an additional 14,000 physicians became employed with an additional 8000 physician practices acquired. Therefore, other combined joint venture models may be more functional.

2. **Physicians and management company.** The demands of a successful practice render it nearly impossible to care for patients and simultaneously perform the administrative tasks of business operations. As such, physicians can partner with Management Services Organizations (MSOs) to assist with the nonmedical burdens of an endovascular surgical center. These include, but are not limited to, billing, coding, supply purchasing, inventory control, human resource management, collections, quality, marketing, accounting and bookkeeping, technological and informational support systems, and so forth. The added expertise of an MSO is advantageous in the physician-management company model. However, in such a venture, the physicians relinquish a certain portion of their equity. Traditionally, MSOs may own a greater than 50% share in the endovascular center.

Arrangements between physicians and MSOs must be carefully crafted and implemented, due in part to the "Corporate Practice of Medicine" (CPOM) laws that most states have. The CPOM prohibition, which applies to MSOs, prohibits nonlicensed individuals or unauthorized entities from practicing medicine, or owning, investing in, or controlling professional medical practices; this is in contradistinction to physician practices—which are typically structured as professional corporations and professional limited liability companies.[18]

Although such MSOs can provide administrative and other nonclinical support to physician practices, the CPOM prohibition forbids such an MSO from controlling or swaying a physician's clinical judgment and independent medical decision-making—which is reserved solely for the physician and the physician practice.

3. **Physicians and hospital.** An increasingly common structure in the industry is the joint venture structure involving joint ownership by physicians and hospitals. This type of venture is generally very popular with the hospital entity as it allows an opportunity for hospitals to provide a better coordination of care through rekindling relationships with physician investors who wish to remain independent.

The trend toward this model has been fueled primarily by the hospital's more robust negotiating power and leverage to attract, engage, and maintain managed care populations. The hospital can command considerably higher rates than physician-owned centers. Although there exist large variations in which either the hospital or physicians own a majority share in the venture, when the hospital has a majority investment interest, it can increase the center's reimbursement by negotiating stronger payer agreements. Furthermore, despite less overall control, this seems to be welcomed by physicians due to substantially higher per share returns on their equity.[19] As with MSOs, this type of joint venture model should be structured and implemented carefully in order to ensure that the hospital and the endovascular center are not considered competitors where they are unable to coordinate their activities without violating antitrust laws (e.g., the *Copperweld* Doctrine).

4. **Physicians, management company, and hospital.** This joint venture model, while resulting in less equity per involved group, may produce a more successful venture overall, due to the economic inputs from each group (i.e., a smaller piece of a larger pie). For instance, the management company may provide the managerial and nonclinical aspects of daily tasks while the hospital partner may help the joint venture gain access to managed care contracts and diffuse tension in the community by recruiting other physicians or physician groups outside the venture.

The management company and hospital partner may form a separate company for the purposes of their investment in the OEC joint venture. This separate "holding company" owns a majority share in the OEC joint venture, usually between 51% and 60%, with the physicians owning the remainder (either individually or through their own physician joint venture company). Within the holding company itself, however, it is the hospital partner that owns the majority (e.g., hospital 51% and management company 49%), as the management company's primary motivation is the provision of management services, for which they are compensated a management fee.

5. **Physicians and hospital-operated outpatient departments.** The hospital-level reimbursement offered by the Outpatient Prospective Payment System (OPPS) fee schedule, along with the cost-efficiency of an outpatient center, offers increased reimbursement, which may go directly to the

bottom line. Acquisition of off-campus surgery centers therefore became commonplace until reimbursement reductions introduced by the Balanced Budget Act of 2015, as well as subsequent OPPS payment update adjustments, slowed that trend. In such a venture, endovascular surgery center physicians function as independent contractors of the hospital, obtaining a flat-fee compensation with some bonuses, as their compensation cannot consider the value or volume of physician referrals. This arrangement is at the other end of the joint venture spectrum, as it is completely owned by the hospital, but managed as an outpatient center, and the hospital enjoys all the reward, but also bears all the risk.

WHY FORM JOINT VENTURES?

A joint venture involves two or more entities that enter into a formal agreement with one another for a specific business project or strategy. In the healthcare field, this can include physicians, physician groups, commercial outfits such as property developers (Surgical Care Affiliates, AMSURG, ASCOA), hospitals, hospital systems, and others. The benefits and risks depend on the parties involved. Clearly, the most difficult obstacle to overcome in having multiple parties involved is to come to an agreement on the strategic plan for the venture.

For the hospital, the advantages are numerous. Hospitals, most of which are tax-exempt, have a mission to provide benefit to the community. Such ventures strengthen the surgeon (interventionalist)/hospital relationship and increase coordination of care, avoiding costly duplication of services. A joint venture also helps with appropriate use of inhospital resources; for instance, procedures that do not need to be performed in an inpatient hospital operating room, interventional radiology suite, or the cardiac Cath lab can be shifted to the lower-cost, OEC, freeing up these spaces for higher-acuity cases. The OEC will provide the hospital with increased efficiency, high-quality, and low-cost capabilities. This is of specific interest to populations with cost-sensitive payers. Eventually, it should be of concern to all parties involved in healthcare to decrease the cost of providing healthcare.

For the physicians, advantages include access to the available capital of the hospital, risk sharing, managed care contracting experience, technology infrastructure, and the fact that financial stability with hospital involvement may attract more investors (Table 26.2). With the trend toward increasing physician employment by hospitals, an OEC joint venture may increase

TABLE 26.2
Pros and Cons of Hospital Partnership.

	Pros of Hospital Partnership	Cons of Hospital Partnership
Efficiency	Partly physician owned; quicker decision-making	More bureaucracy; multiple decision points
Financial	- Access to capital - More financing leverage with lenders - Favors investors if needed - Risk sharing - Cost sharing	- Size dependent - Easier for multispecialty or large numbers - Personal guarantees of physician - Profits must be shared with partner
Quality of care	Peer review required in hospital-owned facilities; quality important to hospitals	Peer review not required although most physician-owned office-based endovascular centers (OECs) would encourage it; physician-owned OECs are usually more focused on outcomes
Contracting	Hospitals with more managed care contracting and favorable reimbursement rates	Physician may have little control or input in this regard
Politics	More influence with regulators, legislators, hospital associations, and insurers	Hospital politics may slow down decision-making; if > 1 dominant health system in market area, physician group likely to be excluded from nonpartners
Technology	Infrastructural upgrades more affordable with "deep pockets"	All data available to the hospital administration

physician participation. Notably, however, there are some risks associated with antitrust laws if the hospital is seen as coordinating activities including reimbursement with a competitor such as an OEC.

Disadvantages of the joint venture include bureaucratic delays in decision-making, tension created by disputes in management decisions, reduced control and possible physician autonomy, hospital and community politics, divergent emphasis on quality issues, sharing any profits with the partner, and, if an MSO is involved, paying a management fee. Another joint venture result may be the status of physician independence, which may be questioned by the other hospitals and healthcare providers excluded from the joint venture.

For interventionalists, a frustrating problem has been the inability to negotiate favorable managed care contracts for their OEC. They lack the market power (volume or exclusivity) to leverage payers to achieve the payment rates often given to hospitals for the same services. If a large health system or hospital has a major investment in the OEC, it is likely that much stronger payer agreements can be negotiated. Physician owners then must decide if the advantages for partnership are enough to make up for dilution of their interest in the OEC.

Another problem for interventionalists may be dealing with noncompliant physician owners. What can be done if one or more physicians invest in, but fail to use and support, the venture? This often leads to resentment among fellow physician investors, especially those who actively support the endovascular center and feel as though they are subsidizing investment returns to physicians who choose not to do cases in the facility. While it is not advisable to simply require a physician to redeem his or her interests in the facility for a lack of referrals, it is possible to use the aforementioned extension of practice requirements to remove a noncompliant physician; in some cases (ASCs but not in OECs), this may be done by requiring physician investors to perform at least one-third of their outpatient cases at the center each year, and further, certify their compliance on a regular basis. Because the so-called "one-third test" is a safe harbor requirement for ASC ownership interests, an ASC is free to impose this obligation on each ASC physician investor. Failure to meet this requirement can be caused to repurchase any noncompliant physician investor's interests in the ASC. This safe harbor is not available for OECs, however, and as such, specific contracting requirements should be discussed as well as ensuring that those involved have defined roles and responsibilities and whose business cultures match.

WHAT OPTIONS DO INTERVENTIONALISTS HAVE TO FORM AN OEC?

There are several options, as noted previously, including an individual or group forming their own OEC, partnering with a management company experienced in OECs or ASCs, sharing ownership with a health system, or even in a tripartite structure with a hospital and management company, and health system investing in and owning the OEC but also accepting a contract to comanage the OEC. The latter may involve predetermined flat compensation for specified activities with or without incentive bonuses.

Specifically, for physicians, forming an OEC with partners has a variety of benefits and risks, as noted in Table 26.3.

QUESTIONS TO ASK BEFORE ENGAGING IN A JOINT VENTURE

Do Our Cultures Match?

Any company's culture is its personality and provides a clue to the interaction between the employees and the

TABLE 26.3
Risks and Benefits of Partnering to Form an OEC.

Benefits	Risks
Risk sharing	Coping with different organizational cultures and management styles
Cost sharing	Decreasing flexibility
Entering markets that previously had high barriers to entry	Bureaucracy
Collective intelligence	Redundancy of management
Collaboration with people with different perspectives	Risk of downsizing due to duplication of resources
Increased opportunities for growth	Lack of commitment or combined vision and mission
Leverage existing technologies from partners	Decreasing autonomy
Investment potential	Navigating bureaucracy
Governance	Decreased equity
Expansion of services	Potential conflicts of interest
Less initial financial capital	
Involved in strategic decisions	
Cost and risk sharing	
Leveraging hospital negotiations such as managed care contracts	
Leveraging hospital technology	
Equipment sharing	
Entering different markets	

manner in which things get accomplished. Since a joint venture is essentially a merger of two different cultures, there are likely to be differences between leaders and employees of the two parties about the joint venture's values. It may take time to merge the two cultures.

Patient safety is one area which deserves the most emphasis and collaboration in the joint venture. The joint venture must emphasize patient safety and the quality irrespective of other considerations. Physician partners may address problems differently compared with hospital leadership. Hospital representatives may lean more toward innovation, external customers, and team performance metrics.[20] Physicians may focus on internal operation, process improvement, and accountability. Regardless, staff must be fully cognizant of the organization's values and safety principles, which must be repeatedly taught to all employees. A formal committee composed of employees from several disciplines should regularly meet and report to the board or executive committee.

Are Roles and Responsibilities Clearly Defined?

An OEC's facility operations may be defined as the "services, competencies, processes, and tools required to assure the built environment will perform the functions for" the OEC, including "the day-to-day activities necessary for the building ... its systems and equipment, and ... users to perform their intended function".[21]

The rules setting forth those operations and assigning the party responsible for each of the delineated operations should be determined up front, and clearly defined in a written agreement (*note that, both Stark Law and Anti-Kickback Statute exceptions/safe harbors require any arrangement to be set forth in writing and signed by the parties*).

The respective responsibilities of the physicians and the hospital (and even a third party) in operating the OEC will likely fall somewhere on a spectrum, ranging from no involvement in the day-to-day activities (i.e., functioning as a passive investor) to conducting the majority or all the facility operations. Often, the scope of each party's responsibilities is codified in a management services agreement, wherein the hospital or a third-party management company assumes some (or all) of the nonclinical, administrative responsibilities, and the physicians undertake the clinical responsibilities (e.g., patient care, physician recruiting, etc.).

Where each party falls on that spectrum of responsibility may be dictated by federal/state regulations, e.g., fraud and abuse laws (to ensure the arrangement complies with applicable exceptions/safe harbors), and state corporate practice of medicine laws. These laws may dictate that certain tasks be conducted by licensed physicians, such as the recruitment and employment of medical staff. In addition to legal considerations, there may be practical issues requiring the delegation of duties, e.g., physicians may want to retain control over operations, in order to maintain their independence.[22] Regardless of the delegation of responsibilities regarding facility operations, those determinations should be thoroughly considered and determined at the outset, and codified in a written agreement, in order to maintain regulatory compliance, and, if applicable, determine any fair market value remuneration for the facility operation services provided. The administrative structure, ideally a "dyad," must be clearly enunciated with roles for the physician and administrator on an equal footing. Administrative and clinical employees should be similarly aware of their supervisors, and dispute resolution mechanisms laid out in formal written policies must be followed. Communication is an important part of the roles assigned to each of the joint venture partners. Regular and frequent methods of communication must be available to allow active participation by all physicians in the joint venture entity. Dispute resolution mechanisms such as arbitration must also be outlined in any agreement.

Are Governance Rules for Facility Operations Clear?

A joint operating committee (board/executive committee) with a clearly designated governance structure is necessary. If possible, the interventionalist must be the chief executive, but if desired, a yearly rotating chairperson may be acceptable to both parties. Other officers can also be rotated. Financial information should be transparent to all partners and shared without restrictions. Buy and sell agreements should be part of the contract signed by both parties. Experienced legal consultations are mandatory due to the thicket of laws governing physician-hospital cooperative endeavors.

What Constitutes "Due Diligence" for Physicians Looking for a Partnership?

It is imperative that physicians looking for a partnership evaluate both the mission and vision of the partnership, in addition to a discussion of strategic goals, the timeline to achieve these, and the metrics by which they can be evaluated. Ask questions and do not assume anything (Table 26.4).

Due diligence can be separated into the following:

TABLE 26.4
Due Diligence Topics to Consider Before Partnering.

Corporate and general operations	- Description - Location - History
Financial	- Audited financial statements - Long-term financial projections - Assets and liabilities - Revenue cycle - Policies regarding bad debt and charity - Third-party payer mix and reimbursement cycle
Legal and compliance	- Investigations - Sanctions - Risk management - Worker's compensation
Material contracts	- Existing and proposed contracts
Personal property	- Fixed assets - Maintenance contracts - Debts and obligations
Licenses and accreditation	- Planning permits and certificates of need - Copies of licenses and permits
Labor and employment	- Personnel policies - Employee handbooks and communication material - Employee terminations
Environmental compliance	- Solid and hazardous waste - Radioactive materials storage - Infectious material waste
Information technology	- Software licenses - Security breaches
Physician matters	

VALUATION CONSIDERATIONS

In addition to considerations for forming an organization, capitalization and ownership structure are subject to regulatory scrutiny. Capitalization, for the purposes of this discussion, is the acquisition of assets for the operation of the OEC. Capitalization needs for a start-up venture may include build-out, equipment, supplies, and working capital, and such requirements may exceed $1 million. The parties to the joint venture typically contribute capital to fund the start-up costs. These capital contributions define the ownership of each of the parties in the joint venture, i.e., capital contributions from each party toward the total capitalization of the project determine the ownership percentage of each party.

Funding may come in the form of cash, assets, or services. Examples of assets contributed may include use of office space, equipment, and intangible assets, such as the use of a trade name or intellectual property. Examples of services contributed may include the use of personnel staff and management services. If capital contributions are in a form other than cash, a determination of the fair market value of those contributions is required to comply with several applicable AKBS safe harbors.

If the OEC is already an ongoing business in operation at the time of the joint venture formation, ownership buy-in amounts are also determined by the fair market value of the existing OEC, using a highly specialized valuation technique. In this case, the OEC is part of an existing medical practice that, in most cases, does not have a separate legal entity or financial statements that isolate the in-office ancillary services provided by the soon-to-be joint venture OBL from the professional services (i.e., physician services not part of the joint venture OBL) of the medical practice. Therefore, a thorough analysis to properly isolate the revenues, as well as the operating and capital expenses of the OEC, from the rest of the practice must be performed. In addition, the fair market value determination must be calculated without the consideration of any increased volume and/or revenue that may be projected to result from the addition of the specific joint venture partners.

CONCLUSION

The current healthcare environment has seen a dramatic shift toward outpatient care and the rendering of such services. In order to mitigate a variety of concerns, chiefly financial, vascular surgeons and others have looked to partner with larger organizations through a joint venture in order to achieve strategic goals of efficient healthcare delivery while concurrently containing cost and sharing risk. Multiple partnership models exist besides solo practice, and the success is based on a combined vision and mission among the stakeholders. Clearly there are benefits and risks to each opportunity, as well as specific legal implications. Ultimately, by reviewing such pros and cons, the vascular surgeon or other specialist will be able to make a comprehensive and informed decision, after appropriate due diligence, as to whether a joint venture opportunity is in his or her best interest.

REFERENCES

1. Goldsmith J, Kaufman N, Burns L. The tangled hospital-physician relationship. *Health Aff.* 2016. https://doi.org/10.1377/hblog20160509.054793.
2. Samson R, Nair D. Outpatient endovascular suites: are they good for the patient or the doctor. *Vasc Specialist;* 2012. www.mdedge.com/vascularspecialistonline/article/83856/outpatient-endovascular-suites-are-they-good-patient-or.
3. Jain KM, Munn J, Rummel M, Vaddineni S, Longton C. Future of vascular surgery is in the office. *J Vasc Surg.* 2010;51(2):509–513.
4. Limitation on Certain Physician Referrals" 42 U.S.C. § 1395nn(a).
5. Limitation on Certain Physician Referrals" 42 U.S.C. § 1395nn(h)(6)(A).
6. The Regulations Specifically Note that "DHS Do Not Include Services that Are Reimbursed by Medicare as Part of a Composite Rate (For Example, SNF Part A Payments or ASC Services Identified at §416.164(a)), except to the Extent that Services Listed in Paragraphs (1)(i) through (1)(x) of This Definition Are Themselves Payable through a Composite Rate (For Example, All Services provided as Home Health Services or Inpatient and Outpatient Hospital Services Are DHS)." "Definitions" 42 C.F.R. § 411.351.
7. Criminal Penalties for Acts Involving Federal Health Care Programs" 42 U.S.C. § 1320a-7b(b)(1).
8. *Re: OIG Advisory Opinion No. 15-10" by Gregory E. Demske, Chief Counsel to the Inspector General, Letter to [Name Redacted]*; July 28, 2015:4–5. U.S. v. Greber" 760 F.2d 68, 69 (3d Cir. 1985) http://oig.hhs.gov/fraud/docs/advisoryopinions/15/AdvOpn15-10.pdf.
9. Re: OIG Advisory Opinion No. 15-10" By Gregory E. Demske, Chief counsel to the Inspector General, Letter to [Name Redacted], July 28, 2015, http://oig.hhs.gov/fraud/docs/advisoryopinions/15/AdvOpn15-10.pdf (Accessed 12/9/15), p. 5.
10. Medicare and state health care programs: fraud and abuse; clarification of the initial OIG safe harbor provisions and establishment of additional safe harbor provisions under the anti-kickback statute. *Final Rule Federal Register.* November 19, 1999;64(223):63518–63520.
11. Re: Malpractice Insurance Assistance. *By Lewis Morris, Chief Counsel to the Inspector General.* Letter to [Name redacted],. United States Department of Health and Human Services; January 15, 2003. http://oig.hhs.gov/fraud/docs/alertsandbulletins/MalpracticeProgram.pdf.
12. *Exceptions: Ambulatory Surgery Centers" 42 C.F.R. § 1001.952(r).* 2015.
13. "Definitions" 42 U.S.C. § 416.2.
14. See "facts about office-based surgery accreditation. *Joint Commission;* February 16, 2018. https://www.jointcommission.org/facts_about_office-based_surgery_accreditation/.
15. Becker S, Pallardy C. Surgery center joint venture models. *Becker's ASC Rev;* 2013. www.beckersasc.com/asc-transactions-and-valuation-issues/5-surgery-center-joint-venture-models.html.
16. Hollingsworth JM, Ye Z, Strope SA, Krein SL, Hollenbeck AT, Hollenbeck BK. Physician-ownership of ambulatory surgery centers linked to higher volume of surgeries. *Health Aff.* 2010;29(4):683–689.
17. Cheney C. Hospital-physician consolidation growth trends moderate. *HealthLeaders;* 2019. www.healthleadersmedia.com/clinical-care/hospital-physician-consolidation-growth-trends-moderate.
18. Shtern Y, Lipsky L. Physician practice management. *Phys Pract;* 2017. www.physicianspractice.com/practice-models/5-things-know-about-physician-practice-management/page/0/1.
19. Strode RD. The resurgence of the ambulatory surgery center: seven considerations for ownership. *Health Care Law Today;* 2018. www.healthcarelawtoday.com/2018/05/24/the-resurgence-of-the-ambulatory-surgery-center-seven-considerations-for-ownership/.
20. Katzenbach J, Zhou A. You can't benchmark culture. *Strategy+Business;* 2019. www.strategy-business.com/article/You-cant-benchmark-culture?gko=4e9e7&utm_source=itw&utm_medium=20190226&utm_campaign=resp.
21. Sapp D. Facilities operations & maintenance – an overview. *Whole Building Design Guide;* 2017. www.wbdg.org/facilities-operations-maintenance.
22. Cross DS. Office-Based labs: getting started. *Cardiac Interventions Today;* 2018. https://citoday.com/2018/02/office-based-labs-getting-started/.

CHAPTER 27

Wound Care

CHARLES E. ANANIAN, BS, DPM

The philosophy of wound care requires a multidisciplinary approach for healing complex chronic wounds. Wounds cause significant morbidity in a person's daily life since most wounds require daily treatments and can be painful. While some wounds can be painless, the patients must keep the wound dry and not be able to shower, adding a level of discomfort to their lives. Other patients live with the constant fear that a wound may lead to amputation. Wounds can result in multiple hospitalizations, long-term intravenous antibiotics, and the use of assistive devices like crutches or a walker to remain nonweight-bearing. There is also a hardship to the family who, due to short comings of home health agencies, become responsible for daily dressing changes that perhaps should be the responsibility of a healthcare professional, not an untrained family member. Some wounds require total contact casting or compression wraps that are uncomfortable. Management of wounds like sacral and trunk wounds, as well as hospital-acquired decubitus ulcers can be expensive adding to the high cost of care in our healthcare system. Complications from diabetes alone cost more than 225 billion dollars a year. The average diabetic wound can take up 52 weeks to heal.[1] Studies show that 29% of venous stasis ulceration can reoccur 5 years.[2] Proper diagnosis and treatment by wound care physician, vascular interventionalist, infectious disease specialist, pedorthist, nutritionist, podiatrist, plastic surgeon (to name just a few) play a big role in healing wounds. Healing wounds quickly and effectively is the key to reducing a patient's morbidity, improving lifestyle, and lowering healthcare costs.

ETIOLOGY

Determining the etiology of the wound is of paramount importance. Treating the underlying cause early will improve a wound's outcome. Not all wounds have an obvious etiology: some are mixed wounds. The following list of wound care–related issues is presented in descending order of importance to wound healing: infection status, vascular status, basic wound care, advanced wound care, and offloading. Baseline blood work should be done at the onset of caring for a patient with a wound. This should include complete blood count with differential, a chemistry panel, albumin and pre-albumin level, complete metabolic panel, bleeding time, PT, and PTT. Liver function test should be ordered when considering antibiotic therapy. If a vasculitis type wound is suspected, blood should also be drawn for a rheumatoid panel and autoimmune markers.

Infection

Controlling infection is the first concern every doctor should have when evaluating a new patient. Obvious infections such as abscess, cellulitis, and osteomyelitis must be treated aggressively before any healing can take place. It would behoove wound care centers to refer patient to an infectious disease specialist when appropriate. Subclinical infection and colonization can impede wound closure and should be addressed appropriately. Blood work should include a complete blood count with differential, erythrocyte sedimentation rate, and c-reactive protein. An MRI can differentiate between osteomyelitis and Charcot changes in the insensate patients. Bone biopsy is the gold standard for diagnosing osteomyelitis. It should be done in an operating room. The Infectious Disease Society of America guidelines have called for a longer duration of intravenous antibiotics in immunocompromised patients such as those having diabetics. The duration should be at least 8 weeks rather than the previously recommended 6 weeks in nondiabetic patients. There should be strict surveillance while the patient is on intravenous antibiotics to monitor renal function and blood dyscrasias. Many of the antibiotics are nephrotoxic. Abscess should be drained and infected exposed tissues such as bone, tendon, fat, ligament, or necrotic tissues that can be a nidus for infection should be removed urgently and aggressively. Blood cultures and proper wound cultures with soft tissue, if possible, should be taken to direct the

Office-Based Endovascular Centers. https://doi.org/10.1016/B978-0-323-67969-5.00027-7
Copyright © 2020 Elsevier Inc. All rights reserved.

antibiotic treatment and to rule out bacteremia or sepsis. Many hospitals have a code sepsis protocol in place as extremity wounds can cause limb and/or life-threatening infections.

Ischemic Ulcers

This section will address the importance of prompt vascular intervention being paramount to wound healing. The most common vascular wounds are ischemic wounds due to atherosclerotic occlusive disease. Many illnesses lead to small vessel disease as seen in our diabetic and end stage renal disease population. This is the leading causes of gangrene and amputation in this patient population. Patients with atherosclerosis in larger vessels can be treated to improve circulation in the limb with nonhealing ulcer or gangrenous changes. Many of the interventions in the office-based endovascular center (OEC) consist of limb-saving angioplasty, atherectomy, and stenting to improve arterial blood flow to the affected limb and wound. These procedures are of paramount importance, as it is impossible to heal a lower extremity wound without adequate arterial blood flow.

Baseline exams and screening tests include arterial Doppler ultrasound with ankle brachial index. Skin perfusion test using sensilase (corVascular, Wayzata, MN) is a good predictor of local wound healing since it measures the oxygen tension at the tissue level in the area of the wound. New techniques such as LUNA fluorescence angiography give a good picture of the microcirculation in the wound bed area and are performed in the clinical setting. Traditional angiogram is done in the OEC. Other imaging studies such CT and MR angiography are available.

Once the level of disease is identified, there are many new and innovative techniques available to improve blood flow (Chapter 31). Atherectomy with various devices such as microblade, burr, and Laser are all being used routinely, and each device has its own advantage, depending on the level of disease and type of plaque being treated. The advent of drug-coated balloons has come into use and has cut down on restenosis rates. Stents are not routinely used below the knee due to the normal torsional stress put on the stents during normal gait.

Venous Ulceration

Venous ulceration is the most common type of wound in the United States today. Theses wounds are chronic and can be extremely painful and debilitating. Typically, they are found at the ankle area near the medial or lateral malleolus. They tend to be highly exudative, large, and edematous. The ulcers are caused by incompetent venous valve systems in superficial veins as well as the perforating veins or venous hypertension caused by obstructive deep venous disease. A venous ultrasound with reflux and venous mapping is the necessary imaging study to identify the level of disease. In case of reflux, the interventionalist can perform endo vein ablation in the OEC and prevent reflux which was causing the wound (Chapter 29). Surgical vein ligation and stripping are not the preferred method since the advent of ablation, given that stripping is a more painful procedure and is more expensive. Compression therapy is a common treatment using paste boots or multilayer compression bandages. Compression stockings are the first-line of treatment in preventing venous ulceration. Venous stockings come in various pressures and lengths, allowing a patient to customize their treatment. New venous pumps exist, which have a smaller, discreet battery-powered unit that can be worn under pants, without reducing effectiveness.

Deep venous obstruction angioplasty and stenting can be carried out with good results (Chapter 30).

Lymphedema

Wounds caused by lymphedema cause significant morbidity and have a poor prognosis. The lymph vessels do not lend themselves to surgical repair as seen in the arterial and venous systems. Very few centers around the country perform surgery on the lymph vessels. These wounds cause severe and sometimes permanent edemas and cause brawny induration and tissue fibrosis in the latter stages of lymph edema. The edema often causes the skin to tear easily with light pressure. The underlying cause could be a parasite infection or pressure on a lymph vessel secondary to a mass. These should be identified and treated. Milroy's disease is the most common cause and is a congenital disorder. Treatments include massage, exercise, lymph edema pumps, and compression garments as well as compression bandages in the acute phases.

Neuropathic Ulceration

Neuropathic ulceration, as seen in most diabetic wounds, is very common and may result in hospitalization and amputation. Neuroarthropathy can be limb-threatening in this patient population. The sorbitol pathway is the leading cause of neuropathy in the diabetic patient. Hansen's disease, medication-induced neuropathy, as well as alcoholic neuropathy can also cause wounds. The diabetic neuropathic wound is further complicated by peripheral vascular disease and microvascular disease. These wounds are usually on the plantar surface of the insensate foot but can be on the ankle and dorsum of the foot as well. These wounds need to be treated aggressively since they can quickly lead to amputations. This wound population is further complicated by being immunocompromised. Noncompliance is also common since these patients cannot feel the pain at the wound site. These wounds usually require weekly sharp debridement and offloading: both surgical and traditional. A diabetic wound that does not reduce in area by 50% in 4 weeks is classified as a chronic wound and has a poor prognosis. Over 91% of the wounds remain open at 12 weeks.[3] Sixty percent of all nontraumatic amputations occur in patients with diabetes. Other treatments include advanced wound care techniques which will be discussed later in this chapter. Lavery and his group at University of Texas reduced amputation rate by 33%[4] using hyperbaric oxygen in the treatment plan. This treatment takes place in a monochamber or a multiperson chamber. This technique uses 100% oxygen at 1.5–2 atm of pressure. This results in the bone marrow to produce white blood cells to help combat chronic osteomyelitis and increase oxygenation in the microcirculation, thereby promoting healing. Other indications for the use of hyperbaric chamber include crush injuries, necrotizing fasciitis, and flap failures. The treatments usually last an hour and 30 min daily over few weeks.

Pressure Wounds

Pressure wounds can occur anywhere on the body because of abnormal pressure on the tissue caused by contracture or paralysis. They can be due to neuropathic and/or vascular etiology. For example, a patient who has suffered a cerebral vascular accident with contracture and paralysis can have an insensate limb that stays in the same position and increased pressure results in skin break down. The patient usually presents with blisters and deep tissue injuries that progress to eschar that can involve the bone, resulting in osteomyelitis. Some of these wounds can be prevented with proper offloading (i.e., air mattress or multimodal splints) and/or changing the patient's position at timely intervals. Many of these patients may be candidates for primary amputation. Sacral and trunk wounds are another group of complicated wounds due to pressure at the hip trochanter and sacrum. Osteomyelitis in these locations can be life threatening. Rotational flaps are beneficial in these types of wounds but have a high rate of failure and reoccurrence due to lack of proper offloading. Also, this patient population tends to have poor nutritional status and healing potential. In addition to other treatment modalities, negative pressure wound therapy may be helpful.

Charcot Arthropathy

Charcot arthropathy is a complication in the diabetic patient that is a major cause of wound-related hospitalization and amputation. This occurs as a direct result of neuropathy. This disease state causes the bone to be demineralized and the normal bodyweight during gait can cause fracture across the joints in the affected limb. This is a synovial tissue disease, and there is a debate about its etiology: the neurovascular theory versus the neurotraumatic theory. The result of this fracture usually results in a wound that often requires surgical correction and stabilization of heal, as well as postoperative bracing for life.

Pyoderma Gangrenosum

Pyoderma gangrenosum is an inflammatory skin disorder that can cause severe painful and hard to heal ulceration. This begins with red or brown blisters that swell causing full thickness ulceration. The exact cause is unknown but is thought to be an autoimmune disorder that can manifest in conjunction with other inflammatory diseases such as inflammatory bowel disease, Crohn's disease, and ulcerative colitis. It is rare: affecting 1 in 100,000 in the United States. It is usually a diagnosis by exclusion. Soft tissue biopsy can help confirm the diagnosis in some cases. Sharp debridement is not indicated and can cause worsening of the wound. Treatments include antibiotics to treat infection, oral steroids, and topical steroid creams. Dapsone has also shown improvement in these wounds as well as immune suppressive treatments such as cyclosporin or azathioprine. Some emerging therapies include Elidil (pimecrolimus) cream and use of intravenous immunoglobin.

Wounds with malignant degeneration

Malignant degeneration should be suspected in wounds with normal clinical appearance, but failure to heal after 3 months. Punch biopsies are the preferred method for these types of wounds. Squamous cell, basal cell carcinomas have been identified in nonhealing wounds with normal appearing wound bed and wound margins. Malignant melanoma can be seen in wounds that fail to heal in a timely manner as well, but usually these wounds have abnormal pigmentation. These patients should be referred to oncologist for treatment and staging.

Phases of wound healing:

- The inflammatory phase occurs at day 0 to 4–6 days postinjury. During this phase, neutrophils are recruited to remove infectious agents and prevent infection. In a diabetic patient when the blood sugar exceeds 200 mg/dL, white blood cells lose their normal function. This is one of the main reasons why diabetics are at high risk for infection.

- The proliferative phase occurs between day 2 and 3 weeks postinjury. During this phase, cell recruitment, migration and proliferation of epithelial cells, fibroblasts, endothelial cells, and stem cells occur. Angiogenesis occurs during this phase as well.
- The remodeling phase begins 3 weeks postinjury with matrix deposition and reorganization followed by wound closure or scar formation.

Basic Wound Care

As the infection is being brought under control, and the vascular status is optimized, aggressive wound care should continue. Documentation in wound care is important. Reimbursements are also tied to proper documentation. If no wound specific electronic medical record is available, the following elements should be included in the weekly wound visits. Pictures, before and after debridement of the wound, are recommended. Documentation of wound type, location, and duration are also parts of the wound care visit. Logging the area of the wound is required, documentation of the volume of the wound is similarly recommended. An inside out approach is recommended when describing a wound, start by describing the wound base. Color of the wound base, i.e., red, pink, pale, gray, black, and yellow, is used commonly in proper documentation. Next describe the quality of tissue, granular, slough, presence of eschar. Is it friable, cicatrix, or bullous? Proper documentation also requires a description of the wound edges: Are they regular annular, irregular, smooth, or rough. Are the wound edges lifting, macerated, dry, keratotic, or hypertrophic? Then describe the periwound area. Is there edema, erythema, induration, fluctuance, or is it boggy. It is important to describe the wound exudate. Describe the amount of drainage. Is there mild, moderate, or heavy exudate? Is the exudate clear, serous, sanguineous, yellow, brown, or purulent?

Debridement

Debridement in its various forms is essential to wound healing. The debridement is important in removing infection and bacterial waste products that halt wound healing because of bioburden. Debridement reduces the time to heal as well.

Sharp excisional debridement is usually done using a scalpel, a sharp dermal curette, scissors, and rongeur. Anesthetic management depends on the wound location, and the type of wound being debrided. Arterial and venous wounds tend to be painful and would require injection of local anesthetic or regional block prior to debridement. Wounds on the trunk and upper extremity would need local anesthesia as well. Diabetic foot wounds are usually the result of neuropathy and are insensate thus may only need topical anesthetic such as lidocaine gel or EMLA cream (Astra Zeneca, Sweden). Since most debridements are done weekly in the clinic, analgesia is an important step in patient care. Studies have shown weekly debridement improved wound healing time.[5] Wilcox looked at frequency of debridement and found that a group of patients that were debrided weekly healed faster than groups that were debrided every other week and even faster than the ones debrided every 3 weeks. This type of debridement aids in removing the senescent cells at the wound periphery that helps stimulate the wound healing pathway. There is often a large amount of bleeding, so hemostasis is essential. In the clinical setting this becomes more of a challenge, in the operating room electrocautery and tying off the vessel is used most often as well as hemostatic agents like surgicel, thrombin, and floseal. In the clinic we use silver nitrate and surgicel. There are disposable single-use cautery pens that are effective as well. It may be advisable to invest in an electrocautery.

Selective debridement is another type of debridement done mainly in the clinic setting, as well as in the operating room. The Versajet (Smith & Nephew, Andover, MA) hydro scalpel uses water pumped at extreme speed into a wand that creates a cutting surface because of Venturi effect. This device is used to remove adherent slough and eschar from chronic wounds and is more forgiving than sharp debridement as it removes tissue layer by layer sparing the deeper healthy tissue that can be violated with a scalpel. Other types of selective debridement technique uses ultrasonic scalpel (Misonix, Farmingdale, NY) to debride the tissue. Other techniques use local dressings for debridement. Debrisoft (Lohmann-rauscher, Milwaukee, WI) is course gauze material that can be used on certain wounds to remove loose slough and film from granular wound beds that do not require sharp debridement. Cleaning the wound with moist gauze is a similar type of debridement. Mechanical debridement falls under this category of selective debridement as well but is seldom used. A wet to dry dressing applied to wound and removed next day results in removing the dead tissue adhering to the gauze that results in mechanical debridement.

Enzymatic debridement is used to loosen eschar and adherent slough from all types of wounds. Santyl

(Smith & Nephew, Andover, MA) is a collagenase that breaks down unwanted wound bed contaminants. Medical honey has been used for enzymatic debridement but has not been found to be effective. Maggot therapy is in this category since the enzyme found in this type of fly larva is a strong collagenase. There are laboratories that sell these larvae in a dressing form and have had good results in clinical trials. Patients tend to shy away from this type of therapy given it is an organism on their wound and is not pleasant from their perspective.

Dressing Selection

Dressings are used to mitigate exudate, prevent infection, reduce pain, and stimulate wound healing. Selecting the appropriate dressing starts with the wound etiology and there should be a balance between dry and moist dressing. Dressings should be exchanged as needed depending on the character of the wound. Antimicrobial creams are often used to reduce infection in wounds, silver sulfadiazineine is the one used in diabetic wounds at our clinic. Bactroban (GlaxoSmithKline, Philadelphia, PA) is a topical antimicrobial cream which is effective against methicillin-resistant *Staphylococcus aureus* (MRSA). Hydrogel is used to hydrate the wound area. Iodosorb (Smith & Nephew, Andover, MA) is a cadexomer iodine–based gel that is used for infected draining wounds. Silver dressings such as Acticoat (Smith & Nephew, Andover, MA) are used to fight infection and are found to be affective against MRSA. The silver ions have been shown to have an analgesic affect by blocking local pain receptors in the wound bed. Alginates and silver alginates are used in highly exudative infected wounds. Sachet type dressing is used to capture moister in wounds with copious amount of drainage. Collagen dressings are used with or without silver to help promote wound healing by assisting in collagen deposition and binding to fill in the wound. Collagen granules are used as well. It should be noted that using silvers and iodine-based dressings can slow down wound healing if used for extended periods. Once the wound bed is free of slough, infection moist dressing should be used to promote wound healing. For wounds that require compression such as venous ulcers and wounds due to lymphedema, paste boots like the Unna boot is used in conjunction with the dressings mentioned above. There are also 4-layer and 2-layer compression wraps that are good at reducing edema in the extremities. Compression stockings such as Tubigrip are a good alternative as well and come in various levels of pressure.

Advanced Wound Care

These techniques are employed if the basic wound care measures are not working in promoting wound healing after 4 weeks or to close a surgically created wound. Again, the wound etiology will dictate the type of wound care needed.

Negative pressure dressing is used on a variety of wounds. Many different manufactures produce devices that produce varying negative pressure with foam dressing under occlusive dressing and a reservoir to capture exudate. Most wound vacuums run on an electric motor. There are new smaller devices that create negative pressure with a spring-loaded apparatus. These can be used with surgical wounds with exposed tendon and bone. Venous wounds are treated with wound vacuums but can cause pain and are not easily tolerated. Contact layers like Adaptic help reduce pain while using these devices. Compliance issues arise with this treatment due to the need to have a machine attached to the body at all times. These devices are portable. There are also issues of malodor and the need for skilled nursing personnel for dressing change on a regular basis. This is expensive treatments but can be highly effective and prevent hospitalization.

Skin substitutes have become an integral part of wound care. They come in two categories: living and nonliving. Each category has its own indication. The nonliving skin substitutes can be a xenograft as produced by Oasis (Smith & Nephew, Andover, MA), Puraply (Organogenesis, Canton, MA), and Kerascis (Keracis, Arlington, VA). The porcine intestinal submucosa can act as a scaffold in wound healing and can create an inflammatory response in the wound bed which helps the wound environment move from chronic to acute stage. Oasis is such a product and has been used for many years. Puraply is a similar tissue with a different manufacturing process and an optional antimicrobial layer which helps remove biofilm from the wound bed. Biofilm has been shown to be an impediment to wound closures. Keracis is a newer skin xenograft and is made from cod fish skin. The proposed mechanism of action is the deposition of high amount of omega-3 fatty acids in the wound that promote healing. Other bovine collagen preparations such as Primatrix (Integra Lifesciences, Plainsboro, NJ) is also used in the wound management. These products usually have a head to toe indication and are cheaper to produce, thus larger size grafts can be used for larger wounds. Depending on the product it may not be used if the patient is allergic to fish, pork, or bovine products. As with any wound care product, each type of skin substitute has different thickness and handling characteristics. The therapy needs to be individualized. These products are usually steri-stripped into place on the wound and do not lend themselves to suturing. The Primatrix collagen could be sutured or stapled into place. Other nonliving therapies can be derived from the amniotic tissues. Products such as EpiFix (Mimedex, Marietta, GA) and Neox are amniotic tissues that are harvested during scheduled cesarean sections. These products provide extracellular matrix and growth factors to the wound bed. Epi fix is dehydrated and has a shelf life of 2 years. This makes it user-friendly in the clinic. Neox (Amniox, Miami, FL) is a frozen product and has a shorter shelf life. Both companies have amniotic tissue allografts which tend to be thinner like a membrane. Under CMS guidance, these products should only be used for diabetic foot ulcers and venous leg ulcers. Coverage should be verified on case by case bases with other health insurances. There is an umbilical cord product also made by Amniox that is 10 times thicker than the amniotic tissue. These tissues are good for use in deeper wounds and are absorbed by the patient at a slower rate. The umbilical cord has the same extracellular matrix and growth factors as amniotic tissue but is rich in hyaluronic acid which adds an anti-inflammatory component to the treatment. Regrnaex gel (Smith & Nephew, Andover, MA) delivers human platelet–derived growth factors to the wound bed. It comes in a gel preparation which is applied to the wound bed for 12 h and has shown good outcomes in clinical trials.

Living cell therapies are not as common since the preparation and preservation are more costly. These products deliver the same extracellular matrix and growth factors with the added advantage of human mesenchymal stem cells to the wound bed. Grafix (Smith & Nephew, Andover, MA) is an amniotic product that has been proven to have 70% living stem cells. These cells are important in modulating wound healing in all three phases of normal wound healing process. There is a cryopreserved product and a lyophilized product available. In randomized clinical trials, use of these products has been shown it to be an effective treatment. Affinity (Organogenesis, Canton, MA) is another amniotic membrane product with viable stem cells and is stable for up to 30 days. Dermagraf (Organogenesis, Canton, MA) is another living cell product that is bioengineered using human-derived fibroblast grown on a suture mesh and is shipped cryopreserved at −80 Celsius and has a 6-month shelf life. Apligraf (Organogenesis, Canton, MA) is a bilayer skin substitute that is grown on agar plate with dermal matrix and has fibroblasts and keratinocytes. It has a shelf life of 10 days. Both products have been derived from donated neonatal foreskin. Both products have shown safety and efficacy in large randomized clinical trials.

Skin grafting has a place in wound healing as an autograft. This can be done for many wound types but has a poor outcome in venous wound due to the amount of exudate and lack of achievable intimal contact needed for the graft to take. Skin graft on diabetic foot wounds on the plantar insensate foot is not recommended since the plantar skin is usually 10 times thicker than the transplanted donor skin. If the graft does take, the lack of native skin can breakdown when weight-bearing resumes. Skin flaps, free myocutaneous, and pedicle grafts are technically difficult but have shown success in the management of traumatic and chronic wounds with large defects and bone involvement. All the abovementioned products have different levels of effectiveness, ease of use, coverage, and deliver a variety of cellular products in the wound bed. In my practice, I look for products with level one evidence and safety. I interchange modalities based on changing character of the wound. There is not one product that is a cure for all, at any given time.

Nutritional status is an area not to be neglected in any wound care program. Serum albumin, pre albumin level, and vitamin D level should be checked. A nutrition consultant should be considered for most patients. All the wound care modalities will have an improved outcome if the patient is optimized from a nutritional standpoint. Vitamin and mineral supplements should be given with zinc and vitamin C as these are important in wound healing.

Offloading is an integral part of the diabetic foot wounds care. The gold standard for offloading is the total contact cast. This treatment has improved with the advent of fiberglass impregnated socks being used rather than the rolled fiber glass cast that can cause irritation and skin breakdown since the pressure is not equally distributed and the contour of the leg is not as well conformed as seen in the new sock-type cast. Total contact padding with felt and foam are an alternative and even when combined with a controlled ankle motion (CAM) walker boot are not as effective as the total contact cast. It has been shown in studies done by Armstrong[6] that a patient who takes 10 steps can halt wound healing in a plantar wound. Compliance is improved with casting rather than the use of CAM walker boots that can be removed. One issue with total contact cast is that negative pressure therapy is hard to use with these casts and dressing changes cannot be done daily since most casts are only changed once a week. We tend to use dressings that can keep the wound clean for up to 7 days such as silver combined with collagen. Diabetic shoes are important in preventing recurrence of ulcer in the diabetic foot. The diabetic shoe can have custom insoles made to offload pressure points and accommodate partial foot amputations. Custom braces and boots are readily available for amputations and charcot deformities. Many surgical wounds should be offloaded with postsplints or boots.

Conclusion

In my wound care practice over several years, I have learned that it requires perseverance and patience as well as compassion and knowledge. We become a big part of the patients' lives since they see us weekly for many months and need constant reassurance. I still rely on continuous learning by attending wound care conferences to make sure my patients get the most advanced and effective treatments available. A multidisciplinary approach is essential.

REFERENCES

1. American Diabetes Association. Economic costs of diabetes in the U.S. in 2012. *Diabetes Care.* 2013;36(4):1033–1046.
2. Ince P, Garne FL, Jeffcoate WJ. Rate of healing of neuropathic ulcers of the foot in diabetes and its relationship to ulcer duration and ulcer area. *Diabetes Care.* March 2007; 30(3):660–663.
3. Mayberry JC, Moneta GL, Taylor JLM, Porter JM. Fifteen-year results of ambulatory compression therapy for chronic venous ulcers. *Surgery;* 1991. europepmc.org.
4. National organization of rare diseases.
5. Wound Healing Phases Heather A. Wallace; P.M. Zito.
6. Off-loading the diabetic foot wound: a randomized clinical trial. *Diabetes Care.* June 2001;24(6):1019–1022.

CHAPTER 28

Limb Preservation Center

KRISHNA JAIN, MD, FACS

INTRODUCTION

There are close to 2 million people living with a major amputation in the United States. In 54% of patients, amputations result from diabetes and vascular disease followed by trauma.[1] According to Owings et al., approximately 185,000 amputations occur in the United States every year.[2] In 2009, amputation-related hospital costs totaled more than $8.3 billion.[3] For individuals with diabetes who have an amputation of one leg, 55% will have an amputation of the other leg.[4] For patients with diabetes and vascular disease a limb preservation center (LPC) is essential to provide patients with all aspects of preventative care to avoid the detrimental outcome of loosing a limb.

The goal of an LPC is to prevent amputation and improve lifestyle. In the literature, the phrase, "limb salvage" is used much more often than limb preservation, suggesting that most patients present for medical care when the limb is already threatened, rather than at a time when it could be preserved. Additionally, limb salvage requires invasive procedures, instead of the preventive measures that could be used earlier on in the disease process. An LPC aims to decrease the number of patients who present with limb-threatening pathology and to help preserve the limb when it becomes threatened. In addition, many patients have debilitating limb-related issues that need to be resolved to improve their quality of life such as chronic venous disease and lymphedema. An LPC can be a free-standing entity, be a part of a hospital, be a part of a practice, or be centered around an office-based endovascular center (OEC). It is logical for the LPC to be centered around an OEC since most of the invasive procedures required for limb preservation can be performed in the OEC.

In an article by Center of Disease Control and prevention, three levels of prevention are defined[5]:

1. **Primary prevention**—Intervention before health effects occur, through measures such as vaccinations, altering risky behaviors (poor eating habits, tobacco use), and eliminating substances known to be associated with a disease or health condition.
2. **Secondary prevention**—Screening to identify diseases in the earliest stages, before the onset of signs and symptoms, through measures such as mammography and regular blood pressure testing.
3. **Tertiary prevention**—Managing disease post-diagnosis to slow or stop disease progression through measures such as chemotherapy, rehabilitation, and screening for complications.

LPCs should provide a comprehensive multidisciplinary approach to prevent limb loss and improve quality of life by developing specific measures to prevent limb loss at every level of prevention during the disease process (Fig. 28.1). The most common causes of limb loss are complications of diabetes, ischemia with or without infection, osteomyelitis, trauma, venous disease, and other minor causes like frostbite or tumors.[1]

The term LPC is not governed by any agency and thus has become synonymous for some with a center providing wound care or invasive therapy for arterial occlusive disease. Various centers have called themselves an LPC or limb salvage center based on the services they are providing. The name may be nothing but a marketing tool. A true LPC should provide comprehensive services for the whole spectrum of disease processes that can result in limb loss. Above all, the center should focus on the patient rather than the limb alone.

MULTIDISCIPLINARY TEAM

A multidisciplinary team is required for the diverse array of care needed to treat patients with primary, secondary, and tertiary prevention measures. The team should include the following specialists:

Diabetologist/endocrinologist/internal medicine physician
Podiatrist

Office-Based Endovascular Centers. https://doi.org/10.1016/B978-0-323-67969-5.00028-9
Copyright © 2020 Elsevier Inc. All rights reserved.

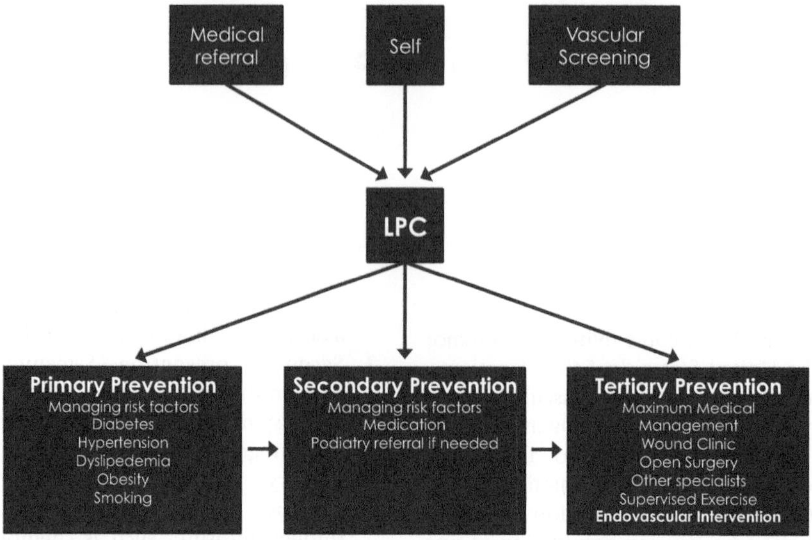

FIG. 28.1 Types of care targeted by prevention level at a limb preservation center.

Infection disease specialist
Nephrologist
Cardiologist
Neurologist
Rheumatologist
Interventionalist (vascular surgeon, interventional cardiologist, interventional radiologist)
Orthopedic surgeon
Plastic surgeon

Diabetologist: Since the most common cause of limb loss is related to diabetes mellitus, it is crucial that the center offers management of diabetes and other risk factors. The center should employ or have a close working relationship with internists and endocrinologist to help patients manage diabetes and other risk factors like hypertension, dyslipidemia, and smoking cessation. However, a focused diabetes clinic is extremely desirable. In a study by Ho et al., it was shown that patients attending a diabetes clinic received better quality of diabetes care compared with those attending a general medical clinic.[6] A diabetic clinic will focus on helping patients maintain a healthy lifestyle. A nutritionist may focus on diet alterations and promote daily exercise to aid patients in reaching their ideal weight, blood pressure and blood sugar levels. Good foot care may help prevent ulcers, and may be provided in cooperation with a podiatrist. This includes daily foot checks for blisters and redness or discoloration by the patient or someone else, and periodic checks for sensation and footwear issues. Smoking cessation is an important component of this clinic. Armstrong et al. showed the benefit of quitting smoking on limb survival.[7] In their study, patients who quit smoking had lower mortality and improved amputation-free survival than patients who continued to smoke. Through the diabetic clinic, patients may be able to get psychological support as well as pharmacological therapy to quit smoking. These services can be provided through a vascular medicine clinic.

Podiatrist: Podiatrists should form an integral part of the team since they may be the first to see patients with foot ulcers and may also be involved in wound care centers.[8] There are several studies demonstrating the benefits of a podiatrist as an integral part of the diabetic limb salvage team.[9] Podiatrists play a very important part in preventing ulcers by using offloading techniques and improving overall care of the foot. Sloan et al. found that having a podiatrist on the healthcare team managing diabetes in Medicare-eligible patients decreased the likelihood of a lower extremity amputation.[10] Patients presenting with an ulceration were 36% less likely to have a lower extremity amputation when a podiatrist was involved in the care. Podiatrists who specialize in surgical care of the foot can perform foot sparing amputations, perform complex debridement, and correct foot deformities. Ideally, they should be physically present at the center for seamless care, if not, they should make it easy for the patients to see them for timely care needed to prevent amputation.

Infectious disease specialist: Many patients at risk of limb loss present with complicated wound infections. This is especially true in patients with diabetic ulcers.

Easy access to an infectious disease expert will result in timely treatment of infection. In a study by Brennan et al., there was a direct positive correlation between the geographic density of infectious disease physicians and limb preservation in patients with diabetic foot ulcers.[11] Treatment of infection may require inpatient or outpatient antibiotic therapy. For long-term outpatient intravenous therapy, a peripherally inserted central catheter can be placed in the LPC. The specialist should also have inpatient privileges at a local hospital in case the treatment requires hospital admission.

Nephrologists: Patients with end stage renal disease have a higher incidence of peripheral artery disease and poorer outcomes after intervention. Nephrologists play an integral part in managing kidney disease as well as hypertension. Gilhotra et al., in a systematic review, showed increased incidence of amputation in patients with end stage renal disease on dialysis.[12] In an article by Garimella and Hirsch, the authors suggest that clinical quality care metrics are essential in order to improve peripheral artery disease-chronic kidney disease outcomes. Standards can and should be set within the LPC to ensure optimal outcomes for patients.[13] Providing comprehensive care within the LPC with multiple specialists on site, including a nephrologist is one giant step toward improving the standard of care for these patients.

Cardiologists: Cardiologists can help optimize the cardiac function, thereby improving peripheral perfusion. For patients in a supervised exercise program, it is important to maximize the cardiac function so that the patient can meet their exercise goals. Management of congestive heart failure is critical to wound healing, since edema causes decrease in microcirculation, limiting clearance of bacteria from the wound. In LPCs where the interventionalist is a cardiologist, they may manage the cardiac care or collaborate with a non-interventional cardiologist.

Neurologists: Many patients with diabetes have peripheral neuropathy that can be best managed by neurologists, which may help diminish the incidence of neuropathic diabetic ulcers. Patients presenting to the center may actually have pain in the lower extremities resulting from degenerative spine conditions. A neurologist could better manage these patients. In addition, many patients with leg symptoms like weakness and pain are initially seen by a neurologist and if found to have vascular disease can then be managed by the LPC.

Rheumatologists: Patients with vasculitis and rheumatoid-associated ulcers will benefit from the care provided by a rheumatologist. Many ulcers in lower extremity are not related to vascular disease. These patients may have an underlying autoimmune disease like lupus erythematosus resulting in an ulcer. These conditions are best diagnosed and managed by a rheumatologist.

Interventionalists: Once the patient becomes symptomatic due to underlying peripheral artery disease, diabetes-related ulcers, or venous disease, the interventionalist can begin tertiary prevention measures. Intervention may be completed by a vascular surgeon, interventional cardiologist, or interventional radiologist. However, the role of interventionalist should not be limited to intervention; once the patient is symptomatic every medical measure should be taken to avoid intervention. When intervention is indicated and performed, it is important to prevent further complications and manage the underlying disease during follow-up. Endovascular intervention consists of balloon angioplasty, stent placement, and atherectomy when indicated. New devices are being developed and tested; however, prior to use, the interventionalist should feel confident that use of the devices is warranted based upon available data. With improving technology, endovascular procedures have become the first-line treatment for arterial disease. As new procedures become available the interventionalist should learn the procedures as per FDA/manufacturer's recommendation before offering them to patients.

Vascular surgeon: If the interventionalist is not a vascular surgeon, a strong working relationship should be developed with a surgeon who has vascular privileges in a nearby hospital. It is inevitable that there will be complications resulting in bleeding and pseudoaneurysms. It is not desirable to just send the patient to local emergency room and let them take care of the complication. Once there is established relationship with a vascular surgeon, the surgeon should be directly called to manage the complication. Endovascular treatment is gradually becoming the first line of therapy for peripherally arterial occlusive disease; however, some patients will suffer from failure of endovascular therapy, necessitating bypass surgery. In certain patients a bypass may be the first option. For these reasons, it is important that a vascular surgeon be an integral part of the multidisciplinary team.

Orthopedic surgeon: Orthopedic surgeons and the podiatrist should work together to offer all the surgical options that can be used to save the limb. The surgical experience of these two specialists differs and can be complimentary. It may not be necessary to have the orthopedic surgeon geographically at the same site as LPC.

Plastic surgeon: Plastic surgeons, though needed sparingly, can perform complex debridement and various flaps to cover defects in the foot. The ultimate goal for patients with foot issues is to save as much functional foot as possible to have a satisfactory gait.

MULTIDISCIPLINARY SERVICES

Similar to providing a multidisciplinary team of healthcare providers, patients should also have access to a number of services.

Wound clinic
Vascular screening
Vascular noninvasive laboratory
Imaging studies
Exercise
Office-based endovascular suite
Hospital access
Lymphedema clinic
Social services
Nutritionist
Rehabilitation

Wound clinic: A great number of patients lose a limb because of diabetic ulcers with or without underlying arterial occlusive disease. Management of the wounds is critical to saving limbs. The wound should be assessed for the size, appearance, type of exudate, and the wound edge. Appropriate cultures should be performed. Diagnostic studies like a bone scan, MRI, or noninvasive arterial studies should be ordered as indicated. Treatment may include surgical debridement, enzymatic debridement, and biosurgical debridement (using maggots). Various dressings can be used that include hydrogels, hydrocolloids, calcium alginate, antimicrobials, film, and foam. Various growth factors and tissues can be used for appropriate wounds. Hyperbaric oxygen therapy has been used for nonhealing diabetic and radiation ulcers. Vacuum-assisted closure has been used successfully to close large wounds. The wound clinic needs to work closely with a vascular surgeon/interventionalist. If the wound is not healing because of underlying ischemia, appropriate procedures need to be performed to revascularize the extremity. In patients with nonhealing venous ulcers, a venous procedure may be indicated to eliminate venous reflux due to superficial vein incompetence or deep venous reflux because of obstruction. The wound clinic may be a part of the LPC or have a strong relationship with the LPC. If separate, the medical directors from the wound clinic and LPC should develop protocols for referral between the two entities.

Vascular screening: In 2013, the US Preventive Services Task Force (USPSTF) did not recommend ankle brachial index (ABI) screening in asymptomatic adults who do not have a known diagnosis of peripheral arterial disease, cardiovascular disease, severe chronic kidney disease, or diabetes based upon insufficient evidence (rating I).[14] In the past, the recommendation was D, which was against screening individuals without symptoms. However, for patients with the aforementioned comorbidities, an abnormal ABI is indicative of cardiovascular disease, and appropriate treatment strategy should be used. Vascular screening should be a part of secondary prevention in this group of patients.

Vascular noninvasive laboratory: A noninvasive vascular laboratory is an important part of the center. The laboratory should have a state-of-the-art color flow duplex scanner as well as equipment to perform physiological studies. The laboratory should be certified by the Intersocietal Accreditation Commission (IAC). The laboratory should have capability of performing ultrasound imaging and physiological studies. In metropolitan areas surrounded by rural community and rural hospitals, a mobile vascular laboratory can provide access to technology that may not be readily available at local level. If the clinical exam indicates arterial or venous disease, a noninvasive study is required to plan the treatment. After intervention, follow-up noninvasive studies are required. All invasive procedures should be performed based on clinical exam and noninvasive studies to decrease the use of invasive studies which are expensive, painful, and have possible complications and side effects.

Imaging: A noninvasive vascular laboratory as mentioned above is an integral part of LPC. Many patients will need other imaging studies using CT angiography (CTA) and magnetic resonance angiography (MRA). The LPC should have good working relationship with centers providing these services so the studies can be done in a timely manner. The decision to proceed with an endovascular revascularization procedure can almost always be made based on clinical and ultrasound findings. CTA and MRA should be used sparingly, and in most circumstances these studies are not required. If there are anatomical reasons to avoid a catheter angiogram or if an open procedure is planned, a CT angiogram can be used.

Supervised exercise: Exercise is the most effective noninterventional treatment to improve pain and increase ambulation distance in patients with intermittent claudication. It also decreases cardiovascular morbidity. This would be part of tertiary prevention to treat patients once they have become symptomatic. Patients may enroll in a community or home-based structural exercise program or a supervised exercise program. Many patients are not able to participate in a supervised program because of transport issues or access to these programs. Directly supervised exercise programs consist of at least three walking sessions per week (30–60 min each) for a minimum 12 weeks. A systematic review by Fakhry et al., examining the benefit of supervised walking therapy, demonstrated an increase in pain free and maximum walking distance.[15] In the CLEVER study (Claudication: Exercise Versus Endoluminal Revascularization), 111 patients with aortoiliac disease receiving optimal medical care were randomly assigned to medical care alone, medical care and supervised exercise, or medical care and revascularization using balloon angioplasty and stent.[16] Both groups with additive care (exercise or revascularization) had better 18-month outcomes than medical care alone and were statistically indistinguishable in their outcomes from each other. There was an increase in claudication onset time for supervised exercise but not for stent revascularization in comparison with control. Supervised exercise therapy though ideal for patients with claudication is not always possible because of underlying medical problems including cardiovascular disease, patients with rest pain, ulcers or gangrene, previous amputation, and other major comorbidities. These types of patients may benefit from other forms of exercise including cycling, strength training, and arm cranking. In one review of exercise modalities, there were no significant differences between other training methods and supervised walking exercise on pain-free walking and maximum walking distance.[17] However, more data is required to make this the treatment of choice. Other alternatives to supervised exercise program use clinician-supported and instruction-based techniques. These programs can be community- or home-based. A metaanalysis by Golledge et al. suggests that structured home exercise programs were effective at improving walking performance and physical activity in the short term for patients with peripheral arterial disease (PAD).[18] Participation in supervised or a monitored exercise programs may avoid or delay interventional therapy for claudication. Atherosclerosis is a progressive disease. Even after intervention, patient needs to continue to exercise to delay clinical symptoms that may result from progressive atherosclerosis.

Office-based endovascular suite: Patients with arterial occlusive disease or venous disease needing intervention have multiple site options for endovascular procedures. The procedure can be carried out in various settings that include hospital inpatient, hospital outpatient, ambulatory surgery center, or OEC. There are strengths and weaknesses for each location; however, the OEC has a number of benefits for patients within the LPC. The key to limb preservation is quick access to the endovascular suite. There are several drawbacks to hospital-based inpatient or outpatient labs. Most of the hospital-based endovascular labs cannot schedule a procedure quickly enough because of underlying inertia of the system, as schedules are difficult to change once in place. The hospital laboratories are not patient-friendly, as patients meet multiple personnel they have never seen before. Additionally, it is more expensive to have a procedure performed in the hospital system. Ambulatory surgery centers (ASCs) may be independent or in partnership with the hospital. Very few of these centers are accredited to perform endovascular procedures. Most ASCs are geared toward taking care of patients with issues related to gastroenterology, ophthalmology, orthopedics, or pain management. If the ASC is designed to take care of patients with threatened limbs, it could serve the need of the patients since it shares the multiple benefits provided by the OEC. OECs are a safe and patient-friendly option (Table 28.1). Patient satisfaction consistently runs above 95%. Patient outcomes for an OEC are similar to hospital-performed procedures. The patient interacts with the same personnel they have

TABLE 28.1
Outcomes in Various Office-based Endovascular Centers.

	Procedures	Complications	Transfer to Hospital	30-day Mortality	Procedure-Related Mortality
Jain et al.[21]	6458	54	26	18	0
Lin et al.[22]	5134	73	22	9	0
Oskui et al.[23]	500	7	1	Not reported	Not reported
Total	12,092	134 (1.2%)	49 (0.4%)	27 (0.2%)	0

been seeing during their office visits. It is cheaper than the hospital. The procedure can be scheduled rapidly since it is the same surgeon or group that owns the OEC and also controls the schedule. With increasing patient deductibles, the patient has to pay less out of pocket. Various procedures that can be performed in the office include diagnostic angiograms, balloon angioplasty, balloon angioplasty and stent, atherectomy and balloon angioplasty. Nationally, venous ablation is almost exclusively done in the office setting. Venous stenting for venous obstruction is being performed at an increasing rate in the office.

Hospital access: Many LPCs are affiliated with a hospital. However, a growing number of centers are freestanding. In contrast to an ASC, the Centers for Medicare and Medicaid services (CMS) does not require transfer agreements between the OEC and the hospital. However, it is critical that the vascular surgeon performing procedures in the office also have privileges in a nearby hospital. If the procedure is performed by a cardiologist or a radiologist, they should have a working relationship with a vascular surgeon or have a hospital transfer agreement for the safety of the patient. Patients should receive care where it is appropriate. A patient may need to be admitted for intravenous antibiotics for complex foot infection, or an extensive debridement. Complex flaps and foot saving operations may need to be performed in a hospital operating room. Though endovascular procedures have significantly improved over the years, many patients will need an open procedure in the hospital. This may include an endarterectomy or bypass procedure. There may be a need for a hybrid procedure, which includes an endovascular procedure and an open procedure simultaneously. Due to the nature of endovascular procedures there are bound to be complications that will need emergency or urgent admission to the hospital. These complications mostly consist of bleeding, embolization, or are cardiac in nature.

Lymphedema clinic: Though most patients with lymphedema do not lose a limb, patients will be invariably referred to the center. A comprehensive LPC should provide care to patients with lymphedema. The care consists of manual lymph drainage (light pressure massage), compression therapy, dietary consultation, management of obesity, elevation of legs, and home use of lymphedema pumps. Patients with recurrent cellulitis may need prophylactic antibiotics on a routine basis. There are very few surgical options for these patients.

Social services: The current healthcare system is extremely difficult to negotiate for a layperson. Social workers can help patients and their families cope with the psychological and social problems that may arise during their care at the center. They may help in identifying rehabilitation facilities, skilled nursing facilities, and home care. Social workers may also offer following services: (a) answering questions related to health insurance, (b) best living arrangements for patient after leaving the center after a procedure, (c) supportive and adjustment counseling, (d) financial assessment and referral services, (e) education and consultative services, and (f) access to community resources.

Nutritionist: The expertise of a nutritionist is valuable during all phases of prevention. Obesity, diabetes, and dyslipidemia are all risk factors for peripheral arterial disease. All these risk factors can be modified under the direction of a nutritionist. In a review article by Nosova et al., the authors advocated "an intensified use of diet in PAD therapy, and ... specifically recommend following eating patterns that are rich in nutrients with anti-inflammatory and anti-oxidant properties."[19] However, Brostow et al. suggests that the data needed to evaluate the impacts of nutrition on the progression of PAD are limited.[20] Irrespective of lack of scientific data related to nutrition and PAD, there are individual data that show the effect of diet on obesity, diabetes mellitus, and dyslipidemia. Proper nutrition is also required for wound healing.

Rehabilitation: The goal of therapy is to have the patient return to the activity level prior to the ailment being treated. Rehabilitation plays an important part in it. Even if the patient does not lose a limb, underlying medical conditions can compromise the activity level. In patients who lose part of a limb or whole limb appropriate gate training, foot ware, and prosthesis are required. The patient may need physical therapy and/or occupational therapy. It may not be possible to provide all these modalities at the LPC. The center should facilitate access to these services.

CERTIFICATION AND REGISTRY

LPCs do not currently require certification. However, there are parts of the center that need to be certified (Chapter 36). Wound care clinics with hyperbaric chamber may need certification. OECs do not need to be certified to receive reimbursement from CMS; however, some states may require the center to be certified. If part of the care is being provided in an ASC, certification of ASC is mandatory. Even if there is not a requirement for the certification of an OEC it may be desirable to do so, as the certification process ensures a safe environment. It requires the center to have policies and procedures that are followed. It ensures proper credentialing, radiation safety, and maintenance of quality. It may also help improve and maintain high patient satisfaction. Registries, containing care outcomes, are offered by various organizations that can be used to compare data with other local and regional centers. Participation in a qualified registry (Chapter 19) further ensures high quality.

PATIENT ENCOUNTERS

Patients should have easy access to the LPC. Patients may be referred through several means, and there should be a common flow of patients through the system as seen in Fig. 28.2. Some general principles apply. Patients with limb-threatening ischemia should be seen within 48–72 h. Patient with infected ulcers should be seen within 24 h. If the patient presents on a weekend, initial treatment may be in the hospital. The revascularization if required should be done as soon as possible depending on the degree of ischemia. Some patients may need revascularization within 24–48 h after presentation. Patients with acute ischemia may be preferentially treated in the hospital. If some of the services are geographically not at the same site as the LPC, the center should arrange for timely appointments. Some specialists may see patients in a weekly satellite clinic at the center so that the patient can possibly be seen at the same location on a weekly basis.

MEDICAL DIRECTOR

The LPC should have a medical director (MD) who works with the clinical director for smooth running of the center. The MD is responsible for the quality of the medical care provided at the center. The MD should work with clinical director in developing policies and procedures related to medical care and make sure they are followed. The MD should review the qualifications of all employees providing direct medical care, be responsible for any patient-related issues and strive to achieve the highest quality at the center. The MD should work with other specialists providing service either at the center or from their respective offices to create a smooth seamless care structure for the patient. Finally, the MD should encourage research at the center and help with marketing.

MARKETING AND COMMUNITY OUTREACH

Marketing the OEC is described in detail in Chapter 20. Specific to LPC the marketing campaign should emphasize the comprehensive nature of the program.

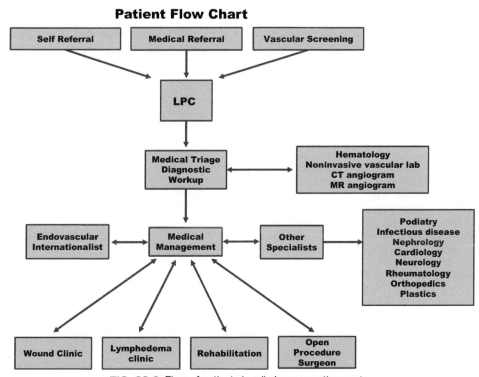

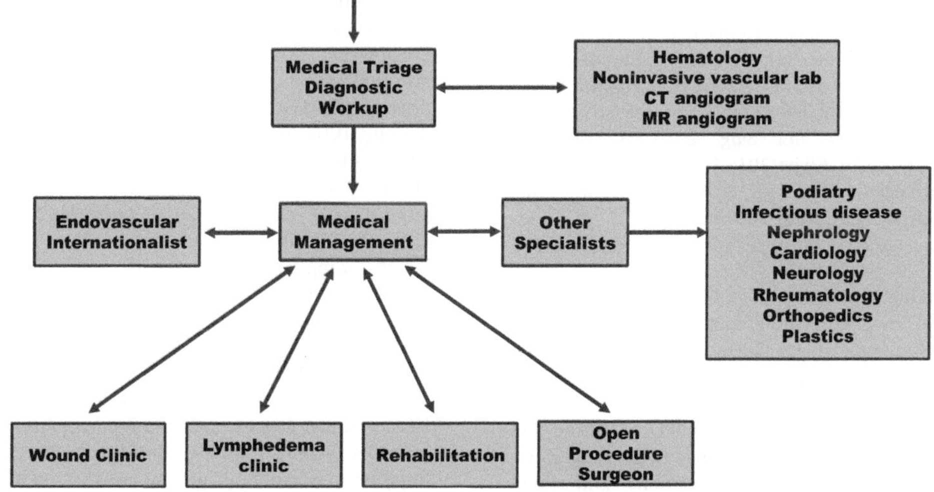

FIG. 28.2 Flow of patients in a limb preservation center.

The marketing effort should be directed toward preventive care as well as the therapeutic aspects of the center. Ease of scheduling appointments with various specialists should be emphasized. The providers within the LPC should seek opportunities to participate in community activities to increase patient awareness. This can be done by participating in health fairs, vascular screening sessions, and other community outlets, using print, audio visual, and digital media.

REFERENCES

1. Ziegler-Graham K, MacKenzie EJ, Ephraim PL, Travison TG, Brookmeyer R. Estimating the prevalence of limb loss in the United States: 2005 to 2050. *Arch Phys Med Rehabil.* 2008. https://doi.org/10.1016/j.apmr.2007.11.005.
2. Owings MF, Kozak LJ. Ambulatory and inpatient procedures in the United States, 1996. *Vital Health Stat.* 1998;13.
3. Healthcare cost and utilization project (HCUP), Nationwide inpatient sample (NIS). *Agency Healthc Res Qual;* 2018. www.hcup-us.ahrq.gov/db/nation/nis/nisdbdocumentation.jsp.%0A.
4. CA Fisher ES, Goodman DC. *Disparities in Health and Health Care Among Medicare Beneficiaries: A Brief Report of the Dartmouth Atlas Project.* 2008.
5. Picture of America: Prevention. https://www.cdc.gov/pictureofamerica/index.html.
6. Ho M, Marger M, Beart J, Yip I, Shekelle P. Is the quality of diabetes care better in a diabetes clinic or in a general medicine clinic? *Diabetes Care.* 1997;20(4):472–475. https://doi.org/10.2337/DIACARE.20.4.472.
7. Armstrong EJ, Wu J, Singh G, Chen D, Amsterdam E, Laird J. Association OF smoking cessation with decreased mortality and improved amputation-free survival among patients with peripheral arterial disease. *J Am Coll Cardiol.* 2014;63(12):A1361. https://doi.org/10.1016/S0735-1097(14)61361-9.
8. Hingorani A, LaMuraglia GM, Henke P, et al. The management of diabetic foot: a clinical practice guideline by the society for vascular surgery in collaboration with the American podiatric medical association and the society for vascular medicine. *J Vasc Surg.* 2016;63(2):3S–21S. https://doi.org/10.1016/j.jvs.2015.10.003.
9. Kim PJ, Attinger CE, Evans KK, Steinberg JS. Role of the podiatrist in diabetic limb salvage. *J Vasc Surg.* 2012; 56(4):1168–1172. https://doi.org/10.1016/j.jvs.2012.06.091.
10. Sloan FA, Feinglos MN, Grossman DS. Receipt of care and reduction of lower extremity amputations in a nationally representative sample of U.S. Elderly. *Health Serv Res.* 2010; 45(6p1):1740–1762. https://doi.org/10.1111/j.1475-6773.2010.01157.x.
11. Brennan MB, Allen GO, Ferguson PD, McBride JA, Crnich CJ, Smith MA. The association between geographic density of infectious disease physicians and limb preservation in patients with diabetic foot ulcers. *Open Forum Infect Dis.* 2017;4(1). https://doi.org/10.1093/ofid/ofx015.
12. Gilhotra RA, Rodrigues BT, Vangaveti VN, Malabu UH. Prevalence and risk factors of lower limb amputation in patients with end-stage renal failure on dialysis: a systematic review. *Int J Nephrol.* 2016;2016:1–7. https://doi.org/10.1155/2016/4870749.
13. Garimella PS, Hirsch AT. Peripheral artery disease and chronic kidney disease: clinical synergy to improve outcomes. *Adv Chronic Kidney Dis.* 2014;21(6):460–471. https://doi.org/10.1053/j.ackd.2014.07.005.
14. Moyer V. Screening for peripheral artery disease and cardiovascular disease risk assessment with the ankle–brachial Index in adults: U.S. Preventive services task force recommendation statement. *Ann Intern Med.* 2013;159(5): 342–348.
15. Fakhry F, van de Luijtgaarden KM, Bax L, et al. Supervised walking therapy in patients with intermittent claudication. *J Vasc Surg.* 2012;56(4):1132–1142. https://doi.org/10.1016/j.jvs.2012.04.046.
16. Murphy TP, Cutlip DE, Regensteiner JG, et al. Supervised exercise, stent revascularization, or medical therapy for claudication due to aortoiliac peripheral artery disease. *J Am Coll Cardiol.* 2015;65(10):999–1009. https://doi.org/10.1016/j.jacc.2014.12.043.
17. Lauret GJ, Fakhry F, Fokkenrood HJ, Hunink MGM, Teijink JA, Spronk S. Modes of exercise training for intermittent claudication. *Cochrane Database Syst Rev.* 2014;7: CD009638. https://doi.org/10.1002/14651858.CD009638.pub2.
18. Golledge J, Singh TP, Alahakoon C, et al. Meta-analysis of clinical trials examining the benefit of structured home exercise in patients with peripheral artery disease. *Br J Surg.* 2019;106(4):319–331. https://doi.org/10.1002/bjs.11101.
19. Nosova EV, Conte MS, Grenon SM. Advancing beyond the "heart-healthy diet" for peripheral arterial disease. *J Vasc Surg.* 2015;61(1):265–274. https://doi.org/10.1016/j.jvs.2014.10.022.
20. Brostow DP, Hirsch AT, Collins TC, Kurzer MS. The role of nutrition and body composition in peripheral arterial disease. *Nat Rev Cardiol.* 2012;9(11):634–643. https://doi.org/10.1038/nrcardio.2012.117.
21. Jain K, Munn J, Rummel MC, Johnston D, Longton C. Office-based endovascular suite is safe for most procedures. *J Vasc Surg.* 2014. https://doi.org/10.1016/j.jvs.2013.07.008.
22. Lin PH, Yang K-H, Kollmeyer KR, et al. Treatment outcomes and lessons learned from 5134 cases of outpatient office-based endovascular procedures in a vascular surgical practice. *Vascular.* 2017;25(2):115–122. https://doi.org/10.1177/1708538116657506.
23. Mesbah Oskui P, Kloner RA, Burstein S, et al. The safety and efficacy of peripheral vascular procedures performed in the outpatient setting. *J Invasive Cardiol.* 2015;27(5):243–249. http://www.ncbi.nlm.nih.gov/pubmed/25929301.

CHAPTER 29

Management of Superficial Venous Disease (Venous Center)

EDWARD G. MACKAY, MD

SUPERFICIAL VENOUS DISEASE

A large number of patients with arterial and venous diseases are asymptomatic. For example, 50% of patients with arterial occlusive disease are totally asymptomatic.[1] Patients with superficial venous diseases are, by and large, no exception. Although 80% of the US population is afflicted by some form of venous disease, most of it is simply of cosmetic concern caused by superficial telangiectasia, popularly known as spider veins. Though the spectrum of venous disease is broad, deep vein thrombosis (DVT), and venous ulcerations receive the most attention. The annual cost of treating venous ulcers to the US healthcare system is estimated to be at $2.5–3.5 billion.[2]

The deep venous circulatory system usually runs parallel to the arterial system. In the infrainguinal region, smaller superficial veins terminate into the small and great saphenous veins. The small saphenous vein drains into the popliteal, and the great saphenous vein drains into the common femoral vein, which is part of the deep venous system. Blood flows cephalad into the iliac veins, to the vena cava, toward the right atrium of the heart. The blood in the veins moves cephalad as a result of contraction of the lower extremity skeletal muscles, while intravenous valves prevent the blood from flowing caudally. The saphenous veins communicate with the deep veins through saphenofemoral or saphenopopliteal junctions and multiple perforator veins. Perforator veins are defined as veins that communicate between superficial and deep veins by "perforating" the deep fascia. Tributaries drain into the saphenous system or directly into the deep system through perforators as well.

Failure of the valves in the superficial veins results in increased pressure in the veins causing vein dilatation and elongation. Pressure is highest when failure occurs at a saphenofemoral or saphenopopliteal junction. Venous reflux can also occur as a result of deep vein obstruction (Chapter 30). As pressure increases, this leads to changes in vein wall and microcirculation, including the activation of matrix metalloproteinases, leukocyte infiltration, and endothelial activation. Clinically, this manifests itself as inflammation and edema.

PATIENT PRESENTATION

Patients arrive at vein centers with various symptoms. These can range from simple cosmetic concerns to venous ulceration. Patients quite often present with the complaint that they do not like the looks of their legs because of prominent veins. The treatment of these veins for cosmetic reasons should be considered. Treatment of varicose veins for cosmetic reasons will not be covered by most insurances, so an approach that considers each patient's finances should be taken.[2]

The presenting symptoms can be extremely vague. A thorough medical history and physical exam can help diagnose the problem. For example, if varicose veins are the cause of symptoms, then standing or sitting should worsen symptoms—and leg elevation should alleviate them. During physical exam if the veins are found to be on medial aspect and the symptoms are on the lateral aspect of the leg, the veins could not be the cause of the symptoms. Some symptoms, like bleeding and superficial thrombophlebitis, can be dramatic. Anyone will be alarmed when blood shoots out of the leg. Venous pressure at the ankle level may reach or surpass 150 mmHg. Elevating the leg above the heart and compression will stop the bleeding quickly and effectively, but panic ensues, and patients

Office-Based Endovascular Centers. https://doi.org/10.1016/B978-0-323-67969-5.00029-0
Copyright © 2020 Elsevier Inc. All rights reserved.

end up in the emergency room. Patient may present with thrombosis in the varicosities resulting in the diagnosis of superficial venous thrombosis (SVT). This can be very painful. These episodes are usually treated with compression stockings, heat, antiinflammatory drugs, and if the SVT is significant, anticoagulation may be required.

Patient may present with "skin changes' a phrase that is broadly used and describes various symptoms, such as redness, discoloration, scarring, and ulceration. History of deep venous thrombosis would suggest venous origin of the symptoms. As a rule of thumb, after taking the history and conducting a physical exam the diagnosis may be made in most cases. Physical examination should be comprehensive including the examination of arterial system.

PREOPERATIVE EVALUATION

The essential preoperative evaluation for superficial venous procedures consists of the duplex ultrasound (DU) evaluation with color flow and mapping of the veins. "The goal of the preoperative evaluation is to identify modifiable risk factors, coordinate a treatment plan with other members of the perioperative care team, and optimize the patient's medical condition to shift the balance of risk/benefit ratio before proceeding with non-emergent surgery."[3] If use of conscious sedation is planned, the risk of anesthesia should be evaluated (Chapter 12).

The DU exam is divided in two parts. The evaluation for occlusion is generally done with the patient in supine position to facilitate compression of the veins. The entire deep and superficial system is scanned. Augmentation with color flow is done to assess complete filling of the vessel with color and generally done in the longitudinal view. The description of all segments should be described in detail: findings of partial compression, noncompressible segment, echogenicity, wall thickening, dilatation, and/or contraction should be documented.

The second portion of the examination is performed to assess venous valvular insufficiency. DU is currently the most inexpensive and effective diagnostic tool to diagnose venous incompetence. "With the patient standing, the saphenofemoral junction (SFJ), common femoral vein (CFV), and the origin of both femoral veins are identified, and manual compression of the calf or thigh is performed to assess reflux."[4] The IAC (Intersocietal Accreditation commission) defines significant reflux in the deep veins for >1 s, in the superficial veins >500 ms, and in the perforators >350 ms. Many insurance companies look at these values to authorize treatment for venous insufficiency.

Beyond ultrasound examination very little other testing is routinely required.

PRE- AND POSTOPERATIVE SCORING

"Preoperative evaluation and risk stratification in surgery patients, and especially vascular surgery patients, should be performed by all practicing surgeons."[5] In order to follow the results of treatment, classification and scoring methods have been developed to quantify the results of treatment. The CEAP classification is the most well-known system for evaluating the venous system.

In CEAP classification, C stands for clinical stage and the range is 0–6. E stands for etiology, A for anatomy, and P for pathophysiology.

C0 No disease
C1 Telangiectasia
C2 Presence of varicose veins
C3 Venous edema
C4 Skin changes
C4a Only inflammation or pigmentation
C4b Lipodermatosclerosis or atrophie blanche present
C5 Healed venous ulcers
C6 Active ulcers

An "a" or "s" can be added if the patient is asymptomatic or symptomatic, respectively, for example, a patient with asymptomatic spider veins would be a C1a.

The E stands for etiology and is given the nomenclature of congenital (c), primary (p), or secondary (s). A stands for anatomy: superficial (s), deep (d), perforator (p). Finally, P stands for pathophysiology: obstruction (o), or reflux (r). For example, a patient with painful varicose veins of the saphenous vein and no deep vein or perforator pathology would be a C2sEpAsPr.

Vein clinical severity score (VCSS) is another effective assessment primarily based on symptoms. This test scores 10 different attributes at a scale of 0–3 for venous disease. For example, while quantifying pain, score of (0) indicates no pain, (1) occasional, (2) daily, (3) severe or daily needing medications. Next measure is the presence of varicose veins with 0 (none) to 3 (extensive). Other factors include presence of edema, pigmentation, inflammation, and induration. For ulcers, score is given for the number, size, and duration. Finally, a score is given for the use of compression.

Using the VCSS is advantageous when following a patient for improvement. For example, using the C in the CEAP system may indicate only mild improvement when an ulcer is healed going form a C6s to C5a. The

VCSS score accounts for improvement in pain, inflammation, induration, and edema, thus it would show potentially a significant clinical improvement, which would more accurately portray the effectiveness of treatment.

The Aberdeen Varicose Vein Questionnaire (AVVQ) is a quality-of-life (QOL) measure that is commonly used for studies and determines the effectiveness of varicose vein treatments.

This questionnaire measures the direct effects of varicose vein treatment, the psychological impact, appearance, and the impact on work and pleasure.

AXIAL VEIN TREATMENT

Prior to any invasive treatment, it is mandatory that medical treatment be used to alleviate symptoms of venous disease. This treatment includes reduction of body weight if the patient is obese, use of compression stockings while awake and elevation of legs during sleep. If there is a venous ulcer it should be treated with Unna boot or compression dressings. The medical treatment should be tried at least for 3 months before considering invasive therapy. Invasive treatment may be required sooner if the ulcer is not healing. Percutaneous procedures can be carried out if patient is on anticoagulation without interrupting the anticoagulants. Axial vein treatment begins with mapping of the vein to be treated prior to the procedure. This is also the opportunity for "time out." Make sure you have the right patient, the right ultrasound map, and the correct leg. Draw the intended vein to be treated on the skin using ultrasound imaging and a marker. For the GSV and ASSV treatment, the patient is generally supine with the leg slightly externally rotated and for treating the SSV generally in prone position. The leg is then prepped and draped, and access into the axial vein is achieved using small amount of local anesthesia and a micropuncture needle using ultrasound guidance. Now we will discuss the treatments offered by different modalities.

Thermal Treatment

Thermal treatment uses one of the two different heat sources available: laser and radio frequency. For any type of heat treatment, tumescent local anesthesia is required. There are several formulations used for fluid used for tumescence. The most common solution contains 1% lidocaine with or without epinephrine (1: 100,00) in 500 cc of saline. Usually epinephrine is recommended as it slows the absorption of lidocaine and thus increases the safety margin. Some patients do not tolerate the epinephrine well, in which case it should not be used. Buffering the solution with sodium bicarbonate is recommended as it has been shown to reduce the discomfort caused by the solution.[6] Very superficial veins should not be treated using thermal treatment. A general rule is to have at least 1 cm of distance between the skin and the vein. Thermal treatment using laser energy is called "endovenous laser ablation." The laser fiber may be positioned in the axial vein using micropuncture and a short sheath, or a fiber placed through the introducer catheter. This is sometimes necessary if the fiber will not travel through the axial vein due to tortuosity, tributaries, or valve leaflets obstructing its path. The tip of the fiber is then placed approximately 2 cm from the source of the reflux (usually the saphenofemoral or saphenopopliteal junction). It may be placed caudal to the epigastric vein to allow flow through the junction and prevent thrombus extension (see complications). Previously prepared solution is infiltrated along the vein under ultrasound guidance for tumescent anesthesia. A pump can be used for infiltration. Pump is recommended if several procedures are going to be carried out on the same day to prevent hand fatigue of the operator. Infiltration of fluid produces local anesthesia, compresses the vein around the fiber to increase the surface area being heated, and shields any surrounding tissue from damage. Once the fiber is positioned and tumescent is adequate, the fiber is attached to the laser generator. Laser generator settings vary, but the usual energy delivery consists of delivery of continuous 7–12 Watts with a pullback of 1–2 cm/10 s resulting in a linear endovenous energy delivery of 60–100 j/cm. The literature suggests a higher percentage of vein ablation and more pain with delivery of higher energy, while lower energy delivery results in lower percentage of ablation rates and less pain.[7] Once the vein has been ablated, the laser energy is turned off, catheters and fiber are removed. Color duplex ultrasound can then be performed to make sure no thrombus has formed at the junction. A small bandage is placed at the puncture site and a compression stocking is placed on the treated leg.

There are decisions that must be made before performing endovenous laser ablation regarding laser equipment to be used. Multiple generators exist on the market, that produce laser in different wavelengths measured in nanometers. Various available wavelengths are 810, 940, 980, 1064, 1319, 1320, and 1470. The most popular wavelengths being used are 1319 and 1470 nm. The literature suggests that the use of longer

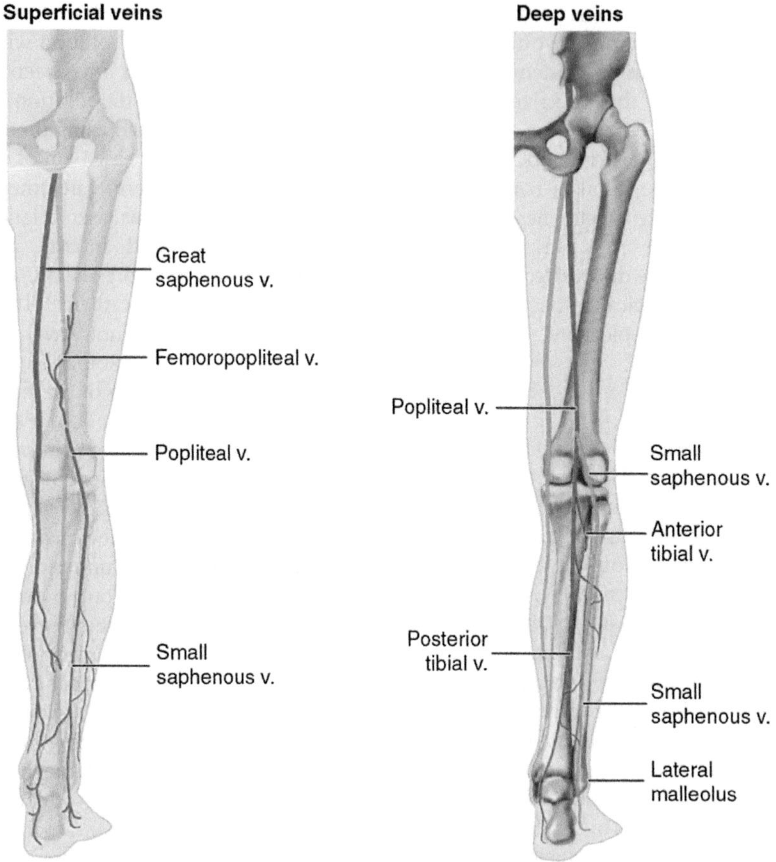

wavelengths results in less pain and bruising. The three basic types of fibers are the bare tip, the jacketed tip, and the radial fiber. There is some evidence that suggests that the bare tip fibers reduce pain and bruising after the procedure.[8] The overall ablation rates between different lasers and different fibers do not seem to be significantly different from each other.

Thermal ablation by radiofrequency (RF) energy uses a catheter with a coil at the end. This procedure is almost identical to endovenous laser ablation. Once access is obtained with an introducer catheter, the RF catheter is placed through the introducer catheter where the tip is placed approximately 3 cm from the SFJ or SPJ. Fluid for tumescent anesthesia is infiltrated around the axial vein being treated using ultrasound guidance.

The generator shows temperature, watts, time, and cycles and is attached to the RF catheter via a cable. There is a button on the catheter that activates the generator, and heat is directed to the coil at the end of the catheter. The generator brings the temperature to a preset level (usually 120°F) and the wattage required to maintain that temperature. If the catheter fails to reach the temperature, an alarm sounds and the generator shuts down. It is generally recommended that two cycles be run at the junction. This is repeated until the desired length of axial vein has been treated. It is important not to pull the RF catheter into the introducer catheter to prevent catheter from burning. Also note that the RF catheter can cause skin burns if too close to the skin. Once the catheter is removed, a bandage is applied along with a compression hose.

There are only two RF devices available. The first is Medtronic's Venefit system. RF catheters are available in 3 cm treatment length and 7 cm treatment length. This system requires a 7 French introducer sheath to gain access. The second choice is the Venclose (Venclose Inc, San Jose, CA) system. This system has one catheter providing 10 cm treatment length. It is possible to change 10 cm length to 2.5 cm at the tip of the catheter with the touch of a button. This system requires a 6 French sheath to gain access.

NONTUMESCENT AXIAL VEIN TREATMENT

Mechanical chemical ablation is performed using the Clarivein (Merit Medical, South Jordan, UT) catheter which is inserted through a 4 French introducer sheath and placed below the SFJ or SPJ. The mechanical portion of this device is attached to the catheter where a small, postlike angled wire projects outward. At the end of this wire there is a small bead which has great visibility on ultrasound. The bead is placed approximately 2 cm from the junction. A 10-cc syringe with 1.5% sodium tetradecyl sulfate (STS) is placed in the device with a one-way valve to deliver STS at the tip of the catheter. The procedure commences by pulling the trigger on the device, causing the wire to spin to cause damage to the intimal layer of the vein. After approximately 2–3 s, STS injection is commenced while simultaneously pulling the device back. Infusion rate of approximately 0.5–1 cc/10 s is used while the pullback rate is kept at 1–2 cm/10 s. It is important to release the trigger and stop the wire rotation as well as the infusion before the catheter comes out of the vein, approximately 5 cm from the tip. This is marked on the catheter with a white line. The catheter can then be removed, and the puncture site bandaged, and a compression hose is placed on the treated leg.

This is a totally self-contained system. There are no generators to purchase. The only variable is the choice of sclerosants and which micropuncture kit to use. The initial studies have been performed using 1.5% STS, but if there is contraindication to the use of STS, Polidocanol (PDL) could be considered. Note that STS is the only FDA-approved sclerosant for the treatment of varicose veins, whereas PDL has FDA approval for treating small veins < 3 mm in size.

Cyanoacrylate venous occlusion (VenaSeal) uses a proprietary formula of cyanoacrylate which glues the axial vein shut. The VenaSeal kit includes a 0.035 wire, a 7 French introducer catheter, a special proprietary catheter for glue delivery, the cyanoacrylate glue, 3 cc syringe with blunt needles for drawing up the glue, and a gun for the syringe. After entering the vein with a micropuncture needle, the 0.035 guidewire is passed in the axial vein. The introducer sheath then goes over the 0.035 wire and is placed near the junction. The wire and dilator are then withdrawn from the axial vein. Next, the glue gun and its 3 cc syringe are attached to the glue catheter and primed. The glue catheter is then guided all the way through the introducer sheath. Once at the end of the introducer sheath, the glue catheter is unsheathed. The tip of the glue catheter has six hyper echoic beads that make the sheath tip very visible on ultrasound. The tip should be placed 5 cm from the junction. Once there, a trigger pull lasting 3 seconds releases one aliquot of glue. The first glue placement is one aliquot with a pullback of 1 cm, followed by a second aliquot with a 3 cm pullback. This is all done under slight compression, and the glue can set for 3 mins. After the glue sets, another aliquot is placed in the vein, catheter gets pulled back another 3 cm and compressed for 30 s after that. This is repeated until the end of the introducer catheter is reached. Following that the catheters are removed. It is important to pull the catheter immediately after placing the aliquot to keep the catheter from sticking to the vein. Bandages are placed at the puncture site. This too is a totally self-contained system. In addition to the VenaSeal kit, only a micropuncture kit is required.

Polidocanol endovenous microfoam (PEM) (Varithena) is a proprietary foam sclerosant consisting of aqueous Polidocanol solution (1%) and other chemicals, which is FDA approved for the treatment of incompetent axial veins and their tributaries. This can be injected through a catheter, angiocath, or needle.

Oxygen is used to mix with the Polidocanol to create foam in a canister. The final gas mixture consists of oxygen and carbon dioxide in a ratio of 65:35 and < 0.8% nitrogen content. Density and bubble size of the foam is controlled. The foam containing Polidocanol is then transferred to a syringe using the Varithena transfer unit.

After the axial vein is accessed, the foam is drawn up into the syringe and injected into the axial vein. The foam can be followed using ultrasound up to the junction where light pressure is applied to compress the axial vein without compressing the deep vein to prevent injection in the deep vein. Injection may be continued while holding compression to fill the vein distal to the access point. Axial vein may be accessed in other segments for injection and tributaries can also be injected. A maximum of 15cc of PEM can be used at one time. A compression bandage is provided with the canister and is applied after the injection. This includes rolls that are placed over the treated veins to provide eccentric compression. A compression stocking is then placed over the bandage. This is left in place for 48 h, at which point patients should wear compression stocking for 2 weeks. The canister, syringes, and bandages are part of the kit bought from Varithena, and the only additional supplies needed are the vein access kit.

PERFORATOR VEIN TREATMENT

As mentioned earlier, perforator veins are another connection between the deep and superficial veins. Incompetent valves result in flow of blood from the higher presser deep system to the low-pressure superficial system. This causes the superficial system to become dilated and elongated, leading to venous insufficiency. Similar to the axial system we can divide treatment into thermal and nonthermal.

Thermal treatment uses the same technology as discussed above. Laser can be used to treat perforators. This is done with a micropuncture catheter that is placed over a wire into the perforator vein, and a laser fiber placed through the catheter. Tumescent anesthesia is then applied around the perforator vein. The catheter is pulled back exposing the fiber, at which point the fiber is attached to the generator. Energy is applied to the perforator vein with similar settings as for the axial vein. The fiber is pulled back until out of the vein or near the skin. Since RF catheters are relatively long to treat perforators, they can cause burning near the skin, and to prevent it a new RF device have been developed. The RFS (Medtronic, Dublin, Ireland) device is the only FDA-approved device for perforators. It has a very short treatment tip on the end of a stiff 10 cm catheter. Generally, the treatment starts after appropriate marking, prepping, and draping; use of local anesthesia; and accessing the perforator using a micropuncture needle. The wire is passed through the needle. Sometimes the stiff end is used. The RFS catheter goes over the wire, and the tip is placed in the perforator vein just below the fascia. The needle and wire are removed and tumescent applied around the perforator vein again to provide anesthesia, compress the vein, and protect surrounding tissue. Heat is applied for 1 min to each quadrant of the vein. Then the catheter is repositioned in 1 cm increments repeating the treatment in each quadrant for 1 min. Once the catheter is out of the vein or close to the skin it is removed. A bandage is then applied.

As for nonthermal treatment of perforators, ligation and sclerotherapy are the long-standing techniques. Ligation requires marking the perforator vein where it enters the fascia. After appropriate prepping and draping and use of local anesthesia, an incision is made over the perforating vein where it enters the deep fascia. The vein is divided between ligatures and the wound closed. It is easy to ligate a superficial perforating vein. Deeper veins are more amenable to the thermal methods, while a superficial vein might be too close to the skin for the thermal method that may cause a skin burn.

Sclerotherapy is another option for perforator veins. The decision to use sclerotherapy will also depend on the anatomy. Large perforators may not close, and short perforators that enter the deep venous system just after penetrating the fascia may carry too high a risk for DVT. The vein is injected under ultrasound guidance using a fine needle or butterfly needle. The vein should be accessed 3–4 cm from the perforator. Injected foam should be followed until the sclerosant enters the perforator and then stopped. Sclerosants in use today are STS that is foamed with air or CO_2 using the Tessari method. This is referred to as physician compounded foam. The other option is the use of PEM.

SURFACE VEIN TREATMENTS

There are two main options for the treatment of the surface varicosities—sclerotherapy and phlebectomy. Thermal methods are not an option due to the possibility of skin burns, and glue has not been used due to its tendency to leave a palpable cord under the skin. Sclerotherapy uses a sclerosant chemical to damage vein wall. There are currently two FDA-approved sclerosant on the market for the treatment of varicose veins named sodium tetradecyl sulfate (STS) and Polidocanol. Although Polidocanol is FDA approved for small veins, it is rarely used for large veins unless there is contraindication to the use of STS. Sclerosants can be injected as liquids, but usually foam is created using the Tessari method. Foaming the sclerosant provides a couple of benefits. It increases the echogenicity of sclerosant making the vein much more visible on ultrasound. Another advantage is the larger displacement of sclerosant that increases adherence to the vein walls. Injection of the sclerosant produces vasospasm. There are different postoperative protocols for different sclerosants. The PEM protocol recommends 48 h of continuous eccentric compression followed by 2 weeks of continued day time use of compression stockings. Generally, once the entire varicosity is treated, eccentric compression is applied over the varicosity followed by compression stockings. The required duration of compression can vary widely from 24 h to 6 weeks.

The other choice for treating surface veins is phlebectomy. This procedure begins with marking of the surface veins. This is done with the patient standing to make varicosities bulge conspicuously, while a marking pen is used to mark the veins to be removed. After appropriate prepping and draping, the skin over the varicosities can be anesthetized with 0.1% xylocaine with or without epinephrine. An incision about 2–3 mm in size is made over the marked varicosity with any number of instruments such as a #11 blade or 16–18 gauge needles. Using one of the many phlebectomy hooks available, the vein is then grasped with hemostats eased through the incision by tugging back and forth and removed. Sometimes only small portion of the vein is removed. This is continued until all marked varicosities are removed. Incisions may then be closed with steri strips or left open. If the procedure is combined with axis vein treatment using tumescent anesthesia, a bulky compressive dressing is applied as there is usually a fair amount of drainage because of the large volume of fluid used for tumescent anesthesia during thermal ablation of the axis vein. If the procedure is performed as a stand-alone procedure, it can be done using local or tumescent anesthesia.

Equipment needed for phlebectomy includes, knife blades, hypodermic needles, phlebectomy hooks, and hemostats. Occasionally instruments may be needed to close an incision subcutaneously.

COMPLICATIONS

After the procedure, patient should be educated to expect certain things. Bruising should be expected and can vary a great deal depending on the procedure. Post-procedural compression may help minimize the bruising as well as use of ice packs for the first 24 h. Occasionally, there is inflammation along the treated segment of vein, or a tributary of a vein because of superficial thrombophlebitis cussed by the thrombus created by the procedure. This is treated with antiinflammatory medication, heat, and compression. If a large vein is thrombosed and there is trapped blood it can be drained with 18-gauge needle under local anesthesia. Postprocedural pain is usually managed by using antiinflammatory medications.

DVT is a major concern after any venous intervention, in particular when axial veins or perforating veins are treated because of direct communication between superficial and deep venous system. Endovenous heat-induced thrombosis (EHIT) is caused by the use of thermal treatment of veins. The incidence is low. Careful surveillance postprocedure with duplex exam is routinely performed. The timing of developing EHIT is variable. It can occur between 48 h and 4 weeks post-procedure. Small extension of thrombus into the deep vein with minimal to no obstruction may be observed, but extension that causes significant obstruction should be treated with anticoagulation.

Thermal treatments have the potential to injure sensory nerves that are in close proximity to the vein. In particular, the sural nerve near the small saphenous vein and the saphenous nerve in the distal leg near the great saphenous vein are particularly at risk of injury. Moreover, the peroneal nerve where it wraps around the fibular head has been known to be injured from tight compression leading to foot drop.

Intra-arterial injection is a particularly disastrous complication that can occur during sclerotherapy. This should be avoided by careful placement of the needle, removal of the syringe so that any pulsatile flow will be obvious, and careful knowledge of the anatomy.

Treatment of superficial venous disease is almost always performed on an outpatient basis. It can be provided in an OEC with minimal complications and very high patient satisfaction at a very reasonable cost. Appropriate training and attention to detail is mandatory for optimal patient outcomes.

REFERENCES

1. Casserly IP, Sachar R, Yadav JS. *Manual of Peripheral Vascular Intervention*. Philadelphia: Lippincott Williams & Wilkins; 2005.
2. Sen CK, Gordillo GM, Roy S, et al. Human skin wounds: a major and snowballing threat to public health and the economy. *Wound Repair Regen*. 2009;17(6):763–771. https://doi.org/10.1111/j.1524-475x.2009. 00543.x.
3. Manley A, Reck SE. Patients with vascular disease. *Med Clin N Am*. 2013;97(6):1077–1093. https://doi.org/10.1016/j.mcna.2013.05.008.
4. Labropoulos N, Leon LR. Duplex evaluation of venous insufficiency. *Semin Vasc Surg*. 2005;18(1):5–9. https://doi.org/10.1053/j.semvascsurg.2004.12.002.
5. Zarinsefat A, Henke P. Update in preoperative risk assessment in vascular surgery patients. *J Vasc Surg*. 2015;62(2): 499–509. https://doi.org/10.1016/j.jvs.2015.05.031.
6. Matsumoto AH, Reifsnyder AC, Hartwell GD, Angle JF, Selby JB, Tegtmeyer CJ. Reducing the discomfort of lidocaine administration through pH buffering. *J Vasc Interv Radiol*. 1994;5(1):171–175. https://doi.org/10.1016/s1051-0443(94)71478-0.
7. Whiddon LL. Advances in the treatment of superficial venous insufficiency of the lower extremities. In: *Baylor University Medical Center Proceedings*. 20 (2). 2007:136–139. https://doi.org/10.1080/08998280.2007.11928269.
8. Kabnick LS. Varicose veins. *Rutherfords Vasc Surg*. 2010: 871–888. https://doi.org/10.1016/b978-1-4160-5223-4.00056-1.

CHAPTER 30

Management of Deep Venous Diseases

JOSE I. ALMEIDA, MD, FACS, RPVI, RVT

Hospitals possess the complex infrastructure and teams of people necessary to take care of patients with acute life-threatening vascular disorders. However, for the treatment of patients with chronic vascular conditions, hospital care is bloated and expensive. Catheter-based platforms for vascular interventions have created an opportunity for physicians to open comprehensive outpatient vascular centers. The office-based endovascular center (OEC) offers a lower cost alternative for the delivery of streamlined outpatient vascular care. About 20 years ago, we began performing superficial venous procedures in the office using tumescent local anesthesia; shortly thereafter, we implemented a full OEC to enable the treatment of deep venous diseases.

OECs are limited in their scope of service but are easier and less expensive to open and operate than a hospital or ambulatory surgery center. Patients with venous conditions present with a broad range of disease severity including spider telangiectasia, varicose veins, edema, lipodermatosclerosis, and venous ulcers. The procedures to treat these conditions vary from small injections to more complex venous reconstructions. With the exception of extensive postthrombotic central venous occlusions, and venous malignancy, most venous disorders can be safely treated in the OEC. The treatment of acute deep vein thrombosis has a narrower role in the OEC setting, mostly because of safety concerns.

While studies have shown that clinical safety and treatment efficacy can be achieved in OECs, critics have raised various concerns due to inconsistent patient care standards and lack of organizational oversight to ensure optimal patient outcome. Lacking in the ambulatory space are evidence-based practices, appropriate use criteria, and vascular societal oversight. Elsewhere in this textbook, strategies to improve patient care delivery in OECs including accreditations and external validation of processes to ensure patient care and safety are discussed in detail.

It is critical to recognize that venous OECs function as small businesses that require financial investment for initiation and maintenance. Capital expenditure is required, the extent of which depends on the breadth of the practice. For example, a comprehensive venous practice might acquire a duplex ultrasound (DU); laser and radiofrequency devices for truncal vein ablation; medications such as local anesthetics, intravenous sedatives, and sclerosants; and, other imaging equipment such as portable C-ARM fluoroscopy and intravascular ultrasound (IVUS). Cost-benefit analyses are critical prior to consideration of adding on new services. Some interventions require the purchase of a generator, and additional disposable catheters per procedure. Other procedures require only disposable equipment. Yet others may require initial purchase of surgical instruments which can be reused extensively after autoclaving. A front and back office must manage operations such as insurance preauthorizations, billing, collections, payroll, IT and a dynamic regulatory environment. Success is inherently dependent on delivering high-quality care and having the business savvy manage the increasing operating expenses in this era of payment reform.

Several factors are causing a shift of care from inpatient to outpatient, including advances in technology and changes in reimbursement rules. One area that can be both challenging and incredibly confusing to keep up with is the changing rules surrounding reimbursement from the Centers for Medicare & Medicaid Services (CMS). Dedicated CPT codes are available for reimbursement and procedures are covered by most payers; although, medical necessity criteria are incongruent between payers. Payment reform has embraced the idea of moving away from fee-for-service because of perceived perverse incentives which encourage increased volume. The shift to accountable payment models is happening slowly. Reducing demand for high-cost services is a key determinant of success under these risk arrangements, which is the opposite incentive from traditional fee-for-service medicine. Going forward, providers must conform to payment models and care models, ideally in a synchronized manner.

Office-Based Endovascular Centers. https://doi.org/10.1016/B978-0-323-67969-5.00030-7
Copyright © 2020 Elsevier Inc. All rights reserved.

Most vendors will offer reduced pricing on generators in exchange for guaranteed minimum purchase volumes on disposable catheters, fibers, and access kits. This, however, can create a perverse situation where OECs are tied to a high target volume of cases and may cause a misalignment of incentives. Spider vein disease is a cosmetic problem and its treatment is not covered by payers; thus, cash revenue from sclerotherapy services can augment medical practice revenue.

Although this chapter focuses on the management of deep venous diseases, the reader should keep in context that most OECs are equipped to handle a wide array of arterial and venous disorders, depending on the interests of the principals. Our practice in Miami focuses exclusively on venous disorders, therefore, our OEC is equipped appropriately for this focus.

SUPERFICIAL VENOUS DISEASE

Superficial venous disease will be addressed in detail in Chapter 29. The two most popular methods of thermal saphenous vein ablation presently in use are radiofrequency (RF) ablation and endovenous laser (EVL) ablation. Both RF and EVL are catheter-based endovascular interventions which use electromagnetic energy to occlude (ablate) the treated vein by heat transfer. Both require a disposable catheter and power source (generator) and can be performed using local tumescent anesthesia with sonographic guidance. For elimination of ropey varicose veins stab phlebectomy can be performed concomitantly. Newer nonthermal ablation therapies are also available for truncal vein ablation. Sclerotherapy involves the injection of a chemical into a vein to achieve endoluminal fibrosis and has been used for almost a century. Sclerotherapy can be used to treat a large range of vein sizes from telangiectasias to large varicose veins. Foam sclerotherapy involves the addition of air to a detergent sclerosing agent by means of agitation to produce tensioactive properties.

DEEP VENOUS DISEASE

Iliac Vein Obstruction

The etiology of venous obstruction can be primary (nonthrombotic) or secondary (postthrombotic), with roughly equal prevalence in patients with chronic venous disease (CVD). Signs and symptoms of chronic venous obstruction can overlap with signs and symptoms of reflux, with some differences. Limb swelling beyond ankle edema is rare with superficial reflux alone. Primary obstruction, often referred to as nonthrombotic iliac vein lesions (NIVLs), usually arises from compression of the left common iliac vein by crossing of the overlying right common iliac artery and may cause more extensive edema, and/or symptoms of venous claudication. Compression at the caval confluence most commonly occurs by the overlying aortic bifurcation, or at the external and internal iliac vein confluence by compression from the bifurcation of external and hypogastric arteries.[1] The common femoral vein (CFV) can be compressed by the inguinal ligament or common femoral artery. Postthrombotic disease can occur anywhere along the length of the femoro-iliocaval outflow tract and the intraluminal changes are readily seen with DU.

While traditional venous corrective surgery concentrated on the correction of superficial and deep venous reflux below the inguinal ligament, the introduction of minimally invasive endovascular venous stenting using venography and IVUS provides the ability to treat the "obstructive" component of the disease above the inguinal ligament. The emphasis on IVUS as the key diagnostic tool was promulgated by Raju and Neglen[2] who have shown that iliac venous stenting alone is sufficient to control symptoms in the majority of patients with combined outflow obstruction and deep reflux.

Endovascular treatment of iliocaval obstruction includes traversing the obstruction with a guide wire (occlusions need to be recanalized), followed by balloon angioplasty and placement of a stent to maintain patency of the obstructed vein segment. Self-expandable stents with a high radial force and sufficient flexibility should be used. Multiple centers report off-label use of braided stents made of elgiloy (cobalt, chromium, and nickel). Recently, several vendors have developed dedicated venous stents of nitinol (nickel and titanium), and FDA approval is expected soon.

Diagnostic testing

The endovenous treatment of iliocaval obstruction in the OBL setting requires adequate space, capital purchase of imaging equipment, and a variety of disposables. IVUS imaging is invaluable for diagnosis and as an intraoperative tool in stent placement. The poor diagnostic sensitivity of venography was well documented by Negus et al.;[3] up to half of significant venous compression cases can be missed if frontal projection venograms alone are relied on for diagnosis. Although anterior-posterior and oblique views may suggest some "pancaking" of the proximal iliac vein, oftentimes, the common iliac vein appears normal. Therefore, IVUS imaging is critical. The IVUS coaxial system allows the operator to examine the target lesion as sound waves are emitted from the catheter tip transducer, usually in the 10–20 MHz range. A real-time ultrasound image of a thin section of the blood vessel is

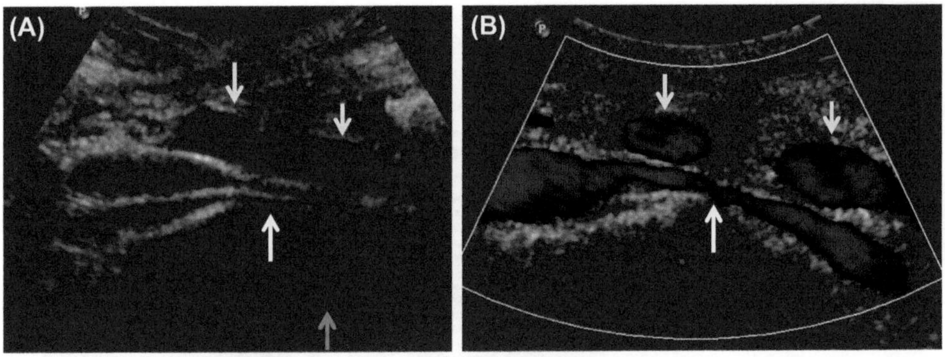

Left common iliac vein compression (white arrows)
Right and Left Iliac Arteries (yellow arrows)
Lumbar vertebrae (blue arrow)

FIG. 30.1 Duplex ultrasound demonstrating compression of the left iliac vein with **(A)** Gray Scale Image With Chroma Tint and **(B)** Power Doppler image.

generated without the use of radiation or nephrotoxic contrast.

During preoperative planning, an imaging study which precisely characterizes the severity of the pathologic lesion(s) is ideal. In the case of iliac vein occlusive disease, this is often not possible. Accurate quantification of a hemodynamically significant venous stenosis using a variety of tests such as velocity measurements,[4,5] waveform contour,[6] venography,[3] hand-foot pressure differential,[1] and plethysmography with limb volume measurements[1] has been challenging because of relatively low diagnostic sensitivity and specificity. DU is the gold standard for the diagnosis of infrainguinal venous disease; however, duplex imaging of the retroperitoneal iliac veins and vena cava has been slow to be adopted. Now equipped with more capacity for deeper depth of penetration and improved image resolution, current DU instruments provide satisfactory iliocaval imaging. The gold standard to determine the threshold for iliocaval stenting relies on IVUS planimetry.[2] Computed tomography and magnetic resonance imaging provide good cross-sectional information but are expensive, operator dependent, and not readily available in the OEC.

Proper use of gray scale, color flow, and pulsed wave Doppler modalities can optimize the evaluation of the femoro-iliocaval outflow tract with DU. Normal venous flow is phasic with respiration and is augmented with distal compression or arrests with the Valsalva maneuver. Asymmetry in flow velocity and waveform patterns at rest and during flow augmentation in the CFVs indicates proximal obstruction. The presence of stenosis is recognized by a narrowed vein diameter, mosaic color pattern that denotes poststenotic turbulence, abnormal Doppler waveform through the area of stenosis, slow flow, and vein dilatation proximal to the stenosis.[4] Additional tools such as Chroma tint, power Doppler, penetration harmonics are useful for image optimization (Fig. 30.1).[7]

Venous diameter can be calculated with the insertion of an IVUS catheter and is the gold standard to determine lesion severity. However, noninvasive DU using gray scale with Chroma tint and optimized harmonic frequency can provide a satisfactory image to measure vein lumen size with ultrasound calipers. The abnormalities seen with color flow and pulsed wave Doppler are useful, but are also limited value for the quantification of lesion severity. Our protocol suggests that a 50% reduction in vein caliber measured with DU calipers (CIV<8 mm, EIV < 7 mm, or CFV < 6 mm) with or without the presence of an abnormality in color flow or Doppler waveforms described herein may give the operator enough information to move directly to IVUS with venography without further testing.[7] Omitting the risks of radiation and/or contrast associated with computed tomographic venography, and the risk of gadolinium deposition disease associated with magnetic resonance venography, is a safer option for patients.

DU, C-ARM fluoroscopy, and IVUS are readily available at the OEC site of service (Fig. 30.2A). Deep venous interventions require a variety of basic disposables which are known to all endovascular specialists (Fig. 30.2B and Table 30.1). Other necessary equipment necessary for patient safety in all medical environments

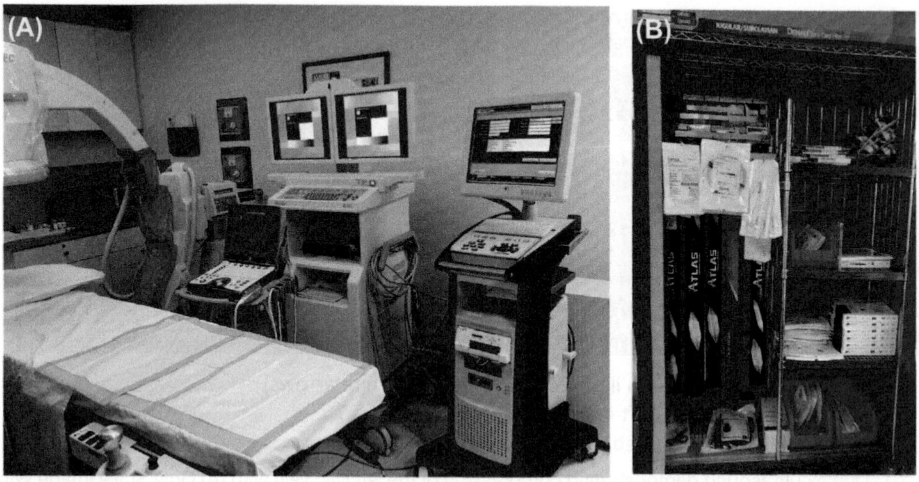

FIG. 30.2 Photographs of Miami Vein angiosuite and catheter cart. **(A)** Office-based lab (OBL) angiosuite with C-ARM fluoroscopy and intravascular ultrasound; **(B)** OBL angiosuite supply cart.

TABLE 30.1
Endovascular Instrumentation Requirements for Iliac Vein Intervention.

4 or 5 FR stiff micropuncture access kit (0.018″ platform)
11F sheath
Nonionic contrast
High-pressure tubing for power injector
0.035″ J-tip of floppy tip guidewire
0.035″ super stiff guidewire
0.035″ angled hydrophilic Glidewire and Glide catheter
6–20 mm noncompliant angioplasty balloons
Balloon insufflators
14–24 mm Wallstents
20–25 mm Z-stents
Imaging
Duplex ultrasound for percutaneous access
Intravascular ultrasound
C-ARM or wall-mounted fluoroscopy for contrast venography

are a full crash cart, emergency medications, supplemental oxygen, etc. All accreditation agencies for OECs have a complete listing of the requirements which are beyond the scope of this chapter.

Operative steps

The patient is taken to the endovascular suite and prepped and draped in the usual manner. The preferred access site is the femoral vein at the upper third of the thigh with the patient supine and the thigh slightly externally rotated and the knee slightly bent. The femoral vein lies inferior to the superficial femoral artery and slightly lateral in most cases. If access is planned via a popliteal approach, then the prone position is preferable. We rarely use the jugular approach for iliac vein work unless concomitant IVC filter removal is planned, or in cases where the "body floss" technique is required to cross an iliocaval chronic total occlusion (CTO). Pelvic vein embolization is also best performed via the internal jugular vein.

Using ultrasound visualization, a 21-gauge needle is inserted into the femoral vein and a 0.018″ wire placed with Seldinger technique. The 4F microintroducer sheath is placed and used to exchange for a 0.035″ guidewire. Using fluoroscopy the 0.035″ wire is navigated into the inferior vena cava (IVC). If the 0.035′ wire meets resistance and has difficulty entering the IVC, an intravenous contrast injection is performed to generate an anatomic roadmap. Most obstructive lesions can be crossed with a 0.035″ Glidewire.

In order to perform contrast venography, a larger sheath (8 FR, 11 cm in length) is ideal. The power injector is prepared and a digital subtraction contrast run is prepared by connecting high pressure tubing from the injector to the sidearm of the sheath. Eight cc per second for a total of 20cc of nonionic intravenous contrast is injected. The resulting image is examined for areas of stenosis, obstruction, and/or the presence of collaterals. Alternatively, the contrast injections may be done manually and the costs of a power injector omitted.

Nonthrombotic Iliac Vein Lesions

Nonthrombotic iliac vein lesions (NIVLs) are most suitable for the OBL because these cases are quite predictable in terms of complexity. As such, the time required and the disposable equipment needed are consistent. The most common lesion encountered is a stenosis at the confluence of the left common iliac vein with the IVC. Usually a standard 0.035″ J-tipped or Bentson guidewire will cross the lesion easily. In cases where the wire does not cross, a 0.035″ hydrophilic angled Glidewire is selected. After the lesion is crossed, we then advance the wire through the heart with the aid of an angled Glide catheter. We use the Glide catheter to exchange for a 0.035″ Amplatz super stiff wire which is anchored in the subclavian or jugular vein. The super stiff Amplatz wire is ideal for tracking balloons, IVUS catheters, and stents.

The IVUS catheter is brought into the field and mounted onto the 0.035″ super-stiff guidewire. IVUS imaging of the entire iliofemoral vein and vena cava outflow tract is performed. Particular attention is paid to the caliber of the veins as demonstrated by IVUS, in particular, where the right common iliac artery can be visualized as it crosses the left common iliac vein. As mentioned earlier, distal NIVLs can also be seen at the hypogastric artery crosses the external iliac vein, on either the right or left sides. Using the IVUS computerized planimetry software, the area of the stenosis can be calculated pre- and postintervention (Fig. 30.3A and B).

Optimum caliber values described by Raju[8] are used as reference in calculating common iliac vein stenosis. There are no validated criteria to determine what percent area reduction constitutes a hemodynamically significant lesion; however, as a rule of thumb, a 50% area reduction is the treatment threshold. Once the decision to treat is made the patient is anticoagulated systemically with intravenous an unfractionated heparin bolus.

A larger sheath, usually 11 FR, must be placed to accommodate the larger balloons and stent delivery systems. After the exchange length 0.035″ stiff wire is parked in the subclavian or jugular vein, a balloon is brought into the field. Iliac veins are quite compliant and fairly resistant to rupture. A 16–20 mm diameter Atlas balloon is usually chosen to dilate the lesion. The balloon is dilated to profile until the waist is

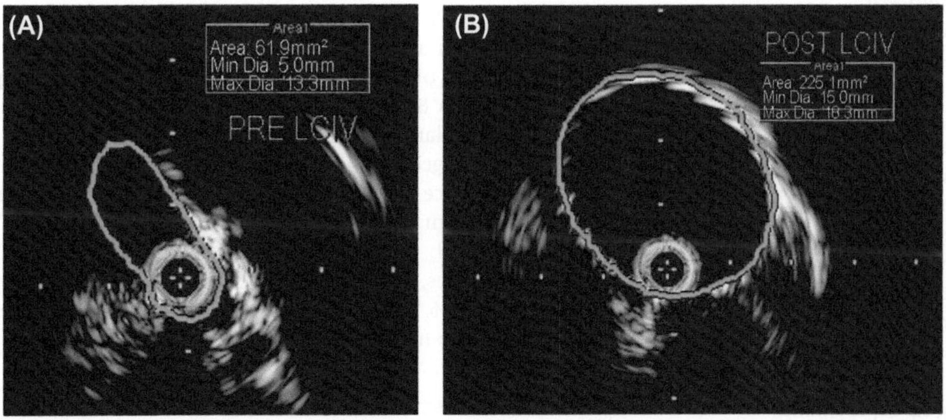

FIG. 30.3 Intravascular ultrasound (IVUS) planimetry images of left common iliac vein compression pre- and posttreatment. **(A)** IVUS image with left common iliac vein stenosis; **(B)** IVUS image post left common iliac vein stenting.

obliterated. Sequential dilatations with larger balloons are rarely required to dilate NIVL lesions, this is not the case for postthrombotic lesions which can be densely fibrotic. Since venous lesions always recoil after dilatation, stent deployment is required. Stent diameters of 16–20 mm are preferred; 20% oversizing of stents is necessary for venous interventions. The most common stents used for iliac vein work are self-expanding braided elgiloy Wallstents (Boston Scientific, Nantucket, MA). Gianturco Z-stents (Boston Scientific, Nantucket, MA) are also used for the vena cava, or for iliac vein interventions when the stent is projected into the vena cava. Murphy et al.[9] found that the use of a Z-stent at the caval confluence protects against contralateral jailing and contralateral iliac vein thrombosis. Note that currently available Wallstents and Z-stents are used off-label in the iliocaval venous system.

IVUS findings

Raju et al.[1] reported that the proximal NIVL was three times more frequently observed on the left side, whereas the distal NIVL was equally distributed bilaterally. The proximal NIVL was typically very focal on the left side and was located at the iliocaval junction; the right proximal NIVL was less focal and was located 1- to 2-cm distal to the iliocaval junction. The median area of the more severe stenosis (proximal or distal), as measured by IVUS, was 0.58 cm^2 (normal, 1.5 cm^2) representing approximately 70% stenosis. Most NIVLs are "soft" with waisting of the balloon often relieved at <2 atm. Postthrombotic lesions on the other hand are fibrotic and much more resistant to balloon dilatation.

Stent deployment

The Wallstent is composed of a thin Elgiloy stainless steel wire mesh, relying on predetermined springlike design to achieve desired expansion. Wallstents are compressed within a delivery catheter, which is an integral part of the delivery system. The external catheter maintains the collapsed state of the stent until its retraction allows for the device to expand. Device deployment is carried out by retracting the outer sheath while holding the stent in place with the inner tube. These stents guarantee precise placement only on the end to be deployed first (Wallstents deploy from distal to proximal). As a rule the leading end of the device is always maneuvered just past the planned landing zone, allowing for fine adjustments during its deployment.

The most dreaded complication is losing a stent and finding it in the heart. The phenomenon results when stents "jump" during deployment. Stents are packaged tightly in delivery sheaths where their potential energy is stored. During deployment, the potential energy converts to kinetic energy as it expands and finds its resting place. The stent will then apply its outward radial force to the vessel wall and maintain an open vessel.

If the stent has the opportunity to find an open area to quickly release its energy, it will. Iliocaval stent deployment for NIVL routinely deploys across a tight iliocaval stenosis into the IVC. The IVC represents a large space where a stent may quickly, and uncontrollably, convert its potential energy into kinetic energy. Thus, the stent could "jump" into the IVC and float into the right ventricle if the operator is not careful. Vessel preparation with balloon dilatation (predilate) may help create space and mitigate stent jumping.

Aside from careful deployment, and stent oversizing, an important maneuver is parking the stiff guidewire into the subclavian or jugular vein prior to stent deployment. This technique will keep the stent "on a rail" or not allow migration into the right atrium, the tricuspid valve, or worse, into the right ventricle. Stent retrieval with a snare, or capturing it with a balloon, and redeploying it in another vessel is much easier when the stent is on a wire.

Hemostasis and anticoagulation

There is no standardization in this area. Most vascular surgeons feel comfortable anticoagulating with standard unfractionated heparin. Whether or not to add antiplatelet therapy is also physician's preference. Postoperatively, antiplatelet therapy with 81 mg aspirin daily is sufficient after stenting of NIVL.

Scientific evidence for NIVL treatment

In four studies, with a total of 1000 lower extremities, NIVL was specifically assessed.[10–13] Technical success was achieved in 96%–100% of cases, with a follow-up of 59 months (6–72 months). Primary patency was 85% (79%–99%), and assisted primary and secondary patency were 100%. Rates of ulcer healing ranged from 82% to 85%,[11,13] with 5%–8% recurrence.[11,12] There was statistically significant improvement at all points of the CIVIQ,[12] and in the VAS and QoL scores.[12,13] Edema decreased in 32%–89% of cases,[11,12] and hyperpigmentation improved in 87%.[11] The influence of site of service on outcomes was not reported in these studies.

Postthrombotic Iliocaval and Femoral Venous Occlusive Disease

Patients presenting with iliac vein occlusive disease secondary to thrombosis are much more difficult to deal with technically, and stent patency is inferior to that of NIVL cases. Recanalization techniques are required. It is important to note that postthrombotic disease can be present at multiple levels. Because of the considerable incidence of iliocaval thrombosis in patients with known DVT, clinical exam should include evaluating pelvic and abdominal components to ensure that more proximal vessels are not involved and contributing to the lower extremity complaints. Duplex US allows for good visualization of lower extremity veins; however, for iliocaval disease, CTV or MRV may help define the landscape and aid planning venography, IVUS, +/− intervention.

Many cases have extensive disease requiring long procedure times just for crossing the occluded lesion(s). Many disposable products are usually required, sometimes even sharp recanalization is chosen for very recalcitrant lesions. Balloon dilatation can be quite aggressive to open densely chronically occluded blood vessels. For these reasons, we prefer the hospital setting and general endotracheal anesthesia. A Foley catheter is placed for urinary drainage as these procedures can become lengthy. A robust hybrid operating room with cone-beam CT capability is ideal for patients with extensive occlusive disease involving long segments of the femoral, iliac, and vena cava systems. Less extensive presentations of postthrombotic obstruction are candidates for recanalization and stenting in the office setting.

It has been shown that in two-thirds of patients with postthrombotic disease it is necessary to implant stents into the groin below the inguinal ligament to improve inflow into the reconstructed iliac veins. In a report by Raju,[14] the CFV was stented to the lower landing zone in 22 cases (56%). When the CFV was occluded or stenosed, inflow from the profunda femoris vein was enough to maintain stent patency. When both the profunda and femoral veins have obstructive lesions, stents may be extended into them, but in this situation, there is a high risk of stent thrombosis due to poor inflow. If the popliteal vein is occluded, it may require tibial vein access in order to recanalize the popliteal and femoral veins to obtain inline flow; these steps are controversial.

Interventions distal to the groin, including endovenectomy or stenting of the femoral vein, are also under investigation and are used in selected cases. Once operative planning has begun, it is important to properly choose an access site. If the femoral vein is patent, it can be used for access to larger vessels. If the femoral vein is occluded then venous access and drainage from the popliteal and profunda femoris veins should be evaluated. If the popliteal and profunda femoris veins are patent, the most proximal segment of an occluded femoral vein may often still be accessed. On occasion, it may be necessary to access the proximal profunda femoris vein, which may be challenging due to its depth.

Femoral vein access under US guidance is preferred at the midthigh level. Midthigh access facilitates shorter-length instrumentation with superior pushability compared with popliteal or internal jugular access sites. We prefer an 11 FR sheath of 11 cm length to allow space cephalad to the sheath and below the inguinal ligament to land a stent into the CFV when necessary. The profunda femoris vein is usually open if the femoral vein is occluded and can be accessed 2–3 cm below the lesser trochanter; stent extension into the profunda femoris vein is performed without impeding inflow from an occluded femoral vein. If the femoral vein is occluded, access is often possible through the upper 3–5 cm of the vein, which tends to remain open.

To cross a CTO an antegrade venogram is performed via the sidearm of the sheath at the midthigh to define the cranial extent of the venous anatomy (groin and pelvis) (Fig. 30.4A). A 0.035-inch soft or stiff Glidewire (Terumo Inc, Ann Arbor, MI) is navigated up to the occlusion. Further progress into the occlusion is made with vigorous rotation of the Glidewire tip with a torque device; the enhanced kinetic energy at the wire tip facilitates wire passage into microchannels present in the organizing fibrous tissue within the vein. Usually a straight or angled support catheter (Quick-Cross support catheter; Spectranetics, Colorado Springs, CO) or CXI support catheter (Cook, Bloomington, IN) is required to facilitate progress. If added support is required we prefer the Triforce system (Cook Medical, Bloomington, IN). This 5 FR braided sheath with tungsten tip adds columnar strength to the inner 4FR CXI support catheter and a nice transition between the two devices placed coaxially.

Glidewire passage must be guided by knowledge of topographic course of the vein. In the frontal projection, the left femoral vein overlies the medial third of the femoral head, coursing up to the lower pelvic brim across the sacroiliac joint joining the IVC variably between the fourth and fifth lumbar vertebral bodies. It is useful to view progress of the recanalization intermittently by rotating the C-ARM gantry into 45 or 60 degrees oblique projections to ensure that the Glidewire does not enter collaterals and tributaries. Interval contrast injections (puff angiograms) will help aid progress into the correct anatomy. An angled-tip catheter is useful in redirecting the Glidewire in the proper direction when it seems to veer off course. Entry into the IVC should be confirmed by injecting contrast

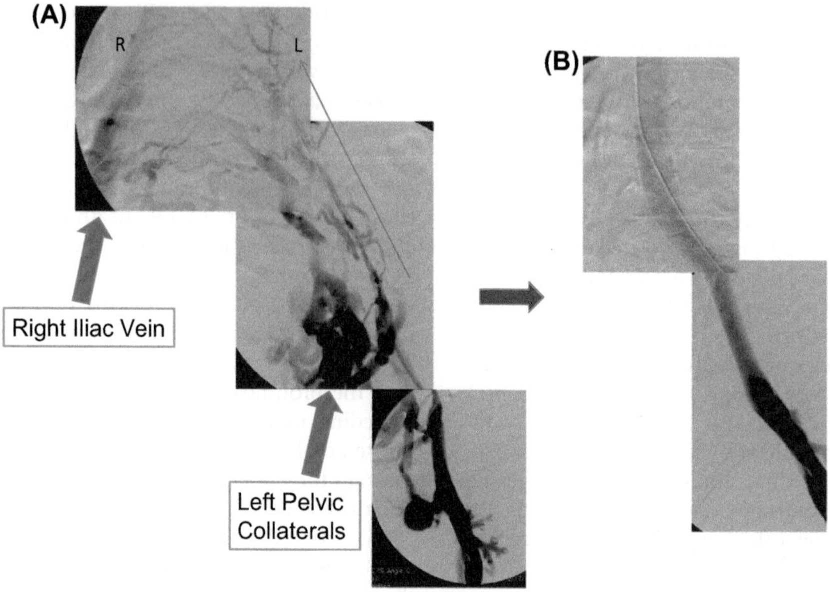

FIG. 30.4 **(A)** Venogram of chronic total occlusion left iliac vein and **(B)** left iliac vein postintervention.

through a catheter placed in the IVC under fluoroscopy, and IVUS.

From this stage of the recanalization procedure, the use of IVUS becomes crucial to assure integrity of the recanalized channel, to select optimal proximal and distal landing sites preferably free of postthrombotic disease, to ensure proper deployment and expansion of the stents, and to minimize radiation exposure.[14] The recanalized channel may be dilated starting with smaller-sized (3-mm) balloons to allow passage of an 8F IVUS catheter and large-caliber balloons. It is useful to use high-pressure balloons (16–18 ATM) expanded at maximum level for at least a minute until the balloon pressure stabilizes at this level. Overdilatation and oversizing of the stent diameter by 2–4 mm for the anatomic location is recommended to compensate for the variable recoil of the recanalized channel. Optimal stent diameters are 18 mm for the common iliac vein, 16 mm for the external iliac vein, and 14 mm for the CFV in normally sized adults.[8] Self-expanding woven braided elgiloy stents (Wallstent, Boston Scientific, Nantucket, Mass) in series with 3- to 4-cm overlap to minimize shelving along the complex course of the iliac vein are used (Fig. 30.4B). A completion IVUS examination and venogram terminate the procedure after noted defects are corrected by repeat ballooning. The sheath is removed and hemostasis is achieved by manual compression and pressure dressing. Occasionally, one may encounter very recalcitrant lesions where sharp recanalization techniques should be considered (i.e., stiff wire, Rosch-Uchida needle). In addition, access from above and below may be required in order to snare a wire to get through and access across the lesion ("body floss" technique).

Anticoagulation

Intraoperatively, unfractionated heparin (5000–10,000 U) is administered and allowed to circulate prior to balloon dilatation. In patients with stents implanted for the treatment of NIVL, usually a daily dose of 81 mg of aspirin is sufficient to maintain stent patency. However, in postthrombotic cases, we have learned that "when in doubt, anticoagulate." In patients who undergo difficult recanalization and lengthy procedures, low-molecular-weight heparin (enoxaparin 1 mg/kg BID subcutaneously) is administered afterward in the recovery room, and daily thereafter for 1–3 months. At this point, we will convert them to an oral agent for long-term anticoagulation. In many patients, especially the ones with inherited or acquired thrombophilias, lifelong oral anticoagulation is indicated to maintain stent patency.

Scientific evidence postthrombotic treatment

In six studies with a total of 921 legs, secondary (postthrombotic) obstruction was specifically examined.[12,15–19] Technical success was achieved in

93%–100% of cases, with a mean follow-up of 46 months (2–72 months). Primary patency was 57% (50%–80%), assisted primary patency 80% (76% –82%), and secondary patency 86% (82%–90%). Ulcer healing ranged from 63% to 67%,[18] with 0%–8% recurrence.[15] There was statistically significant improvement at all points of the CIVIQ[12] and VCSS[16] scores. Edema decreased in 32%–51% of cases.[12,17] The influence of site of service on outcomes was not reported in these studies.

Acute Deep Venous Thrombosis

Although there seems to be a growing interest in treating patients with acute thromboembolic disease of the lower extremities in the OEC, we prefer the hospital setting for most of these cases. Patient safety and comfort, the ability to treat as much thrombus as possible, number of accesses needed, and the ability to deliver appropriate devices are all factors that must be considered before beginning a case. Cross-sectional imaging can often determine the extent of thrombus, relationship to major tributary veins, and, when possible, differentiation of acute from chronic occlusion.

When approaching any acute deep venous thrombosis (DVT) intervention, the procedure can be divided into the thrombus management component and the secondary intervention. If the patient has an acute DVT, thrombus management will be a greater portion of the procedure than the secondary intervention. If the patient has occlusive disease of the deep venous system, there will be little thrombus to manage and a significant amount of secondary interventions being performed. If symptoms are moderate to severe, then venography, angioplasty, and stenting should be considered for relief of occlusive disease in patients with iliocaval involvement. Femoral-popliteal DVT is managed medically with anticoagulation. The most difficult cases are those patients with iliocaval thrombus between 4 and 8 weeks old. If the thrombus is $<$ 4 weeks old and there are no absolute contraindications, it will likely respond well to catheter-directed lytic therapy or thrombectomy. If the thrombus is older than 2 months, it is likely well organized and firmly adherent to the vein wall, and unlikely to respond to catheter-directed lytic therapy (or thrombectomy). Therefore, we prefer anticoagulation for organized thrombus to allow for recanalization to occur.

Rheolytic pharmacomechanical thrombectomy with the AngioJet (Boston Scientific, Nantucket, MA) is our preference for acute iliofemoral DVT. These cases require tissue plasminogen activator (TPA). We infuse 10 mg of TPA in the pulsed mode and another 10 mg of TPA in the thrombectomy mode. These patients are at risk for intraoperative bleeding. In addition, bradycardia and hematuria are common so careful monitoring is required throughout the case. A mobile console and disposable catheter are required for rheolytic thrombectomy, therefore, a cost analysis must be performed if one is considering doing these procedures in the OBL site of service.

Newer technology for clot management continues to evolve. The goal has been to eliminate the bleeding risk from lytic therapy and focus on developing more robust suction thrombectomy platforms. The focus will become more attractive for the OEC site-of-service as the bleeding risk will decrease with the omission of TPA.

Inferior Vena Cava Filter Placement and Retrieval

IVC filter placement and retrieval can technically be performed in an OEC in selected patients; however, these patients are usually found and treated in the hospital setting. IVUS can be used for placement of IVC filters; it is a more accurate method than contrast venography for localizing the renal veins and measuring vena cava diameter. Previously placed IVC filters with short dwell times can be retrieved safely in the office. However, forceful traction is usually required to remove filters with long dwell times which have incorporated themselves into the vena cava wall, and this can be quite painful. IVC filters with long dwell times are therefore best retrieved under general anesthesia in the hospital setting. In some instances, the filter must be displaced sideways or remodeled/fractured by repeated high-pressure balloon dilation to maneuver it off the vena cava wall.

Current evidence-based guidelines do not support systematic use of IVC filters to prevent PE recurrence, unless there is absolute contraindication to anticoagulation or recurrent PE despite therapeutic anticoagulation. We adhere to these guidelines and do not place IVC filters for softer indications (such as prior to bariatric surgery), hence IVC filters are placed rarely in our OEC.

Pelvic Venous Disorders

The venous circulation of the pelvis consists of three interconnected venous systems—(1) the left renal and ovarian veins; (2) the iliac veins (common, external, and internal); and (3) the lower extremity veins. Iliac vein obstruction has already been discussed.

The spectrum of pelvic venous disorders includes four clinical presentations—(1) chronic pelvic pain, (2) pelvic source varices of the leg, (3) symptoms related to renal venous hypertension, and (4) leg swelling.

Primary ovarian/internal iliac venous incompetence

The development of varicose veins in the pelvis may cause disabling symptoms, mainly in women of childbearing age; the disease is known as pelvic congestion syndrome. Transabdominal/vaginal DU or CT/MR venography can be performed to confirm ovarian vein reflux into a plexus in the broad ligament that forms pelvic varicose veins. Endovascular therapy relies on coil embolization alone or in conjunction with foam sclerotherapy.

It is important to exclude a Nutcracker syndrome as the cause of the left ovarian vein enlargement. This condition is diagnosed by an elevated pullback or simultaneously measured renocaval gradient. The gradient in this region should normally be 1 mm Hg or less and is typically greater than 5 mm Hg in patients with Nutcracker syndrome.[20]

A variety of medical, surgical, and endovascular approaches have been proposed for the treatment of primary ovarian and internal iliac venous incompetence. A variety of percutaneous embolization approaches have been reported including simple coil embolization of the refluxing trunks, glue embolization, and a combination of sclerotherapy and coil embolization. The percutaneous transcatheter treatment can be performed from either the femoral or jugular approach. We prefer the jugular technique as it allows a more natural angle into the left renal vein. Selection of the left as well as the right ovarian vein can be very difficult from the femoral approach because of the acute angle at the origin of the right ovarian vein with the inferior vena cava. Injection of the left renal vein will usually depict the presence of a dilated (6–10 mm) left ovarian vein which is incompetent. There are usually cross-filling pelvic collaterals filling the right ovarian vein system. In a percentage of cases the reflux causes filling of the internal iliac vein tributaries. Venography can be done during the valsalva maneuver if the resting venogram does not demonstrate an enlarged ovarian vein.[21]

The procedure begins with catheterization of the left renal vein and subsequently the left ovarian venogram (Fig. 30.5). The left ovarian vein is easily catheterized from a jugular approach with a multipurpose shaped catheter and either a soft-tipped guidewire or a hydrophilic guidewire. The ovarian vein arises proximally from the left renal vein usually around a centimeter lateral to the vertebral body. Initial imaging may demonstrate a single, simple ovarian vein or in many instances it may demonstrate numerous collaterals which are of great importance because if left untreated they may provide collateral flow to the pelvis. Once the decision to treat the patient is made, a long 6 French sheath or guide catheter can be advanced, if the ovarian vein is large, into the vein for the purpose of using occluding devices and catheters in a coaxial fashion. If a sheath or guiding catheter cannot be placed into the ovarian vein, a standard 5 French catheter can be used to negotiate the vein. It is important to place the catheter in the pelvis down into the broad ligament. Treatment of the incompetence in the ovarian vein and deep pelvic vessels is usually sufficient to reduce the pressure load on these vessels.

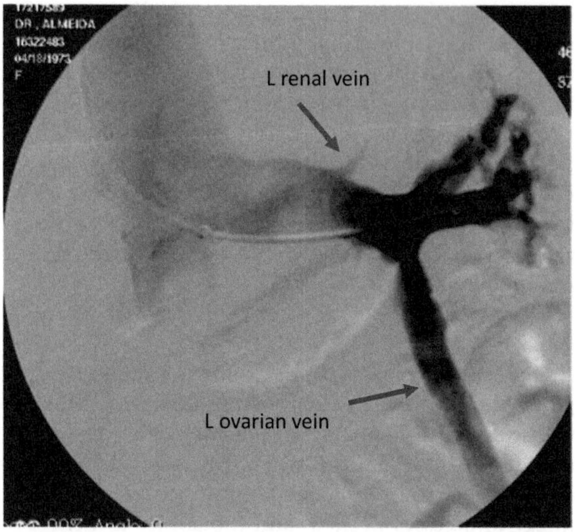

FIG. 30.5 Venogram of left renal vein and reflux of contrast into dilated left ovarian vein.

We usually treat the left ovarian vein and will study and then treat the right ovarian vein. The right ovarian vein is usually more challenging to catheterize because it arises from an acute angle slightly anterior and inferior to the right renal vein. From the femoral approach, a reverse curve catheter may be helpful and from the jugular approach a multipurpose or cobra-shaped catheter often is ideal.

Treatment involves a combination of coil embolization of the ovarian vein and sclerotherapy of the small vessels and collaterals. With the catheter in the vessels below the pelvic brim sclerosants and liquid embolics are used.[22] Sclerotherapeutic agents that are used are "off label" for this indication and include 1.5% STS (sodium tetradecyl sulfate) or 2% Aethosxysklerol (Polidocanol) foam. Prior to injecting any liquid sclerosant or embolic agent it is advisable to determine the volume of agent needed as well as the rate in which the agent should be injected. This is achieved by testing with small contrast injections to determine how much contrast is needed to fill a group of collaterals and to evaluate the presence of reflux. Care must be taken to avoid overinjection and refluxing into the IVC via collaterals. The ovarian vein may have a number of accessory veins requiring the packing of coils at several levels throughout the course of the left ovarian vein. Coils are oversized in order to prevent embolization into the central venous system.[23] We usually will not treat concomitant internal iliac incompetence at the time of ovarian vein intervention. The published literature has demonstrated symptomatic response in greater than 80% of patients treated.[24,25] Only a small subset of patients will require subsequent embolization of internal iliac veins. Complications may include ovarian vein perforation and coil migration. Despite a growing body of evidence that these interventions benefit properly selected patients, the medical necessity criteria among payers is inconsistent—some go as far as to call the interventions "experimental."

Left renal vein compression (Nutcracker syndrome)

Many patients with Nutcracker syndrome (compression of the distal left renal vein between the superior mesenteric artery and the aorta) are asymptomatic and can be managed conservatively. However, for those patients with disabling symptoms, both surgical and endovascular approaches have been proposed. The standard-of-care remains open surgery (left renal and gonadal vein transposition); while left renal vein stenting remains very controversial with multiple reports of stent migration into the vena cava and/or heart.[24] We currently do not offer left renal vein stenting in our OBL; perhaps this will change with future improvements in stent technology.

CONCLUSION

OECs are efficient and streamlined and have been well received by patients. Now in our 20th year of operating a dedicated OEC focused on venous disease in downtown Miami, FL—it is clear that this is the best environment for treating venous disease. However, we are facing payers who have steadily implemented convoluted and capricious coverage policies to curb utilization and, reimbursement is cut annually. The preauthorization process has become quite labor-intensive, requiring us to employ extra staff. Every year we are doing a similar volume—with less reimbursement and more overhead costs.

REFERENCES

1. Raju R, Neglen P. High prevalence of nonthrombotic iliac vein lesions in chronic venous disease: a permissive role in pathogenicity. *J Vasc Surg*. 2006;44:136–144.
2. Raju S, Darcey R, Neglén P. Unexpected major role for venous stenting in deep reflux disease. *J Vasc Surg*. 2010; 51(2):401–408.
3. Negus D, Fletcher EWL, Cockett FB, Thomas ML. Compression and band formation at the mouth of the left common iliac vein. *Br J Surg*. 1968;55:369–374.
4. Labropoulos N, Borge M, Pierce K, Pappas PJ. Criteria for defining significant central vein stenosis with duplex ultrasound. *J Vasc Surg*. 2007;46:101–107.
5. Metzger PB, Rossi FH, Kambara AM, et al. Criteria for detecting significant chronic iliac venous obstructions with duplex ultrasound. *J Vasc Surg Venous Lymphat Disord*. 2016;4:18–27.
6. Kayılıoglu SI, Köksoy C, Alaçayır I. Diagnostic value of the femoral vein flow pattern for the detection of an iliocaval venous obstruction. *J Vasc Surg Venous Lymphat Disord*. 2016;4:2–8.
7. Sloves J, Almeida JI. J Venous duplex ultrasound protocol for iliocaval disease. *Vasc Surg Venous Lymphat Disord*. 2018;6(6):748–757.
8. Raju S, Buck WJ, Crim W, Jayaraj A. Optimal sizing of iliac vein stents. *Phlebology*. 2018;33:451–457.
9. Murphy EH, Johns B, Varney E, Buck W, Jayaraj A, Raju S. Deep venous thrombosis associated with caval extension of iliac stents. *J Vasc Surg Venous Lymphat Disord*. 2017; 5(1):8–17.
10. Lou WS, Gu JP, He X, et al. Endovascular treatment for iliac vein compression syndrome: a comparison between the presence and absence of secondary thrombosis. *Korean J Radiol*. 2009;10:135–143.
11. Meng QY, Li XQ, Qian AM, et al. Endovascular treatment of iliac vein compression syndrome. *Chin Med J*. 2011; 124:3281–3284.
12. Neglén P, Hollis KC, Olivier J, et al. Stenting of the venous outflow in chronic venous disease: long-term stent-related outcome, clinical, and hemodynamic result. *J Vasc Surg*. 2007;46:979–990.
13. Ye K, Lu X, Li W, et al. Long-term outcomes of stent placement for symptomatic nonthrombotic iliac vein compression lesions in chronic venous disease. *J Vasc Interv Radiol*. 2012;23:497–502.
14. Raju S, Neglen P. Percutaneous recanalization of total occlusions of the iliac vein. *J Vasc Surg*. 2009;50:360–368.
15. Raju S, Hollis K, Neglen P. Obstructive lesions of the inferior vena cava: clinical features and endovenous treatment. *J Vasc Surg*. 2006;44:820–827.
16. Rosales A, Sandbaek G, Jorgensen JJ. Stenting for chronic post-thrombotic vena cava and iliofemoral venous occlusions: mid-term patency and clinical outcome. *Eur J Vasc Endovasc Surg*. 2010;40:234–240.
17. Alhadad A, Kolbel T, Herbst A, et al. Iliocaval vein stenting: long term survey of postthrombotic symptoms and working capacity. *J Thromb Thrombolysis*. 2011;31:211–216.

18. Nayak L, Hildebolt CF, Vedantham S. Postthrombotic syndrome: feasibility of a strategy of imaging-guided endovascular intervention. *J Vasc Interv Radiol.* 2012;23:1165–1173.
19. Oguzkurt L, Tercan F, Ozkan U, et al. Iliac vein compression syndrome: outcome of endovascular treatment with long-term follow-up. *Eur J Radiol.* 2008;68:487–492.
20. Kim HS, Malhorta AD, Rowe PC, Lee JM, Venbrux AC. Embolotherapy for pelvic congestion syndrome: long-term results. *J Vasc Interv Radiol.* 2006;17:289–297.
21. Freedman J, Ganeshan A, Crowe PM. Pelvic congestion syndrome: the role of interventional radiology in the treatment of chronic pelvic pain. *Postgrad Med J.* 2010;86:704–710.
22. Gandini R, Chiocchi M, Konda D, Pampana E, Fabiano S, Simonetti G. Transcatheter foam sclerotherapy for symptomatic female varicocele with sodium-tetradecl-sulfate foam. *Cardiovasc Intervent Radiol.* 2008;31:778–784.
23. Liddle AD, Davies AH. Pelvic congestion syndrome: chronic pelvic pain caused by ovarian and internal iliac varices. *Phebology.* 2007;22:100–104.
24. Scultetus AH, Villavicencio L, Gillespie DL. The nutcracker syndrome: its role in the pelvic venous disorders. *J Vasc Surg.* 2001;34:812–819.
25. Maleux G, Stocks L, Wilms G, Marchal G. Ovarian vein embolization for the treatment of pelvic congestion syndrome: long term technical and clinical results. *J Vasc Interv Radiol.* 2000;11:859–864.

CHAPTER 31

Lower Extremity Arterial Procedures in an Office-Based Endovascular Center

ALI KHALIFEH, MD • MOTAHAR HOSSEINI, MD • RAFAEL SANTINI DOMINQUEZ, MD • KHANJAN H. NAGARSHETH, MD, MBA, FACS

PATIENT SELECTION

Over the past several years, there has been growing interest in ambulatory endovascular lower extremity arterial procedures. Safety and effectiveness of the procedures in an office-based endovascular center (OEC) have been reported, in addition to possible economic benefits.[1–3] Some authors reported that preformation of outpatient peripheral arterial procedures in hospitals may actually have an unintended effect of increasing cost and higher rates of reinterventions.[4,5] However, these studies had several limitations including inability to stratify for geographic regions and extent of patient disease. In our experience, lower extremity arterial procedures in an OEC are safe, and efficient in offloading busy tertiary centers' operating rooms.

In selecting patients suitable to undergo invasive procedures for lower extremity revascularization in an OEC, there are several factors that need to be considered. First and foremost, the patient should have failed maximum medical therapy. Intermittent claudicants should be encouraged to stop smoking, have exercise therapy, and should be on optimal antihypertensive, lipid lowering therapy, and glycemic control. In a literature review, Parvar et al. found that nicotine replacement, bupropion, and varenicline are more effective than placebo[6] when used for smoking cessation. The authors note that although supervised exercise therapy is ideal, there can be several barriers preventing patients from attaining such benefit. In addition, despite need for further studies, blood pressure and glycemic control provide a large benefit. Caution must be drawn to some hypoglycemic agents that have shown an increased incidence of lower limb amputation. Furthermore, they conclude that dual antiplatelet therapy and even low-dose rivaroxaban are beneficial in decreasing perioperative complications.

Once a decision has been made to intervene, the influencing factors can be divided into the factors related to the patient, and factors related to the procedure. In addition to thorough evaluation of the patient comorbidities, the surgeon must be able to recognize issues that might prevent the patient from lying flat for procedures under conscious sedation such as orthopnea, severe back pain, akathisia, or history of not tolerating procedures under sedation.

During procedures, the surgeon needs to maintain communication with the patient, alerting them to needle sticks, injection of local anesthetics and prior to any action that may cause discomfort, e.g., when the balloon is inflated to perform angioplasty there can be significant discomfort. These maneuvers may result in sudden movement of the limb resulting in possible complications.

Furthermore, if the surgeon anticipates complex and lengthy procedure or possibility of an open procedure which may require deeper sedation, or general anesthesia, the procedure may be more appropriately performed in hospital operating room. In the end, the ultimate goal is patient safety, comfort, and favorable outcome for lower extremity arterial interventions.

APPROACHES AND CLOSURE DEVICES

Ever since the introduction of the Seldinger technique, arterial access for angiography has evolved at exponential rates with newer sheaths, catheters, wires, and closure devices. This is much better for the patient as compared to the more traumatic cutdown access. In addition to common femoral artery access, both "up and over" and antegrade approach, radial artery (RA), popliteal artery (PA), and pedal artery access have gained popularity for both diagnostic and therapeutic lower extremity angiography and intervention.

Office-Based Endovascular Centers. https://doi.org/10.1016/B978-0-323-67969-5.00031-9
Copyright © 2020 Elsevier Inc. All rights reserved.

Closure Devices

In the early 1990s, pressure devices such as Femostop (RADI Medical Systems) and more recently TR Band (Terumo Interventional Systems) have been introduced to replace digital pressure. The introduction of vascular closure devices (VCDs) transformed access site closure especially while using larger access sheaths. VCDs can be placed into three general groups: collagen-based, suture-based, and staples and clips.[7,8]

Collagen sealant products utilize exposed arterial wall smooth muscle and promote clot formation over absorbable collagen plug. Commercially available VCD include Angio-Seal, VasoSeal, Vascade. Other products such as Mynx and Exoseal have a sealant or gel-based plug. These products aid in closure of arterial hole caused by 5 to 8 French sheaths. In addition to the risk of device failure there is risk of possible distal embolization of the plug.

Suture-based VCDs involve the use of a pair of needles to deploy a suture with a preplaced knot. Multiple stitches can be deployed depending on the size of the sheath. At the end of the procedure, the knots are cinched and immediate hemostasis is expected. Available devices include Perclose ProGlide, Xsite, and SuperStitch. These devices can help in closing larger holes in the artery and thereby a sheath up to 21 French in size can be used. Multiple devices are used for larger holes.

Finally VCDs that employ a clip such as StarClose deploy an extravascular clip to close up to an 8 French arterial hole. After deployment, manual pressure might be needed. In the setting of OEC where the sheath size is not expected to exceed 8 Fr, we commonly use collagen or sealant-based VCDs for common femoral artery access. For alternative access sites, manual compression remains the preferred technique for hemostasis. While using axillary or PA access a VCD is rarely used due to vessel diameter and proximity to vein.[9]

The lower extremity arterial system can be approached using different access points. Following approaches are commonly used.

COMMON FEMORAL ARTERY

The most common access point for lower extremity intervention is the common femoral artery using the "up and over" technique also known as contralateral retrograde access. Prior imaging of the aortoiliac angulation and knowledge of prior surgeries allows for better preparation for access. Ultrasound-guided access of the common femoral artery to avoid "high" or "low" sticks is highly recommended.[10] Additionally, use of ultrasound for access enables visualization of calcific plaque and helps in planning the use of appropriate closure device.

Challenges to the "up and over" approach include steep bifurcation angle, tortuous or calcific iliac arteries, history of aortobifemoral bypass or iliac stents. Several techniques have been employed to meet these challenges.[11] However, if all fails, ipsilateral antegrade femoral artery allows the use of shorter length devices and wires to target lesions.[12]

RADIAL ARTERY

Radial artery access for coronary angiography has been established by cardiologist as a safe, feasible, and affords more patient comfort than femoral artery access.[13,14] There has been growing interest in RA for peripheral vascular interventions.[15–17] Patient evaluation and physical exam is fundamental in this approach. All patients need to undergo Allen and or Barbeau tests to delineate hand perfusion prior to access. Again, ultrasound evaluation of vessel caliber and calcific burden along with ultrasound-guided access is recommended to avoid possible complications. RA access can prove helpful when performing a diagnostic angiography for operative planning when the patient is morbidly obese, has a hostile groin or challenging iliofemoral anatomy. This approach is vital for upper extremity intervention; however, it may be limited in treating lower extremity occlusive disease because of device length. Unless the patient is very short, the device may not reach lower extremity target lesions. In appropriately selected patients some interventions can be performed using radial approach.[15] Furthermore, the use of RA may be limited because of the need for larger sheaths required for balloon or stent angioplasty.[16] There have been reports of use of the GlideSheath Slender (Terumo Interventional Systems) during the transradial approach. Due to its thinner wall and hydrophilic coating it allows use of larger devices in smaller size sheaths.[18,19] Hemostatic pressure bands have been utilized and allow for early patient mobility postprocedure.

POPLITEAL ACCESS

In recent years, femoropopliteal disease management has been reevaluated and there is more acceptance of an "endovascular first" approach.[20] Chronic occlusion of the superficial femoral artery (SFA) and proximal PA has been amenable to angioplasty, atherectomy, and stent placement[20]. When contralateral or antegrade femoral access proves challenging, retrograde PA has been reported with success in revascularization in selected patients.[21] Using ultrasound guidance, a patent's supragenicular segment of the PA is identified and accessed percutaneously from the medial approach and cannulated with a 6–7 Fr sheath. After atherectomy and stent angioplasty of the occluded stasis is obtained with manual compression for 15–20 min. There are promising data as well for more distal PA access through an anterolateral approach through the anterior compartment of the lower extremity either under ultrasound or fluoroscopic guidance.[22] This approach allows retrograde access to distal PA (P3 segment), as well as tibioperoneal trunk. Hemostasis is achieved by inflating a pressure cuff to 10 mmHg higher than the systolic blood pressure for at least 5 min. In a large vascular quality improvement database analysis, Komshian et al. recommended that retrograde PA access should only be used when common femoral artery access has failed.[23]

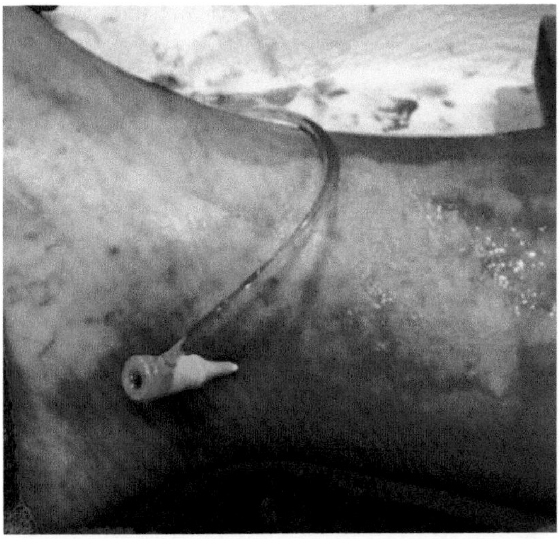

FIG. 31.1 Pedal access sheath (Cook Medical). (Image courtesy: KH Nagarsheth.)

PEDAL ACCESS

The increasing prevalence of diabetes mellitus and end stage renal disease in patients presenting with chronic limb ischemia has resulted in an increase in lesion complexity. A retrograde tibial-pedal access is useful and safe in patient with severe peripheral artery disease, unsuccessful antegrade access, or unable to tolerate common femoral access due to body habitus or comorbidities.[24] Combination of antegrade and retrograde access yields higher success rates, up to 90%–100% of patients.[25] Retrograde revascularization is an important technique to improve the limb salvage rates especially in patients with TASC C class or higher. As a consequence, transpedal access has emerged as a vascular access site for the management of complex PAD.[26] When there is failure to cross the lesion in an antegrade manner, the lesion can be crossed in retrograde manner using one of the tibial vessels. At this point the wire can be snared and target lesion can be treated in an antegrade or retrograde manner depending on operator's preference (Fig. 31.1).

Under ultrasound guidance, one of the pedal arteries is visualized and accessed using a short 21 G needle, and a 4 Fr microsheath is inserted over a microwire. Wire location is confirmed either using US or flouroscopy. Retrograde atherectomy, stenting, and balloon angioplasty can be performed with a 4 Fr sheath or upsizing to a 6 Fr GlideSheath Slender (Terumo Interventional Systems). Our preferred wire to cross lesions is a 0.018-inch v18 wire. But a vast range of wires have been used and reported in the literature. Hemostasis of the puncture site can be achieved either with manual compression or the use of a transradial band in selected patients.

Ultrasound guidance remains an important tool for the access of the tibial and pedal vessels. In a review paper, Marmagkiolis et al. reported that US guidance was used in 60% and flouroscopy in about one-third of the cases.[26] The anterior tibial and dorsalis pedis arteries were the most commonly accessed vessels (54.7%), followed by the posterior tibial artery (28.0%) and peroneal artery (7.5%). Ninety-three percent of the patients had an occlusion and the average occlusion length treated was 206.0 ± 125.0 mm. A recent report from Lai et al. demonstrated the safety of retrograde tibial access,[27] with the access vessel remaining patent for possible future bypass. The vessels most commonly treated were infrapopliteal vessels in 67.1%, the popliteal in 18.7%, and the SFA in 43.0% of cases.

Multiple techniques have been reported during pedal access including subintimal arterial flossing with antegrade-retrograde intervention (SAFARI) technique[28], controlled antegrade and retrograde subintimal tracking (CART),[29] and tibiopedal arterial minimally invasive retrograde revascularization (TAMI) technique (Figs. 31.2–31.4).[30]

In a recent study, D'Souza et al. did not find any statistically significant difference in outcomes comparing office-based versus in-hospital transpedal access interventions.[31]

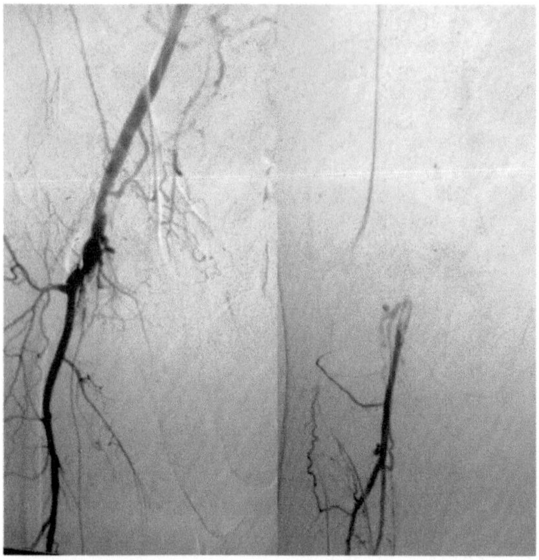

FIG. 31.2 Subintimal arterial flossing with antegrade-retrograde intervention (SAFARI) technique preintervention. (Image courtesy: KH Nagarsheth.)

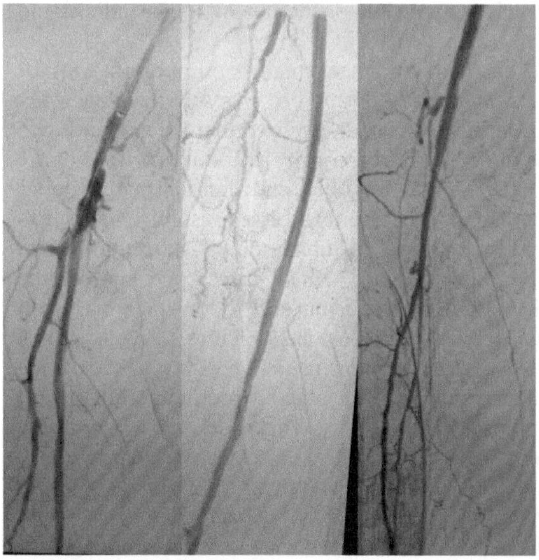

FIG. 31.3 Subintimal arterial flossing with antegrade-retrograde intervention (SAFARI) technique postintervention. (Image courtesy: KH Nagarsheth.)

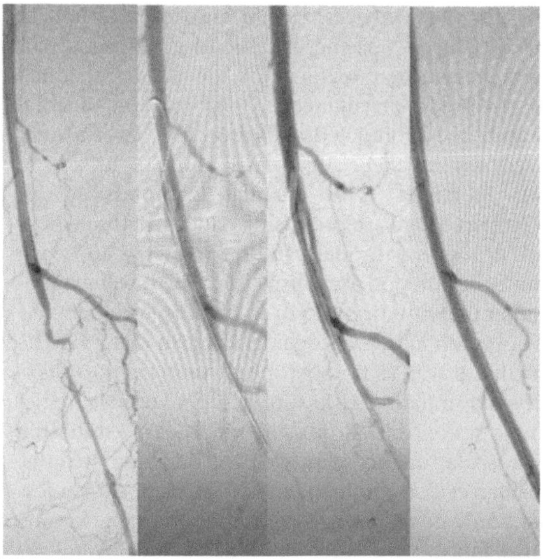

FIG. 31.4 Controlled antegrade and retrograde subintimal tracking (CART) technique. (Image courtesy: KH Nagarsheth.)

TREATMENT MODALITIES

Balloon Angioplasty

Percutaneous transluminal angioplasty or balloon angioplasty has been traditionally used for treatment of focal lesions. Once the lesion is traversed by the balloon catheter, the balloon is expanded and the plaque is displaced and compressed against the artery wall. As a stand-alone approach, this technique can cause flow-limiting dissections and elastic recoil of lesions. In addition, there is a high rate of early restenosis related to negative remodeling and neointimal proliferation. To address the short-term complications, several variations and additions to standard balloon angioplasty have been introduced.

Cutting balloons may have three to four cutting blades mounted longitudinally on the balloon. The blade directly penetrates this vessel wall on first inflation disrupting the lamina and decreasing inflammation, reducing elastic recoil, and theoretically reducing rates of restenosis.[32] However, in several randomized controlled trials there was no benefit of cutting balloons compared with conventional angioplasty in treating femoropopliteal vessels and vessels with restenosis. More distal vessels may have worse outcomes with cutting balloons.[33]

Cryoplasty balloons are of only historical interest as they are no longer available.

Radiation in the form of gel or beads is also utilized in conjunction with balloon angioplasty. The radiation is thought to decrease the risk of intimal hyperplasia; however, it may compromise a vessel healing in the area of disrupted surfaces. There has been some evidence supporting the use of brachyplasty to decrease femoropopliteal stent restenosis; however, this approach remains unpopular.[34]

The use of drug coated balloons (DCBs) has gained popularity recently. The most common DCB have various doses of paclitaxel, an antimitotic agent, coupled with an accipient to help deliver the drug to the vessel wall. This technique involves the use of a standard balloon angioplasty to predilate the stenotic portion of a vessel. This allows the DCB to provide optimal drug delivery to the vessel wall. Ninety percent of the drug is presumed to be lost in the bloodstream, 6% retained on the surface of the balloon, and 4% is delivered to the vessel wall.[35] Compared with standard balloon angioplasty, DCB has been shown to have lower rates of lumen loss.[36] A recent systematic review and metaanalysis from Katsanos et al.,[37] revealed an increased risk of death following the use of paclitaxel-coated balloons and stents. This report has caused the FDA to issue a letter to providers alerting them to use such therapies with caution. In addition, two large trials using paclitaxel were halted.

ATHERECTOMY

Atherectomy is a procedure performed to debulk the atherosclerotic plaque from diseased arteries. It has been used effectively in the treatment of both coronary and peripheral arterial disease. It provides the theoretical advantage of debulking plaque, instead of crushing it against the vessel wall by balloon angioplasty. Following atherectomy, balloon angioplasty or stenting can be utilized. Atherectomy should not be used when crossing a lesion in a subintimal plane or when the vessel diameter is smaller than indicated in device instructions for use.

Atherectomy devices are grouped by their mechanism of action: directional, rotational, orbital, and photoablative or laser atherectomy. There are also devices designed for crossing complete occlusions.[38] Some advantages of directional atherectomy may include treating a targeted eccentric plaque in severely calcified lesion. However, these devices cause vessel wall trauma, discharge debris, require multiple passes and are time-consuming. Rotational atherectomy is effective in severely calcified lesions and is faster in general. The tip of the device or "burr" has a set of blades that rotate removing plaque. The operator, however, is not able to moderate the depth of atherectomy. In contrast, orbital atherectomy has a special configuration that allows an increase in debulking area with increasing rotational speed. Laser or excimer atherectomy utilizes Laser to remove atheroma at thickness of 10 mm with each pulse. Total occlusion crossers with atherectomy capabilities are available and utilize high frequency wire vibrations. Multiple ongoing randomized controlled studies are underway comparing multiple devices and combination therapies.[38] A variety of these devices have been and continue to be used in the OEC setting. Despite the paucity of evidence showing benefit of atherectomy over angioplasty,[39] there has been increasing use of these devices especially in the OEC setting.[40] In a recent study by Lai et al atherectomy was shown to have satisfactory results when performed in an OEC. The primary patency in 571 vessels was 90% at 12 months and 84% at 29 months.[40a]

Some atherectomy devices, such as Pathways Jetstream (Boston Scientific), Peripheral Roblator (Boston Scientific), and Rotarex S(Straub Medical) have aspiration mechanisms that may decrease the risk of distal embolization of fractured plaque. There are several other mechanisms that can be employed for embolic prevention. These include filter embolic prevention device (EPD), proximal occlusive balloon with or without flow reversal, and distal occlusive balloon. Use of any EPD is dependent on vessel caliber and plaque anatomy. Although there has been some evidence showing the benefit of EPD in carotid and renal artery interventions, there are currently no studies suggesting increased benefit in lower extremity interventions.[41] If a major embolic event occurs in LE interventions, catheter aspiration or thrombolysis can be used to reestablish flow. Rarely, an open procedure may be necessary.

STENT

Self-expanding stents (SESs) have proven efficacy when used for femoropopliteal disease. General recommendations advocate the use of SES in treating shorter lesions or when a dissection flap appears to be flow limiting. Although some studies have suggested better patency rates of femoropopliteal lesions treated with SES versus balloon angioplasty alone, large metaanalysis have failed to demonstrate clinical significance.[42,43] These studies are difficult to analyze because the patient population remains heterogeneous. In addition, stents are made from a variety of materials and have variable risks of fracture, thrombosis or in-stent restenosis. In our experience, if a short-segment lesion in the femoro PA fails to improve after balloon angioplasty or if there is evidence of flow limiting dissection flap, we recommend the use of SES. When comparing drug-eluting stents (DESs) to bare metal stents (BMSs) in femoropopliteal disease, some authors showed benefit to DES in patency rates; however, large metaanalysis showed similar outcomes.[44]

For infrapopliteal disease, studies have shown equivocal outcomes when comparing balloon angioplasty alone to BMS. Several authors inspired by coronary data have reported favorable outcomes with DESs in infrapopliteal disease.[45,46] With these favorable reports, it appears that DES for infrapopliteal arterial disease is a safe and efficient approach.[47] For more distal infragenicular arterial disease, there are ongoing trials assessing safety and efficacy of DES use. In addition, there is currently rising concern regarding DESs that contain paclitaxel.[37]

CO_2 ANGIOGRAPHY

Patients with PAD tend to have multiple comorbidities, including advanced kidney disease which places the patient at increased risk for contrast-induced nephropathy (CIN) after fluoroscopic interventions. The incidence of CIN in patients with baseline chronic kidney disease (CKD) undergoing peripheral interventions has been reported up to 5.1%.[48] In an effort to reduce the risk associated with contrast, carbon dioxide is used for lower extremity angiography. The main benefit of CO_2 as a contrast agent is the lack of renal toxicity and anaphylactic response. Carbon dioxide angiography is an accurate, safe, and effective technique that can be utilized to guide endovascular interventions in patients with baseline CKD[49].

We report our technique as initially described by Cho et al.[50]

- Use any shape of distal catheter bend and any size of catheter. An end-hole catheter can be used for both CO_2 infrarenal aortography and vena cavography.
- Use the plastic bag system, CO2mmander with AngiAssist (AngioAdvancements, FL, USA), or the handheld syringe method for CO_2 delivery to prevent explosive gas delivery and air contamination.
- Connect the catheter directly to the CO2mmander through the sterile bag. The CO_2 cartridge should have been attached to the CO2mmander prior to procedure.
- Close the stopcock of the CO_2-filled handheld syringe until injection to prevent air contamination.
- Purge the catheter with 5 mL of CO_2 immediately prior to a CO_2 angiogram to prevent explosive gas delivery.
- Increase CO_2 volumes to improve CO_2 imaging quality.
- Separate CO_2 injections by 2–3 min.
- Elevate the area of interest (15° for the lower extremity imaging and 45° for renal artery imaging).
- Inject 100 mg of nitroglycerin intraarterially prior to a lower extremity CO_2 arteriogram.
- Perform selective injection when imaging a dilated, tortuous artery.
- Use the CO_2 reflux technique for better imaging the iliac and femoral arteries with CO_2 injection into the SFA.
- If motion is a problem for CO_2 imaging, use rapid exposure (4–7.5 frames/sec) with additional mask images for better subtraction, pixel shifting, and image stacking.

Complications related to CO_2 use for angiography are uncommon. Air contamination of the CO_2 delivery system, injection of gases other than CO_2, delivery of excessive volume of CO_2, and neurotoxicity related to an inadvertent injection of CO_2 into the cerebral circulation are some adverse effects related to the use of CO_2. CO_2 angiography should be limited to imaging under the diaphragm.

POSTPROCEDURE MANAGEMENT AND RECOVERY

After common femoral artery catheterization, the patient lays flat for 1–3 h if there is successful deployment of closure device. Following that, the patient is allowed to elevate the head of the bed to 30 degrees and then 45 degrees for 30 min each. The patient is allowed to ambulate after 2 h. The groin site is inspected at each interval for hematomas. If any are detected, the patient is laid flat and manual compression is applied for at least 15 min. The cycle is repeated after obtaining hemostasis. Any further concerns for pseudoaneurysm should be evaluated with an arterial duplex ultrasound.

Radial access patients can ambulate as soon as able to walk with compression device on radial artery puncture site. In our practice, we utilize a pneumatic wrist compression device that is sequentially deflated at 15 min intervals while inspecting puncture site for hemostasis.

Patients with pedal access are positioned with head of the bed at 45 degrees and are kept on bed rest for 2 h.

Early mobilization is safe after angioplasty procedure, and up to 90% of patients are able to walk after 4 h of procedure.[51] Groin checks and Doppler ultrasound of ankle arteries in both feet are performed every 15 min for the first hour and then every 30 min until discharge. The amount of observation time will depend on the size of the sheath and complexity of the case. For 4F sheath a 2 h observation time is safe according to an early report from Millward et al.[52] For 5F sheath we recommend a 4-h observation time following report of Kraus et al.[53] For larger sheaths, we recommend arbitrary observation time depending on the complexity of case and risk factors for complications.

COMPLICATIONS

The complications as a result of the procedure can be prevented but not completely eliminated by using proper selection criteria. When the patients are selected appropriately the complication rate in general will be the same as in inpatient setting.

CONCLUSIONS

Lower extremity arterial interventions can be safely performed in the office-based laboratory. There are a variety of techniques that can be used to revascularize patients with lower extremity ischemia including angioplasty, stenting, and atherectomy. Alternative access points such as radial, popliteal, and pedal arteries can be used to avoid the need for femoral puncture in many cases and carbon dioxide is a valuable adjunct in patients with contrast allergies or CKD. Complications in the OEC can be mitigated by selecting the correct patient, using proper technique, ultrasound guidance for access and appropriate postprocedural monitoring. Overall, the management of lower extremity arterial revascularization in the OEC is efficient, effective, and safe.

REFERENCES

1. Albert B, Davaine JM, Chaillet MP, et al. Clinical and economic evaluation of ambulatory endovascular treatment of peripheral arterial occlusive lesions. *Ann Vasc Surg.* 2014. https://doi.org/10.1016/j.avsg.2013.06.008.
2. Safety T. The safety and efficacy of peripheral vascular procedures performed in the outpatient setting. *J Invasive Cardiol.* 2019:1–9.
3. Peterson ED, Patel MR, Curtis LH. Trends in settings for peripheral vascular intervention and the effect of changes in the outpatient prospective payment system. *J Am Coll Cardiol.* 2015;65(9). https://doi.org/10.1016/j.jacc.2014.12.048.
4. Jones WS, Mi X, Qualls LG, et al. Trends in settings for peripheral vascular intervention and the effect of changes in the outpatient prospective payment system. *J Am Coll Cardiol.* 2015. https://doi.org/10.1016/j.jacc.2014.12.048.
5. Turley RS, Mi X, Qualls LG, et al. The effect of clinical care location on clinical outcomes after peripheral vascular intervention in medicare beneficiaries. *JACC Cardiovasc Interv.* 2017;10(11). https://doi.org/10.1016/j.jcin.2017.03.033.
6. Parvar SL, Fitridge R, Dawson J, Nicholls SJ. Medical and lifestyle management of peripheral arterial disease. *J Vasc Surg.* 2018;68(5):1595–1606. https://doi.org/10.1016/j.jvs.2018.07.027.
7. Noori VJ, Eldrup-Jørgensen J. A systematic review of vascular closure devices for femoral artery puncture sites. *J Vasc Surg.* 2018;68(3):887–899. https://doi.org/10.1016/j.jvs.2018.05.019.
8. Hon LQ, Ganeshan A, Thomas SM, Warakaulle D, Jagdish J, Uberoi R. An overview of vascular closure devices: what every radiologist should know. *Eur J Radiol.* 2010;73(1):181–190. https://doi.org/10.1016/j.ejrad.2008.09.023.
9. Sheth RA, Ganguli S. Closure of alternative vascular sites, including axillary, brachial, popliteal, and surgical grafts. *Tech Vasc Interv Radiol.* 2015;18(2):113–121. https://doi.org/10.1053/j.tvir.2015.04.009.
10. Seto AH, Abu-Fadel MS, Sparling JM, et al. Real-time ultrasound guidance facilitates femoral arterial access and reduces vascular complications: FAUST (Femoral Arterial Access with Ultrasound Trial). *JACC Cardiovasc Interv.* 2010;3(7):751–758. https://doi.org/10.1016/j.jcin.2010.04.015.
11. Vatakencherry G, Gandhi R, Molloy C. Endovascular access for challenging. *Tech Vasc Interv Radiol.* 2016;19(2):113–122. https://doi.org/10.1053/j.tvir.2016.04.004.
12. Kang WY, Campia U, Ota H, et al. Vascular access in critical limb ischemia. *Cardiovasc Revasc Med.* 2016;17(3):190–198. https://doi.org/10.1016/j.carrev.2016.02.001.
13. Jolly SS, Yusuf S, Cairns J, et al. Radial versus femoral access for coronary angiography and intervention in patients with acute coronary syndromes (RIVAL): a randomised, parallel group, multicentre trial. *Lancet.* 2011;377(9775):1409–1420. https://doi.org/10.1016/S0140-6736(11)60404-2.
14. Michael TT, Alomar M, Papayannis A, et al. A randomized comparison of the transradial and transfemoral approaches for coronary artery bypass graft angiography and intervention: the RADIAL-CABG Trial (RADIAL versus femoral access for coronary artery bypass graft angiography and intervention). *JACC Cardiovasc Interv.* 2013;6(11):1138–1144. https://doi.org/10.1016/j.jcin.2013.08.004.
15. Kumar AJ, Jones LE, Kollmeyer KR, et al. Radial artery access for peripheral endovascular procedures. *J Vasc Surg.* 2017;66(3):820–825. https://doi.org/10.1016/j.jvs.2017.03.430.
16. Sanghvi K, Kurian D, Coppola J. Transradial intervention of iliac and superficial femoral artery disease is feasible. *J Interv Cardiol.* 2008;21(5):385–387. https://doi.org/10.1111/j.1540-8183.2008.00384.x.
17. Patel T, Shah S, Pancholy S. Transradial bilateral common iliac ostial stenting using simultaneous hugging stent (SHS) technique. *Cardiovasc Revasc Med.* 2016;17(3):202–205. https://doi.org/10.1016/j.carrev.2015.12.009.
18. Aminian A, Dolatabadi D, Lefebvre P, et al. Initial experience with the glidesheath slender for transradial coronary angiography and intervention: a feasibility study with prospective radial ultrasound follow-up. *Catheter Cardiovasc*

Interv. 2014;84(3):436–442. https://doi.org/10.1002/ccd.25232.
19. Aminian A, Saito S, Takahashi A, et al. Impact of sheath size and hemostasis time on radial artery patency after transradial coronary angiography and intervention in Japanese and non-Japanese patients: a substudy from RAP and BEAT (Radial Artery Patency and Bleeding, Efficacy, Adverse evenT) randomized multicenter trial. *Catheter Cardiovasc Interv.* 2018;92(5):844–851. https://doi.org/10.1002/ccd.27526.
20. Jaff MR, White CJ, Hiatt WR, et al. Special article an update on methods for revascularization and expansion of the TASC lesion classification to include below-the-knee arteries : a supplement to the inter-society consensus for the management of peripheral arterial disease (TASC II) Ann Vasc Dis. doi:10.1002/ccd.26122.
21. Dumantepe M. Retrograde popliteal access to percutaneous peripheral intervention for chronic total occlusion of superficial femoral arteries. *Vasc Endovascular Surg.* 2017;51(5):240–246. https://doi.org/10.1177/1538574417698902.
22. Silvestro M, Palena M, Manzi M, Gómez-jabalera E. Anterolateral retrograde access to the distal popliteal artery and to the tibioperoneal trunk for recanalization of femoropopliteal chronic total occlusions. *J Vasc Surg.* 1824;68(6): 1824–1832. https://doi.org/10.1016/j.jvs.2018.05.231.
23. Komshian S, Cheng TW, Farber A, Schermerhorn ML. Retrograde popliteal access to treat femoropopliteal artery occlusive disease. J Vasc Surg. 68(1):161-167. doi: 10.1016/j.jvs.2017.12.022.
24. Montero-baker M, Schmidt A, Bra S, Botsios S, Bausback Y, Scheinert D. Retrograde approach for complex popliteal and tibioperoneal occlusions. *J Endovasc Ther.* 2008:594–604.
25. Hua WR. Popliteal versus tibial retrograde access for subintimal arterial flossing with antegrade e retrograde intervention (SAFARI) technique. *Eur J Vasc Endovasc Surg.* 2013. https://doi.org/10.1016/j.ejvs.2013.05.007.
26. Marmagkiolis K, Sardar P, Mustapha JA, et al. Transpedal access for the management of complex peripheral artery disease. *J Invasive Cardiol.* 2017.
27. Lai SH, Fenlon J, Roush BB, et al. Analysis of the retrograde tibial artery approach in lower extremity revascularization in an office endovascular center. *J Vasc Surg.* 2019:1–9. https://doi.org/10.1016/j.jvs.2018.10.114.
28. Gandini R, Pipitone V, Stefanini M, et al. The "Safari" technique to perform difficult subintimal infragenicular vessels. *Cardiovasc Intervent Radiol.* 2007. https://doi.org/10.1007/s00270-006-0099-3.
29. Chou HH, Huang HL, Hsieh CA, et al. Outcomes of endovascular therapy with the controlled antegrade retrograde subintimal tracking (CART) or reverse CART technique for long infrainguinal occlusions. *J Endovasc Ther.* 2016. https://doi.org/10.1177/1526602816630533.
30. Mustapha JA, Saab F, McGoff T, et al. Tibio-pedal arterial minimally invasive retrograde revascularization in patients with advanced peripheral vascular disease: the TAMI technique, original case series. *Catheter Cardiovasc Interv.* 2014; 83(6):987–994. https://doi.org/10.1002/ccd.25227.
31. Souza SMD, Stout CL, Krol E, et al. Outpatient endovascular tibial artery intervention in an office-based setting is as safe and effective as in a hospital setting. *J Endovasc Ther.* 2018. https://doi.org/10.1177/1526602818806691.
32. Cejna M. Cutting balloon: review on principles and background of use in peripheral arteries. *Cardiovasc Intervent Radiol.* 2005. https://doi.org/10.1007/s00270-004-0115-4.
33. Amighi J, Cejna M, Schlager O, et al. De novo superficial femoropopliteal artery lesions: peripheral cutting balloon angioplasty and restenosis rates—randomized controlled trial. *Radiology.* 2008. https://doi.org/10.1148/radiol.2471070749.
34. Hansrani M, Overbeck K, Smout JJ, Stansby GP. Intravascular brachytherapy for peripheral vascular disease. *Cochrane Database Syst Rev.* 2003;1:2–4. https://doi.org/10.1002/14651858.cd003504.
35. Waksman R, Pakala R, Lemesle G, Bonello L, De Labriolle A, Scheinowitz M. Paclitaxel-eluting balloon: from bench to bed. *Catheter Cardiovasc Interv.* 2008. https://doi.org/10.1002/ccd.21895.
36. Diehm NA, Hoppe H, Do DD. Drug eluting balloons. *Tech Vasc Interv Radiol.* 2010;13(1):59–63. https://doi.org/10.1053/j.tvir.2009.10.008.
37. Katsanos K, Spiliopoulos S, Kitrou P, Krokidis M, Karnabatidis D. Risk of death following application of paclitaxel-coated balloons and stents in the femoropopliteal artery of the leg: a systematic review and meta-analysis of randomized controlled trials. *J Am Heart Assoc.* 2018;7(24). https://doi.org/10.1161/JAHA.118.011245.
38. Katsanos K, Spiliopoulos S, Reppas L. Debulking atherectomy in the peripheral arteries: is there a role and what is the evidence? *Cardiovasc Intervent Radiol.* 2017: 964–977. https://doi.org/10.1007/s00270-017-1649-6.
39. Ambler GK, Radwan R, Hayes PD, Twine CP. Atherectomy for peripheral arterial disease. *Cochrane Database Syst Rev.* 2014;2014(3). https://doi.org/10.1002/14651858.CD006680.pub2LK. http://vh5ge7rw9u.search.&stitle=Cochrane+Database+Syst.+Rev.&title=Cochrane+Database+of+Systematic+Reviews&volume=2014serialssolutions.com?sid=EMBASE&sid=EMBASE&issn=1469493X&id=doi:10.1002%2F14651858.CD006680.pub2&atitle=Atherectomy+for+peripheral+arterial+disease&issue=3&spage=&epage=&aulast=Ambler&aufirst=Graeme+K.&auinit=G.K.&aufull=Ambler+G.K.&coden=&isbn=&pages=-&date=2014&auinit1=G&auinitm=K.
40. Mukherjee D, Hashemi H, Contos B. The disproportionate growth of office-based atherectomy. *J Vasc Surg.* 2011. https://doi.org/10.1016/j.jvs.2016.08.112.
40a. Lai SH, Roush BB, Fenlon J, Munn J, Rummel M, Johnston D, Longton C, Bauler LD, Jain KMJ. Outcomes of atherectomy for lower extremity ischemia in an office endovascular center. *Vasc Surg.* 2019 Sep 10;(19):31794-X. https://doi.org/10.1016/j.jvs.2019.06.198. pii: S0741-5214 [Epub ahead of print].
41. Roffi M, Mukherjee D. Current role of emboli protection devices in percutaneous coronary and vascular interventions. *Am Heart J.* 2009;157(2):263–270. https://doi.org/10.1016/j.ahj.2008.09.008.

42. Hofmann M, Hockings A, Sieunarine K, Mwipatayi BP, Garbowski M. Balloon angioplasty compared with stenting for treatment of femoropopliteal occlusive disease: a meta-analysis. *J Vasc Surg.* 2007;47(2):461–469. https://doi.org/10.1016/j.jvs.2007.07.059.
43. Chowdhury MM, McLain AD, Twine CP. Angioplasty versus bare metal stenting for superficial femoral artery lesions. *Cochrane Database Syst Rev.* 2014;2014(6). https://doi.org/10.1002/14651858.CD006767.pub3 LK. http://vh5ge7rw9u.search.serialssolutions.com?sid=EMBASE&sid=EMBASE&issn=1469493X&id=doi:10.1002%2F14651858CD006767.pub3&atitle=Angioplasty+versus+bare+metal+stenting+for+superficial+femoral+artery+lesions&stitle=Cochrane+Database+Syst.+Rev.&title=Cochrane+Database+of+Systematic+Reviews&volume=2014&issue=6&spage=&epage=&aulast=Chowdhury&aufirst=Mohammed+M.&auinit=M.M.&aufull=Chowdhury+M.M.&coden=&isbn=&pages=-&date=2014&auinit1=M&auinitm=M.
44. Cai L, Ding Y, Shi Z, Wang Y, Zhou M. Comparison of drug-eluting stent with bare-metal stent implantation in femoropopliteal artery disease: a systematic review and meta-analysis. *Ann Vasc Surg.* 2018;50(March):96–105. https://doi.org/10.1016/j.avsg.2017.12.003.
45. Huang ZS, Schneider DB. Endovascular intervention for tibial artery occlusive disease in patients with critical limb ischemia. *Semin Vasc Surg.* 2014;27(1):38–58. https://doi.org/10.1053/j.semvascsurg.2014.12.003.
46. Ndrepepa G, King L, Cassese S, et al. Drug-eluting stents for revascularization of infrapopliteal arteries. *JACC Cardiovasc Interv.* 2013;6(12):1284–1293. https://doi.org/10.1016/j.jcin.2013.08.007.
47. Rana MA, Gloviczki P. Endovascular interventions for infrapopliteal arterial disease: an update. *Semin Vasc Surg.* 2012;25(1):29–34. https://doi.org/10.1053/j.semvascsurg.2012.03.003.
48. Fujihara M, Kawasaki D, Shintani Y, et al. Endovascular therapy by CO2 angiography to prevent contrast-induced nephropathy in patients with chronic kidney disease: a prospective multicenter trial of CO2 angiography registry. *Catheter Cardiovasc Interv.* 2015. https://doi.org/10.1002/ccd.25722.
49. Palena LM, Diaz-Sandoval LJ, Candeo A, Brigato C, Sultato E, Manzi M. Automated carbon dioxide angiography for the evaluation and endovascular treatment of diabetic patients with critical limb ischemia. *J Endovasc Ther.* 2016. https://doi.org/10.1177/1526602815616924.
50. Cho KJ. Carbon dioxide angiography: scientific principles and practice. *Vasc Spec Int.* 2015. https://doi.org/10.5758/vsi.2015.31.3.67.
51. Butterfield JS, Fitzgerald JB, Razzaq R, et al. Early mobilization following angioplasty. *Clin Radiol.* 2000. https://doi.org/10.1053/crad.2000.0595.
52. Millward SF, Marsh JI, Peterson RA. Outpatient transfemoral angiography with a two-hour observation period. *Cardiovasc Intervent Radiol.* 1989. https://doi.org/10.1007/BF02575419.
53. Kruse JR, Cragg AH. Safety of short stay observation after peripheral vascular intervention. *J Vasc Interv Radiol.* 2000:3–5.

CHAPTER 32

Management of Dialysis Access

AZHER IQBAL, MD • ASAD BAIG, MD

INTRODUCTION

As an internal medicine physician in 1966, James E. Cimino had patients who needed dialysis, and at the time, the Scribner shunt was being used. It was a Teflon tube inserted in an artery and a vein. The shunt would last for only a few days to a few weeks. Cimino thought back to his days at Bellevue hospital in New York City in the 1950s where he worked as a phlebotomist. He remembered how easy it was to repeatedly get vascular access in patients who had fought in the Korean War and had traumatic arteriovenous fistula (AVF). Cimino convinced Dr Kenneth Appell to try to create a fistula in a chronic kidney disease patient to achieve the same effect. The first Cimino fistula was born, later renamed to AVF. Cimino, Appell, and Brescia successfully created the first AVF and used it for hemodialysis. This set the standard in dialysis care.[1–4]

KEY DEFINITIONS OF VASCULAR ACCESS

In patients with the need for long-term vascular access, there are two major types of permanent access: AVF and arteriovenous graft (AVG). Tunneled central venous catheters (TCVCs) can be used for temporary access while the AVF or AVG matures. As the name suggests, an AVF is an arteriovenous access created by connecting an autologous artery and vein (e.g., radial artery linked to cephalic vein) where the vein serves as the accessible conduit. An AVG is similar to an AVF but it is an artificial prosthetic segment that connects a vein to an artery. The purpose of both AVF and AVG is to provide stable access for dialysis patients to receive their repeated high-pressure blood exchange dialysis for a long period of time.[5]

COMMON LOCATIONS OF VASCULAR ACCESS

The location of AVF/AVG is important. The ideal locations for vascular access is in the forearm; radial artery to cephalic vein fistula or less commonly ulnar artery to basilic vein fistula.[1,6] In the upper arm a brachial-cephalic, brachial-antecubital vein, or brachial-transposed basilic vein fistula can be created. The AVG can be created in the forearm or upper arm using brachial artery and one of the outflow veins. Patients with failed permanent vascular access in the upper extremity can either switch to peritoneal dialysis or have arterial venous access in the lower extremity.[7]

Lower extremity vascular access is not the ideal option, and physicians are reluctant to pursue it for several reasons, including patient preference, lack of available surgical expertise, fear of complications, inadequate information in nephrology literature, and limited knowledge/familiarity among dialysis providers. Several patient factors, such as diabetes, peripheral arterial disease, and/or morbid obesity, make planning and selecting a site in lower extremity access difficult.[8] If neither upper nor lower extremity is amenable for long-term permanent vascular access through AVF/AVG, a femoral TCVC may be considered as a last resort option.[8] Axillar artery and vein can also be used to create AVG access.

The right internal jugular vein is the preferred site for TCVC followed by the subclavian vein, which is an option that is not frequently used or preferred.[6] As the access site matures, TCVC should be avoided being placed on the same side of a maturing venous access.[6] Additionally, multiple TCVC placement can cause potential loss of upper extremity access sites because of endothelial injury and central vein stenosis.[1] If necessary, femoral dialysis catheters can be placed; however, they should not be placed on the same side as a future renal transplant.[6]

AVF VERSUS AVG

AVF vascular access is preferred to AVG because of its superior long-term patency and morbidity/mortality outcomes as compared with a synthetic AVG or a tunneled central venous catheter (CVC). AVF is considered the

Office-Based Endovascular Centers. https://doi.org/10.1016/B978-0-323-67969-5.00032-0
Copyright © 2020 Elsevier Inc. All rights reserved.

preferred type of vascular access in hemodialysis patients.[9] Once they have matured sufficiently to be cannulated for hemodialysis, AVFs have secondary patency that is superior to that of AVGs, and require less frequent interventions to maintain long-term patency.[10] Timely creation of AVFs has been shown to reduce the mortality rate by 1.72 times.[11,12] Early evaluation of patients with CKD for an AVF placement and avoidance of initiation of hemodialysis with a CVC to reduce morbidity, mortality, and healthcare costs is recommended as per the guidelines set by several national renal societies.[9,13]

PROBLEMS WITH VASCULAR ACCESS

Among end stage renal disease patients, vascular access dysfunction is one of the leading causes of morbidity and mortality.[11,12] The complications include postdialysis hemorrhage, low venous flow or hematoma, infections, the development of an aneurysm and/or pseudoaneurysm, stenosis, congestive heart failure, steal syndrome, ischemic neuropathy, and thrombosis.[8,12] Lack of maturation is an additional cause of vascular access dysfunction. Some of these causes and their treatment will be discussed.

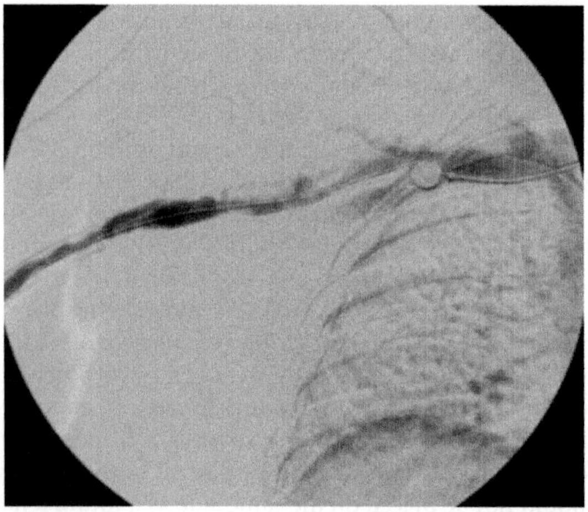

Right upper extremity Angiogram/Fistulogram demonstrating multiple areas of stenoses.

STENOSIS

Hemodynamically significant stenosis is defined as >50% reduction of normal AVF or AVG diameter with one or more clinical, functional, or hemodynamic abnormality, not explained by other reasons.[14] Various surveillance measures used to diagnose the stenosis include abnormal duplex ultrasound, decreased blood flow (blood pump or intra-access flow), elevated venous pressure, elevated negative arterial pressures that prevent acceptable blood flow, unexplained decreases in hemodialysis efficacy, and elevated access recirculation.

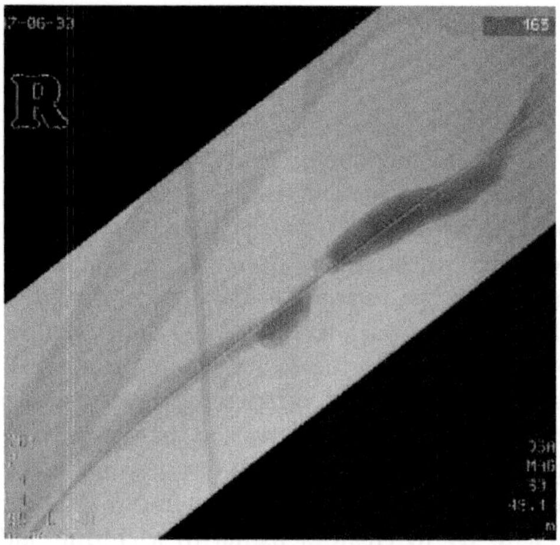

Right upper extremity Fistulogram demonstrating a focal area of stenosis.

Signs and symptoms of AVF or AVG stenosis include prolonged bleeding after needle withdrawal, altered pulse or thrill in the fistula or graft, altered bruit in the fistula or graft, and persistent extremity swelling.[15]

An intervention should not be performed on patients with only a reduction in diameter measurement. Clinical correlation is required. It is suggested that one or more signs/symptoms and one or more abnormal surveillance measures should be present for stenosis to be considered hemodynamically significant.[8]

THROMBOSIS

A complete absence of a bruit or thrill on palpation and auscultation at least 8 cm proximal to the arteriovenous anastomosis is considered to signify complete thrombosis.[14] A complete access thrombosis is indicative of loss of clinical, hemodynamic, and anatomic patency. A weak thrill or bruit may be identified in access with nonocclusive/incomplete thrombosis, especially if clots are observed at the time of cannulation. If patency cannot be restored and the access can no longer be used for dialysis following mechanical or chemical thrombectomy/thrombolysis, it is considered terminal access thrombosis.[8]

LACK OF MATURATION

In the literature there is variability regarding the definition of a functional AVF. If an AVF can be used with two-needle cannulation for two-thirds or more of all dialysis runs for 1 month and an average blood flow rate (total blood processed over duration of hemodialysis) of 300 mL/min in a 3.5-hour hemodialysis session or 250 mL/min overnight during a 7-hour hemodialysis session, it is safe to say the AVF is successful. The same criteria can be applied to AVG.[8,14–16] It is assumed that the healthcare providers cannulating the vein are experts. If an inexperienced operator attempts to cannulate and the fistula does not appear to function properly, it may or may not be because of poor fistula maturation. Because of this reason, it is recommended that the first time an AVF or AVG is accessed, it should be done by an experienced technician using the appropriate blood pump rate and needle size.

Within approximately 3 days of AVF or AVG creation, if there is no bruit or thrill, this may be due to technical causes, such as an intraprocedural thrombosis, small vein or artery, angulation of the vein, undiagnosed venous intimal disease, poor technique, etc. Immediate loss of access in this timeframe may also be due to iatrogenic causes, for example, emergent ligation of and AVF or AVG due to steal syndrome.[8]

Early failure is classified as failure of an AVF or AVG to be used successfully for dialysis by 3 months following its creation despite radiological or surgical intervention. Early failure is usually due to stenosis or presence of accessory or collateral veins. For this reason, accesses should not be deemed a failure unless endovascular or open surgical techniques have failed to correct these problems. A high success rate for use for dialysis has been reported following intervention.[17]

Late failure describes unsuccessful dialysis for 6 months following vascular access procedure despite intervention.[15] The descriptions as described above pertain to new fistulas and those used for new cannulation.

INFECTION

As mentioned previously, AVF is preferred to AVG. One of the reasons is the significant difference in infection rates. AVG is 10 times more likely to get infected than AVF. Infection accounts for approximately 20% of all AVF complications.[18,19] Peri-fistula cellulitis, which may manifest as localized erythema and edema can be treated using antibiotics. Much more serious is an infection associated with anatomical abnormalities, such as aneurysms, hematomas, or abscesses, which require surgical excision and drainage.[20] If the access is infected, clinical signs of inflammation are present at the vascular access puncture site (pain, erythema, swelling, heat, etc.) with or without systemic manifestations. Localized infections occurring at AVF access sites are treated with appropriate antibiotics based on the results of swab and blood cultures. AVF infections are rare and, in most cases, respond well to antibiotic treatment, lasting 4–6 weeks. A ligature and excision of the AVF is required only when it becomes a source of recurrent septic pulmonary embolism.[18–20] If the AVG gets infected it may need to be surgically removed if local treatment and systemic antibiotic treatment fails. The whole graft should be removed and artery reconstructed.

INDICATIONS FOR PROCEDURE

After vascular access is created, it must be monitored routinely. As mentioned previously, monthly physical exams, quantitative measurement of flow within the vascular access with duplex ultrasound, and/or static venous dialysis pressures should be routinely performed.

Patients should be referred for evaluation and treatment of vascular access when flow rates fall below 400–500 mL/min in fistulas or below 600 mL/min in grafts, the static venous dialysis pressure to mean arterial pressure ratio is greater than 0.5, the arterial dialysis pressure to mean arterial pressure ratio is greater than 0.75, or if any other abnormal trends are noted during routine surveillance.[2] Additionally, if there is, thrombosis, increased venous pressures, increased bleeding postdialysis aneurysms/pseudoaneurysms formation, low clearance during dialysis, extremity swelling, or arterial steal, the patient should be evaluated by an interventionalist. The dialysis unit should routinely monitor the patient's access and refer the patient when indicated (Fig. 32.1).

THE ROLE OF ULTRASOUND

The selection of vessels to be used for constructing an AVF at one time was based exclusively on physical examination of the upper limbs; however, the literature has demonstrated that physical examination alone is insufficient.[21–23] Ultrasound, which is noninvasive, repeatable, and safe, offers real-time dynamic information and visualization of anatomy as well as blood flow in the deep and superficial veins and the arteries. The physician performing the procedure should utilize ultrasound guidance to his/her advantage in preparation for the procedure. International guidelines recommend the use of ultrasound in all patients who are candidates

Access Referral Form

Date______________________ DOB: _______________

Patient Name: _________________________________

Weight: ___________________

Phone #:___________________________

Dialysis Days: ☐ Monday, Wednesday, Friday or Tuesday, Thursday, Saturday

Dialysis Time: _________ Last dialysis Treatment. Date: _______________

Dialysis Facility: ☐

Access Type: ☐ Right ☐ Left ☐ Graft ☐ Fistula ☐ Catheter ☐ Permanent Catheter

Access Flows:

Previous Result Date: ____________

Access Flow Rate: ______________________

Current Result Date: _____________

Access Flow Rate: _______________________

Access Problem: ☐ Clotted ☐ Poor Flows ☐ Infection ☐ Increase Venous Pressure

☐ KT/V<1.4 or URR <60 ☐ Cannulation difficulty ☐ Pain ☐ Prolonged bleeding

Referral Indication: At least 1 item **MUST** be checked

- ☐ Elevated Venous Pressure >200mmHg on a 200cc/min pump
- ☐ Elevated recirculation time of 12% or greater
- ☐ Low Urea Reduction Rate (URR) <60%
- ☐ An access with a palpable highly pulsatile thrill or "water hammer" pulse on exam (indicates outflow stenosis)

Explanation:

____

____

____

____

Urgency: ☐ Hyperkalemia ☐ Fluid overload ☐ Other (explain) (call office with any urgent needs)

____

____

____

Nephrologist: ___________________________________

RN Name/Signature: ________________________________

FIG. 32.1 Outpatient Vascular Access Referral Form.

for an AVF.[21,24] If an AVF does not appear to be mature based on physical examination, the ultrasound examination and assessment of hemodynamic parameters can help determine the suitability for cannulation. It can also help determine if the AVF has failed to mature or has a low flow.[25] In certain patients, well-developed vein can be difficult to visualize or palpate because of the depth of the vein. In these cases, ultrasound can determine the maturity of fistula. US mapping of the outflow veins can facilitate the first cannulation and simplify subsequent punctures.[26] "The rule of 6's" may provide some clarification regarding whether a fistula is ready for use/mature; an outflow vein diameter of $\geq$6 mm, an outflow vein depth of $\leq$6 mm below the skin surface, and a flow volume of >600 mL/min.[9,27] If the vein is very deep, it may need to be surgically elevated.

INDWELLING AND TEMPORARY DIALYSIS CATHETERS

In patients who need acute dialysis, a nontunneled hemodialysis catheter (NTHC) or tunneled central venous catheter (TCVC) may be placed.[28] Common locations for NTHC include the internal jugular vein, subclavian vein, or less preferred, femoral vein. TCVC is inserted in the right or left internal jugular veins. NTHC is usually used in acute settings where a patient needs it for lifesaving dialysis. TCVC, while also temporary, can be used for longer period of time, and may be placed if a patient requires dialysis while the AVF is maturing. If a TCVC is placed, it should be placed on the opposite side of the AVF or planned AVF.[29] Both NTHC and TCVC have associated complications. Bleeding, catheter-related infections/central line–associated bloodstream infection, cardiac arrhythmias, and central venous stenosis are complications associated with NTHC.[30–33] TCVC patients may experience prolonged bleeding/oozing at the insertion site. Patients should be made to sit upright and pressure should be held at the site. Occasionally, the patient may require admission to the hospital and administration of desmopressin (DDAVP).[34] Another risk is infection, although at a lower rate than with NTHC.[31–33] Catheters should be locked with heparin or sodium citrate solutions.[35]

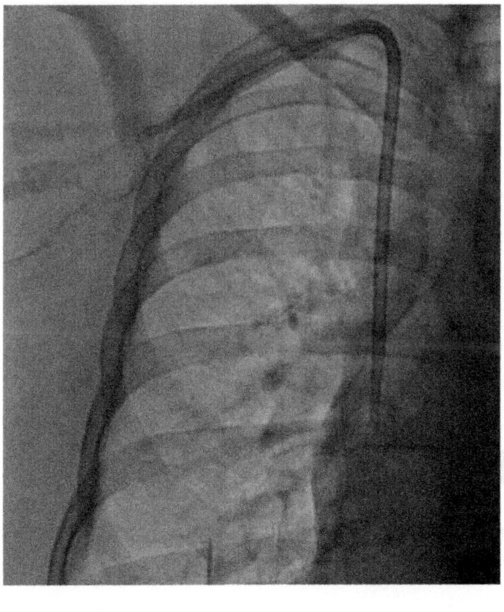

Tunneled central venous hemodialysis cathether in the right internal jugular vein terminating at the atrial/caval junction.

In the OEC, the catheters should always be inserted using ultrasound guidance. Since the procedure is carried out under fluoroscopy a chest X-ray at the end of the procedure is not required. The tip of the catheter should be appropriately placed. Right internal jugular vein is the ideal access site. If the thrombectomy procedure for a clotted AVF or AVG is unsuccessful in an OEC, a catheter can be inserted at the same time so that the patient does not miss dialysis. If the creation of new access is going to be delayed a tunneled catheter should be inserted.

MANAGEMENT OF CENTRAL VEIN STENOSIS

Increased venous curvature/tortuosity may result in increased contact between the catheter and the vein wall. It is suggested that this is the reason that catheters in right subclavian and internal jugular veins may carry less risk of stenosis compared with left-sided ones.[30] There is a strong association of central venous stenosis with pacemaker wires and previous central catheter placement, especially in the subclavian veins.[36–41] Patients with central vein stenosis may be asymptomatic, or may display venous hypertension and/or edema in the corresponding breast and/or extremity if the stenosis occurs in the subclavian vein. There may also be erythema, tenderness, pain, and/or swelling, which may lead clinicians to think of cellulitis.[42] Patients may also experience vascular access dysfunction or may present with superior vena cava syndrome, which requires emergent treatment. On ultrasound, there will be polyphasic arterial waves as well as absence of normal respiratory variation in the diameter of central veins.[43–45]

Treatment options for central vein stenosis include bare metal stent (BMS) placement and percutaneous transluminal angioplasty (PTA), with PTA being the initial recommended intervention.[46] One of the drawbacks of PTA is that it requires repeated interventions.[42] BMS may be used at sites that do not respond well to PTA. They function well with elastic stenosis post PTA, kinked stenosis, and maintaining patency of chronic central venous stenosis. BMSs do have the potential to shorten, migrate, or fracture on a subacute or delayed basis and placing a BMS may threaten future endovascular procedures or surgical revision. Additionally, BMS incite intimal hyperplasia, leading to recurrent stenosis resulting in multiple repeat interventions to maintain patency.[47] The use of BMS has increased greatly in recent years, leading the Society of Interventional Radiology to recommend BMS be reserved for central vein lesions in which PTA has failed, that recur within 3 months after initially successful PTA or to treat rupture after PTA.[48]

TREATMENT OF MALFUNCTIONING DIALYSIS ACCESS

Angiogram (fistulogram) is performed prior to intervention. The access vein or graft is accessed and contrast is injected to evaluate the vasculature from the created vascular anastomosis to the right atrium-superior vena cava junction (hemodialysis vascular access circuit). A fistulogram is performed to determine the patency of the hemodialysis vascular access circuit and the central veins. Any stenosis, aneurysms, pseudoaneurysm, collaterals, or large tributaries are identified. A digitally subtracted angiogram is the gold standard to evaluate the hemodialysis vascular access circuit. Recently, it has been demonstrated that in patients with advanced chronic kidney disease, not on hemodialysis, AVF can be evaluated and salvaged successfully using small contrast volumes with a low incidence of contrast-induced nephropathy.[49,50] Ultrasound-guided techniques can also be used (Chapter 15). Many times colloquially an angiogram may be referred to as a fistulogram even when imaging an AVG.[8] There is no indication for an angiogram/fistulogram if at least one of the clinical criteria is not met.

ANGIOPLASTY

Endovascular interventional techniques have been successful in treating stenosis within AVF and AVG.[51–55] Angioplasty is a minimally invasive procedure performed by interventionalists in the treatment of vascular access stenosis that improves function and prolongs survival in patients with shorter lesions (<1 cm). Even in longer segment stenosis, there is a high success rate in patients with failing fistulas that undergo angioplasty. If there is greater than 50% stenosis in AVG or venous limb of an AVF or at arterial venous stenosis, angioplasty should be performed. The commonest site of stenosis in an AVG is at the graft vein anastomosis. The entire hemodialysis vascular access circuit and the central veins should be visualized. Any significant stenosis should be subjected to angioplasty. The central venous stenosis may need angioplasty using high-pressure balloons. It is not uncommon to use pressure above 20 atm during angioplasty of the central vein stenosis. The treated lesions should have <30% residual stenosis.[6] Angioplasty may be used to assist in maturation of a poorly developing fistula. There are randomized single-center studies which demonstrate the benefit of drug-coated balloon angioplasty compared with non-drug-coated balloon angioplasty.[56–60] Another procedure that may be performed along with angioplasty is coil embolization of accessory veins.[61,62] Even with interventions, restenosis remains a potential problem. Collaboration between nephrologists, interventionalists, and surgeons is key to maintaining and prolonging function of the vascular access.[63–65]

STENTS

Studies have shown that the routine use of stents as a first-line treatment of either venous stenosis or recurrence of stenosis after angioplasty is unnecessarily costly.[66,67] After angioplasty, it is necessary to clinically monitor patients. If there is persistent >50% stenosis after angioplasty or if restenosis occurs within 3 months of angioplasty, stent placement should be considered.[6] Other indications for stent placement include angioplasty-induced venous rupture, and kinked outflow veins.[66] The stents can be either covered or non-covered BMSs.[5] Studies have shown that covered stents (CS) improve patency with little residual stenosis.[68] Conceptually, CS could provide a relatively inert and stable intravascular matrix for endothelialization while providing the mechanical advantages of a BMS.[42]

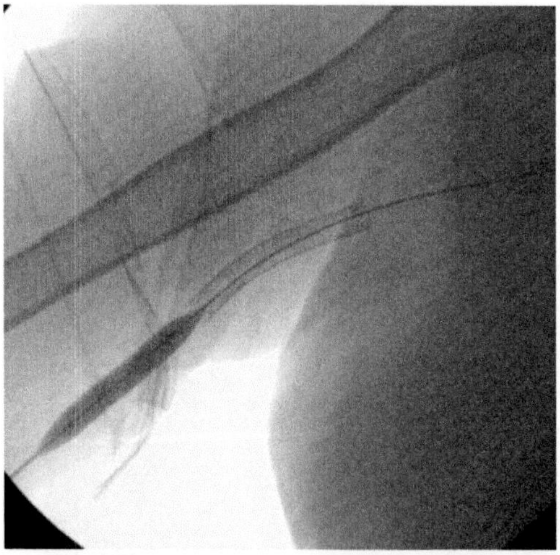

Balloon angioplasty and stenting of a long segment of stenosis in a right upper extremity AV fistula.

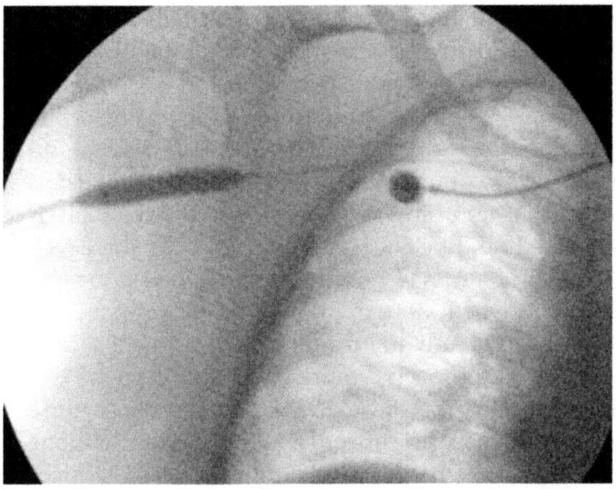

Balloon angioplasty of a stenosed right upper extremity AV fistula.

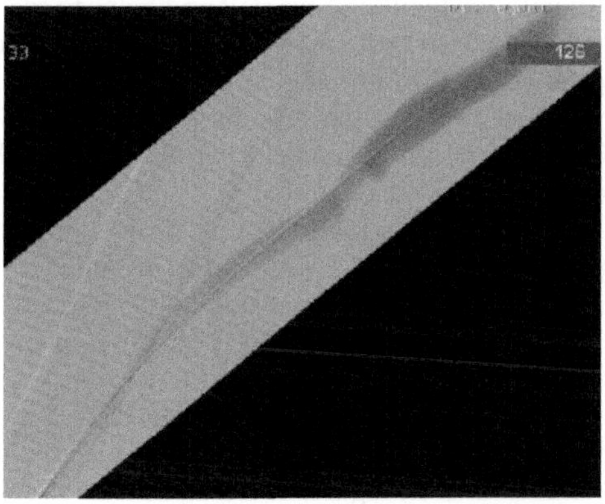

Status post balloon angioplasty of a focal area of stenosis in an AV fistula. Fistulogram demonstrates improvement in the stenosis, and increased patency and flow.

Stents coated with an antiproliferative agent represent the most significant advance in the treatment of venous neointimal hyperplasia. Studies have shown nearly a complete absence of stenosis in patients with coronary angioplasty using sirolimus-treated stents.[69,70]

CS are also used commonly in treating pseudoaneurysms that may occur due to repeated puncturing at the site of vascular access. These defects may threaten the viability and function of the AVF or AVG. After angiogram, a sheath is placed, and the diameter of the graft is measured using a calibrated guidewire. The approximate CS diameter and length are chosen by allowing approximately 15% oversizing for a good seal, and then the CS is deployed. The CS will exclude the aneurysm sac and treat any underlying stenosis.[71]

THROMBOLYSIS/THROMBECTOMY

When thrombosis is suspected based on clinical signs and symptoms, thrombolysis/thrombectomy should be considered. The options are pharmacologic thrombolysis, mechanical thrombectomy, and a combination of the two. In pharmacologic treatments, a thrombolytic agent is used to lyse the thrombus located at any level of the hemodialysis vascular circuit.[1] If thrombosis is detected, mechanical thrombectomy should be performed as early as possible.[2] Percutaneous mechanical thrombectomy by aspiration of thrombosed dialysis AVF or AVG with a vacuum-assisted thrombectomy catheter is a safe procedure with a low complication rate and effective method for restoring patency before hemodialysis.[37] Mechanical thrombectomy uses a mechanical device to fragment or macerate a thrombus located at any level of the hemodialysis vascular circuit.[1] The thrombectomy of an access can also be carried out cannulating the graft with 6 French sheaths twice. The sheaths should point toward each anastomosis. Fistulogram is performed to confirm thrombosis. Two milliliter of tissue plasminogen activator is instilled and left in place for 15 min. After that over the wire Fogarty catheter (Edwards lab, Irvine, CA) is used to carry out the thrombectomy. Angioplasty with or without stenting of underlying stenosis causing the thrombosis is invariably needed to keep the access functional.

EMBOLIZATION

If there is an AVF that is not maturing, one of the causes may be excessive outflow into the side branches. A treatment to help increase the probability of maturation is coil embolization of these side branches, thereby improving flow in the main vein. The embolization should be done carefully since these vessels are arterialized and the coils have the potential of embolization. Using embolization technique, coils are placed in the venous side branches, obliterating them. This method has been shown in studies to be a safe and effective treatment for a nonmaturing AVF.[72]

PRACTICAL APPLICATIONS IN AN OFFICE-BASED INTERVENTIONAL SUITE

Deficit reduction act of 2005 included the provision for CMS to reimburse for endovascular procedures in the office setting (Site 11). The endovascular procedures related to dialysis access were reimbursed by Medicare and Medicaid. This was the birth of office-based endovascular center also known as OBL. The migration of the procedures from the hospital setting to office has revolutionized the care of these patients. The timeliness of care for these patients is of utmost importance. Vascular access is the lifeline of hemodialysis patients. In an OEC, any failing access is managed in a timely manner before the access thromboses. It is much more difficult to carry out thrombectomy as compared to angioplasty. Using appropriate protocols for management of the access, the number of procedures carried out per access per year to keep it functional can be decreased. A study published by Jain et al. demonstrated decreasing intervention rate with the group performing 2.62 procedures per dialysis patient per year, followed by 2.16 procedures the following year, and 1.93 procedures 2 years after the study started.[73]

Thrombectomy of a dialysis access also known as declot procedure can be done on the same day as the day of thrombosis. The patient may not miss a dialysis day.

An indwelling dialysis catheter can be removed on the same day as the day when it is decided that the access is working well and catheter is not needed. This decreases the number of days the patient has a catheter which is a potential cause of infection. It also helps meet the kidney disease outcome quality initiative (KDOQI) guidelines. It was not unusual that the dialysis access–related cases were done in the middle of the night because that is the only time hospital operating rooms could accommodate these patients. Now the procedures get done between 8 a.m. and 5 p.m., which is good for the patient, patient's family, and the operator.

Patient's care in an office-based endovascular suite is streamlined and is timely, resulting high patient satisfaction. End stage renal disease patients spend many hours attached to dialysis machine multiple times a week, and they look forward to speedy resolution of AV access problems and return to their lives. Office-based interventional suite location and parking are generally more convenient as compared to a hospital complex. Risk of nosocomial infections is reduced by avoiding the hospital. In an office-based setting, same clinical staff takes care of patients from the moment they step in until the moment they are discharged providing smooth and easy transition. This allows for efficiency and return to hemodialysis unit on the same day for dialysis treatment. Patients feel welcome and become a part of an extended family or community. They receive education about maintenance and management of their AV access allowing them to become involved in their care. As a result, the patient will often call in seeking advice on a potential problem before it is picked up by the dialysis staff, thus becoming an important participant in their own AV access surveillance. It is very common to see patients becoming your best advocate to other fellow dialysis patients and their physicians about the quality of service that they have experienced.

Having a good relationship with the referring nephrologist is imperative. There should also be an open line of communication between the physicians and the dialysis unit. The nephrologist and the dialysis unit staff should be encouraged to call with any developing issues such as poorly maturing newly created AV fistula, patient developing ischemic hand pain due to arterial steal, and any concerns related to AV access.

Proactive approach requires that an AV access surveillance program is created. The practice charge nurse or a designee could be assigned to undertake telephone follow-up with hemodialysis unit on each patient treated, 8–12 weeks after the procedure, to make sure there are no access-related issues such as prolonged bleeding, reduced clearances, increased venous pressures, arterial steal, arm swelling, etc. This helps build a rapport with the hemodialysis staff and helps to identify access-related issues for early treatment thereby preventing AV access thrombosis. Central venous stenosis and specific stenosis such as cephalic vein genu/origin tend to recur at about 3-month interval; they usually require treatments in that time.

To run an efficient hemodialysis access program through the office-based endovascular center, it is important that the center designate one person as the access coordinator. This person, in a full-time or part-time capacity should keep track of all the accesses and catheters being managed by the center. The coordinator should also work closely with the dialysis center charge nurses and the nephrologists. The dialysis unit should be able to call one number and schedule the patient to be seen in a timely manner and have the procedure done on the same day. OECs have revolutionized the care of patients on hemodialysis and have helped numerous patients live longer happier lives.

REFERENCES

1. Quinton WE, Dillard DH, Scribner BH. Cannulation of blood vessels for prolonged hemodialysis. *Trans Am Soc Artif Intern Organs*. 1960;6:104–113.
2. Konner K. History of vascular access for haemodialysis. *Nephrol Dial Transplant*. 2005;20:2629–2635.
3. Allon M. Current management of vascular access. *Clin J Am Soc Nephrol*. 2007;2:786–800.
4. Brescia MJ, Cimino JE, Appel K, Hurwich BJ. Chronic hemodialysis using venipuncture and a surgically created arteriovenous fistula. *N Engl J Med*. 1966;275(20):1089–1092. https://doi.org/10.1056/NEJM196611172752002. PMID 5923023.

5. Parekh VB, Niyyar VD, Vachharajani TJ. Lower extremity permanent dialysis vascular access. *Clin J Am Soc Nephrol.* 2016;11(9):1693–1702. https://doi.org/10.2215/CJN.01780216.
6. Navuluri R, Regalado S. The KDOQI 2006 vascular access update and fistula first program synopsis. *Semin Intervent Radiol.* 2009;26(2):122–124. https://doi.org/10.1055/s-0029-1222455.
7. AV fistula first breakthrough coalition. National Vascular Access Improvement Initiative (NVAII).
8. Lee T, Mokrzycki M, Moist L, et al. Standardized definitions for hemodialysis vascular access. *Semin Dial.* 2011;24(5): 515–524. https://doi.org/10.1111/j.1525-139X.2011.00969.x2.
9. KDOQI clinical practice guidelines and clinical practice recommendations for vascular access 2006. *Am J Kidney Dis.* 2006;48(suppl 1):S176–S322.
10. Allon M. Current management of vascular access. *Clin J Am Soc Nephrol.* 2007;2:786–800.
11. Rehman R, Schmidt RJ, Moss AH. Ethical and legal obligation to avoid long-term tunneled catheter access. *Clin J Am Soc Nephrol.* 2009;4:456–460.
12. Ortega T, Ortega F, Diaz-Corte C, Rebollo P, Ma Baltar J, Alvarez-Grande J. The timely construction of arteriovenous fistulae: a key to reducing morbidity and mortality and to improving cost management. *Nephrol Dial Transplant.* 2005;20:598–603.
13. Feldman HI, Held PJ, Hutchinson JT, Stoiber E, Hartigan MF, Berlin JA. Hemodialysis vascular access morbidity in the United States. *Kidney Int.* May 1993; 43(5):1091–1096.
14. Dember LM, Dialysis Access Consortium Study Group, et al. Effect of clopidogrel on early failure of arteriovenous fistulas for hemodialysis: a randomized controlled trial. *J Am Med Assoc.* May 14, 2008;299(18):2164–2171.
15. Lok CE, Allon M, Moist L, Oliver MJ, Shah H, Zimmerman D. Risk equation determining unsuccessful cannulation events and failure to maturation in arteriovenous fistulas. *J Am Soc Nephrol.* November 2006;17(11): 3204–3212.
16. Feldman HI, Kobrin S, Wasserstein A. Hemodialysis vascular access morbidity. *J Am Soc Nephrol.* April 1996; 7(4):523–535.
17. Beathard GA, Arnold P, Jackson J, Litchfield T. Aggressive treatment of early fistula failure. *Kidney Int.* 2003;64:1487–1494.
18. Stolic R. Infection of arteriovenous graft for hemodialysis. *Praxis Medica.* 2007;35:113–115.
19. Schild AF, Perez E, Gillaspie E, Seaver C, Livingstone J, Thibonnier A. Arteriovenous fistulae vs. arteriovenous grafts: a retrospective review of 1,700 consecutive vascular access cases. *J Vasc Access.* 2008 Oct-Dec;9(4): 231–235.
20. Saxena AK, Panhotra BR, Al-Mulhim AS. Vascular access related infections in hemodialysis patients. *Saudi J Kidney Dis Transpl.* 2005 Jan-Mar;16(1):46–71.
21. Ferring M, Henderson J, Wilmink A, Smith S. Vascular ultrasound for the pre-operative evaluation prior to arteriovenous fistula formation for haemodialysis: review of the evidence. *Nephrol Dial Transpl.* 2008;23:1809–1815. https://doi.org/10.1093/ndt/gfn001.
22. Malovrh M. Native arteriovenous fistula: preoperative evaluation. *Am J Kidney Dis.* 2002;39:1218–1225. https://doi.org/10.1053/ajkd.2002.33394.
23. Wong V, Ward R, Taylor J, Selvakumar S, How TV, Bakran A. Factors associated with early failure of arteriovenous fistulae for haemodialysis accesses. *Eur J Vasc Endovasc Surg.* 1996;12:207–213. https://doi.org/10.1016/S1078-5884(96)80108-0.
24. Tordoir J, Canaud B, Haage P, et al. EBPG on vascular access. *Nephrol Dial Transpl.* 2007;22(Suppl 2):ii88–ii117.
25. Zamboli P, Fiorini F, D'Amelio A, Fatuzzo P, Granata A. Color doppler ultrasound and arteriovenous fistulas for hemodialysis. *J Ultrasound.* 2014;17:253–263.
26. Davidson I, Chan D, Dolmatch B, et al. Duplex ultrasound evaluation for dialysis access selection and maintenance: a practical guide. *J Vasc Access.* 2008;9:1–9.
27. Rayner HC, Pisoni RL, Gillespie BW, et al. Creation, cannulation and survival of arteriovenous fistulae: data from the dialysis outcomes and practice patterns study. *Kidney Int.* 2003;63:323–330. https://doi.org/10.1046/j.1523-1755.2003.00724.x.
28. Clark EG, Barsuk JH. Temporary hemodialysis catheters: recent advances. *Kidney Int.* 2014;86(5):888–895.
29. Clark E, Kappel J, MacRae J, et al. Practical aspects of non-tunneled and tunneled hemodialysis catheters. *Can J Kidney Health Dis.* 2016;3, 2054358116669128.
30. Miller L, MacRae JM, Kiaii M, et al. ; On behalf of the Canadian society of nephrology vascular access work group. Hemodialysis tunneled catheter noninfectious complications. Can J Kidney Health Dis. (in press).
31. Vats HS. Complications of catheters: tunneled and nontunneled. *Adv Chronic Kidney Dis.* 2012;19(3):188–194.
32. Maki DG, Kluger DM, Crnich CJ. The risk of bloodstream infection in adults with different intravascular devices: a systematic review of 200 published prospective studies. *Mayo Clin Proc.* 2006;81(9):1159–1171.
33. Taylor G, Gravel D, Johnston L, et al. Prospective surveillance for primary bloodstream infections occurring in Canadian hemodialysis units. *Infect Control Hosp Epidemiol.* 2002;23(12):716–720.
34. Hedges C. Research, evidence-based practice, and quality improvement. *AACN Adv Crit Care.* 2006;17(4):457–459.
35. Moran JE, Ash SR. Locking solutions for hemodialysis catheters; heparin and citrate—a position paper by ASDIN. *Semin Dial.* 2008;21(5):490–492.
36. Agarwal AK, Patel BM, Farhan NJ. Central venous stenosis in hemodialysis patients is a common complication of ipsilateral central vein catheterization. *J Am Soc Nephrol.* 2004;15:368A–369A.
37. Barrett N, Spencer S, McIvor J, Brown EA. Subclavian stenosis: a major complication of subclavian dialysis catheters. *Nephrol Dial Transplant.* 1988;3(4):423–425.
38. Cimochowski GE, Worley E, Rutherford WE, Sartain J, Blondin J, Harter H. Superiority of the internal jugular over the subclavian access for temporary dialysis. *Nephron.* 1990;54(2):154–161.

39. Schillinger F, Schillinger D, Montagnac R, Milcent T. Post catheterisation vein stenosis in haemodialysis: comparative angiographic study of 50 subclavian and 50 internal jugular accesses. *Nephrol Dial Transplant.* 1991;6(10):722–724.
40. Vanherweghem JL, Yassine T, Goldman M, et al. Subclavian vein thrombosis: a frequent complication of subclavian vein cannulation for hemodialysis. *Clin Nephrol.* 1986;26(5):235–238.
41. MacRae JM, Ahmed A, Johnson N, et al. Central vein stenosis: a common problem in patients on hemodialysis. *ASAIO J.* 2005;51:77–81.
42. Kundu S. Central venous obstruction management. *Semin Intervent Radiol.* June 2009;26(2):115–121.
43. Baker GL, Barnes HJ. Superior vena cava syndrome: etiology, diagnosis, and treatment. *Am J Crit Care.* 1992;1(1): 54–64.
44. Khanna S, Sniderman K, Simons M, et al. Superior vena cava stenosis associated with hemodialysis catheters. *Am J Kidney Dis.* 1993;21:278–281.
45. Rose SC, Kinney TB, Bundens WP, Valji K, Roberts AC. Importance of Doppler analysis of transmitted atrial waveforms prior to placement of central venous access catheters. *J Vasc Interv Radiol.* 1998;9(6):927–934.
46. Glanz S, Gordon D, Butt KMH, Hong J, Adamson R, Sclafani SJ. Dialysis access fistulas: treatment of stenoses by transluminal angioplasty. *Radiology.* 1984;152(3): 637–642.
47. United States Renal Data System USRD 2003. *Annual Data Report: Atlas of End-Stage Renal Disease in the United States.* Bethesda, MD: National Institutes of Health, National Institute of Diabetes and Digestive and Kidney Diseases; 2003.
48. Aruny JE, Lewis CA, Cardella JF, Standards of Practise Committee of the Society of Cardiovascular & Interventional Radiology, et al. Quality improvement guidelines for percutaneous management of the thrombosed or dysfunctional dialysis access. *J Vasc Interv Radiol.* 2003; 14:S247–S253.
49. Asif A, Cherla G, Merrill D, et al. Venous mapping using venography and the risk of radiocontrast-induced nephropathy. *Semin Dial.* 2005;18(3):239–242.
50. Kian K, Wyatt C, Schon D, Packer J, Vassalotti J, Mishler. Safety of low-dose radiocontrast for interventional AV fistula salvage in stage 4 chronic kidney disease patients. *R Kidney Int.* April 2006;69(8):1444–1449.
51. Trerotola SO, Stavropoulos SW, Shlansky-Goldberg R, Tuite CM, Kobrin S, Rudnick MR. Hemodialysis-related venous stenosis: treatment with ultrahigh-pressure angioplasty balloons. *Radiology.* April 2004;231(1):259–262.
52. Roy-Chaudhury P, Melhem M, Husted T, Kelly BS. Solutions for hemodialysis vascular access dysfunction: thinking out of the box!. *J Vasc Access.* 2005;6:3–8.
53. Roy-Chaudhury P, Sukhatme VP, Cheung AK. Hemodialysis vascular access dysfunction: a cellular and molecular viewpoint. *J Am Soc Nephrol.* 2006;17:1112–1127.
54. Lee T, Roy-Chaudhury P. Advances and new frontiers in the pathophysiology of venous neointimal hyperplasia and dialysis access stenosis. *Adv Chronic Kidney Dis.* 2009;16:329–338, 34. Lee T. Hemodialysis vascular access dysfunction. In: Carpi A, Donaldio C, Tramonti G, editors. Progress in Hemodialysis – From Emergent Biotechnology to Clinical Practice. Rijeka: InTech; 2011. pp. 365–388.
55. Schild AF. Maintaining vascular access: the management of hemodialysis arteriovenous grafts. *J Vasc Access.* 2010;11:92–99.
56. Lai CC, Fang HC, Tseng CJ, Liu CP, Mar GY. Percutaneous angioplasty using a paclitaxel-coated balloon improves target lesion restenosis on inflow lesions of autogenous radiocephalic fistulas: a pilot study. *J Vasc Interv Radiol.* 2014;25:535–541. pmid:24529550PubMedGoogle Scholar.
57. Katsanos K, Karnabatidis D, Kitrou P, Spiliopoulos S, Christeas N, Siablis D. Paclitaxel-coated balloon angioplasty vs. plain balloon dilation for the treatment of failing dialysis access: 6-Month interim results from a prospective randomized controlled trial. *J Endovasc Ther.* 2012;19: 263–272. pmid:22545894CrossRefPubMedGoogle Scholar.
58. Kitrou PM, Katsanos K, Spiliopoulos S, Karnabatidis D, Siablis D. Drug-eluting versus plain balloon angioplasty for the treatment of failing dialysis access: final results and cost-effectiveness analysis from a prospective randomized controlled trial (NCT01174472). *Eur J Radiol.* 2015;84:418–423. pmid:25575743PubMedGoogle Scholar.
59. Kitrou PM, Spiliopoulos S, Katsanos K, Papachristou E, Siablis D, Karnabatidis D. Paclitaxel-coated versus plain balloon angioplasty for dysfunctional arteriovenous fistulae: one-year results of a prospective randomized controlled trial. *J Vasc Interv Radiol.* 2015;26:348–354. pmid:25542635PubMedGoogle Scholar.
60. Kitrou PM, Papadimatos P, Spiliopoulos S, et al. Paclitaxel-coated balloons for the treatment of symptomatic central venous stenosis in dialysis access: results from a randomized controlled trial. *J Vasc Interv Radiol.* 2017;28:811–817. pmid:28434662PubMedGoogle Scholar.
61. Nassar GM, Nguyen B, Rhee E, Achkar K. Endovascular treatment of the 'failing to mature' arteriovenous fistula. *Clin J Am Soc Nephrol.* 2006;1:275–280.
62. Morris ST, McMurray JJ, Rodger RS, Jardine AG. Impaired endothelium-dependent vasodilatation in uraemia. *Nephrol Dial Transplant.* 2000;15:1194–1200.
63. Van Tricht I, De Wachter D, Tordoir J, Verdonck P. Hemodynamics and complications encountered with arteriovenous fistulas and grafts as vascular access for hemodialysis: a review. *Ann Biomed Eng.* September 2005;33(9):1142–1157.
64. Turmel-Rodrigues L, Pengloan J, Blanchier D, et al. Insufficient dialysis shunts: improved long-term patency rates with close hemodynamic monitoring, repeated percutaneous balloon angioplasty, and stent placement. *Radiology.* April 1993;187(1):273–278.
65. Kanterman RY, Vesely TM, Pilgram TK, Guy BW, Windus DW, Picus D. Dialysis access grafts: anatomic location of venous stenosis and results of angioplasty. *Radiology.* April 1995;195(1):135–139.

66. Lorenz JM. Use of stents for the maintenance of hemodialysis access. *Semin Intervent Radiol.* 2004;21(2):135–140. https://doi.org/10.1055/s-2004-833688.
67. Hoffer EK, Sultan S, Herskowitz MM, et al. Prospective randomized trial of a metallic intravascular stent in hemodialysis graft maintenance. *J Vasc Interv Radiol.* 1997;8:965–973.
68. Anaya-Ayala JE, Smolock CJ, Colvard BD, Naoum JJ, et al. Efficacy of covered stent placement for central venous occlusive disease in hemodialysis patients. *J Vasc Surg.* 2011;54:754–759.
69. Stolic R. Most important chronic complications of arteriovenous fistulas for hemodialysis. *Med Princ Pract.* 2013; 22(3):220–228. https://doi.org/10.1159/000343669.
70. Rotmans JI, Pattynama PM, Verhagen HJ, et al. Sirolimus-eluting stents to abolish intimal hyperplasia and improve flow in porcine arteriovenous grafts: a 4-week follow-up study. *Circulation.* March 29, 2005;111(12): 1537–1542.
71. Ryan JM, Dumbleton SA, Doherty J, Smith TP. Technical innovation. Using a covered stent (Wallgraft) to treat pseudoaneurysms of dialysis grafts and fistulas. *AJR Am J Roentgenol.* 2003;180:1067–1071. https://doi.org/10.2214/ajr.180.4.1801067.
72. Effect of venous side branch obliteration for nonmaturing arteriovenous fistulas Altieri Matthew et al. J Vasc Surg, Volume 65, Issue 3, e7
73. Jain K, Munn J, Rummel MC, Johnston D, Longton C. Office-based endovascular suite is safe for most procedures. *J Vasc Surg.* 2014;59:186–191.

FURTHER READING

1. Clinical practice guidelines for vascular access. Vascular Access 2006 Work Group. *Am J Kidney Dis.* July 2006;48(Suppl 1):S176–S247.
2. Paulson WD, Moist L, Lok CE. Vascular access surveillance: an ongoing controversy. *Kidney Int.* January 2012;81(2): 132–142.

CHAPTER 33

Inferior Vena Cava Filters and Ports

JESSE CHAIT, BS • ANIL HINGORANI, MD • ENRICO ASCHER, MD, FACS

CHAPTER OVERVIEW

Placement of inferior vena cava (IVC) filters (IVCFs) and totally implantable venous-access devices (TIVADs), like many other interventions covered in this text, are safely and effectively being performed in the office setting. This chapter will cover the office-based considerations of these procedures including indications, device selection, evidence-based technique, and postoperative care, including potential complications and their associated management. Since these aspects are unique to each intervention, they will be covered separately.

PREOPERATIVE EVALUATION

All patients should undergo proper preoperative medical assessment and optimization before insertion of an IVCF or TIVAD. We recommend routine laboratory studies including a complete blood count, metabolic panel, prothrombin time, and an international normalized ratio (INR). In order to reduce bleeding-related complications, all patients should have an INR <1.6 for TIVAD placement and <3.0 for IVCF insertion. In all cases, local anesthesia should be utilized to reduce pain associated with obtaining venous access. For patients undergoing TIVAD placement, we offer monitored anesthesia care (MAC) with intravenous sedation; however, the authors do not routinely employ this practice for uncomplicated IVCF insertions.

INFERIOR VENA CAVA FILTERS

Overview

In the past, the number of IVCF insertions performed in the United States experienced a marked increase often postulated to be due to an increase in retrievable filters placed for prophylactic indications.[1,2] Contemporarily, due to questionable efficacy, negative views regarding long-term safety, and increased rates of litigation,[3,4] IVCF placement has been decreasing. This overall downward trend in filter insertion has been accompanied by increases in IVCF placement in the outpatient setting, a rise in the volume of insertions by nonsurgeon insertions, and increased retrieval rates.[5,6]

Indications for Filter Insertion

IVCF placement is indicated for patients who have experienced—or are at high risk—pulmonary embolism (PE), who have an absolute contraindication or experienced complications to anticoagulation therapy, or who suffered from deep vein thrombosis (DVT) or PE despite maintaining therapeutic anticoagulation. IVCF insertion should be avoided unless absolutely indicated, as implantation increases incidence of DVT without proven mortality benefit.[7,8] Furthermore, IVCFs should not be used as an adjunct to prevent recurrent PE in patients who are able to tolerate anticoagulation.[9]

Technique for Filter Insertion

Ultrasound-guided percutaneous access is typically obtained via the common femoral vein; however, in cases where this is not feasible, the internal jugular and upper extremity veins remain viable options.[10,11] A single access site is typically adequate for successful IVCF placement; however, some providers prefer two access sites when utilizing intravascular ultrasound (IVUS).[12,13] The authors recommend an oversized (6 or 7Fr) sheath, as opposed to a typical 4Fr, in order to allow for rapid injection of contrast bolus without the need for an expensive power injector. Fluoroscopic guidance is used to identify bony landmarks that guide proper anatomic deployment, typically inferior to the renal veins. In most patients, the L2-L3 vertebral level marks the approximate level of the renal veins, and a 20-mL contrast bolus can be utilized to properly demarcate the renal veins. While an IVUS pullback technique from the right atrium can also be used to identify the renal veins,[13] this may be cost-prohibitive in the office-based setting. Suprarenal filter placement is a safe alternative typically indicated when infrarenal

Office-Based Endovascular Centers. https://doi.org/10.1016/B978-0-323-67969-5.00033-2
Copyright © 2020 Elsevier Inc. All rights reserved.

deployment is inadequate, such as in the presence of thrombus, compression, or pregnancy.[14]

Transabdominal ultrasound (TAUS) also remains a viable option for filter insertion—a practice that has been utilized at the bedside for patients deemed too unstable for the operating room or interventional suite.[14] This technique may also be used in the office-based setting. Proper probe positioning at the right flank to identify the confluence of the right renal vein (RRV) and IVC allows for safe and effective deployment.[15]

The authors recommend a postdeployment venogram to ensure proper filter deployment within the desired IVC segment and to identify any immediate complications such as filter malposition.[16] Patients are encouraged to return to the office within 1 week of filter placement for follow-up examination with duplex ultrasonography (DUS). In order to increase filter retrieval rates and decrease complications related to prolonged dwell time, the authors recommend quarterly follow-up visits.

Complications of Filter Insertion

Placement of IVCFs is a relatively low-risk intervention that can be safely performed in both hospital and office settings.[17] As with any endovascular procedure, there is always a risk of access site complications; however, the majority of issues related to filters are attributed to the device itself. Filter complications can increase the risk of PE and prevent or complicate attempts at retrieval. Filter tilt is a common complication defined as >15 degrees angulation, which increases the risk for PE and some have suggested that this may be an indication for insertion of a second filter.[16,18] Filter migration, defined as >2 cm movement from the initial deployment site, most commonly occurs >30 days after insertion.[18] Struts can fracture and embolize, or pierce the caval wall. Thrombosis of the IVC can lead to edema, pain, PE, or even renal failure if the thrombus propagates to the level of the renal veins.[18] Management of these complications is often complex, must be tailored to the exact needs of the patient, and therefore are out of the scope of this text.

Indications and Strategies for Filter Retrieval

An increase in awareness of complications associated with long-standing IVCFs has led to widespread efforts to develop effective retrieval campaigns and techniques. All retrievable filters should be removed unless an indication for permanent filtration is present assuming there is no anticipated return to a high-risk status. Operator-dependent barriers to filter retrieval, such as difficult anatomy or prolonged dwell time, should not be considered contraindications to a retrieval attempt.

Risk factors for nonretrieval of retrievable filters include advanced age, presence of an acute bleed, and current malignancy.[19] Patients are often unaware of the retrievable status of their filter, and some may not be aware one is present at all, and therefore healthcare providers must be vigilant in their follow-up.[20] Development of a documented retrieval algorithm (Fig. 33.1), along with the creation of a multidisciplinary team or dedicated clinic, and access to an office-based endovascular center have all been shown to significantly increase filter retrieval rates.[21–24]

Technique for Filter Retrieval

As with many endovascular interventions, a variety of tools are available for the retrieval of vena cava filters.[25] Preoperatively, abdominal X-ray or computed tomography (CT) should be performed in order to determine filter location, degree of angulation, the presence of any strut fractures. Preintervention planning is paramount for efficient and safe filter retrieval, and DUS should be used liberally in order to confirm filter location and ensure access can be safely obtained. Typically, percutaneous access is obtained via the right IJV; however, some authors report the use of a femoral or upper extremity approach.[26] In complex cases, multiple access sites may be utilized in order to facilitate the use of several retrieval devices. Unlike filter insertion, retrieval necessitates the use of fluoroscopic guidance, and complex scenarios may lead to both prolonged case times and increased radiation exposure.

In simple cases, a combination of sheath and snare is used to hook, collapse, and remove the filter. This approach has a high success rate when attempting to retrieve filters with limited dwell time. However, retrieval of IVCFs that have remained in vivo for an extended period of time can often be complicated by filter malposition, wall penetration, endothelialization, or IVC thrombosis.[25] In more complex cases, the use of endobronchial forceps and excimer lasers to dissect and free embedded filters and fractured components has been described with high levels of success.[27] Adjunctive techniques such as grasping the hook with the endobronchial forceps, wire loop snare, and deflection of the filter hook with a balloon placed from the groin can also be helpful.

Rationale for Office-Based Placement and Retrieval

The majority of IVCF insertion and retrieval procedures are simple, safe, and require a limited amount of equipment, making them ideal interventions to be performed

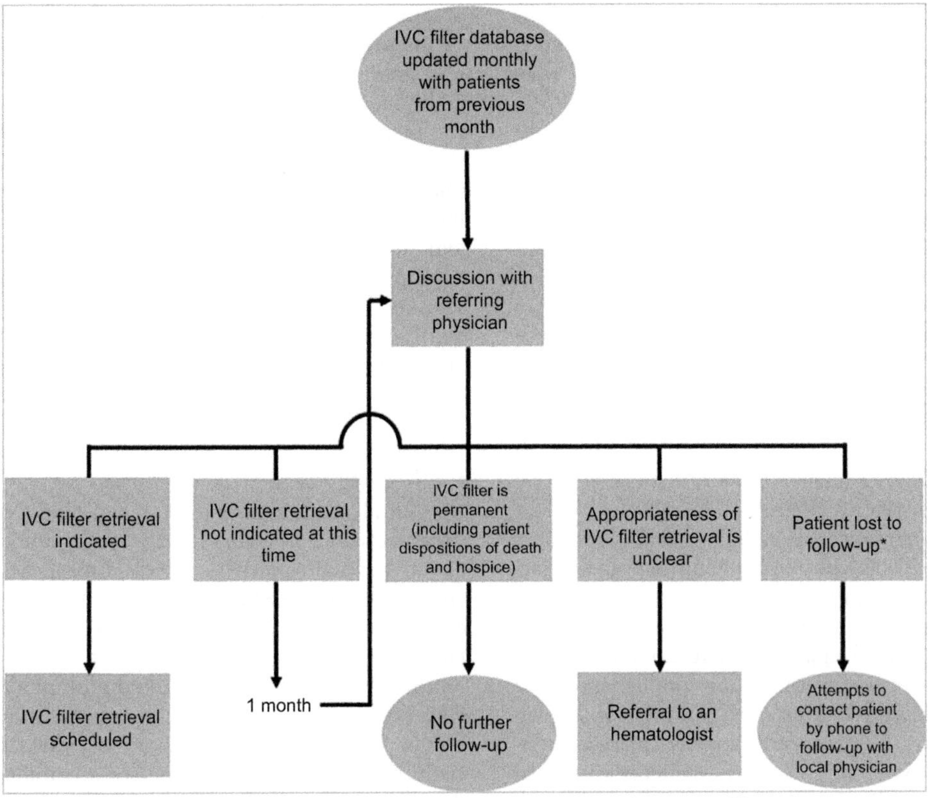

FIG. 33.1 Inferior vena cava (IVC) filter retrieval algorithm.[23]

in the office. Retrospective analyses have confirmed the safety and efficacy of both filter insertion[17] and removal in the office-based setting, with an increased retrieval rate associated with access to an office endovascular center.[24]

Furthermore, the continuity of care, physician-patient rapport, and presence of dedicated support staff associated with office-based centers make it an ideal environment for development of a culture dedicated to IVCF retrieval. All staff should be made aware of this effort and motivated to educate patients on their filter status. All patients who receive filter insertion in the office, report a history of filter placement, or have evidence of an IVCF on imaging should have their information placed in a registry that allows for continuous follow-up and evaluation of the necessity of the filter.

TOTALLY IMPLANTABLE VENOUS ACCESS DEVICES

Overview

TIVADs, commonly referred to as "ports," provide reliable access for patients who require long-term, intermittent intravenous therapy, typically in those with chronic hematologic disease and malignancy.[28] While device selection and technique vary greatly between providers, the general principle of TIVAD placement is reliable central venous access through a subcutaneous port. Most modern ports are magnetic resonance imaging (MRI)-safe, able to endure thousands of repeat Huber needle punctures and can withstand high pressures and infusion volumes associated with intravenous contrast studies. The catheters attached to these ports may be double, single, or lumen, the latter allowing for simultaneous infusions, such as chemotherapy alongside total parenteral nutrition (TPN).[29]

Indications

Ports are often necessary for those with chronic diseases, such as malignancy or hematologic disorders, who require intermittent infusion of venotoxic agents or exchange transfusions. The most common indications for TIVAD placement include solid and hematologic malignancies, and a long-term need for apheresis.

In general, two options exist for long-term venous device-aided access: tunneled or subcutaneous catheters. Whereas a tunneled device is preferable when venous access is needed on a constant basis, TIVADs are better suited for intermittent access, such as for chemotherapy, TPN, or routine transfusions.[28] Tunneled catheters are typically preferred for short-term use, whereas TIVADs are more suitable for long-term access, such as in patients with chronic disease.

The subcutaneous port aspect of the TIVAD design is the factor most associated with fewer complications, a lower infection rate, higher quality of life, and increased patient satisfaction, when compared with tunneled, nontunneled, and peripherally inserted central venous catheters.[30,31]

Technique

We recommend routine administration of a prophylactic, preoperative antibiotic. Our preferred agent is cefazolin; however, for patients with allergy or sensitivity to beta lactam antibiotics, we utilize clindamycin or vancomycin. Initial venous access can be obtained percutaneously or via an open surgical approach. A recent metaanalysis showed a higher successful primary implantation rate with the Seldinger technique when compared with open venous cutdown; however, percutaneously placed subclavian catheters were more likely to experience complications. These complications, however, were not related to pneumothorax (PTX) or infection.[32]

Classically, a two-incision method has been the standard procedure for TIVAD placement[33]; however, a single-incision technique has also been described.[34,35] Ultrasound-guided catheter placement into the internal jugular vein is preferred due to the ease of access and ability for direct visualization. Unless contraindicated due to prior surgery, wound, or history of ipsilateral device placement, some authors prefer insertion of the TIVAD catheter in the right subclavian or cephalic vein, as these options necessitate the shortest catheter length and least amount of angulation for proper positioning.[36] Other options include branches of the thoracoacromial vein.[37] The femoral vein is an alternative TIVAD site for patients with unsuitable upper extremity access, which can be due to central venous stenosis, thrombosis, inadequate vasculature, or superior vena cava syndrome. Regardless of insertion site, all office-based centers should have electrocautery available, as extensive axillary, pectoral, or femoral venous collaterals may cause bleeding during pocket creation.

As with all percutaneous endovascular procedures, systematic reviews have demonstrated that ultrasound (US) guidance improves safety outcomes when obtaining venous access via the femoral, subclavian, or internal jugular vein (IJV).[38,39] In the office, high-resolution DUS should be available for both diagnosis and image-guided intervention. US guidance allows for preprocedural identification of nonviable access sites, such as a thrombosed IJV, or a small caliber cephalic vein. Use of the routine US guidance reduces the incidence of iatrogenic PTX and prevents inadvertent arterial injury. Due to the lower incidence of hemopneumothorax, the authors prefer placement of TIVADs in the right IJV. This also eliminates the rare occurrence of "pinch off" syndrome with interaction and possible obstruction of the catheter due to compression at the costoclavicular junction with placement via the subclavian route.[40–42]

Follow-Up

As with all intravascular devices and long-term access sites, frequent follow-up evaluation is paramount in order to maintain patency, prevent complications, and ensure removal—when indicated. We recommend evaluation with physical exam within 7 days of implantation, and every 3 months thereafter. New onset neck or upper extremity swelling should prompt a thorough DUS examination. If sonogram cannot identify a culprit lesion, a contrast port study may be indicated, especially since the tip of the catheter—a common site of thrombus—is not able to be visualized due to its location at the caval-atrial junction.

Complications

Pneumothorax

Complications associated with TIVAD placement are rare. In many centers, routine postprocedural chest X-ray (CXR) is required after obtaining central venous access via the IJV and subclavian veins, in order to evaluate for iatrogenic PTX and proper catheter tip placement. However, some authors have suggested that this practice may be unnecessary due to a variety of reasons. First, the incidence of PTX is exceedingly low when utilizing US guidance to assist with TIVAD placement.[43] Second, CXR has poor diagnostic capabilities in terms of both identifying postoperative PTX[43] and catheter malposition.[44] Third, postprocedure US can be used to assess for iatrogenic PTX and catheter malposition with similar or better efficacy when compared with CXR.[45,46] Nevertheless, we still recommend a postinsertion chest radiograph following any type of central catheter placement. Some authors forgo formal radiographs in lieu of postinsertion fluoroscopic assessment; however, some infusion centers mandate confirmatory CXR prior to initial TIVAD access.

Suspected postprocedure PTX is suggested by dyspnea, tachycardia, and decreased oxygen saturation and should be evaluated with prompt CXR or US and managed initially oxygen supplementation. The authors suggest having some type of pleural decompression device available in the office setting, such as a large gauge intravenous cannula, in the case of a tension PTX. All patients with suspected PTX should be sent to the nearest emergency department for further evaluation and monitoring.

Infection

As with the placement of any indwelling catheter, the risk of infection is of paramount concern. The strongest risk factors for TIVAD-associated infections include presence of a hematologic malignancy, frequent device utilization, young age, difficulty obtaining proper needle insertion, concomitant steroid use, and infusion of TPN through the port.[47–49] Ports placed in the office have a lower incidence of infection and dehiscence when compared with those placed in the inpatient setting.[50]

Suspected port infection should be expeditiously evaluated, first by differentiating between local and bloodstream infection. Since local infections often occur due to extraluminal contamination, concomitant bloodstream infection is rare, and local signs are rarely seen with disseminated disease. Whereas local infection can be confirmed by tissue culture, bloodstream infection attributed to a contaminated TIVAD can be confirmed by positive, matching cultures withdrawn from both a native peripheral vein and the device itself. The management of TIVAD-related infection depends on location and severity. In some cases, local infections can be managed conservatively; however, in the majority of cases of catheter-associated bloodstream infection, the TIVAD should be explanted along with systemic antimicrobial therapy.[47] In select scenarios, conservative management of systemic antimicrobial therapy with close observation and repeated cultures may be warranted.

Rationale for office-based placement and removal

A large percentage of endovascular and vascular access procedures have migrated from the hospital to the outpatient and office setting,[51] owing to reduced costs and increased preference by both patient and provider.[52] As indications for port placement typically include chronic disease and cancer, TIVAD implantation is not emergent and can be scheduled as an elective, office-based procedure.

The benefits of office-based TIVAD placement are multifaceted. Compared with implantation in the hospital setting, office-based placement results in fewer infections,[51] decreased costs,[52] and increased patient satisfaction. As healthcare expenditures continue to rise, providers should be cognizant of all options that reduce costs, especially for high-utilization patients, such as those with chronic disease who require TIVAD insertion or removal.

REFERENCES

1. Duffett L, Carrier M. Inferior vena cava filters. *J Thromb Haemost.* 2017;15(1):3–12.
2. Duszak R, Parker L, Levin DC, Rao VM. Placement and removal of inferior vena cava filters: National trends in the medicare population. *J Am Coll Radiol.* 2011;8(7): 483–489.
3. Phair J, Denesopolis J, Lipsitz EC, Scher L. Inferior vena cava filter malpractice litigation: Damned if you do, Damned if you don't. *Ann Vasc Surg.* 2018;50:15–20.
4. Oh K, Hingorani A. Outcomes and associated factors in malpractice litigation involving inferior vena cava filters. *J Vasc Surg.* 2018;6(4):541–544.
5. Morris E, Duszak R, Sista AK, Hemingway J, Hughes DR, Rosenkrantz AB. National trends in inferior vena cava filter placement and retrieval procedures in the medicare population over two decades. *J Am Coll Radiol.* 2018;15(8): 1080–1086.
6. Ahmed O, Wadhwa V, Patel K, Patel MV, Turba UC, Arslan B. Rising retrieval rates of inferior vena cava filters in the United States: insights from the 2012 to 2016 summary medicare claims data. *J Am Coll Radiol.* 2018;15(11): 1553–1557.
7. Decousus H, Leizorovicz A, Parent F, et al. A clinical trial of vena caval filters in the prevention of pulmonary embolism in patients with proximal deep-vein thrombosis. *N Engl J Med.* 1998;338(7):409–416.
8. Jiang J, Jiao Y, Zhang X. The short-term efficacy of vena cava filters for the prevention of pulmonary embolism in patients with venous thromboembolism receiving anticoagulation: meta-analysis of randomized controlled trials. *Phlebology.* 2016;32(9):620–627.
9. Mismetti P, Laporte S, Pellerin O, et al. Effect of a retrievable inferior vena cava filter plus anticoagulation vs anticoagulation alone on risk of recurrent pulmonary embolism. *J Am Med Ass.* 2015;313(16):1627–1635.
10. Lambe BD, Bedway JJ, Friedell ML. Percutaneous femoral vein access for inferior vena cava filter placement does not cause insertion-site thrombosis. *Ann Vasc Surg.* 2013; 27(8):1169–1172.
11. Stone PA, AbuRahma AF, Hass SM, et al. TrapEase inferior vena cava filter placement: use of the subclavian vein. *Vasc Endovasc Surg.* 2004;38(6):505–509.
12. Gunn AJ, Iqbal SI, Kalva SP, et al. Intravascular ultrasound-guided inferior vena cava filter placement using a single-

puncture technique in 99 patients. *Vasc Endovasc Surg.* 2013;47(2):97–101.
13. Passman MA, Dattilo JB, Guzman RJ, Naslund TC. Bedside placement of inferior vena cava filters by using transabdominal duplex ultrasonography and intravascular ultrasound imaging. *J Vasc Surg.* 2005;42(5):1027–1032.
14. Kalva SP, Chlapoutaki C, Wicky S, Greenfield AJ, Waltman AC, Athanasoulis CA. Suprarenal inferior vena cava filters: a 20-year single-center experience. *J Vasc Interv Radiol.* 2008;19(7):1041–1047.
15. Qin X, Lu C, Ren P, et al. New method for ultrasound-guided inferior vena cava filter placement. *J Vasc Surg.* 2018;6(4):450–456.
16. Rajasekhar A. Inferior vena cava filters: current best practices. *J Thromb Thrombolysis.* 2015;39(3):315–327.
17. Alsheekh A, Hingorani A, Marks N, Ascher E. The next frontier of office-based inferior vena cava filter placement. *J Vasc Surg.* 2016;4(3):283–285.
18. Grewal S, Chamarthy MR, Kalva SP. Complications of inferior vena cava filters. *Cardiovasc Diagn Ther.* 2016;6(6): 632–641.
19. Siracuse JJ, Al Bazroon A, Gill HL, et al. Risk factors of nonretrieval of retrievable inferior vena cava filters. *Ann Vasc Surg.* 2015;29(2):318–321.
20. Aurshina A, Brahmandam A, Zhang Y, et al. Patient perspectives on inferior vena cava filter retrieval. *J Vasc Surg.* 2019. Article in press.
21. Inagaki E, Farber A, Eslami MH, et al. Improving the retrieval rate of inferior vena cava filters with a multidisciplinary team approach. *J Vasc Surg.* 2016;4(3):276–282.
22. Minocha J, Idakoji I, Riaz A, et al. Improving inferior vena cava filter retrieval rates: impact of a dedicated inferior vena cava filter clinic. *J Vasc Interv Radiol.* 2010;21(12): 1847–1851.
23. Litwin RJ, Huang SY, Sabir SH, et al. Impact of an inferior vena cava filter retrieval algorithm on filter retrieval rates in a cancer population. *J Vasc Surg.* 2017;5(5):689–697.
24. VanderVeen N, Friedman J, Rummel M, et al. Improving inferior vena cava filter retrieval and success rates utilizing an office endovascular center [Abstract]. *J Vasc Surg.* 2018; 67(6):e225.
25. Kuyumcu G, Walker TG. Inferior vena cava filter retrievals, standard and novel techniques. *Cardiovasc Diagn Ther.* 2016;6(6):642–650.
26. Posham R, Fischman AM, Nowakowski FS, et al. Transfemoral filter eversion technique following unsuccessful retrieval of option inferior vena cava filters: a single center experience. *J Vasc Interv Radiol.* 2017;28(6):889–894.
27. Chen JX, Montgomery J, McLennan G, Stavropoulos SW. Endobronchial forceps-assisted and excimer laser-assisted inferior vena cava filter removal: the data, where we are, and how it is done. *Tech Vasc Interv Radiol.* 2018;21(2): 85–91.
28. Walser EM. Venous access ports: indications, implantation technique, follow-up, and complications. *Cardiovasc Interv Radiol.* 2011;35(4):751–764.
29. Teichgräber UK, Nagel SN, Kausche S, Streitparth F, Cho CH. Double-lumen central venous port catheters: simultaneous application for chemotherapy and parenteral nutrition in cancer patients. *J Vasc Access.* 2010; 11(4):335–341.
30. Fang S, Yang J, Song L, Jiang Y, Liu Y. Comparison of three types of central venous catheters in patients with malignant tumor receiving chemotherapy. *Patient Prefer Adherence.* 2017;11:1197–1204.
31. Coady K, Ali M, Sidloff D, Kenningham RR, Ahmed S. A comparison of infections and complications in central venous catheters in adults with solid tumours. *J Vasc Access.* 2014;16(1):38–41.
32. Hsu CC, Kwan GN, Driel ML, Rophael JA. Venous cutdown versus the Seldinger technique for placement of totally implantable venous access ports. *Cochrane Database Syst Rev.* 2011.
33. Funaki B, Szymski GX, Hackworth CA, et al. Radiologic placement of subcutaneous infusion chest ports for long-term central venous access. *Am J Roentgenol.* 1997; 169(5):1431–1434.
34. Charles HW, Miguel T, Kovacs S, Gohari A, Arampulikan J, Mccann JW. Chest port placement with use of the single-incision insertion technique. *J Vasc Interv Radiol.* 2009; 20(11):1464–1469.
35. Cheng H, Ting C, Chu Y, Chang W, Chan K, Chen P. Application of an ultrasound-guided low-approach insertion technique in three types of totally implantable access port. *J Chin Med Assoc.* 2014;77(5):246–252.
36. Wei W, Wu C, Wu C, et al. The treatment results of a standard algorithm for choosing the best entry vessel for intravenous port implantation. *Medicine (Baltim).* 2015; 94(33):e1381.
37. Su T, Wu C, Fu J, et al. Deltoid branch of thoracoacromial vein: a safe alternative entry vessel for intravenous port implantation. *Medicine (Baltim).* 2015;94(17).
38. Brass P, Hellmich M, Kolodziej L, Schick G, Smith AF. Ultrasound guidance versus anatomical landmarks for subclavian or femoral vein catheterization. *Cochrane Database Syst Rev.* 2015.
39. Brass P, Hellmich M, Kolodziej L, Schick G, Smith AF. Ultrasound guidance versus anatomical landmarks for internal jugular vein catheterization. *Cochrane Database Syst Rev.* 2015.
40. Aitken DR, Minton JP. The "pinch-off sign": a warning of impending problems with permanent subclavian catheters. *Am J Surg.* 1984;148(5):633–636.
41. Orsi F, Grasso RF, Arnaldi P, et al. Ultrasound guided versus direct vein puncture in central venous port placement. *J Vasc Access.* 2000;1(2):73–77.
42. Tamura A, Sone M, Ehara S, et al. Is ultrasound-guided central venous port placement effective to avoid pinch-off syndrome? *J Vasc Access.* 2014;15(4):311–316.
43. Brown JR, Slomski C, Saxe AW. Is routine postoperative chest X-ray necessary after fluoroscopic-guided subclavian central venous port placement? *J Am Coll Surg.* 2009; 208(4):517–519.
44. Salimi F, Hekmatnia A, Shahabi J, Keshavarzian A, Maracy MR, Jazi AH. Evaluation of routine postoperative chest roentgenogram for determination of the correct

position of permanent central venous catheters tip. *J Res Med Sci*. 2015;20(1):89–92.
45. Smit JM, Raadsen R, Blans MJ, Petjak M, Ven PM, Tuinman PR. Bedside ultrasound to detect central venous catheter misplacement and associated iatrogenic complications: a systematic review and meta-analysis. *Crit Care*. 2018;22(1).
46. Ablordeppey EA, Drewry AM, Beyer AB, et al. Diagnostic accuracy of central venous catheter confirmation by bedside ultrasound versus chest radiography in critically ill patients. *Crit Care Med*. 2017;45(4):715–724.
47. Lebeaux D, Fernández-Hidalgo N, Chauhan A, et al. Management of infections related to totally implantable venous-access ports: challenges and perspectives. *Lancet Infect Dis*. 2014;14(2):146–159.
48. Zhang S, Kobayashi K, Faridnia M, Skummer P, Zhang D, Karmel MI. Clinical predictors of port infections in adult patients with hematologic malignancies. *J Vasc Interv Radiol*. 2018;29(8):1148–1155.
49. Wang TY, Lee KD, Chen PT, et al. Incidence and risk factors for central venous access port-related infection in Chinese cancer patients. *J Formos Med Assoc*. 2015;114(11): 1055–1060.
50. Pandey N, Chittams JL, Trerotola SO. Outpatient placement of subcutaneous venous access ports reduces the rate of infection and dehiscence compared with inpatient placement. *J Vasc Interv Radiol*. 2013;24(6):849–854.
51. Patel N, Hingorani A, Ascher E. Office-based surgery for vascular surgeons. *Perspect Vasc Surg Endovasc Ther*. 2008; 20(4):326–330.
52. Feo CF, Ginesu GC, Bellini A, et al. Cost and morbidity analysis of chest port insertion in adults: outpatient clinic versus operating room placement. *Ann Med Surg*. 2017;21: 81–84.

CHAPTER 34

Other Endovascular Procedures and Embolization

DAVID C. SPERLING, MD, FSIR

What procedures can and should be performed in your office-based endovascular center? Irrespective of the specialty, this is a common question asked by the owners of the endovascular centers. Whether you are establishing a new center, or have an established center and are looking for new procedures to incorporate into your menu of offered services you provide, knowing your choices and understanding the risks and benefits, as well as the financial implications, are of paramount importance. Embolization procedures fall into an area of debate for some. Can these procedures be done at a high level and if it is appropriate to perform these procedures in an office setting? The questions center around the technical aspects of the procedure and regarding recovery after the procedure. Here we will discuss embolization procedures as they pertain to the office-based endovascular center (OEC).

Embolization procedures generally fall into two major categories: arterial and venous. Technically, there is a third category of embolization, lymphatic embolization, specifically thoracic duct embolization. Thoracic duct embolization, as most embolization procedures, are traditionally performed in a hospital setting using fixed fluoroscopy units. The procedure involves injecting a lower extremity lymph node or lymphatic duct with ethiodized oil, waiting for the ethiodized oil to reach the cisterna chyli in the upper abdomen, puncturing the cisterna chyli under fluoroscopic guidance, gaining wire and catheter access into the thoracic duct, and embolizing with microcoils. This procedure is somewhat complex, requiring multiple access points, superior quality fluoroscopy and can take several hours to complete. It is a safe procedure, with little downside and a benign recovery, however, for the reasons specified above, I do not perform these procedures in the OEC. I will limit the discussion to procedures that are typically performed in less than 2 h, and can be performed using mobile C-ARMs, as this is the most common piece of fluoroscopic equipment present in current OEC.

ARTERIAL EMBOLIZATION

Arterial embolization procedures are the most common type of embolization procedures performed by endovascular specialists. When a layperson and many referring physicians think of EP, they think of treatment of gastrointestinal bleeding. Typically, arterial GI bleeds in both the upper and lower GI tracts are brisk and cause significant hemodynamic compromise. These patients are almost always inpatients in an acute care facility, many times admitted to an ICU. These patients by definition will not come to an OEC, and therefore will not be discussed. However, there are many other arterial embolization procedures that can be performed on an outpatient basis in your OEC. These procedures include uterine fibroid (uterine artery) embolization, chemoembolization (liver), Y90 radioembolization (liver), angiomyolipoma embolization, and prostate embolization.

Uterine Fibroid (Uterine Artery) Embolization

Uterine fibroid embolization (UFE) is a procedure that is used to treat symptomatic fibroids. Patients with fibroids in the uterus can present with significant symptoms, including bleeding and symptoms caused by the bulk and mass effect of the fibroids. Bleeding can present as menorrhagia and bleeding between menstruation, sometimes leading to significant anemia. Symptoms because of the bulk can include pain, pelvic pressure, bloating, constipation, and increased urinary frequency. When these symptoms occur, they can significantly affect a woman's quality of life and women will frequently go to their gynecologist seeking treatment. The treatment options include no treatment (essentially waiting until the patient goes into menopause, at which time fibroid symptoms typically resolve), oral contraceptives, leuprolide (a monthly injection that is a gonadotropin-releasing hormone agonist that effectively stops menstruation), endometrial ablation (thermal ablation that can treat fibroids near the

Office-Based Endovascular Centers. https://doi.org/10.1016/B978-0-323-67969-5.00034-4
Copyright © 2020 Elsevier Inc. All rights reserved.

endometrial canal), MRI-guided high-frequency ultrasound treatment, UFE, myomectomy, and hysterectomy.

UFE was first performed in France in 1995,[1] and in the United States in 1997.[2] The procedure consists of gaining access to the arterial system using the femoral or radial artery, with placement of a catheter into the left common iliac artery, followed by the internal iliac artery, the anterior division of the internal iliac artery, and then the uterine artery. With the catheter safely located well within the uterine artery, embolization is performed (Fig. 34.1). Permanent embolization with particles is performed, utilizing 500–700 micron particles or starting with 500–700 micron particles and increasing to 700–900 micron particles, to achieve near arterial stasis (Fig. 34.2). Care must be taken to prevent embolic particles from refluxing back into the proximal vessels where nontarget embolization can occur. Additionally, not uncommonly, communication between the uterine artery and the ovarian artery may be present. Overembolizing the uterine artery in these situations will also cause embolization of the ovarian artery and place the patient at risk of premature ovarian failure. Once the left side is embolized, similar steps are taken to embolize the right uterine artery (Figs. 33.3 and 33.4). Bilateral uterine artery embolization is mandatory, as there are frequent cross-filling vessels. In certain instances, if there is difficulty finding one or both of the uterine arteries, it is necessary to find and catheterize and embolize the ovarian arteries, as these may be the only source of blood supply to the uterus and fibroids. Since this scenario is accompanied by a high risk of premature ovarian failure, the patient should be aware of it before signing the informed consent.

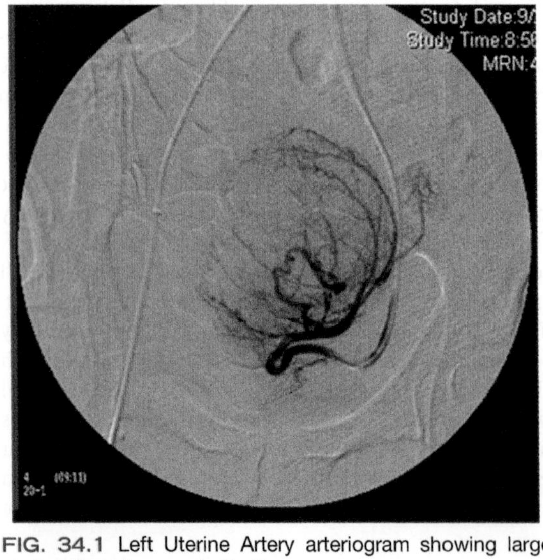

FIG. 34.1 Left Uterine Artery arteriogram showing large uterine fibroid, preembolization.

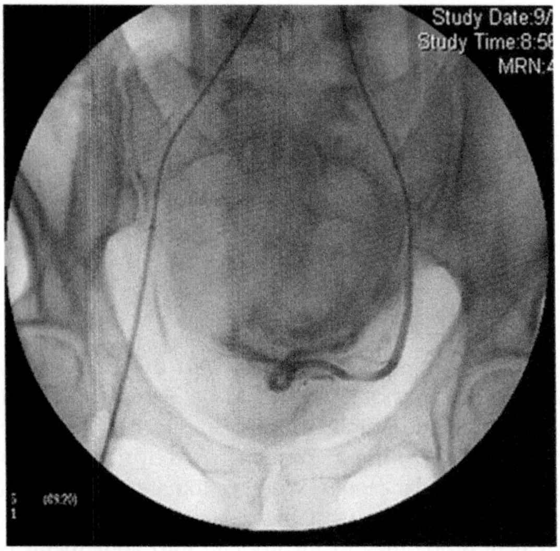

FIG. 34.2 Left Uterine Artery arteriogram showing stasis following embolization.

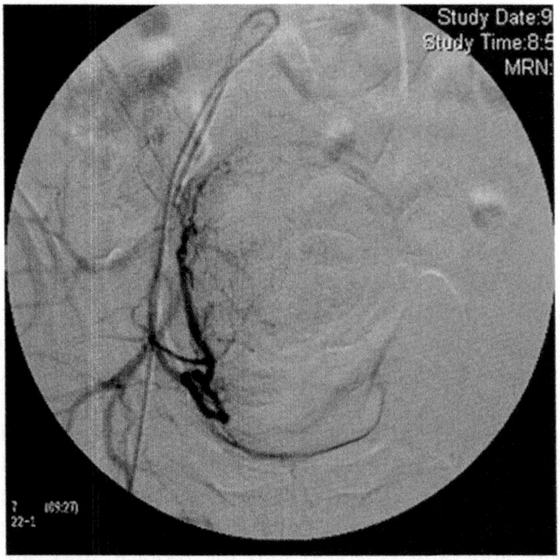

FIG. 34.3 Right Uterine Artery arteriogram showing large uterine fibroid, preembolization.

UFE can easily be performed in an OEC. The procedure does not cause any more discomfort than any other arterial case, and during the procedure, intravenous conscious sedation is certainly adequate to maintain patient comfort. Mobile C-ARM units provide adequate

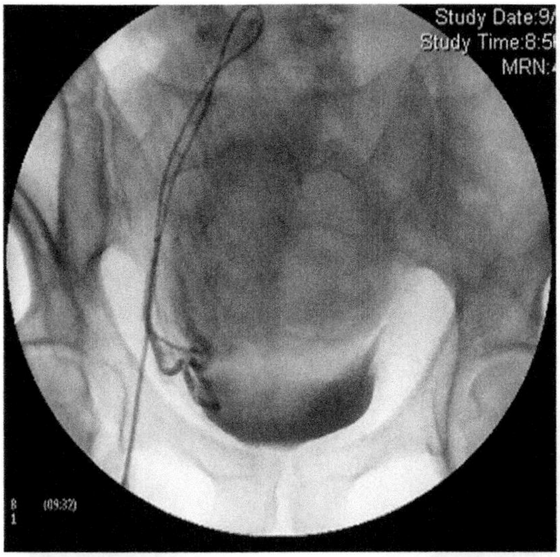

FIG. 34.4 Right Uterine Artery arteriogram showing stasis following embolization.

penetration and resolution to see all the required vessels in most patients. To have a successful office-based UFE practice, the operator needs to have a comprehensive postprocedure pain control protocol. In my experience, the pain experienced by the patient post UFE is more severe than any other procedure done in the office. We are inducing ischemia to the fibroids resulting in death of the cells, and this results in pain. When UFE began to become popular, many physicians kept their patients in the hospital at least overnight, and sometimes longer for pain control. Patient-controlled analgesia pumps were routinely ordered, and patients would recall and report terrible crampy pelvic pain on a level somewhere between the worst menstrual cramps of their life and labor pains. In order to be able to perform this procedure in an OEC followed by discharge of the patient 4–6 h postprocedure, the pain control protocol needed to be significantly improved. For more than 20 years, protocols to control the postprocedure pain have continued to evolve. Some operators have incorporated spinal anesthesia, superior hypogastric nerve blocks, transdermal fentanyl patches, or IV acetaminophen into their "usual" pain control regimen. My protocol relies on an *extensive conversation* with the patient during the consultation regarding expected pain after the procedure. Most importantly, the patient needs to understand that the pain following the procedure is expected in the setting of killing the fibroids, and that nothing life threatening is happening. Once the fear of the pain signifying, "something terrible might be happening inside of me" is gone, I have found that patients actually tolerate all aspects of the procedure well, and are more willing to follow instructions, take their medications as prescribed, and understand that they just need a little time to feel better. My typical pain control protocol is summarized.

1. Before arterial access, ketorolac 30 mg IV
2. Immediately after arterial access is obtained, 1 mg midazolam IV and 50 mcg fentanyl IV
3. After the left uterine artery is embolized, 1 mg midazolam IV and 50 mcg fentanyl IV are given and 5 mg of lidocaine 1% is injected into the embolized uterine artery
4. After the right uterine artery is embolized, 1 mg midazolam IV and 50 mcg fentanyl IV are given and 5 mg of lidocaine 1% is injected into the embolized uterine artery
5. After percutaneous closure of the arterial access site, 1 g acetaminophen IVPB is given
6. In the recovery room, the nurses have prn orders written for meperidine 25 mg IV q 2h, morphine sulfate 4 mg IV q 2h, hydromorphone 1 mg IV q 2h, ketorolac 30 mg X 1, acetaminophen/oxycodone 5/325 mg tabs 1-2 q 4h, as well as antiemetics

The nurses in the recovery play a very important role in pain control. They monitor the patients very closely and are instructed to prevent the pain levels of the patient to get too high. Analgesics in recovery should be given early rather than late. Reviewing our data in 174 UFE patients who were discharged home the same day as their procedure, using this protocol, we found that the average International Pain Scale Score at the time of discharge was 4.1 out of 10.[3]

Our prescribed medications after discharge for our UFE patients are as follows:

1. Acetaminophen/oxycodone 5/325 mg tabs, 1–2 every 4 h prn
2. Ketorolac 10 mg tabs, 1 every 4 h prn

During the first 24 h after the procedure, I recommend that the acetaminophen/oxycodone and the ketorolac can be alternated with each other every 2 h for tighter pain control, if needed.

3. Ibuprofen 600 mg tabs, every 8 h prn

The ibuprofen is typically not needed until day 4–5 after the procedure, once the other prescribed analgesics are no longer needed.

4. Prochlorperazine 10 mg tabs, every 6 h as needed for nausea or vomiting

Since pain control is probably the single most prominent reason to consider whether or not UFE should be performed in the office instead of a hospital environment, admission rates to the hospital after discharge from our office were tracked. The charts of the first 423 patients who had UFEs in the office setting were reviewed. Using the pain control regimen described above, only one patient needed to go to the hospital for pain control (1/423 = 0.2%) following the procedure. Complications of UFE include fibroid expulsion, vaginal discharge, endometritis, ovarian failure, contrast allergy, and groin site complications. The site of service does not have any impact on the incidence of complications. UFE can be successfully performed in the OEC, as long as there is a plan to control the post-procedural pain. The patients undergoing this procedure in the office will be able to go home and will rarely need hospital admission.

Chemoembolization

Chemoembolization is a procedure that is used to treat liver tumors. Primarily, chemoembolization is used to treat hepatocellular carcinoma. However, it is also used to treat cholangiocarcinoma, and metastatic adenocarcinomas to the liver. Chemoembolization is an umbrella term that is used to describe a set of procedures that involve selective catheterization of the hepatic arteries, with the injection of some combination of embolization particles and chemotherapy drugs. When the embolization agent is injected without the drugs, the procedure is called "bland embolization." The embolization of a mixture of chemotherapy drugs and gelatin sponge particles was the first chemoembolization procedure developed in Japan in 1977 by Yamada et al.[4] When the embolization agent is mixed with ethiodized oil, an iodine-based poppy seed oil, and the chemotherapy drug, this is called "conventional trans arterial chemoembolization," or "conventional TACE." This was developed in Japan in the 1980s by Konno et al.,[5] and Nakamura et al.[6] In its current iteration, we mix a powdered form of doxorubicin (50 mg) with 10 cc of iodinated contrast, and 10 cc of the ethiodized oil. In the mid-2000s, new technology was developed that allowed the chemotherapy drugs to be absorbed into embolization beads, and once injected into the arterial bed of the tumors, the drug would be delivered by eluting out of the beads into the tumors.[7] This technique is now called DEB TACE, where DEB is an acronym for drug-eluting beads.

The basic premise behind liver embolization procedures is that the tumors can be killed, while the liver tissue is preserved. The main reason for the success of this technique in the liver is due to the fact that the liver has a dual blood supply from the hepatic artery and the portal vein. In hypervascular tumors, such as hepatocellular carcinoma, the tumor is predominantly supplied by the hepatic artery (Figs. 34.5 and 34.6). The surrounding liver is mainly supplied by the portal vein. Therefore, in the setting of a hypervascular tumor with arterial enhancement, embolizing the feeding artery or arteries should decrease the size of the tumor significantly, while the underlying liver remains viable and minimally affected.

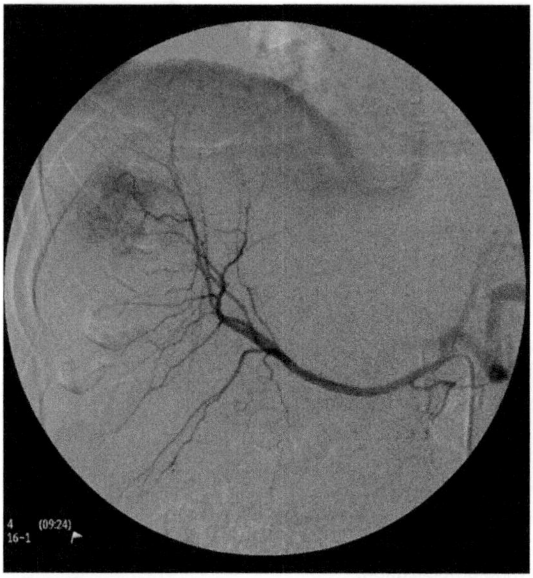

FIG. 34.5 Replaced Right Hepatic Artery arteriogram with enhancement of a solitary hypervascular liver mass.

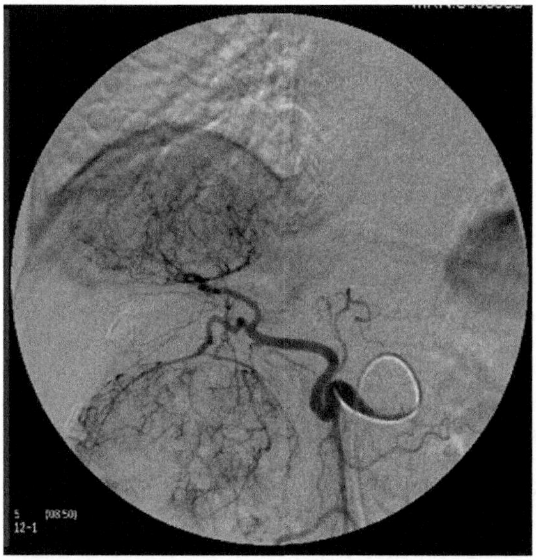

FIG. 34.6 Right Hepatic Artery arteriogram showing two large hypervascular hepatocellular carcinomas.

Complications of liver tumor embolization procedures include hepatic arterial dissection, femoral artery (access site) pseudoaneurysm, liver rupture, liver abscess, cholecystitis, biloma, tumor lysis syndrome, liver infarction, nontarget embolization (gastric or duodenal ulcer), pulmonary embolus, alopecia, leukopenia, anemia, bacteremia/sepsis, hepatic failure, hepatic encephalopathy, variceal bleeding, renal failure, allergic reactions, and the release of neurohumoral factors (in the setting of neuroendocrine tumors). Complication rates vary based on the underlying medical comorbidities of the patient. For instance, the vast majority of patients with hepatocellular carcinoma have cirrhosis. The degree of cirrhosis will therefore determine the level of risk to the patient for hepatic decompensation following a procedure that can compromise the liver's blood supply. Patients who have an adenocarcinoma that is metastatic to the liver may have completely normal underlying liver function. However, if the patient has received a significant amount of systemic chemotherapy over the course of their treatment, the liver may be compromised due to the effect on the liver by the drugs used during systemic chemotherapy. Due to these factors, there is a wide variety of complication rates quoted in the literature for hepatic tumor embolization procedures, with an overall adverse event rate occurring in approximately 10% of patients.[8]

Our complication rate in the first 425 chemoembolization procedures performed in our office endovascular suite was 1.8%. A significant fact to note is that all of the complications and admissions to a hospital following the procedure related to chemoembolization occurred between 6 and 17 days after the procedure. If these patients had their procedures in a hospital, they most likely would have been discharged home from the hospital before 6 days. Therefore, the complications and subsequent admission to the hospital would have occurred regardless of the site of service. We believe that these procedures are safe to be performed with same day discharge in an OEC.

The recovery from a chemoembolization procedure is typically well tolerated by the patient. These patients are either pain free following a typical 2- to 4-hour recovery period, or, if they have any pain, it is well managed with a standard use of analgesics. In comparison with UFE, the liver embolization patients feel much less pain and have less nausea and vomiting.

The important factor in performing chemoembolization procedures safely in the outpatient endovascular office is having a thorough knowledge of the patient's history, anatomy, and ultimate disposition. Catheterizing as subselectively as possible to treat the tumor completely, but sparing portions of the liver that do not need to be affected by embolization, is a primary goal. If patients are too large to get high-quality diagnostic arteriograms in your OEC, then perhaps not treating the patient in the office is the wisest choice. Proper patient selection is of crucial importance. High-risk patients who have significantly elevated bilirubin levels, biliary ductal dilation, or portal vein invasion or occlusion should perhaps be better treated with different modalities or in a more acute care setting. It is also extremely important to perform these procedures within the context of a strong multidisciplinary approach. Many hepatocellular carcinoma patients are under consideration for, or are in a program awaiting, liver transplant. These procedures should not be performed independent of the knowledge and management of their liver transplant physicians.

Yttrium 90 Radioembolization

Yttrium 90 (Y90) selective internal radiation therapy is one of the newer arterial-based EP that is being performed in an OEC. Y90 was approved by the FDA in 2002 for the treatment of metastatic colorectal cancer to the liver. Utilizing the same rationale as chemoembolization, the treatment involves delivery of the tumoricidal agent through the hepatic arterial tree. This procedure, however, involves the delivery of a carrier device (resin or glass spheres) that have been loaded with radioactive particles. These radioactive particles are the yttrium 90. In this radioactive form, Y90 emits radiation as a pure β radiation particle, which in essence is a high-energy, high-speed electron. The delivery device (the resin or glass particles) is slightly larger than red blood cells. These particles are injected into the hepatic artery supplying the tumor, and the particles get wedged into the capillary bed within the tumor causing ischemia. Additionally, once in this location, the Y90 continues to emit its high-energy radiation. The half-life of Y90 is 2.68 days, meaning that approximately 95% of the radioactive energy is emitted over a 12-day period. Pure β emitters such as Y90 have an average range of effect in tissue size of 2.5 mm, so the radiation effect is truly local at the tumor capillary level. This results in selective tumor cell death. The liver is a relatively radiation resistant organ, so the effect on the surrounding liver is much less than the tumor. The tumor types that are selected for treatment tend to be historically radiosensitive tumor that have metastasized to the liver, such as colorectal, neuroendocrine, hepatocellular, bile duct, breast, pancreas, melanoma, lung, sarcoma, stomach, small intestine, esophagus, urothelial, renal, ovarian tumors, and others.

Patient selection for eligibility to be treated with Y90 radioembolization include the following:

- Patients with inoperable liver metastases, not surgical candidates with intent to cure

- Liver only or liver-dominant disease
- Percent liver involvement <60
- Eastern Cooperative Oncology Group (ECOG) 0-2
- Life expectancy > 3 months
- Adequate renal, hepatic and pulmonary function
- Bilirubin <2.0
- Liver-lung shunt <20%

Part of the evaluation process includes the performance of a "mapping" procedure. In this procedure, diagnostic angiography is performed in order to determine which vessels are supplying the tumors. Additionally, vessels that would ordinarily be within the delivery field, but feed either stomach or duodenum, are identified. If it is determined at the time of the mapping that these vessels would possibly get radioactivity within their distribution, this is typically addressed with coil embolization of the vessel. This serves as a protective measure against nontarget embolization and nontarget delivery of radioactive material. In particular, the gastroduodenal artery can originate very close to the right or left hepatic artery origin. If this is the case, coil embolization of the gastroduodenal artery, which supplies the duodenum, would be performed to mitigate against the risk of a radiation induced ulcer. The same logic is used for a fairly common anatomic variant, the right gastric artery that originates from the left hepatic artery. This artery typically supplies a portion of the greater curvature of the stomach, and radiation-induced gastric ulcers can occur if the vessel is not preemptively embolized.

Once the vessel to be treated is chosen, a test dose of radiation is injected in the form of Technetium 99m MAA particles. These particles are the same particles that are injected during a ventilation-perfusion scan (V/Q scan) for the diagnosis of pulmonary embolism. These particles are similar in size to the Y90 particles. By injecting this innocuous form of radiation, we can mimic where the Y90 will go by getting a nuclear medicine study (typically a SPECT CT) following the delivery of these particles into the artery. This maps out the potential radiation delivery in the liver and outside the liver. Importantly, it gives us the percentage of the particles that will travel through the capillary bed of the tumor, and enter the systemic circulation. The amount of radiation delivered to the liver is compared with the radiation delivered to the lung. Excessive radiation delivered to the lung can cause radiation pneumonitis. The threshold is 20%. If after the mapping, more than 20% of the radiation is delivered to the lungs, alternative measures need to be considered for treatment.

If the mapping goes as planned and the patient remains eligible for Y90 treatment, a second procedure is scheduled for dose delivery. The radiation dose is calculated (via various methods beyond the scope of this chapter), ordered, and Y90 is delivered in the exact same artery to mimic the mapping parameters. Postdelivery scans (either an SPECT CT or a PET CT) are obtained for documentation of delivery and its distribution (Figs. 34.7–34.12).

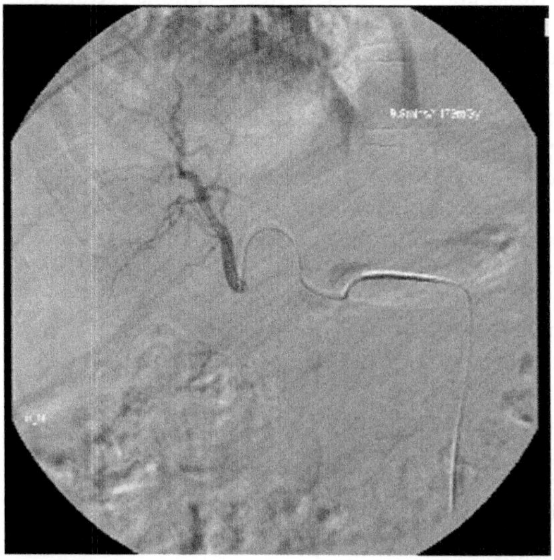

FIG. 34.7 Right Hepatic Artery arteriogram during Y90 mapping procedure. Patient was known to have tumor in this vascular distribution.

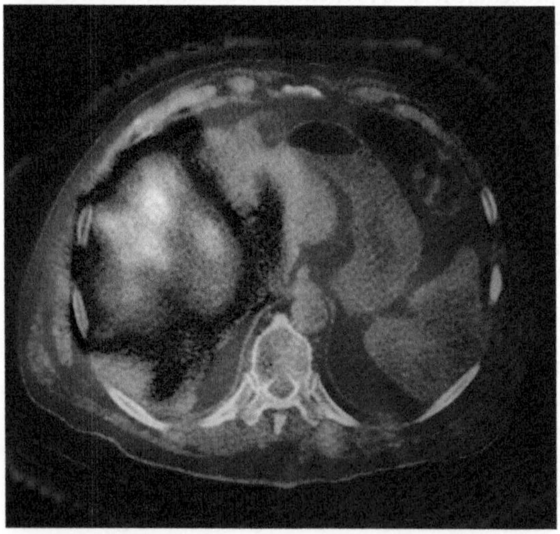

FIG. 34.8 SPECT CT image following injection of Tc99m MAA into the right hepatic artery shown in Fig. 34.7. The colored areas are showing the distribution of the radioisotope within the liver.

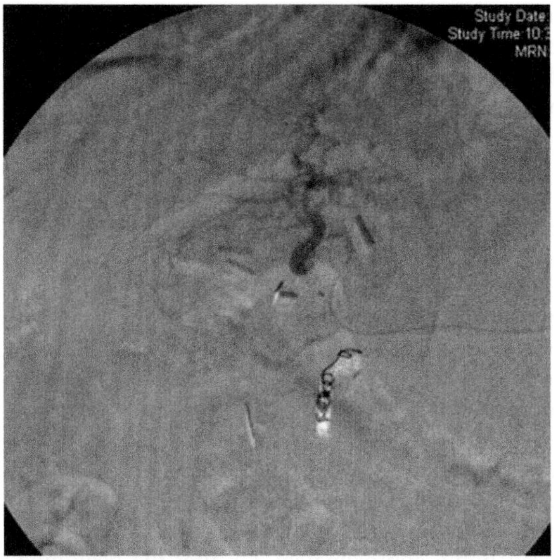

FIG. 34.9 Right Hepatic arteriogram on the day of Y90 treatment in the office.

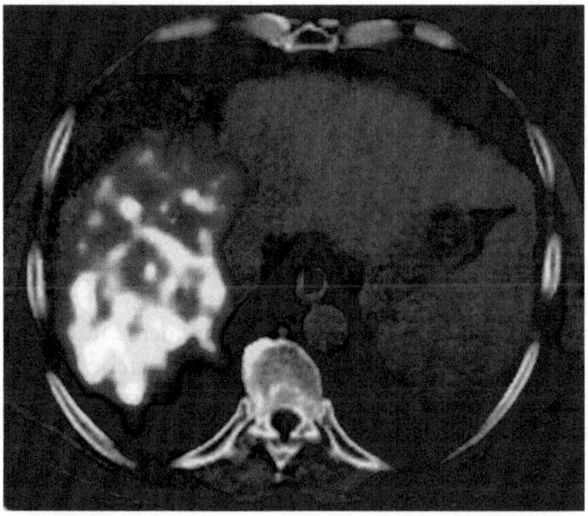

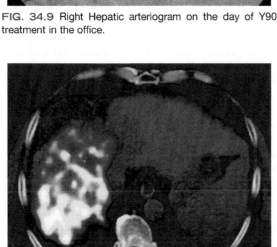

FIG. 34.10 PET CT image of the liver following injection of a therapeutic dose of Y90 into the right hepatic artery shown in Fig. 34.9. Colored area denotes the area of liver treated.

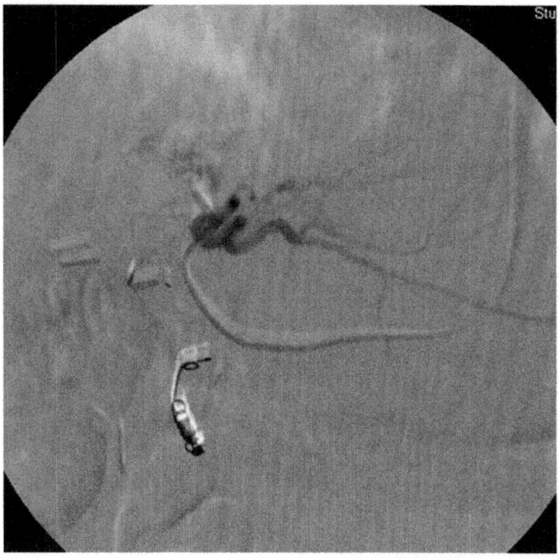

FIG. 34.11 Left Hepatic arteriogram during Y90 treatment.

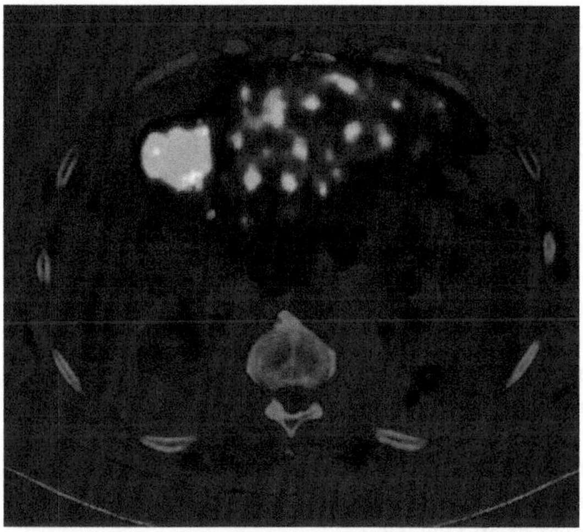

FIG. 34.12 PET CT following injection of a therapeutic dose of Y90 into the left hepatic artery distribution. Note the colored area of treatment within the left lobe of the liver, as well as the dense yellow-orange area of extremely hot uptake within the tumor.

If treatment with Y90 is to be considered in your OEC, there are many steps that need to be taken in planning. The procedure, since its inception, has always been an outpatient procedure. In fact, the procedure typically is not reimbursed if performed on an inpatient basis. The side effects are minimal. The mapping has almost no side effects other than access site complications. The most common side effects and complications that occur after the delivery of the Y90 are fatigue, mild pain, mild nausea, duodenal or gastric ulceration (as described above), and radiation-induced liver disease (RILD). The ulcers, if they occur, typically occur several weeks after treatment. The site of service is certainly not an issue for a complication that occurs that far removed from the procedure. Additionally, proton pump inhibitors are typically prescribed to be taken for 4 weeks after treatment to reduce the possibility of this complication. RILD occurs 6–8 weeks after treatment and is manifested by elevated liver enzymes and liver decompensation. While the liver is relatively radiation resistant, it is not immune to the side effects of radiation. Should the underlying liver be somewhat compromised, either by cirrhosis or exposure to many rounds of systemic chemotherapy, it can be at risk of developing RILD. In these cases, a reduction of the prescribed radiation dose is sometimes warranted. However, since this effect would possibly occur almost 2 months after the treatment, and there would be no difference in how the procedure is performed in a hospital or an office setting, there should be no difference in the rate of occurrence based on the site of service.

Several issues need to be considered if you would like to perform radioembolization in your OEC. Will you be performing the mapping and the delivery of the Y90 at your facility, or just the delivery of the Y90? The mapping procedure involves locating, sometimes 1–2 mm sized right gastric arteries to embolize prior to dose delivery. Most OECs utilize mobile C-ARM units. It can be difficult to identify these very small arteries with confidence while using a mobile C-ARM. If you have a fixed angiography unit at your office facility, this will not apply to you. While this may fall under a personal preference of the operator, we have chosen to perform our mappings on a fixed unit in the hospital, and our dose delivery in the office. The mapping also requires major diagnostic imaging equipment like an SPECT CT. Either you have a unit on the premises, or you have a facility close by that the patient can be sent to following the procedure, but either way, arrangements need to be made to accommodate this major requirement of the procedure. This issue will also come into play following the dose delivery. The Y90 can be visualized using a PET CT or an SPECT CT, so that adds a little flexibility to your arrangements. The technetium used during mapping can only be seen on standard nuclear medicine equipment such as a gamma camera or an SPECT CT.

Due to the fact that both the procedures require radioactive materials, there will be regulatory requirements that will come into play. Regulations can differ in different localities and municipalities. Acquiring the knowledge of these regulations should be one of the first steps taken during planning. In order to have radioactivity in your office, you will need a Radioactive Materials License. Additionally, you will need to find out if you require a "hot lab," a place to receive and store radioactive material. Specialized delivery and disposal vendors will be necessary, as will contractual arrangements with radiation safety personnel, a radiation safety officer, and radiation physics personnel, all of whom are necessary for safety and security of radioactive materials onsite. An authorized user will be needed to calculate the dose for each patient, as well as to assist in the delivery of the Y90. If you do not have all these people onsite, you cannot perform the procedure. Once all of the regulatory issues have been addressed, the procedure itself is not that difficult. Once a successful mapping procedure has been performed, the anatomy has already been identified, the site of delivery determined, and all other obstacles cleared, the delivery day can be short and relatively painless. We try to perform our Y90 delivery procedures via a radial approach, and because we already know the anatomy, we can usually place the catheter in the desired position relatively quickly. Dose delivery usually takes 15–20 min, and we usually have the radial compression device removed within one to one and a half hours after the procedure. During that time, the postprocedure imaging is performed. The patients typically are discharged home approximately 2 h after the beginning of the procedure, usually with no pain, nausea, or other complaints. Discharge instructions do include prescriptions for pain and nausea control. Patients have told us that they have rarely had to use them. Since the radiation cannot penetrate more than a few millimeters, there is inherent safety for loved ones, pets, and children in terms of proximity to the patient and risk of radiation exposure to others. We advise others to keep a three-foot distance from the patient for 3 days to maximize radiation safety, but this is probably excessive and not necessary based on the radiation physics.

Y90 radioembolization is a safe, extremely well-tolerated procedure. If you can navigate all of the regulatory and personnel issues and requirements in order to be eligible to perform this procedure, it can be incorporated seamlessly into your office endovascular office practice.

Other Arterial Embolization Procedures

There are other arterial embolization procedures that can be done, or may be possible in the future. For instance, embolization of a benign fat containing renal tumor, an angiomyolipoma, can be performed in your OEC. However, it is a relatively rare lesion that is usually asymptomatic. It typically only needs to be treated if it is symptomatic (flank pain, hematuria), or if it is of a certain size (depending on the source, larger than 4 cm or larger than 7 cm), or if it has hemorrhaged into itself. The main caveat I will offer, based on personal experience, is that I will only attempt to embolize an angiomyolipoma if it is arising from either the tip of the upper or lower pole of the kidney. In these scenarios, a single artery can be found that supplies arterial flow to the entire lesion, thus making embolization relatively straightforward. If, however, the lesion is arising from the interpolar regions, many different arteries can be supplying the lesion, and at times, the resolution on a mobile C-ARM may not be adequate to identify tumor feeding vessels and those supplying normal kidney. The kidney is composed of all "end arteries" and the sparing of normal renal parenchyma is extremely important. If you cannot be confident about sparing normal kidney, a fixed unit is a better choice for imaging.

Prostate embolization may be the next arterial embolization to be performed at outpatient facilities. This is because there is very little pain or other side effects after the procedure, and the arterial vasculature is relatively consistent. The procedure is performed for symptomatic benign prostatic hypertrophy. The main concern with this procedure is the potential of nontarget embolization of embolic particles into vessels supplying either the penis or the rectum. These vessels are very small and at times can be difficult to identify using current mobile C-ARMs. If you have a fixed fluoroscopy unit in your office, you may be able to perform these procedures with greater success and safety. It is possible that with experience and better technology, this procedure can be migrated to the OEC in time.

VENOUS EMBOLIZATION

Gonadal Vein Embolization

Gonadal vein embolization is a procedure that is used to address refluxing testicular or ovarian veins in symptomatic patients. When the refluxing vein is in a male patient, the resultant enlargement and accumulation of tortuous veins occurs in the scrotum and is called a varicocele. In a female patient, the refluxing vein causes dilated and tortuous veins in the pelvis, mostly in the periureteral and adnexal regions, but at times, also extending into the deep pelvic recesses, including communication with vulvar and vaginal veins. This conglomerate of veins and the associated set of symptoms result in pelvic congestion syndrome. Both the testicular veins and the ovarian veins are embryologically the same. Each structure, the testes and the ovary, originates in the region of the kidney, where in utero, the gonads begin development. As the fetus develops, the ovary or testes migrate caudally to the pelvis or the scrotum and the gonadal artery and vein migrate caudally along with the gonad. The left gonadal vein typically originates from the left renal vein, and the right gonadal vein originates from the inferior vena cava just below the level of the right renal vein. The pathophysiology of the varicocele or the pelvic varices seen in pelvic congestion syndrome is dysfunctional valves in the gonadal vein. Typically, the valvular dysfunction originates at the highest point of origin in these veins. Reflux causes reversal of flow in the vein, sometimes at rest, but most commonly with gravity-dependent activities, exercise, or sexual activity. The veins fill in retrograde fashion resulting in the pooling of blood in the veins in pelvis or the scrotum. Blood is rerouted to competent veins in the pelvis and returned to normal circulation pattern. The accumulation of enlarged veins in the pelvis or scrotum can cause symptoms. In men, these symptoms include pain, heaviness, a feeling in the scrotum of a "bag of worms," increased sensitivity, and infertility (due to a low sperm count). In women, typical symptoms include pain, heaviness, and achiness in the deep pelvis. Additionally, the dilated veins in the pelvis can irritate adjacent nerves and cause pain in the distribution area supplied by the nerves.

There are medical therapies and surgical therapies to treat each of these entities. Medical therapies are usually not very successful, and a large proportion of patients prefer treatment using minimally invasive techniques. Embolization of the veins in men and women is performed using very similar techniques. Either a femoral or jugular venous approach is chosen, and catheters and wires are placed into the gonadal veins and advanced just past the inguinal ligament in men and to the level of the ovary in women. Coil embolization alone or in conjunction with a flowable embolic agent such as sotradecol foam or glue (n-butyl cyanoacrylate) are commonly used with high technical and clinical success rates. These veins tend to have some branches, therefore, traditional teaching is that in men, embolization should be performed at the level of the inguinal ligament, the bottom of the sacroiliac joint, the top of the sacroiliac joint, and at or near the origin of the gonadal vein. In women, similar multilevel embolization throughout the length of the vein is warranted to maximize effectiveness. Additionally, in women it may be necessary to perform venography of the pelvic veins that arise from the internal iliac veins. This can be performed at rest or by using an occlusion balloon to see if reflux is present or if injection provides visualization of enlarged deep pelvic veins (Figs. 34.13–34.22).

Recovery is typically short for gonadal vein embolization. Patients usually stay in our recovery room for only 1–2 h after the procedure. Patients usually have minimal pain. During recovery at home the patient may experience mild pelvic soreness for a few days. Nonsteroidal antiinflammatory agents are commonly sufficient for pain relief. Symptomatic improvement for pain occurs in approximately 87% of patients.[9] Improvement usually occurs within 1–2 weeks. When

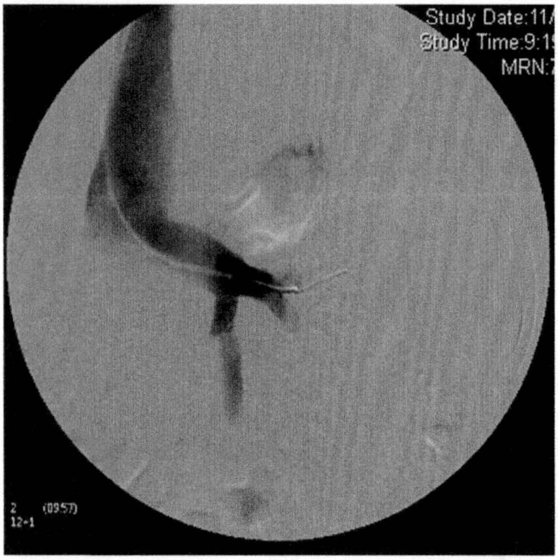

FIG. 34.13 Left renal venogram with opacification of the left renal vein, the inferior vena cava, and spontaneous reflux into the downward flowing left ovarian vein.

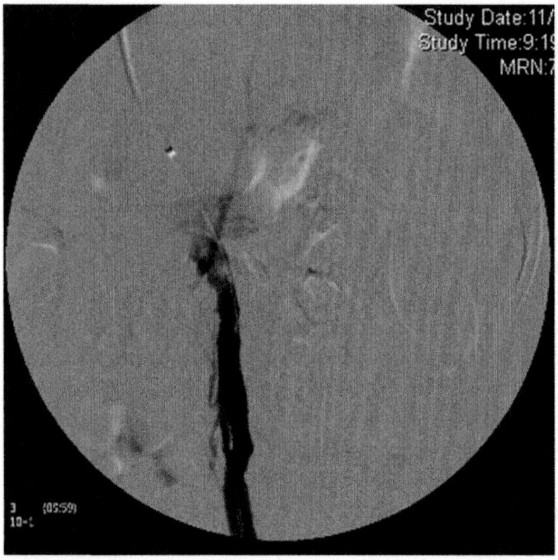

FIG. 34.14 Venogram of the left ovarian vein with the catheter located within the proximal left gonadal vein.

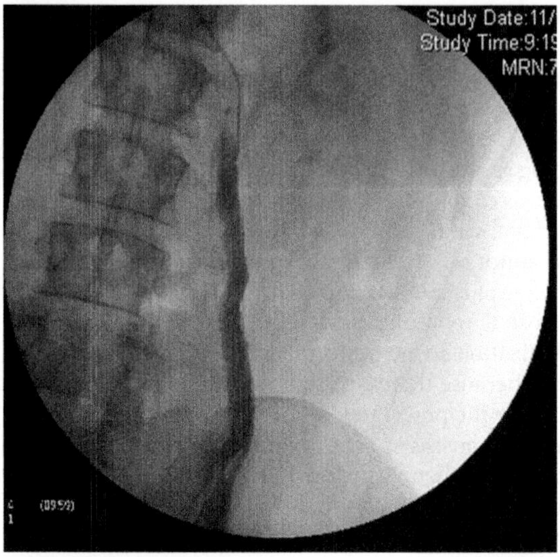

FIG. 34.15 Image showing stasis of flow within the contrast-filled left ovarian vein.

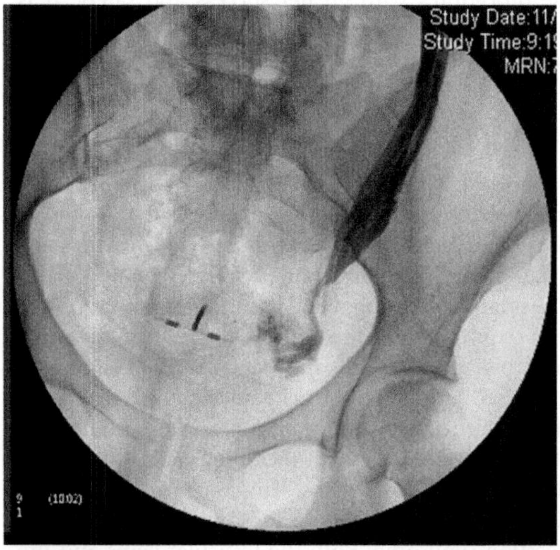

FIG. 34.16 Contrast filling the left ovarian vein to the level of the left ovary.

performed for male infertility, the success rate is approximately 40%–50%.[10] In order to follow sperm count and morphology, a full sperm cycle must occur (approximately 70–80 days) before repeat semen analysis is obtained.

In summary, gonadal vein embolization is an excellent procedure that can easily be performed in the OEC with a high degree of technical and clinical success.

Other Venous Embolization Procedures

There are additional venous embolization procedures that can be incorporated into your office-based practice. Full details of these procedures are beyond the scope of this chapter, but suffice it to say, we perform these procedures rather routinely and patients recover from these procedures quickly and with excellent clinical outcomes. Portal vein embolization (Figs. 34.23–34.24),

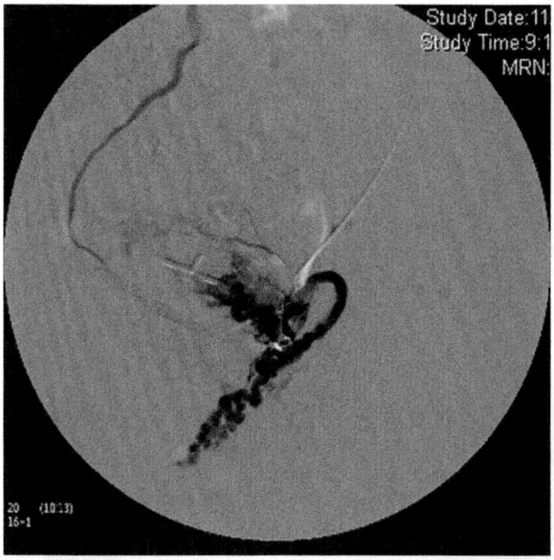

FIG. 34.17 Left ovarian venogram with catheter located at the level of the left ovary. Note contrast flowing retrograde into a large refluxing varix toward the left vulvar region.

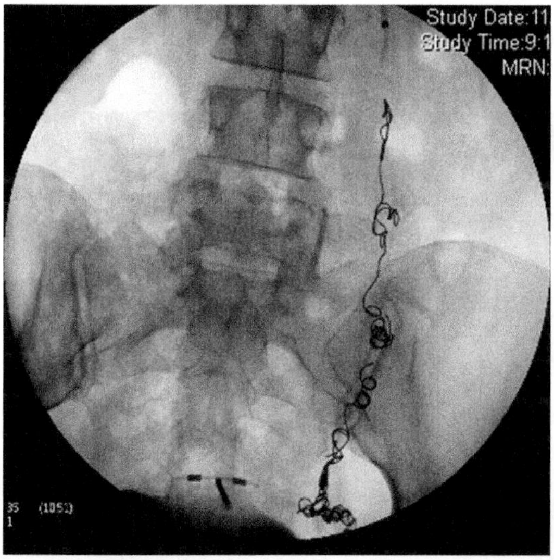

FIG. 34.18 Static image postembolization of the left ovarian vein with metallic coils.

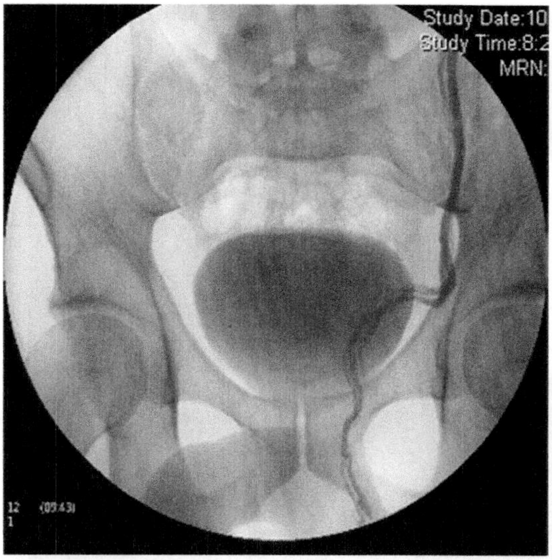

FIG. 34.19 Contrast within the left testicular vein, extending caudally past the inguinal ligament to fill a varicocele within the scrotum.

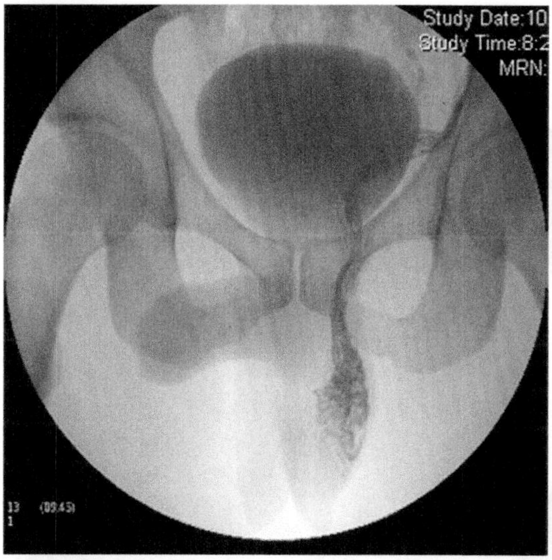

FIG. 34.20 Contrast within the left testicular vein filling a varicocele within the scrotum, slightly later during the injection of contrast, filling dilated veins in the scrotum.

direct stick embolization of lower extremity congenital venous malformations (Figs. 34.25–34.26), and dialysis-related arteriovenous fistula maturation embolization (of competing veins preventing maturation of a primary extremity vein) are examples of venous embolization procedures that can be performed in the OEC with great confidence and excellent results.

In conclusion, embolization procedures in both arterial and venous systems can be performed with regularity in an OEC. Some of the procedures require planning and

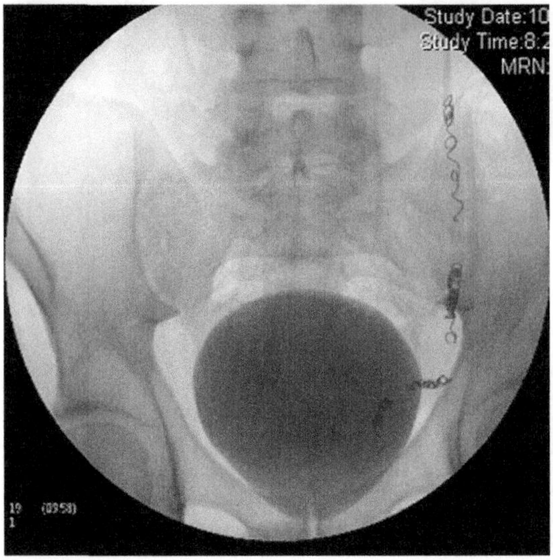

FIG. 34.21 Static image following coil embolization of the left testicular vein from the left inguinal ligament shown in the pelvis near the left inguinal canal.

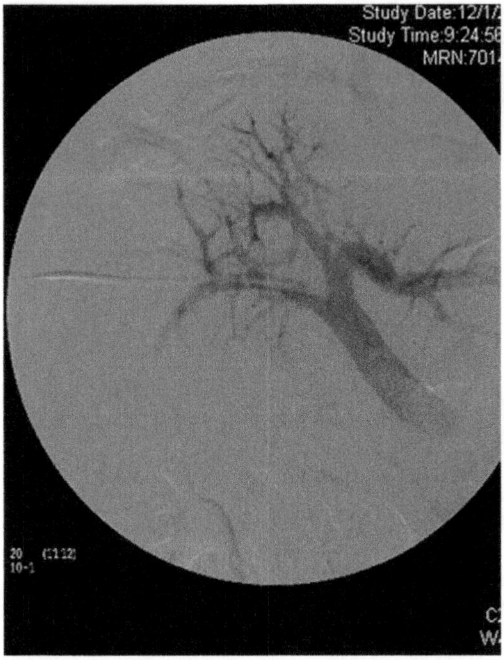

FIG. 34.23 Portal vein venogram with catheter extending from a percutaneous approach into the right portal vein. Catheter tip is located at the origin of the right portal vein as it arises from the main portal vein.

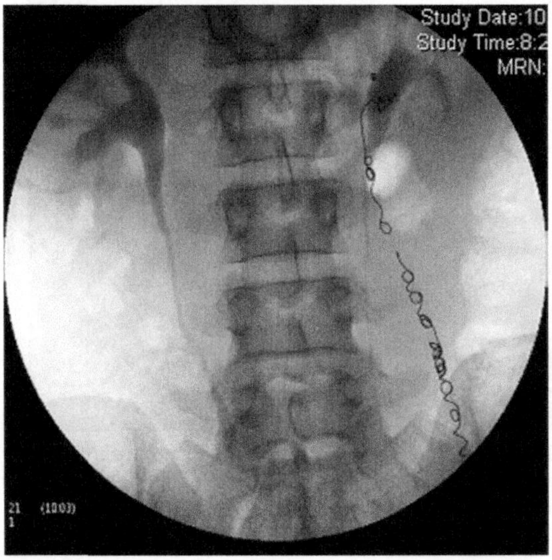

FIG. 34.22 Static image following coil embolization of the left testicular vein, shown higher in the abdomen to the origin of the left testicular vein at the level of the left renal vein.

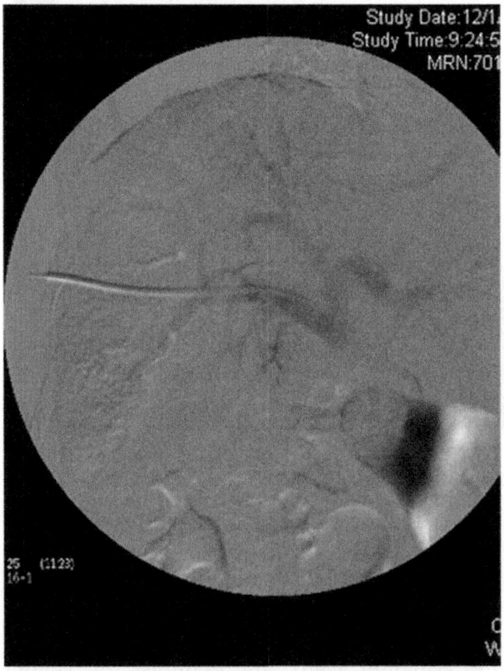

FIG. 34.24 Portal venogram following embolization of the right portal vein. Catheter tip is in the same location as in Fig. 34.23. Note lack of filling of the right portal vein and branches with contrast only filling the left portal vein.

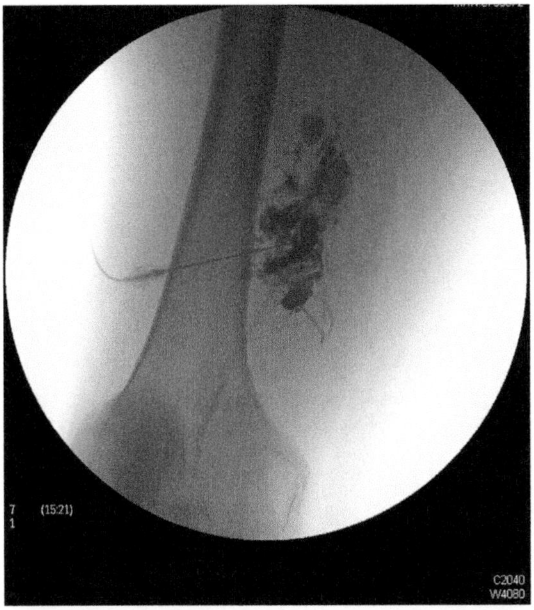

FIG. 34.25 Percutaneous needle placement into a large right lower extremity venous malformation. Contrast fills the innumerable serpentine branches of the malformation and remains static within the veins.

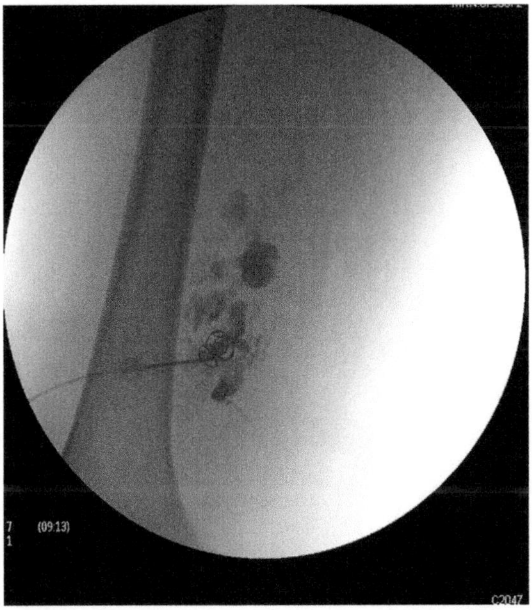

FIG. 34.26 Right leg venous malformation following percutaneous embolization with sotradecol foam and metallic coils.

coordination with other services and specialties. In certain embolization procedures this is extremely important. The clinical results are satisfactory and the procedures can be added to the portfolio of cases performed in the office-based endovascular center.

REFERENCES

1. Ravina JH, et al. Arterial embolization to treat uterine myomata. *Lancet*. 1995;346(8976):671–672.
2. Goodwin SC, et al. Preliminary experience with uterine artery embolization for uterine fibroids. *J Vasc Interv Radiol*. 1997;8(4):517–526.
3. Mar S. *Sperling, Evaluation of Pain Scores Following Fibroid Embolization, Poster Presentation*. Las Vegas, NV: National Meeting for the American Osteopathic College of Radiology; October 2006.
4. Yamada R, et al. Hepatic artery embolization in 120 patients with unresectable hepatoma. *Radiology*. 1983;148: 397–401.
5. Konno T, et al. Effect of arterial administration of high molecular weight anti cancer agent SMANCS with lipid lymphographic agent on hepatoma: a preliminary report. *Eur J Cancer Clin Oncol*. 1983;19:1053–1065.
6. Nakamura H, et al. Transcatheter oily chemoembolization of hepato-cellular carcinoma. *Radiology*. 1989;170: 783–786.
7. Varela M, et al. Chemoembolisation of hepatocellular carcinoma with drug eluting beads: efficacy and doxorubicin pharmacokinetics. *J Hepatol*. 2007;46:474–481.
8. Gaba R, et al. Quality improvement guidelines for transarterial chemoembolization and embolization of hepatic malignancy. *J Vasc Interv Radiol*. 2017;28:1210–1223.
9. Puche-Sanz I, et al. Primary treatment of painful varicocoele through percutaneous retrograde embolization with fibred coils. *Andrology*. 2014;2:716–720.
10. Nabi G, et al. Percutaneous embolization of varicoceles: outcomes and correlation of semen improvement with pregnancy. *Urology*. 2004;63:359–363.

CHAPTER 35

Cardiac Interventions in the Office Interventional Suite

JEFFREY G. CARR, MD, FACC, FSCAI

BACKGROUND AND EVOLUTION

Although the past several decades have demonstrated amazing advances in cardiovascular disease, it remains the number one killer of patients and consumer of healthcare dollars in the United States.[1] In September 1977, Andreas Gruentzig performed the first balloon angioplasty in a coronary artery. This revolutionized minimally invasive coronary interventions, but it took several decades to develop the pharmacologic agents and devices that could be used safely so that the patient can be discharged from the hospital on the same day as the procedure. Early in the percutaneous coronary intervention (PCI) experience, in an attempt to prevent acute thrombosis and vessel closure, patients were placed on high dose heparin, low-molecular-weight dextran, dipyridamole, aspirin, and warfarin loading. The proverbial pharmacologic "kitchen sink" was used in hopes that a hospitalized patient could be safely discharged without a thrombotic coronary event. Patients were routinely hospitalized for 4–7 days at a minimum after undergoing a coronary balloon angioplasty or receiving a first-generation stent usually waiting until a therapeutic INR could be achieved. Additionally, there was a requirement for a level 1 cardiothoracic surgery operating room standby when coronary angioplasty was being performed. This meant that a cardiothoracic surgeon, cardiothoracic anesthesiologist, and experienced staff needed to remain on immediate standby during coronary artery interventions at most hospitals around the country.

Additionally, in the early days, permanent pacemakers (PPMs) and the early automatic implantable cardioverter defibrillators were often implanted in surgical operating rooms. Patients remained in the hospital at least 2–3 days postoperatively to ensure stability of the wound sites and efficacy of the procedure. Rarely, surgical pocket infections or lead problems created significant clinical complications and had economic consequences.

SAME-DAY CARDIOLOGY INTERVENTIONS

Enter the concept of same-day intervention and discharge. In the 1990–2000s, there were significant advances in device and pharmacologic therapies. These advances continue to be made to make coronary intervention safer. This has allowed an unprecedented shift of patient care from the tertiary and quaternary care hospitals to the outpatient and office-based settings. To some degree, Centers for Medicare and Medicaid Services (CMS) has recognized that cost of providing care is significantly less in an outpatient environment. If procedures and quality care can be delivered in an outpatient or office setting in a more cost-effective, appropriate, safe, and patient-preferred manner, then true value for the healthcare system can be realized.

First and foremost, cardiac interventions in the office or freestanding clinic environment have to be done in a safe manner. If a patient is to be discharged home after a cardiac intervention in 2–4 h from an office or an ambulatory surgery center (ASC), then it is paramount that the patient's safety after discharge is ensured. To that end, it is imperative that patients are selected properly for appropriate diagnostic evaluations and interventions. Patients with coronary artery disease (CAD) should undergo diagnostic cardiac catheterizations when they have symptoms based on physiologic testing (stress testing, etc.) suggestive of coronary artery ischemia.

Origin and Evolution of Cardiac Procedures in Free-Standing Labs

Office-based or freestanding labs have been in existence for several decades. Cardiac catheterization labs opened in freestanding facilities detached from a hospital in the late 1980s, and cardiac-related services have been safely performed since. However, due to negative coverage policy issues surrounding independent diagnostic testing facilities (IDTFs), most of the popularity and growth of catheterization labs organized by MedCath Partners

Office-Based Endovascular Centers. https://doi.org/10.1016/B978-0-323-67969-5.00035-6
Copyright © 2020 Elsevier Inc. All rights reserved.

(later MedCath, Inc.) and other groups waned in the beginning of mid-1990s. These early cath labs were solely diagnostic facilities, and cardiac interventions were not performed. The reasons for failure were untenable IDTF coverage, policy changes, and new business models rather than safety concerns. Interesting to note, cardiac interventions in these freestanding facilities at that time would have been premature and possibly unsafe. In the early 2000s, there was a marked growth in physician ownership in specialty heart hospitals in predominately non–Certificate of Need (CON) states. This expansion in heart hospitals occurred until 2003 when the Congress passed the Medicare Prescription Drug, Improvement, and Modernization Act, which amended the Stark Law's whole hospital exception to include an 18-month moratorium on physician ownership in specialty hospitals. The moratorium continued until 2006, when CMS delivered a final report detailing physician ownership in specialty hospitals.[2] More recently, passage of the Patient Protection and Affordable Care Act in March 2010 curtailed growth in physician ownership by effectively prohibiting both the creation of new and the expansion of existing physician-owned hospitals and outpatient facilities after March 2010.[3]

Fast forward to our current era

The marked advances in interventional cardiac devices and pharmacology have resulted in proving the safety and efficacy of performing same-day interventions. To that end, the modern, very low-profile coronary drug-eluting stents are composed of unique metallic alloys and have an extremely low risk of acute thrombotic vessel occlusion. The current balloon and stent designs allow for safe and successful delivery of stents to extremely complex coronary lesions and minimize stent jailing of side branches.[4] Anticoagulant and oral antiplatelet therapies have improved pharmacokinetics for intra- and postprocedure antithrombotic and antiplatelet protection.[5] Covered coronary stents, thrombectomy catheters, distal embolic protection devices, thrombolytics, access closure devices to deal with and prevent complications from cardiac interventions also contribute to the safety of coronary interventions. In addition to stocking these products in the lab, it is essential that cardiologists possess bail-out experience if one is to perform cardiac interventions in a freestanding facility such as the office interventional suite (OIS) or an ASC (Fig. 35.1).

SAFETY AND OUTCOME DATA FOR PCI WITHOUT ON-SITE SURGICAL BACKUP

As the devices, techniques, and experience grew, procedural success rates for PCI also improved for increasingly complex interventions. The need for emergent coronary artery bypass surgery following a failed PCI significantly fell from 1.5% in 1992 to 0.14% by 2000 (Fig. 35.2). Data reported in 2009 from the ACC-SCAI sponsored NCDR CathPCI showed that out of the 308,161patient cohort undergoing PCI from 2004 to 2006, 8736 patients underwent PCI in 60 centers with no surgical backup. These "off-site PCI centers" had similar observed procedure success, morbidity, emergency cardiac surgery rates, and mortality in cases that required emergency surgery compared with centers with backup capabilities. Interestingly, one-fourth of these centers had traveled distances more than 40 miles away or greater than 30 min in transport time (by

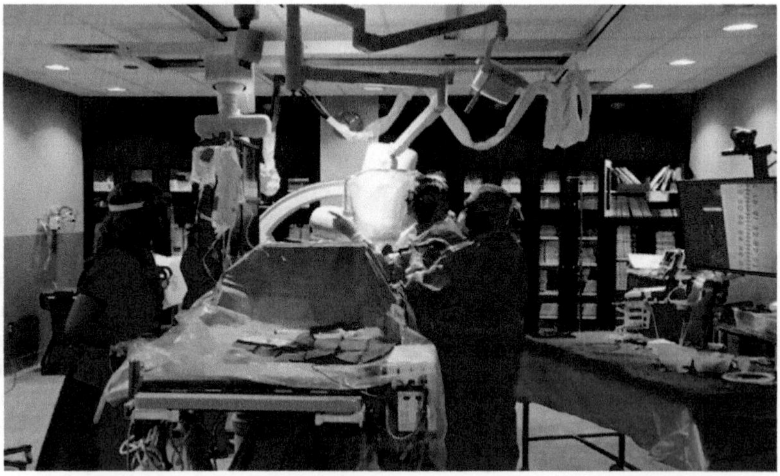

FIG. 35.1 Intervention underway in an office interventional suite.

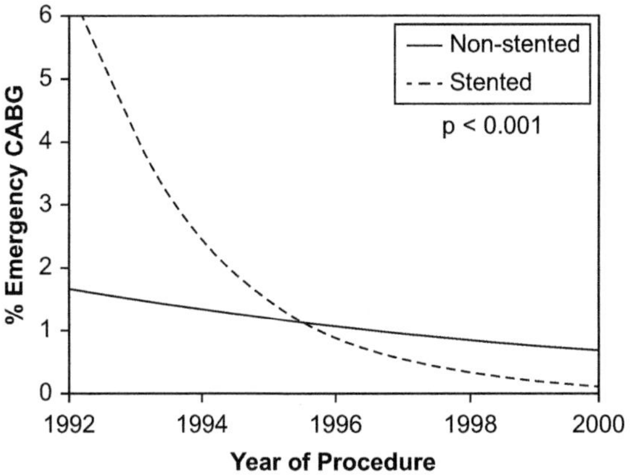

FIG. 35.2 Prevalence of emergency CABG in stented and nonstented patients from 1992 through 2000. (Seshadri N, Whitlow PL, Acharya N, Houghtaling P, Blackstone EH, Ellis SG. Emergency coronary artery bypass surgery in the contemporary percutaneous coronary intervention era. Circulation 2002; 106:2346–2350.)

ground or air) demonstrating that these facilities were truly some distance away from the nearest emergency surgical facilities.[6]

Two large randomized clinical trials assessed the safety of nonemergent PCI procedures in outpatient settings (sites without on-site surgical backup). The Cardiovascular Patient Outcomes Research Team Non-Primary PCI (CPORT-E) trial supported the safety of performing PCI in 60 hospitals in 10 states with or without on-site surgical backup for stable CAD patients from 2006 to 2011. In this study, 18,867 patients with stable CAD or ACS (STEMIs excluded) were randomly assigned in a 3:1 ratio to nonemergent PCI at a hospital with (n = 4718) or without (n = 14,149) on-site cardiac surgery from 2006 to 2011. The investigators found that elective PCI at hospitals without on-site cardiac surgery was noninferior when compared with similar procedures performed at hospitals with surgical capabilities in terms of 6-week mortality (0.9 vs. 1.0%) and 9 months MACE rates (12.1 vs. 11.2%) (Table 35.1).[7]

A second randomized trial to compare PCI between Massachusetts Hospitals with Cardiac Surgery On-Site and Community Hospitals without Cardiac Surgery On-Site (MASS COMM) included 3,691 patients and showed similar safety and efficacy regardless of patients' transfer to a hospital with on-site surgery backup or no backup for a nonemergent PCI. The 30 day and 12 month MACE rates (death, MI, repeat revascularization, and stroke) were not different and the noninferior endpoints were reached.[8]

TABLE 35.1
Nine Month Outcomes for Elective PCIs Performed in Hospitals Without Versus With On-site Surgical Backup in the CPORT-E Trial.

	No On-Site Surgery (n = 14,149)	On-Site Surgery (n = 4,718)	*P* Value
Death	3.2%	3.2%	
TVR	6.5%	5.4%	0.01 (for superiority)
MI	3.1%	3.1%	
MACE	12.1%	11.2%	1.1 (for non-inferiority)

Adapted from C-PORT E, Aversano T, Lemmon CC, Liu L, for the Atlantic CPORT Investigators. N Engl J Med. 2012;366:1792–1802.

Furthermore, commensurate with these safety and efficacy data and indicating trends and outcomes in real-world practices, there was a dramatic shift in numbers of PCIs performed in the United States without on-site surgery. A large retrospective analysis of over 6,900,000 patients undergoing PCI (from 2003 to 2012) showed a sevenfold increase over a 10-year period in the number of PCIs performed in centers without on-site surgery backup (5.7% of the total) and showed no difference in adjusted in-hospital mortality if PCI was performed in centers without on-site surgery backup for patients with acute coronary syndromes (ACSs) and elective procedures.[9]

These trials and registries collectively demonstrate that patients undergoing nonemergent PCI have similar outcomes whether or not they are treated at hospitals that possess on-site cardiac surgery capabilities.

SOCIETAL GUIDELINES AND REGULATORY TRENDS

In response to these studies and multiple other metaanalyses and published reports, the SCAI, ACC, and AHA Expert Consensus Document in 2014 concluded that "performance of PCI without on-site surgery in the US has gained greater acceptance, and questions about its safety in the presence of a proven, well-defined, and protocol driven approach have diminished." This document summarized the available published data and updated guidelines for best practices for sites performing PCI.[10] The state Departments of Health regulate PCI without on-site surgery in 34 states, but it is unregulated in 16 states. A survey by the writing committee for the

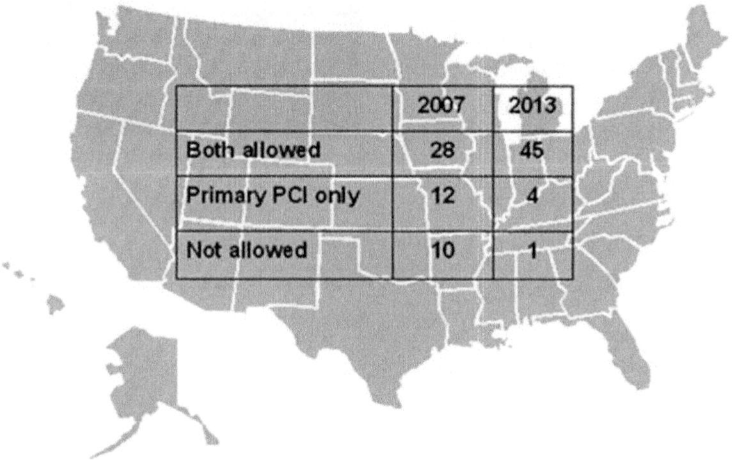

2007
2013
Both allowed 28 45
Primary PCI only 12 4
Not allowed 10 1

FIG. 35.3 Change in the availability of percutaneous coronary intervention (PCI) without on-site surgery from 2007 to 2013. The numbers shown indicate the number of states where primary and nonprimary PCI without on-site surgery were allowed.

Consensus Document determined that there was a significant shift in states' position in allowing PCI without on-site surgery from 2007 to 2013, with 45 states allowing both primary and elective PCI (Fig. 35.3).

PCI ADVANCES, TRANSRADIAL PCI AND SAME-DAY DISCHARGE

Coronary PCI management has advanced in numerous ways in recent years. As a growing trend in many hospitals in the United States, patients are sent home following PCI on the same day and treated as a same-day discharge (SDD) with no differences in outcomes at 7 and 30 days compared with next day discharge.[11] Transradial artery access for coronary interventions continues to grow in popularity and is gradually becoming the standard of care for PCI. Efforts are underway to adopt a "radial first" approach to all coronary interventions.[12] Interventions performed by transradial artery access, although associated with increased radiation exposure, offer a SDD that provides increased safety in terms of reduced bleeding rates compared with transfemoral artery access.[12,13] Additionally, radial artery access prevents the formation of life-threatening retroperitoneal hematoma that can occur after transfemoral access. Vascular closure devices have also reduced postprocedure bed rest times postcatheterization and intervention and have been shown to reduce hematoma rates compared with manual compression in selected cases.[13,14] Current-generation coronary stents are very low profile and allow efficient delivery of stents to lesions that previously had been uncrossable. These stents also have very low acute thrombosis rates and have long-term durability with low target lesion revascularization rates.[4] Improved guide catheter shapes, guidewire design, and support catheters have added to technical success and improved safety. Notable improvements in pharmacology also have led to the acute and long-term safety and efficacy of coronary interventions.[5] Oral antiplatelet therapy with ticagreglor (AstraZeneca, Wilmington, DE) and prasugrel (Eli Lilly, Indianapolis, IN) has been shown to have more rapid, potent, and effective platelet inhibition without pharmacogenetic variability compared with clopidogrel.[15]

EVIDENCE FOR SAME-DAY DISCHARGE AFTER INTERVENTION

As the delivery of PCI and cardiac interventional care continues to evolve, same-day coronary and cardiac interventions have been a growing practice for many institutions incentivized by patient satisfaction and an effort to reduce costs. In addition to the numerous studies showing PCI safety without surgical backup, there have been several studies demonstrating that PCI is safe for selected patients in the setting of SDD. In 2007, the Elective PCI in Outpatient Study (EPOS) Trial randomized 800 patients undergoing elective PCI (using transfemoral approach only) in an outpatient setting to be discharged 4 h after PCI on the same day or after an overnight stay. There was no safety difference (noninferiority) with death, MI, CABG, repeat PCI, or puncture-related complications for SDD compared with hospitalized patients at 24 h and 30 days.[16] Adding to this evidence, the NCDR CathPCI Registry showed no differences in 2- and 30-day outcomes for rates of death or rehospitalization following elective PCI in selected Medicare patients (n = 107,018) whether the patient had SDD (n = 1339) or stayed overnight (n = 105,679). This study analyzed only Medicare patients (>65 years) and concluded that PCI is safe with SDD in properly selected elderly patients. The authors caution that patients' home support systems need to be verified as part of the selection process.[17]

Similar efficacy and safety results were shown for SDD compared with overnight stays in two transradial PCI studies. A single center, observational, Same-Day Trans Radial Intervention and Discharge Evaluation (STRIDE) study of 450 hospitalized stable and ACS patients who underwent transradial PCI showed no difference in complications whether patients were discharged at 6 h (SDD) or in 24 h.[18] Published in 2006, the Early Discharge After Transradial Stenting of Coronary Arteries (EASY) Study randomized 1,005 patients who had undergone a successful transradial PCI to overnight stay into two groups: abciximab bolus (Eli Lilly, Indianapolis, IN) + 12-hour infusion versus SDD-PCI abciximab bolus only. Interestingly, the investigators included a higher-risk cohort of 18% patients with elevated cardiac troponins at baseline. At 30 days and at 1 year, there was no difference in the composite primary endpoint, defined as death from any cause, myocardial infarction, unplanned revascularization, major bleeding, access site complications, or rehospitalization.[19,20] Metaanalyses of randomized trials showed no differences in adverse outcomes including death, MI, MACE, hospitalization, blood transfusions, repeat revascularization, hematoma, and bleeding with selected patients undergoing PCI in SDD compared with overnight stay.[21,22]

OFFICE INTERVENTIONAL SUITE—SAFETY STUDIES

There is also published evidence for the safety of performing a variety of interventions specifically in the OIS and freestanding facilities detached from a hospital. Three single-center, retrospective studies, of predominately peripheral endovascular interventional procedures in an office lab setting, showed low death and emergent hospital transfer rates with no direct procedural deaths. Jain et al. reported their office-based endovascular procedure outcomes in 6,458 procedures including a variety of arterial and venous procedures and dialysis access interventions. In this single-center experience that included a high proportion of dialysis patients, there was a 0.4% hospital transfer rate with 18 deaths at 30-day follow-up (0.28%) but no procedure-related deaths.[23] Oskui et al. reviewed their 500 case experience (335 dialysis access interventions, 148 lower extremity artery endovascular procedure, and 17 miscellaneous—mostly vascular interventions) in their single office lab and reported a 1.4% adverse event, 0.2% emergent transfer rate, and no deaths related to the procedures.[24] Lin et al. reported their series of 5,123 predominately arterial and venous endovascular procedures in a vascular surgery practice at two locations and found a total complication rate of 1.4%, a 0.29% immediate transfer rate, a 1.4% total complication rate, 9 deaths at 30 days (0.18%), and no procedure-related deaths. The authors in this study also distinguished their early versus later case experience to demonstrate overall process and quality improvement resulting in reduction of the total complication rate from 3% in their first 1000 cases to 0.7% in 4000–5000 cases performed in their freestanding facilities.[25] It should be noted that none of these office-based studies reported performing cardiac procedures, and more cardiac specific outcomes data are needed.

SAFE OPERATIONS AND PROCESSES—OEIS SCOCAP

Establishing and ensuring safe cath lab operations and processes is imperative if one is to perform cardiac interventions in the OIS. The ACC, SVS, SIR, and SCAI all have societal guidelines for conducting safe and appropriate interventions related to their specialties, but none have provided guidance based on site of service. The Outpatient Endovascular and Interventional Society (OEIS) has championed six quality initiatives for every intervention specifically performed in an OEC or ASC environment. The acronym SCOCAP encompasses standards of **S**afety, **C**redentialing, **O**utcomes measures, **C**ompliance, **A**ppropriateness, and **P**eer Review. Accreditation is currently offered by several agencies (The Joint Commission, AAAHC, AAAASF) to attest to a lab's safety and efforts are underway to develop a separate, dedicated accreditation pathway specific to the OIS (Chapter 36). At a minimum, policies and procedures should be in place at each facility to mitigate medical errors and standardize the patient experience. It is highly recommended that all freestanding facilities establish emergency transfer agreements with local hospitals in the event that an emergent problem arises and the patient requires hospitalization. All cardiologists in the office lab should be properly credentialed and experienced to perform cardiac interventions. New operators, recently finishing a training program, should demonstrate experience with independent cardiac interventions and bail-out techniques or undergo a period of mentorship or proctorship. The staff involved in the case and aftercare need to have cardiac experience and be skilled to provide care to patients after cardiac procedures. Beyond credentialing, all labs would be well advised to undergo mock "bail-out" drills to remain current and fresh to deal with a potential emergent situation that may rarely occur in the OIS. All patients should have a risk assessment prior to undergoing procedures, such as an American Society of Anesthesiologists (ASA) score. There should be appropriate clinical indications and evaluation of procedural risks and comorbidities to properly select patients for cardiac interventions. A peer-review and quality improvement process in each lab is healthy and advisable. Guideline-driven decision-making is also highly recommended as cardiology-specific appropriate use criteria have matured.

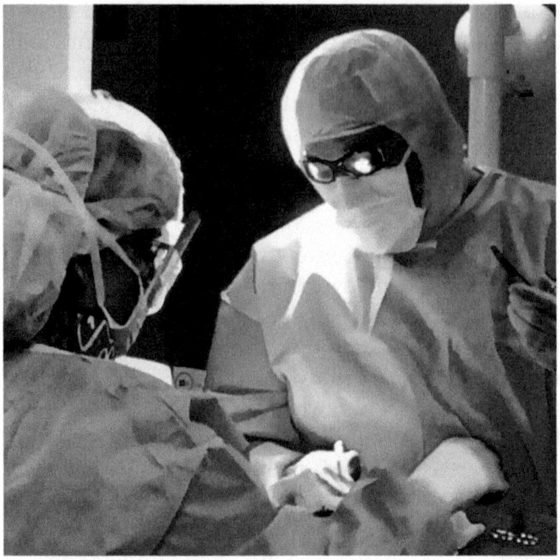

FIG. 35.4 Pacemaker implantation procedure in the office interventional suite.

AVOIDING AND PREPARING FOR COMPLICATIONS

Ensuring excellent procedure outcomes is vital to performing cardiac procedures in the office or ASC labs. Fluoroscopic imaging equipment should at least meet minimum standards to perform coronary angiography, PCI, or cardiac rhythm management (CRM) implants with proficiency. Equipping the lab with bailout and support products such as an intra-aortic balloon pump, covered coronary stents, thrombolytic therapy, thrombectomy catheters, snares, embolic protection devices, pericardiocentesis kits, and pressor agents provides the safest environment for the patient and are justifiable expenses. Post-PCI success means that there is no flow-limiting coronary dissection or thrombus at the treated sites resulting in good blood flow and no significant residual stent stenosis. PCI involving complex lesion morphology such as severely calcified, angulated lesions should be avoided. Side branch closures greater than 2.0 mm during PCI has been associated with MI and death, so deferring high-risk bifurcation cases to the hospital or providing side branch protection should be considered.[26]

ACCESS DECISIONS

The choice of transfemoral or transradial access site should be considered with every patient based on operator experience and patient anatomy. The access site choice continues to be a significant factor in potential major and minor complications. (Fig. 35.5) Although traditionally less popular with cardiologists, ultrasound guidance and micropuncture techniques have been shown to reduce complication rates for femoral access.[27,28] With direct ultrasound visualization, the operator can more likely avoid placing a sheath into a side branch, an unstable or irregular common or superficial femoral artery plaque or a suprainguinal ligament location.[27] These techniques can add a great deal of safety by preventing access complications which are the most common cause of morbidity after any catheterization procedure in any setting. Regardless of the location used, a stable access site following intervention is the prime goal.

PATIENT COMPLIANCE AND SUPPORT SYSTEM

Regardless of the procedural setting and type of cardiac procedure performed, each patient should be assessed for candidacy for a SDD. An assessment of the patient compliance and support system is required if one is to perform same-day cardiac interventions. The operator and staff should understand a priori if a patient will be compliant with dual antiplatelet therapy or if there are potential intolerances or bleeding concerns. A patient must have a reliable driver and support system at home postprocedure should any problems arise. Education for the patient and caregivers as to normal postprocedure care and potential complications is important before the patient leaves the facility. Patients without significant support systems may be better cared for in the inpatient hospital environment.[26]

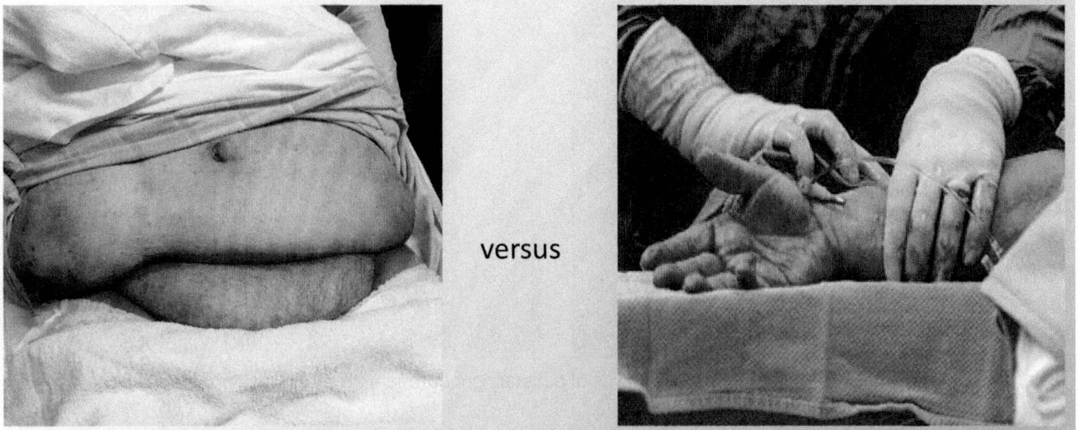

FIG. 35.5 Example of challenging femoral access anatomy (left) compared to straightforward radial access (right).

CASE SELECTION FOR THE CARDIAC PATIENT AND CORONARY LESION CHARACTERISTICS

In light of the significant advances, coronary artery and cardiac interventions in properly selected patients can be safely and effectively performed in the OIS and ASC. To ensure safety, proper case selection is vital. Patients' comorbidities, lesion morphological characteristics, ventricular and valvular function, and ASA class should all be considered prior to performing the case. Evaluation of the patient's renal function, pulmonary and hemodynamic status, and bleeding risks (Chapter 14) are central to the preprocedural planning. Based on these factors a decision can be made about the appropriate site of service.

So how does one select the appropriate coronary lesion type and satisfactory safety profile in patients to be able to perform PCI in an OIS or ASC environment? The 2014 ACC-SCAI consensus document gives some guidance by addressing lesion morphologic risk for intervention in sites without surgical backup. (Fig. 35.6) High-risk lesions with severe angulation, severe calcium, complex bifurcations, thrombus-laden or large ischemic territories with little to no myocardial reserve should be avoided.[10] Additionally, patients with severely compromised ventricular function, severe aortic stenosis, active congestive heart failure, or at increased risk for needing hemodynamic support would be best served in the hospital environment. Both a 2017 multisocietal consensus document for appropriateness of coronary revascularization in stable ischemic disease patients and SCAI offer guidelines and a practical tool kit for guiding ischemia-driven coronary interventions and appropriate decision-making by employing checkpoints on "appropriate, may be appropriate, and rarely appropriate" cases.[29,30]

Undoubtedly, acceptable candidates for PCI based on lesion severity and risk profiles will likely continue to evolve and advance over time, but consideration for patient safety and appropriateness should be

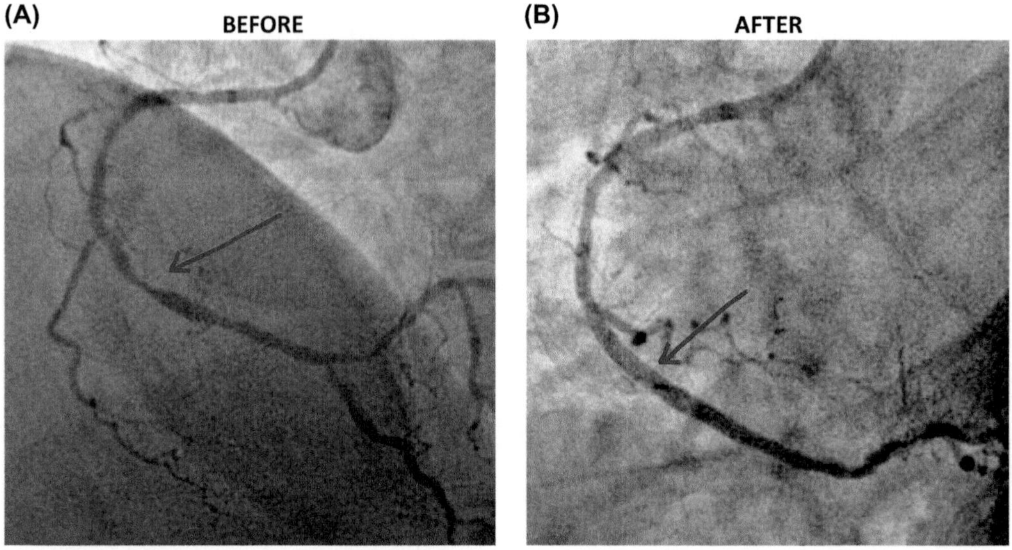

FIG. 35.6 Before (left) and after (right) angiograms of a distal right coronary artery PCI performed in the office interventional suite.

paramount. As the future evidence mounts, there will continue to be a need for updating guidelines for the site of service. This has traditionally been challenging for cardiologists as the rapid changes in technology and device improvements often outpace the published data.

DOCUMENTATION AND REPORTING OF CLINICAL OUTCOMES

Documenting clinical outcomes is increasingly important and is required in our value-based healthcare system. Qualified clinical data registries (QCDR) offer a platform for recording outcomes in a transparent and CMS-certified manner since these registries are mandated to perform random data and reporting audits (Chapter 19). Tracking next day and 30 days postprocedure outcomes is preferred to demonstrate safety and outcomes of all cardiac interventions performed in the office, ASC, or the hospital. Presently, the NCDR Cath-PCI Registry, ICD Registry, and AFib Ablation Registry are able to report outcomes and have been predominately hospital based. The OEIS National Registry (OEIS NR) became operational in 2017 and is a QCDR designed to report outcomes for all office-based interventions. Currently supporting only peripheral vascular interventional module, the OEIS NR plans to offer a single cardiac module specifically focused on all cardiac interventions performed in the OIS and ASC.

CARDIAC RHYTHM MANAGEMENT IN THE OIS AND ASC

CRM which includes device implantations and arrhythmia studies and ablations have been performed for many years in the OIS and ASC. As with coronary intervention, individual states regulate what specifically can be performed in these facilities. PPMs, loop recorders, implantable cardioverter defibrillators (ICDs) and cardiac resynchronization therapy-biventricular pacemakers-ICDs (BiVs) can be safely implanted and the patient discharged within a few hours.[31] Fig. 35.4 Perceived advantages to performing CRM procedures in the OIS or ASC are efficiencies in the service line and the lack of exposure to nosocomial infections that have been a problem for most US hospitals. Additionally, patients appreciate the focused staff and convenient facilities of undergoing CRM procedures in the OIS and ASC.

Equipping the lab to meet ASC standards and strict adherence to sterile technique for physicians and staff are essential operational procedures for all permanent implants. A terminal clean of the procedure room helps mitigate the risk of infection. Patients may undergo ablation or implant procedures using moderate conscious sedation or short-acting general anesthesia under the direction of an anesthesiologist or CRNA. Ensuring safety by stocking pericardiocentesis trays and having the ability to manage a possible perforation or vascular complication is essential. Routine use of postprocedure chest X-ray has not been shown to be a requirement for CRM device implantation by experienced operators,[32] but having processes established to obtain a chest X-ray for suspected pneumothorax is advised. Likewise, routine defibrillation threshold testing (DT) following ICD has not been shown to reduce mortality.[33] A Joint Consensus document recommended not to perform routine DT for left-sided lead implants. "It is reasonable to omit defibrillation efficacy testing in patients undergoing initial left pectoral transvenous ICD implantation procedures where appropriate sensing, pacing, and impedance values are obtained with fluoroscopically well-positioned RV leads" (Class IIa recommendation).[34]

CRM device implant procedures (including PPMs, ICDs, BiV ICD, and loop recorders) have been approved for reimbursement by CMS in the ASC (POS 24) but not in the OIS (POS 11). Many commercial carriers reimburse for CRM device implants as well as electrophysiology studies (EPS) and arrhythmia ablations which are performed in patients with supraventricular tachycardia (SVT) and atrial flutter in the OIS (POS 11). However, as of the time of this publication, CMS does not reimburse EPS and ablations for Medicare beneficiaries in either site of service (POS 11 or 24). As with coronary interventions, individual states regulate what CRM services can be licensed to be performed. Proper patient selection is essential and follow-up with the patient after discharge is important to monitor for any complications, especially within the first week and 30 days postimplant.

Similar to the recommendations for PCI with SDD, each patient should undergo a CRM procedure implant for appropriate indications. When ICDs were initially and more broadly approved by CMS to be implanted for primary prevention of sudden death, there was concern about the potential for overutilization. Thus, an ICD Registry was mandated by CMS through the ACC, NCDR from 2005 through 2018 to collect data about appropriateness of ICD implants. This registry ended and is no longer required, but CMS may revisit registry participation in the future for CRM and possibly all cardiac interventions.

Presently, ablations for atrial fibrillation, ventricular tachycardia, or left-sided SVT (that require transseptal puncture) are not performed in the OIS or ASC due to safety reasons. These procedures are increasingly performed in the hospital with strict protocols for SDD. More data are required to demonstrate safety and case selection criteria need to be developed before these cases can migrate to the OIS or ASC.

COST-EFFICIENT CARE IN OIS AND ASC

One of the prime drivers to shift cardiac interventional care to outpatient status, whether the procedure is done in the hospital or at a freestanding facility, is to reduce cost. Several studies have estimated cost savings if procedures were moved from the inpatient to office or outpatient status. Although published in 2010, Popescu et al. calculated that if half of the coronary PCIs were done as an outpatient compared with an inpatient, there would be an estimated \$200–\$500 million savings per year to CMS.[35] Another study published in 2018 concluded that "greater and more consistent use of SDD could increase the overall value of PCI care and save US hospitals approximately \$577 million in costs if adopted in the United States in the bundled payment era." Interestingly, this approximately \$5000 per case savings only reflected hospital-based cost savings.[36] If a significant portion of the SDD PCIs were to be shifted to the ASC or OIS, further cost-reduction may show incremental potential savings to the healthcare system. Signaling that a reduction in costs is a major initiative by CMS, cost measure development work was initiated in 2018 by CMS through the MACRA program for elective outpatient PCI as one of the eight Cost Episodes of Care.[37] In addition, in the 2020 ASC Payment Systems Final Rule, CMS expanded coverage of 6 PCI codes to be performed in the ASC starting in 2020 in an effort to reduce costs.[38] Further work needs to be done to refine cost analyses and case-lesion risk adjustment. Cost will likely be a major driver to continue the shift from inpatient cardiac work to the outpatient and office or ASC settings.

REGULATIONS AND ADVOCACY

All states regulate the type of cardiac procedures that can be performed in an office or ASC setting. Additionally, in 26 states a CON is required if cardiac interventions are to be performed.[10] There has been a significant shift in state policies. In 2007, only 28 states allowed PCI in settings without an on-site surgical backup. In 2013, 45 states allowed for PCI without requiring surgical backup capabilities. A joint consensus document was published in 2014 by SCAI, ACC, and AHA stating that in properly selected patients, coronary PCI was safe in sites without surgical backup.[10]

As there are procedural regulations regulating procedures in the outpatient, ASC, or office settings, there are also payment and coverage issues which are separate and distinct. CMS has encouraged outpatient and observation status for many cardiac diagnoses and conditions in an effort to save money compared with more costly inpatient services. CMS does not currently cover PCI or CRM implants in the office (POS 11) setting. Many states, however, do allow coverage for coronary PCI and CRM procedures in the office setting but for commercial patients only. CMS has allowed and covered diagnostic coronary angiography but not coronary intervention in the office (nonfacility) setting. This is a significant discrepancy and demonstrates that CMS policies have not kept pace with advances in state regulations and clinical guidelines for coronary PCI. However, in 2019, following years of strategic advocacy, CMS did allow and expand coverage for 17 diagnostic cardiac codes in the ASC setting (POS 24).[39] As noted above, in the Final Rule for 2020, CMS expanded coverage for balloon angioplasty and coronary stenting for Medicare beneficiaries in the ASC. This was a positive first step in bringing policy in line with the evidence base for safety of performing PCI as a SDD and at the same time moved a major step forward toward reducing costs. Fractional flow reserve (FFR) assessments for indeterminate coronary obstructions are part of the coronary interventional guidelines according to the American College of Cardiology (ACC) guidelines on coronary revascularization. FFR is reasonable for the assessment of angiographic intermediate coronary lesions (50% −70% diameter stenoses) and can be useful for guiding revascularization decisions in patients with CAD (Class IIa, Level A).[40] FFR codes (CPT 93571 and 93572) were approved in 2019 for POS 24, but as an N1 designation they are a packaged service item with no separate payment provided. It is hoped that given positive coverage for PCI in the ASC, FFR, intravascular ultrasound and related codes will be separately reimbursed in the future to align all sites of service with the most appropriate and optimal care for cardiac patients.

THE FUTURE OF CARDIAC INTERVENTIONS IN THE OIS

Many well-established and new cardiac procedures continue to evolve and improve with the advances in technology and operator experience. Currently, percutaneous valvular interventions (transcatheter aortic valve replacement and mitral valve repair), atrial septal defect and patent foramen ovale closure, left atrial appendage occlusion, coronary atherectomy, and other structural heart procedures are not covered or reimbursed in POS 11 or 24 and are hospital-based only. However, if one reflects back on the extraordinary advances in cardiovascular care in the past, it is conceivable that with evidence to support it, many of these procedures will someday be performed safely and effectively in an OIS or ASC. Transitions to SDD for any of these or future cardiac procedures will likely be tested in the hospital first. Cardiologists, healthcare providers, industry, health delivery systems, and other stakeholders will continue to innovate, develop, and encourage better devices, medications, and techniques to deliver safe and appropriate care in the most cost-efficient settings. For the patients who will be the primary beneficiary of these advances, the future is exciting and bright for cardiac interventional care in the office and ASC environments.

REFERENCES

1. Centers for Disease Control and Prevention, National Center for Health Statistics. Multiple Cause of Death 1999−2015 on CDC WONDER Online Database, released December 2016. Data are from the Multiple Cause of Death Files, 1999−2015, as compiled from data provided by the 57 vital statistics jurisdictions through the Vital Statistics Cooperative Program. Accessed at http://wonder.cdc.gov/mcd-icd10.html.
2. C. Conway. N.d. Physician Ownership of Hospitals Significantly Impacted by Health Care Reform Legislation (Houston, Tex. University of Houston Law Center). http://www.law.uh.edu/healthlaw/perspectives/2010/(CC)%20Stark.pdf (accessed 5/23/13).
3. Patient protection and affordable care Act. H.R. 3590, Section 6001, Pub. Law No. 111−148. In: *111th Congress*. 2010.
4. Schmidt T, Abbott JD. Coronary stents: history, design, and construction. *J Clin Med*. 2018;7(6):126. https://doi.org/10.3390/jcm7060126. Published 2018 May 29.
5. Matteau A, Bhatt DL. Recent advances in antithrombotic therapy after acute coronary syndrome. *Can Med Assoc J*. 2014; 186(8):589−596. https://doi.org/10.1503/cmaj.130506.
6. Kutcher MA, Klein LW, Ou F-S, et al. Percutaneous coronary interventions in facilities without cardiac surgery on site: a report from the National cardiovascular data registry (NCDR), Albert Woodward, eric D. Peterson, Ralph G. Brindis, National cardiovascular data registry (NCDR). *J Am Coll Cardiol*. June 2009;54(1):16−24. https://doi.org/10.1016/j.jacc.2009.03.038.
7. C-PORT E, Aversano T, Lemmon CC, Liu L, for the Atlantic CPORT Investigators. *N Engl J Med*. 2012;366:1792−1802.
8. Alice K, Jacobs MD, et al. For the MASS COMM investigators*. Nonemergency PCI at hospitals with or without on-site cardiac surgery (MASS COMM). *NEJM*. 2013;368:1498−1508.
9. Outcomes and temporal trends of inpatient percutaneous coronary intervention at centers with and without on-site cardiac surgery in the United States Goel, et. al. *JAMA Cardiol*. 2017;2(1):25−33.
10. Dehmer GJ, et al. SCAI/ACC/AHA expert consensus document 2014 update on percutaneous coronary intervention

without on-site surgical backup. *J Am Coll Cardiol*. June 2014;63(23). https://doi.org/10.1016/j.jacc.2014.03.002.
11. Agarwal S, Thakkar B, Skelding KA, Blankenship JC. Trends and outcomes after same-day discharge after percutaneous coronary interventions. *Cardiovasc Qual Outcomes*. 2017;10. https://doi.org/10.1161/CIRCOUTCOMES.117.003936Circulation.
12. Mason PJ, Shah B, Tamis-Holland JE, et al. An update on radial artery access and best practices for transradial coronary angiography and intervention in acute coronary syndrome: a scientific statement from the American heart association. *Cardiovasc Interv*. September 2018;11. https://doi.org/10.1161/HCV.0000000000000035Circulation. Originally published1 Sep. 2018.
13. Gewalt SM, et al. Comparison of vascular closure devices versus manual compression after femoral artery puncture in women. Gender-based analysis of a large scale, randomized clinical trial. *Circ Cardiovasc Interv*. 2018;11. https://doi.org/10.1161/CIRCINTERVENTIONS.117.006074. Originally published1 Aug 2018.
14. Smilowitz NR1, Kirtane AJ, Guiry M, et al. Practices and complications of vascular closure devices and manual compression in patients undergoing elective transfemoral coronary procedures. *Am J Cardiol*. July 15, 2012;110(2):177–182. https://doi.org/10.1016/j.amjcard.2012.02.065.
15. Yang Y, Lewis JP, Hulot JS, Scott SA. The pharmacogenetic control of antiplatelet response: candidate genes and CYP2C19. *Expert Opin Drug Metab Toxicol*. 2015;11(10):1599–1617. https://doi.org/10.1517/17425255.2015.1068757 17.
16. Heyde GS, Koch KT, Tijssen JGP. Randomized trial comparing same-day discharge with overnight hospital stay after percutaneous coronary intervention: results of the Elective PCI in Outpatient Study (EPOS). *Circulation*. 2007;115:2299–2306. https://doi.org/10.1161/CIRCULATIONAHA.105.591495. Published in Circulation 2007.
17. Rao SV1, Kaltenbach LA, Weintraub WS, et al. Prevalence and outcomes of same-day discharge after elective percutaneous coronary intervention among older patients. *J Am Med Assoc*. October 5, 2011;306(13):1461–1467. https://doi.org/10.1001/jama.2011.1409. JAMA. 2011;306:1461-1467.
18. Jabara R, Gadesam R, Pendyala L, et al. Ambulatory discharge after transradial coronary intervention: preliminary US single-center experience (Same-Day TransRadial Intervention and Discharge Evaluation, the STRIDE Study). *Am Heart J*. 2008;156(6):1141–1146.
19. Bertrand OF, De Larochellière R, Rodés-Cabau J, , et alEarly discharge after transradial stenting of coronary arteries study investigators. A randomized study comparing same-day home discharge and abciximab bolus only to overnight hospitalization and abciximab bolus and infusion after transradial coronary stent implantation. *Circulation*. 2006;114(24):2636–2643.
20. Bertrand OF, Rodés-Cabau J, Larose E, et al. One-year clinical outcome after abciximab bolus–only compared with abciximab bolus and 12-hour infusion in the randomized early discharge after transradial stenting of coronary arteries (EASY) study. *Am Heart J*. 2008;156(1):135–140.
21. Bundhun PK, Soogund MZ, Huang WQ. Same day discharge versus overnight stay in the hospital following percutaneous coronary intervention in patients with stable coronary artery disease: a systematic review and meta-analysis of randomized controlled trials. *PLoS One*. January 9, 2017;12(1):e0169807. https://doi.org/10.1371/journal.pone.0169807.
22. Brayton KM, Patel VG, Stave C, de Lemos JA, Kumbhani DJ. Same-day discharge after percutaneous coronary intervention: a meta-analysis. *J Am Coll Cardiol*. 2013;62(4):275–285.
23. Jain K, et al. Office-based endovascular suite is safe for most procedures. *J Vasc Surg*. January 2014;59(1):186–191.
24. Oskui P, et al. Safety and efficacy of peripheral vascular procedures performed in the outpatient setting. *J Invasive Cardiol*. 2015;27(5):243–249.
25. Lin P., et al. Treatment Outcomes and Lessons Learned from 5134 Cases of Outpatient Office-Based Endovascular Procedures in a Vascular Surgical Practice VASCULAR 2016.
26. Shroff A, Kupfer J, Gilchrist IC, et al. Same-day discharge after percutaneous coronary intervention: current perspectives and strategies for implementation. *JAMA Cardiol*. 2016;1(2):216–223. https://doi.org/10.1001/jamacardio.2016.0148.
27. Seto AH, Abu-Fadel MS, Sparling JM, et al. Real-time ultrasound guidance facilitates femoral arterial access and reduces vascular complications: FAUST (Femoral Arterial Access with Ultrasound Trial). *JACC Cardiovasc Interv*. July 2010;3(7):751–758. https://doi.org/10.1016/j.jcin.2010.04.015.
28. Pitta SR, Gulati R, Mathew V. Ultrasound-guided vascular access: a new tool in the cath lab. Quality improvement toolkit: the society for cardiovascular angiography and interventions. *SCAI QIT*; June 2016. Available online at: http://www.scai.org/QITTip/ultrasound-guided-vascular-access-new-tool-in-cath.
29. Patel MR, Calhoon JH, Dehmer GJ, et al. ACC/AATS/AHA/ASE/ASNC/SCAI/SCCT/STS 2017 appropriate use criteria for coronary revascularization in patients with stable ischemic heart disease. *J Am Coll Cardiol*. May 2017;69(17):2212–2241. https://doi.org/10.1016/j.jacc.2017.02.001.
30. http://www.scaiaucapp.org/auc_welcome.
31. Peplow J1, Randall E1, Campbell-Cole C1, et al. Day-case device implantation-A prospective single-center experience including patient satisfaction data. *Pacing Clin Electrophysiol*. May 2018;41(5):546–552. https://doi.org/10.1111/pace.13324.
32. Edwards NC, et al. Routine chest radiography after permanent pacemaker implantation: is it necessary? *J Postgrad Med*. 2005 Apr-Jun;51(2):92–96. discussion 96-7.
33. Kannabhiran M, et al. Routine DFT testing in patients undergoing ICD implantation does not improve mortality: a systematic review and meta-analysis. *J Arrhythm*.

September 3, 2018;34(6):598–606. https://doi.org/10.1002/joa3.12109. eCollection 2018 Dec.
34. Wilkoff BL, Fauchier L, Stiles MK, et al. HRS/EHRA/APHRS/SOLAECE expert consensus statement on optimal implantable cardioverter-defibrillator programming and testing. *Heart Rhythm*. 2015;13:e50–86, 2016.
35. Popescu AM, et al. *JACC Cardiovasc Interv*. 2010;3(10):1020–1021.
36. Amin A, et al. Association of same-day discharge after elective percutaneous coronary intervention in the United States with costs and outcomes. *JAMA Cardiol*. 2018;3(11):1041–1049. https://doi.org/10.1001/jamacardio.2018.3029.
37. https://qpp.cms.gov/mips/explore-measures/cost.
38. federalregister.gov/d/2019-24138.
39. https://s3.amazonaws.com/public-inspection.federalregister.gov/2018-24243.pdf.
40. Levine GN, Bates ER, Blankenship JC, et al. ACCF/AHA/SCAI guideline for percutaneous coronary intervention: a report of the American College of cardiology foundation/American heart association task force on practice guidelines and the society for cardiovascular angiography and interventions. *Circulation*. 2011;124:e574–651, 2011.

CHAPTER 36

Certification and Accreditation

KRISHNA JAIN, MD, FACS

Office-based endovascular center (OEC) is an extension of a medical practice, so no additional certification or accreditation is required by Centers for Medicare and Medicaid Services (CMS) for Medicare or Medicaid reimbursement. Private insurance companies generally follow the same pattern. However, some states (Chapter 2) and insurance companies may require the OEC to be accredited by a national organization. Currently, there are no organizations established to review the appropriateness and/or outcomes of the care being provided in the OEC. Accreditation and certification are two different processes. The process of accreditation for a healthcare organization involves documenting compliance with a set of standards developed by an official accrediting agency that typically relate to the quality of efficiency of services. Accreditation for institutions and agencies in the United States and Canada is voluntary. Certification is a process used to prove that an organization or individual is competent and skilled in a particular area, typically associated with completion of a training or course. Many specialty areas have professional organizations that provide certification to individual practitioners. National associations may control the process and development of certification examinations conducted by their specialty interest groups. Accreditation is provided by nongovernment agencies, while CMS may certify various health organizations. Private organizations also certify various health-related programs, e.g., American College of Surgeons certifies trauma and bariatric centers in various hospitals.

As mentioned above the CMS does not require the OEC to be accredited or certified. However, accreditation by a national organization provides several benefits like indicating a commitment to quality and patient safety, recognition by insurance companies, improvement in risk reduction and management, help creating an organizational structure, providing standard operating process for the whole organization, competitive advantages, compliance with HIPAA, meeting state requirements (if any), possible reduction in insurance cost, educational opportunities and patient satisfaction.

While there are no accreditation organizations with dedicated framework to accredit an OEC, there are several organizations that provide accreditation for ambulatory surgery centers (ASCs). Accreditation by one of these deemed organizations leads to certification by CMS. This makes the ASC eligible to receive reimbursement from Medicare and Medicaid. Additionally, in almost all states, ASCs must obtain a state license. To obtain Medicare certification, and a state license, an ASC must have a physical inspection conducted by an inspector of the organization that the federal government has deemed fit to conduct that inspection. It may also need an inspection by a state official. Certain states may inspect the OEC or require accreditation by a local state accrediting agency prior to granting the OEC operational status. To accredit the OEC, accrediting bodies in these states have used the same tools that they use to accredit ASC. Many states are struggling with developing guidelines for an OEC and are looking to national societies for guidance. The Society of Vascular Surgery (SVS) in collaboration with American College of Surgeons (ACS) and other societies are developing a certification/accreditation program for OEC.

CURRENT ACCREDITATION ORGANIZATIONS

The following organizations accredit ASC, and several of them are being used by OEC for accreditation.[1]

The American Association for Accreditation of Ambulatory Surgery Facilities (AAAASF)

Office-Based Endovascular Centers. https://doi.org/10.1016/B978-0-323-67969-5.00036-8
Copyright © 2020 Elsevier Inc. All rights reserved.

The Accreditation Association for Ambulatory Health Care (AAAHC)
The Joint Commission
Healthcare Facilities Accreditation program (HFAP)
Institute for Medical Quality (IMQ)

All organizations charge for providing accreditation. The fee schedule varies depending on the size of the facility and number of physicians providing service.

All the organizations use the following process with some variation: (1) application, (2) survey, (3) decision, and (4) reaccreditation.

AAAASF

The American Association for Accreditation of Ambulatory Plastic Surgery Facilities, Inc. was formed in 1980. In 1992, the AAAASF was created to provide accreditation of all American Board of Medical Specialties (ABMS)-certified surgical specialties office-based surgery units. Its program follows the guidelines provided in the 1994 American College of Surgeons publication, "Guidelines for Optimal Office-Based Surgery."[2] The "AAAASF accreditation programs help facilities demonstrate a strong commitment to patient safety, standardize quality, maintain fiscal responsibility, promote services to patients and collaborate with other health care leaders."[3] The AAAASF claims to be the only accrediting organization that mandates 100% compliance with standards that include peer review as a means to demonstrate safety and quality measures in the accredited facilities. The AAAASF holds office-based facilities to hospital standards, requires surgeons (interventionalists) to be board certified and have hospital privileges for any procedure they perform, requires the use of anesthesia professionals for deeper levels of anesthesia, requires a safe and clean surgical environment that meets stringent standards and requires peer review.

Application

As per AAAASF website following list of documentation must be completed for accreditation:
Application Form with payment
Floor plan for facility
A copy of each physician's State Medical License
A copy of each physician's Board Certificate or letter of admissibility by the physician/surgeon certifying board (ABMS, AOABOS, ABOMS, or ABPS as applicable)
A current copy of the delineation of hospital privileges for each physician/surgeon (must state the department of surgical specialty and list the procedures that may be performed at the hospital)
Authorization to Release Information Form signed by each physician on staff
HIPAA Business Associate Agreement
Facility Identification Form
Staff Identification Form
Facility Director's Attestation Form
Random Review Form
Unanticipated Sequela Form
New York OBS Addendum (*New York applicants only*)
Appropriate legal documentation as specified under your entity type on the New York OBS Addendum (*New York applicants only*)

Additional documents may be required after the initial review of documents is completed in 10 business days.

Survey

AAAASF facility surveyors are board-certified medical specialists trained to assess the center in following categories:
Personnel
Medical records
Disaster preparedness
General safety
Quality assurance
Clinical practices

A survey team, whose size and composition are appropriate for the facility, conducts a thorough and unbiased facility survey based upon the surveyor handbook in accordance with the AAAASF guidelines, survey schedule, and checklist. Surveyor reviews the facility plan, reviews any deficiencies, and recommend any corrections needed. Surveys are documented and submitted to the AAAASF central office.

DECISION

Once all the requirements are met the center is accredited. The center must display the sign of accreditation.

REACCREDITATION

To maintain accreditation the facility is reevaluated through a self-survey every year, and an onsite survey every 3 years.

SELF-SURVEY

The following list of documentation must be completed and submitted for the self-survey before the beginning of second and third year.
Facility Identification Form

Staff Identification Form
Facility Director Attestation Form
Completed Standards Manual

If there are deficiencies, a report is sent to the facility director allowing 30 days for correction. If there are no deficiencies a new certificate is issued.

RESURVEY

Before the 3 years are up, the following documents should be completed.

A copy of each physician's State Medical License
A copy of each physician's Board Certificate or letter of admissibility by the physicians certifying board (ABMS, AOABOS, ABOMS, or ABPS)
A current copy of the delineation of hospital privileges for each physician (must state the department of surgical specialty and list the procedures that may be performed at the hospital)
Authorization to Release Information Form signed by each physician on staff
Facility Identification Form
Staff Identification Form
Facility Director's Attestation Form
New York OBS Addendum (*New York OBS applicants only*)
Copy of Floor Plan

The documents are reviewed in 10 business days and a site visit is scheduled. There is a fee charged for recertification.

THE ACCREDITATION ASSOCIATION FOR AMBULATORY HEALTH CARE

AAAHC has been surveying and accrediting ambulatory surgery centers since 1979. The AAAHC was created by six founding members including the American College Health Association, the American Group Practice Association (now known as the American Medical Group Association), the Federated Ambulatory Surgery Association (now known as the Ambulatory Surgery Foundation), the Group Health Association of America (now known as the American Association of Health Plans), the Medical Group Management Association, and the National Association of Community Health Centers.[4] The AAAHC aims to promote the highest level of care for patients of ambulatory healthcare organizations in the most efficient and economic manner. This is accomplished by the operation of a peer-based assessment, consultation, education, and accreditation program. The accreditation process includes submission of an application, survey by qualified surveyors followed by a decision to provide accreditation after all the requirements are met. Reaccreditation is required every 3 years. The AAAHC has also created an institute for quality improvement.

Institute for Quality Improvement

The Institute for Quality Improvement was established in 1999. It is a department within AAAHC.

The Institute provides following activities to support AAAHC:

National benchmarking studies to improve care
Patient safety and disease management toolkits to improve safety
Bernard A. Kershner Innovations in Quality Improvement Award is given to accredited organization for quality improvement
Analyzing and reporting on data from AAAHC surveys through the annual *Quality Roadmap* publication
Present data at national meetings and publish in peer-reviewed journals

Survey

Documentation needed to be submitted prior to onsite survey visit is extensive. Surveyors are physicians, nurses, dentists, and administrators selected and trained by AAAHC. Survey fees are based upon information obtained from the facility's application document. The size and type, as well as the range of services the organization provides, are considered in determining the fee.

Recertification

It is done every 3 years. A facility is eligible for participation if it has been providing healthcare services for at least 6 months before the inspection. There is no annual fee, but there is a fee paid at the time of recertification.

THE JOINT COMMISSION

The Joint Commission (TJC) provides accreditation to healthcare organizations to improve healthcare for the public by ensuring the care provided is safe and effective with the highest quality and value.[4] "In 1951, the American College of Physicians, the American Hospital Association, the American Medical Association, and the Canadian Medical Association joined ACS as corporate members to create the Joint Commission on Accreditation of Hospitals (JCAH), an independent, not-for-profit organization to provide voluntary accreditation. In the late 1980s, the organization name was changed to the Joint Commission on Accreditation of Healthcare Organizations (JCAHO). In 2007, the organization shortened its name to "the Joint Commission."[4] Most physicians know TJC as an organization that accredits hospitals. However, there are only about 5000 acute care hospitals, and TJC accredits more than 21,000 healthcare organizations including ASCs.

Application

TJC gives free 90-day access to online standards manual (e-edition) to review the requirements. When reviewing the standards, a list of areas of compliance and noncompliance can be made and updated to meet the standards. After completing an application, it is submitted with a deposit. If any changes are required they should be completed before the site visit.

Survey

After submitting the application, a survey is commissioned. For comprehensive onsite review, surveyors can consist of physicians, nurses, and other healthcare workers trained to carry out the survey. The surveyor provides the onsite review and a preliminary written report is made available at the end of the survey.

Decision

If any changes are needed, they should be made and usually within 60 days the center is accredited. After receiving "The Gold Seal of Approval," the center should display the gold seal and notify any organizations, insurance companies, State health board requiring the accreditation. Because of accreditation the center may experience reduced rate of insurance.

Reaccreditation

Reaccreditation occurs every 3 years. There may be surprise visits during the 3 years' accreditation period. If there are any major changes within the organization TJC should be informed. There is an annual fee of $1000.00.

HEALTHCARE FACILITIES ACCREDITATION PROGRAM

Healthcare Facilities Accreditation Program (HFAP) is authorized by the CMS to survey hospitals for compliance with the Medicare Conditions of Participation and Coverage. HFAP was originally created in 1945 to conduct an objective review of osteopathic hospitals. CMS was formed in 1965. HFAP has maintained its deeming authority for CMS continuously and meets or exceeds the standards required by CMS/Medicare to provide accreditation to all hospitals and ambulatory care/surgical facilities. In addition to others, HFAP also is recognized by National Committee for Quality Assurance (NCQA), Accreditation Council for Graduate Medical Education (ACGME), State Departments of public health managed care organizations and insurance companies.

Survey

The HFAP standards are based on the Medicare conditions of participation (CoPs) for each facility type.[5] Approximately 80% of HFAP standards are annotated to align with the Medicare CoPs and associated requirements. In addition to Medicare standards, the HFAP standards include criteria proven to improve quality and patient safety. Surveyors are experienced medical professionals. The HFAP claims to be the most cost-effective accrediting body.

INSTITUTE FOR MEDICAL QUALITY

IMQ is a 501(c)3 corporation founded in 1996 by the California Medical Association to improve the quality of care for patients in California.[6] The IMQ was designed to make it easier to provide quality care and eliminate barriers. IMQ puts great emphasis on education, counseling, and direct involvement of practicing physicians. Some IMQ programs require surveys of facilities. Each program is updated on a regular basis to keep it clinically relevant. IMQ is recognized in a number of states.

Mission

"The Institute for Medical Quality's (IMQ) mission is to be an innovative leader in improving the quality of care provided to patients across the continuum of health care by encouraging, developing, and implementing programs which effectively measure and improve the quality of care provided to people in California and beyond. In support of its mission, IMQ will conduct educational programs and will evaluate health care delivery. It will be responsive to diverse constituencies, and its outcomes will be patient-oriented and population-based."[6]

Application

An application is filed along with necessary documents. After reviewing the application and supporting documents the IMQ sends a presurvey analysis to the center, allowing the center to make any necessary revisions before the onsite survey begins.

Survey

As per website the survey focuses on following areas:

Administration: scope of services, patient rights, and administrative policies and procedures

Personnel: staff policies and procedures, physician credentialing in both small group settings and larger settings with an organized medical staff

Quality management and peer review
Medical records: surgery and invasive diagnostic records, HIPAA, and clinical record confidentiality
Care and treatment
Facility and environmental safety: infection control, fire safety, preparation for emergencies, medical equipment, and facility design and access
Surgical, anesthesia, and invasive diagnostics

Decision

This may include full 3-year accreditation or deferred action if the center does not meet the standards.

CERTIFICATION OF OEC IN DEVELOPMENT

All of the accrediting bodies described above do not address the appropriateness of care being provided in the OEC. The accreditation process is mainly related to safety measures taken in providing care to the patients as well as the safety of the workers in the facility. The SVS is working with the American College of Surgeons and some other societies to develop a certification process for the OEC. This process will be modeled after some of the other certification processes ACS has developed in the past, i.e., trauma centers, bariatric centers, etc. The procedures that may be included are endovascular management of arterial disease except carotid stenting and abdominal aortic aneurism, management of superficial and deep venous disease, embolization procedures, management of dialysis access, insertion, and removal of intracaval filters and management of central lines and ports. The certification process is expected to be unveiled in the near future. Initial certification may be limited and not include all the procedures carried out in the OEC.

The certification process developed by American College of Surgeons to certify trauma centers, etc. is based on five phases of care: Preoperative evaluation and preparation, immediate preoperative readiness, intraoperative care, postoperative care, and postdischarge care.[7] The ACS believes in the following principles of care: Shared decision-making between the care provider and patient/family, risk stratification and reduction of risk before the procedure, evidence-based care, and following the safety standards and coordination among team members. When certifying or accrediting the center, adherence to the standard of care in these phases becomes important. The center should strictly follow the written policies and procedures. Let us look at the five phases of care that would have an impact on performing a percutaneous procedure for chronic limb ischemia in an OEC.

PREPROCEDURE EVALUATION

When a patient presents with symptoms of arterial ischemia, the first step is to determine if the symptoms are truly of arterial origin. Patients in older age group may have several causes of pain in the legs, e.g., spinal stenosis, arthritis, etc. The diagnosis is based on history, physical exam and arterial ultrasound findings, and ankle brachial index. In case the patient cannot give reliable history, the patient's family or caretaker may play an important role. The process is carried out in the physician's office. Other tests such as an MRI of the spine may be useful in the diagnosis algorithm. Once the diagnosis of arterial ischemia has been made, the medical management must be instituted. The patient should have the benefit of maximal medical benefit. This includes smoking cessation, modification of risk factors, supervised exercise therapy, and use of antiplatelet and other drugs like cilostazol. Other risk factors should be assessed using lab values and additional tests like cardiac stress test, etc. At this point in managing the patient, the appropriateness of care becomes very important. Appropriateness of care is not addressed by the existing accreditation bodies in a meaningful way. The invasive procedure should be recommended only for the appropriate indication and after the medical therapy has failed. All risk factors should be addressed and optimized. The medications that may have bearing on the procedure should be addressed. For example, if the patient is on anticoagulants, there should be a plan in place to manage these before, during, and after the procedure. Appropriate input should be sought from the primary care physician and any other specialists providing care for the patient. Risk and benefits of the procedure and alternative therapies should be discussed with the patient and the family. An informed consent should be signed by the patient. The patient should be educated about the arterial disease and the planned procedure and after care. If there are any medical insurance–related issues, those should be resolved. Since OEC is an extension of the practice, this phase of care usually will be provided in the same office where the intervention will be carried out. The office should meet all the safety requirements. There are guidelines by various societies in providing care for these patients. The guidelines should be followed.[8,9]

IMMEDIATE PREOPERATIVE CARE

The patient should be examined and the history and physical should be updated. The patient and the family, interventionalist, nurses and other members of the team, and an anesthesia provider if needed should all be involved in care as appropriate. The patient will be seen in the part of the office that is being used as an OEC. The lab values will be rechecked specially for renal function and coagulation perimeters if the patient was on anticoagulants. The procedure should be appropriately discussed with the patient and the family. The informed consent form duly signed by the patient and/or the power of attorney should be in the chart. The surgical site needs to be marked and appropriate groin shaved and prepared. For the arterial procedure, it is preferable to shave both groins and tibial area if tibial approach is contemplated. If the patient is diabetic, blood sugar needs to be checked and the oral intake status needs to be confirmed as per the directions given in advance. If anesthesia is planned, appropriate evaluation needs to be documented (chapter 10). If an anesthesia personnel is not being used, then the interventionalist and the registered nurse giving medication and monitoring the patient during the procedure should be certified in advanced cardiac life support. The patient should be given appropriate drugs as per protocol prior to the procedure and hydrated if there is evidence of renal insufficiency. The availability of patient supervision by a responsible adult for 24 h postprocedure should be confirmed. The area for preprocedure evaluation needs to provide privacy for the patient and be HIPAA compliant. All data should be entered in an EMR.

INTRAOPERATIVE CARE

In the next phase of care, the procedure is carried out in the interventional suite. The interventional suite should have appropriate imaging system, radiolucent table, power injector for contrast, and an ultrasound machine for accessing the vessel. All the disposable equipment like sheathes, wires, and catheters should be available. If there is a plan to use an atherectomy device and/or intravascular ultrasound the appropriate equipment should be available. Appropriate stents and covered stents for a bail out procedure should be available. Availability of these supplies needs to be checked before the procedure is started. There should be an emergency generator in case of power failure. Before the procedure is started an appropriate checklist that includes timeout should be completed. Appropriate personnel should be available and present in the endovascular suite. The personnel should be appropriately dressed and behave professionally.

The patient should be appropriately prepped and draped for the arteriogram. Once the procedure starts, appropriate record should be kept and images stored in PACS. The equipment being used should meet all the manufacture's recommended service requirements. Since these procedures are carried out using local anesthesia and/or conscious sedation, it is important to keep the patient comfortable using verbal assurance and appropriate medications. After the intervention is completed, appropriate measures should be taken for hemostasis at the site of vessel entry using manual compression or a closure device.

POSTPROCEDURE PHASE

Once the patient comes to the recovery room, the patient should be monitored appropriately for vital signs as well as for signs of bleeding at the procedure site. The distal circulation at the pedal level should be checked in both feet. All the findings need to be documented in the EMR. The interventionalist should finish recording the comprehensive procedure note. The interventionalist should be available in case of a complication. Appropriately trained employees should monitor the patient. There should be equipment available for monitoring, like handheld Dopplers. The biological waste and general waste should be disposed of as per the policy. The instruments should be cleaned and sterilized as per the specifications of the autoclave being used.

POSTDISCHARGE PHASE

The patient and the caretaker are given appropriate instructions verbally and in writing. If the patient had medications held prior to the procedure, instructions to restart the medication should be given. It must be ascertained that patient will have caretaker with the patient for at least 24 h postprocedure. A follow-up appointment should be given. If the patient needs follow-up appointment with other specialists or primary care doctor, it should be arranged. If the patient is returning to a facility then the facility should be given appropriate instructions. If needed, social service referrals should be made.

During these phases of care there are various requirement for the building, equipment, and personnel that need to be met. Once the certification/accreditation process being created by SVS/ACS is in place the OEC may use this particular approach to get certified since the process will be geared specifically toward an OEC. Another requirement for getting accredited under this process may be mandatory participation in a quality clinical data registry. There are various registries a center could participate in.

Currently there are several organizations providing accreditation for the OEC. Though not mandated by CMS, it is prudent to get the OEC accredited by one of the national accreditation bodies. Some states mandate it, and some insurance companies will not pay for the procedure if the center is not accredited. A stamp of approval from an outside organization is always looked upon favorably by regulatory bodies and patients alike.

REFERENCES

1. A.S.C. Association, Accreditation Organizations, (n.d.).
2. *Guidelines for Optimal Ambulatory Surgical Care and Office-Based Surgery*. 3rd ed. 2000.
3. American Association for Accredidation of Ambulatory Surgery Facilities, What is Accreditation, (n.d.). https://www.aaaasf.org/who-we-are/what-is-accreditation (accessed April 29, 2019).
4. The Joint Commission, (n.d.). American College Health Association, the American Group Practice Association (now Known as the American Medical Group Association), The Federated Ambulatory Surgery Association (now Known as the Ambulatory Surgery Foundation), The Group Health Association (accessed April 29, 2019)..
5. Healthcare Facilities Accreditation Program (HFAP), (n.d.). https://www.hfap.org/about/overview.aspx.
6. Institute for Medical Quality (IMQ), (n.d.).
7. Hoyt D, Clifford K. *Optimal Resources for Surgical Quality and Safety*. American College of Surgeons; 2017.
8. Aboyans V, Ricco J-B, Bartelink M-LEL, et al. Editor's choice – 2017 ESC guidelines on the diagnosis and treatment of peripheral arterial diseases, in collaboration with the European society for vascular surgery (ESVS). *Eur J Vasc Endovasc Surg*. 2018;55:305–368. https://doi.org/10.1016/J.EJVS.2017.07.018.
9. Olin JW, Allie DE, Belkin M, et al. ACCF/AHA/ACR/SCAI/SIR/SVM/SVN/SVS 2010 performance measures for adults with peripheral artery disease. *Vasc Med*. 2010;15:481–512. https://doi.org/10.1177/1358863X10390838.

CHAPTER 37

Advocacy for Office-Based Intervention

JEFFREY G. CARR, MD, FACC, FSCAI

CHANGES IN HEALTHCARE

There have been seemingly endless changes in healthcare over the years that make it difficult and challenging to continue to offer quality services to patients. Specifically, when it comes to therapies and treatments, policies regarding approved indications for procedures and the payments for these services have changed from the original fee-for-service model and continue to change. Healthcare costs remain high. Fueling the drive to reduce costs are the facts that in 2017 total healthcare expenditures in the United States was $3.5 trillion and total healthcare spending was 17.9% of the gross domestic product.[1] Policies have been put in place that impact physicians' and hospitals' abilities to offer evaluation and therapeutic services to their patients. It first started with the changes in payments to hospitals based on diagnosis-related groups.[2] Subsequently, the reimbursement system for physician services changed and relative value units were created.[3] In the mandate to curb overall spending for the Medicare and Medicaid programs,[4] there are ongoing attempts to maintain spending at a budget neutral level. If there is an increase in payment for services granted in one area of medicine then commensurate cuts need to be made somewhere else. This has led to annual reviews and adjustments to the allowable payments by Centers for Medicare and Medicaid Services (CMS) for every service provided by physicians in hospital, ambulatory surgery center (ASC), and office settings. Since the advent of Medicare Access and CHIP Reauthorization Act of 2015 (MACRA),[5] there has been a significant shift by CMS to compensate services and programs through the Quality Payment Program that advances a value-based model and essentially attempts to eliminate the traditional fee-for-service model of the past. The Merit-based Incentive Payment System (MIPS) and Advanced Alternative Payment Model (APM) programs were designed to incorporate measures of quality, cost, outcomes, electronic integration, episodes of care and risk sharing.[5]

NEED FOR ADVOCACY AND WHAT ROLE IT PLAYS

Patients' access to necessary, lifesaving, or quality of life improving medical services is usually tied to reimbursement. In light of these vast and rapid changes in the past few decades and the mandates to reduce costs, which typically have come in the form of reducing payments for services, there is a great need to advocate for patient access. Physician and other provider groups have relied on various medical societies, patient advocacy groups, and industry to speak out and defend when policy decisions negatively impact patients' access to care as well as physicians' ability to provide care. Significantly curtailing or ending reimbursement for services primarily impacts patients' access and their choices for medical care.

Patients often do not understand the complexities in healthcare systems. CMS is the largest payer of the healthcare services. Thus, they are at the frontline of putting forward policies and regulations that impact patient care. Other insurance companies and payers often follow the policy and coverage leads of CMS. As the healthcare delivery systems continue to evolve, physicians should be at the forefront to advocate for patients. It is incumbent on physicians to take the lead as health advocates not only as agents for patients on an individual level but also on a macro level as activists attempting to effect positive changes in policy. Health advocacy campaigns are needed to bring about institutional, social, economic, and political changes that will help drive systems toward improved access and health. Advocacy, however, does not always have to be reactionary. Advocacy can also play an important role in providing education, guidance, and collaboration in making positive policy and reimbursement changes that will help patients and be cost-effective as well.

In an article, Seklar[6] emphasizes that "Physician involvement in the development of policy and regulations related to the health of patients and communities has been widely, although not universally,[7] recognized as a legitimate activity known as health advocacy." The

Office-Based Endovascular Centers. https://doi.org/10.1016/B978-0-323-67969-5.00037-X
Copyright © 2020 Elsevier Inc. All rights reserved.

FIG. 37.1 OEIS- The Voice of Outpatient Endovascular and Interventional Centers.

Royal College of Physicians and Surgeons of Canada identifies health advocacy as one of the seven competencies required of all physicians.[8] They define health advocacy "as Health Advocates, physicians contribute their expertise and influence as they work with communities or patient populations to improve health. They work with those they serve to determine and understand needs, speak on behalf of others when required, and support the mobilization of resources to effect change."

FORMATION OF AN ADVOCACY VOICE: ORGANIZING A COALITION

Although office-based interventional suites (OISs), also known as office-based endovascular centers (OECs), have been operational for several years, there had been no formal or organized voice to advocate for patient access to this site of service until 2013. Prior to that time, the peripheral artery disease (PAD) sector and stakeholders were fragmented and predominately disengaged. In 2013, the Medicare Professional Fee Schedule (MPFS) Proposed Rule for 2014 threatened steep cuts of up to 56% to lower extremity revascularization codes for nonfacilities, place of service (POS) 11, OECs. Although it appeared that atherectomy codes were targeted, the primary reason for the significant cuts to vascular care services in the Proposed Rule related to a proposal to cap all lower extremity revascularization (LER) codes and other services at the level of the outpatient department (HOPD) or the ambulatory surgical center (ASC) rates, whichever was lower. LER services in the ASC are paid at rates which are significantly discounted as compared with HOPD rates. At that time the medical societies that represent the three main endovascular specialists (vascular surgeons, interventional cardiologists, and interventional radiologists) who perform these procedures were relatively silent on addressing these proposed cuts that threatened to significantly impact atherectomy procedures in the office. Also, at that time, the Outpatient Endovascular and Interventional Society (OEIS) (Fig. 37.1) did not exist, since the landmark and formative meeting was to be held later in August of 2013. An office-based Cath lab management group sought out a healthcare advisory firm in Washington, D.C., to organize a response to CMS during the comment period. At the same time a physician reached out to industry stakeholders to organize a coordinated response to CMS during the comment period and form a grassroots campaign. A physician and an industry stakeholder group were able to meet representatives of CMS to educate them regarding the potential impact of the Rule and procedural variances within their rule making. Representatives from the Society of Interventional Radiology (SIR) and Society for Vascular Surgery (SVS) also met with CMS. This emerging coalition of various stakeholders also helped to marshal a major grassroots effort with numerous letter submissions to CMS during the comment period. As a testament to the actions of this large coordinated voice, CMS rolled back the cuts in the 2014 MPFS Final Rule.

ADVOCACY TO SUPPORT ACCESS TO OFFICE-BASED ENDOVASCULAR CENTERS AND PREVENT LIMB LOSS

Within the crucible of this existential threat and the lessons learned, efforts to formalize an advocacy organization were launched. The Cardiovascular Coalition (CVC) (Fig. 37.2) was formed in 2013 as a 501(c) organization consisting of physician members through the OEIS as well as members from industry, service, and management groups as the founding members. Although in the past, a predecessor PAD coalition existed to serve primarily as a direct to patient advocacy group, this group had dissolved. To serve the unmet

CardioVascular
COALITION
Joining Together for Patient Access

FIG. 37.2 Cardiovascular Coalition.

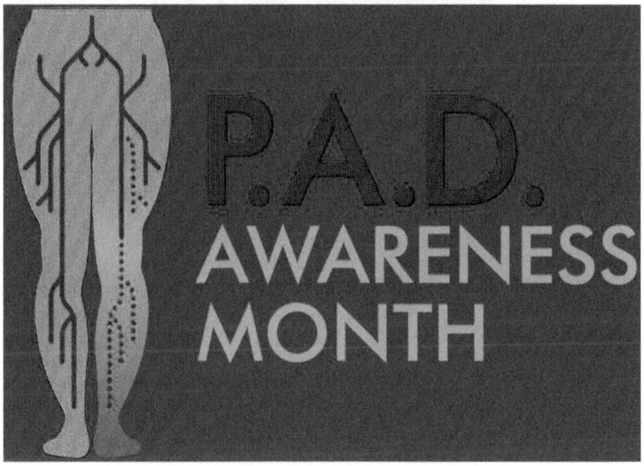

FIG. 37.3 PAD Awareness Month.

need, the CVC was organized independently to represent the broader reach of the cardiovascular (CV) community. Since inception, the focus of the CVC has been to educate CMS and congressional leaders regarding PAD and CV disease. During the CVC's initial visits to CMS and meetings with lawmakers in the House and Senate, it was very clear that policymakers had very little awareness of the impact of PAD and PAD-related amputations as well as the financial burden it caused on the national healthcare budget. There was also a lack of unified advocacy community working together on issues related to PAD. At one meeting, a US senator, who served on the Senate Finance Committee which oversees CMS, advised the CVC members to "get as large possible and come to us with one voice ... this is what makes us move in Congress." So, with the formation of the CVC, a collaborative infrastructure was created to bring stakeholders together and build awareness around PAD.

Since its formation, the CVC has been very active in Washington, D.C., building awareness by publishing dozens of op-ed articles, conducting Capitol Hill briefings, engaging in social media, and relaunching September as the PAD Awareness Month (Fig. 37.3). The CVC has also regularly engaged with CMS and has worked with various committees within the agency to work on access to care, quality measures, and amputation prevention. In 2015, the CVC was represented at the Medicare Evidence Development and Coverage Advisory Committee (MEDCAC) Meeting to present evidence for PAD interventions and access to care and wrote comment letters in coordination with other groups and medical societies.

AMPUTATION PREVENTION AND DISPARITIES IN CARE

Amputation prevention has been a core strategic mission for advocacy in the office interventional and outpatient space. It has been clearly shown that there remains a disparity in amputation rates in the United States based on where one lives.[9] The site map from the year 2013 depicts the marked regional variations in total major amputations and amputation rates as measured by the total number of amputations at hospitals per 100 endovascular procedures performed throughout the United States. Red circles indicate a high rate of amputation and blue, a low rate (Fig. 37.4). There is a direct correlation between access to vascular care and amputation rates.[9] Additionally,

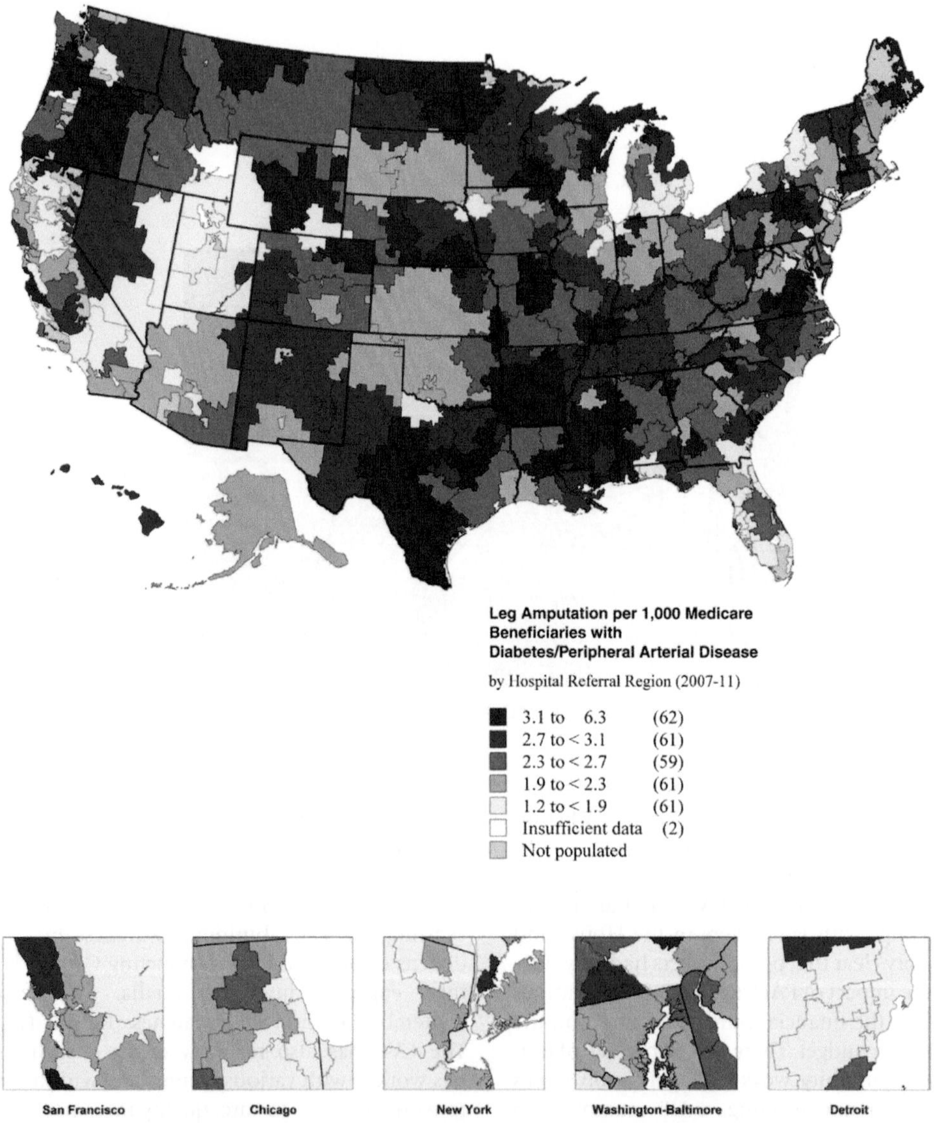

FIG. 37.4 Geographic disparities in leg amputation rates in Medicare beneficiaries with diabetes and PAD in the US (2007-2011). (Source: From Goodney PP, Dzebisashvili N, Goodman DC, Bronner KK. Variation in the Care of Surgical Conditions: Diabetes and Peripheral Arterial Disease. Lebanon, NH: The Dartmouth Institute of Health Policy & Clinical Practice, 2014.)

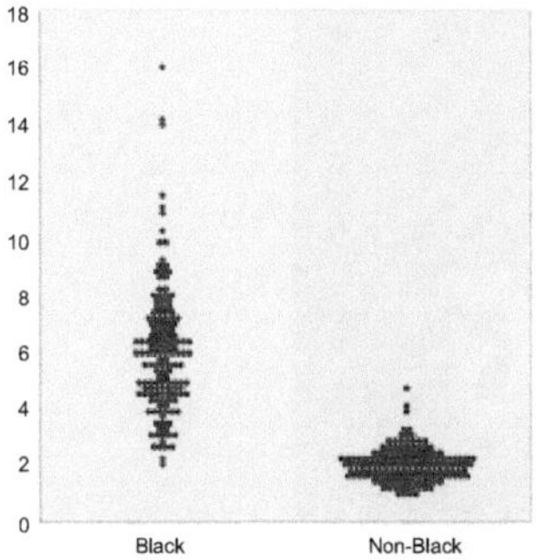

FIG. 37.5 **Leg amputation per 1000 Medicare beneficiaries with diabetes and PAD by race among hospital referral regions (2007–11).** Each blue dot represents the rate of leg amputation among patients with diabetes and PAD in one of 306 hospital referral regions in the United States. Rates are adjusted for age and sex. (Source: Variation in the Care of Surgical Conditions: Diabetes and Peripheral Arterial Disease. A Dartmouth Atlas of Health Care Series. http://www.dartmouthatlas.org/downloads/reports/Diabetes_report_10_14_14.pdf.)

significant variation in care exists with nearly five times higher amputation rates for African Americans and those of lower socioeconomic status.[10] The Dartmouth Atlas data show the markedly high rates of major lower extremity amputations for blacks with diabetes compared with nonblacks (Fig. 37.5). Additionally, Mexican Americans have 75% more risk and Native Americans nearly double the risk of amputation compared with whites.[11] OECs and ASCs together are numerically more prevalent than hospitals in the United States. The provision of dedicated endovascular care in these facilities may offer a local site of service support to combat these geographic and racial disparities in amputation rates.

STANDING TALL AND AMPUTATION PREVENTION CAMPAIGNS

Due to these significant disparities, the CVC founded a Standing Tall campaign to bring a positive message and awareness to the importance of amputation prevention (Fig. 37.6). While lower extremity amputation includes traumatic, oncologic, and nontraumatic amputations, the vast majority are due to arterial vascular insufficiency.[12] The goal and mission of the CVC is to prevent major amputations due to vascular insufficiency. It has been shown that lower extremity revascularization can prevent amputation.[13] Verapumilli showed that 30% of all amputations are performed without noninvasive testing done prior to amputation.[14] It is known that arterial testing can lead to angiography and revascularization that can improve limb salvage. This can also result in significant improvement in mortality and cost savings. Sheehan et al.[15] point out that "the immediate healthcare costs associated with the amputation of a limb, not including prosthetic or rehabilitation costs, total nearly than $8 billion."[16] When the costs of prosthetic care, rehabilitation, and other healthcare costs are accounted for, the economic costs associated with amputation are significantly higher. It is estimated that the 5-year healthcare costs associated with limb loss are more than $500,000 per person, nearly double the lifetime healthcare costs of an average person. In addition, the 5-year prosthetic costs for a person with limb loss are estimated to be as high as $450,000. If patients can avoid a major amputation or be converted to a minor amputation with revascularization, coordinated care and medical therapy, there is a potential for substantial savings to the Medicare system and the broader healthcare industry. This objective of saving limbs while reducing costs resonates with commercial payers, regulatory agencies, and patients.

This has become the significant advocacy battle cry. One aim is to prevent potentially avoidable amputations by pursuing policies that would not reimburse for a major amputation without a documented attempt to identify vascular insufficiency using various tests and an effort to revascularize the limb if there is evidence of vascular insufficiency. The disparities in major amputation in the United States described above are significant. Although there are many reasons for these disparities, there is need for teamwork to include a dedicated community of interventionists, wound care specialists, podiatrists, primary care physicians, and other specialists to eliminate the fragmented care that currently exists (see Chapter 28 on limb preservation). A few hospital systems have embraced a comprehensive care approach to amputation prevention. One model of coordinated care for amputation prevention is the Preservation-Amputation-for-Veterans Everywhere (PAVE) program through the Veteran's Affairs (VA) system. The VA is a closed, contained system that may not relate to the diverse care delivery systems across the United States; but there are several lessons to be learnt from the PAVE program that may be extrapolated to other groups. The PAVE program attempts to identify patients with ischemic wounds or skin changes early. This translates to a timely referral to vascular specialists to provide more definitive evaluation and therapy for arterial ischemia resulting in prevention of painful wounds, debility, and increased downstream cost burden.

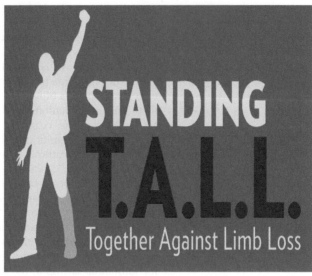

FIG. 37.6 Standing Tall Campaign.

COLLABORATIVE AND COMPREHENSIVE CARE

The CVC has championed a collaborative care approach and early identification of PAD. The CVC advocates for policy changes to improve access to care and quality interventions that make a difference. These interventions not only include important and meaningful revascularization procedures but also lifestyle modification and pharmacologic interventions to prevent CV events such as death, MI, and stroke. These lifestyle modifications include supervised exercise training, tobacco cessation, along with hypertension, lipid, and glycemic control.

PAD AWARENESS AND CONGRESSIONAL SUPPORT

It was clear in meetings with numerous lawmakers and healthcare policy leaders that there was a significant lack of understanding of PAD and its impact on patients and healthcare. What was needed was education for PAD and the toll it takes on patients and the healthcare system. Physicians need to be at the forefront in educating policymakers and lawmakers in their spheres of influence. Physicians may be able to educate and influence their local, state representatives, or an influential congressperson or a senator.

Several congressional Hill meetings with key senators and congressmen were helpful in educating members about the impact of appropriate legislation to help patients with PAD. A PAD awareness campaign was organized and targeted specifically for healthcare policymakers. To that end, the CVC conducted PAD Congressional Hill Briefings in 2016 and 2018. Numerous members of the Congress were individually contacted, and a Congressional letter was written highlighting four key initiatives:

1. PAD awareness is needed, given the prevalence and increasing incidence of the disease
2. A multidisciplinary approach in caring for advanced PAD
3. No amputation without arterial evaluation first
4. PAD screening for high-risk population patients

This letter was originally cosponsored by Rep Paulsen (R-Min) and Rep Payne (D-NJ), and numerous congresspersons signed on. This letter has been influential in ongoing efforts to educate CMS regarding the importance of patient access to definitive vascular care. As a result of these initial efforts, a congressional PAD caucus was convened in 2019 in which additional members of the Congress have signed on to this initiative with plans to provide active support.

NATIONAL AND REGIONAL COVERAGE POLICY CHALLENGES

In addition to advocating at the national level to influence National Coverage Determination policies, the CVC has engaged numerous regional and state policymakers. Local Coverage Determinations and potential regional policy changes have posed substantial threats to office-based interventions over the past few years. The Florida State Department of Health (DOH) proposed to change the policy for procedures performed in OEC in 2017. This was a challenge to coverage for arterial and venous stenting (among other policy changes) in the office labs based on dated statutory language. In 2019, the Florida DOH again revisited regulations governing OECs and redefine ASCs in the state because of a few physicians' outlier behavior in plastic surgery. In both instances, the CVC responded and educated the state policymakers helping in modernizing policies to ensure public safety.

In 2018, the Pennsylvania DOH issued sweeping changes to existing policy for outpatient surgery facilities that threatened the viability of performing most endovascular and dialysis access procedures in ambulatory surgery facilities and office labs. The concern was that the policy would have disallowed any of these procedures outside of the hospital setting. The CVC met with the governor and Medical Director of Quality Assurance. A few key physician advocates representing OEIS, SIR, SVS, and the American Society of Diagnostic and Interventional Nephrology (ASDIN) were able to successfully educate and assist the Director in redrafting improved policies to preserve access to care for LER and dialysis access procedures.

Also, in 2018, the Medicare Administrative Contractor, Novitas proposed eliminating LE venous stenting in the OIS (POS 11). As another example of collaborating with other stakeholders, the CVC reached out to leaders in the American Venous Forum, American Vein and Lymphatic Society, SVS, and other stakeholders to mount a unified message in response to address Novitas' concerns. These collective advocacy efforts and a direct meeting with Novitas leaders were successful in preserving coverage for venous stenting for qualified operators.

On the national front, the proposed 2019 MPFS Physician Fee Schedule would have imposed deep cuts of over 30% to revascularization procedures in the OEC setting. These proposed cuts were due to equipment and supply price updates in the Medicare database. The CVC worked with its members to collect more accurate equipment and supply cost data. The CVC coordinated the message with several specialty societies (SIR, Society for Cardiac Angiography and Interventions, SVS) and other stakeholders. A few CVC physician members met with CMS in person to educate them and address their concerns. As a result of these efforts, the proposed cuts in the Final Rule of the 2019 Physician Fee Schedule were substantially mitigated and reimbursement for some of the codes actually increased.

EXPANSION OF CARDIAC PROCEDURE CODES

Although much of the advocacy efforts have been in defending against proposed cuts in reimbursement and the ability to perform procedures in the office, there was an expansion of cardiac diagnostic and interventional codes in the ASC beginning in 2019. After years of educating CMS about the safety of performing same-day discharge (SDD) for cardiac procedures including percutaneous coronary intervention (PCI), 17 diagnostic cardiac codes were approved in the ASC setting (POS 24). Additionally, in the 2020 ASC Payment Systems Final Rule, CMS further expanded coverage for appropriate PCI (6 codes) in the ASC.[17] These were positive first steps for CMS to acknowledge the advances made in safety and efficacy of cardiac interventions in facilities without on-site surgical backup in a move to also reduce costs. Advocacy efforts continue to educate CMS about significant disparities in cardiac care based on the site of service. The aim is to have CMS further expand coverage for coronary fractional flow reserve, intracoronary ultrasound, appropriate PCI lesion subsets and other cardiac interventions in the ASC or office since many of these procedures are currently being performed safely as a SDD in hospital settings (see Chapter 35 on Cardiac Procedures).

THE CVC POLITICAL ACTION COMMITTEE: PAC WITH A PURPOSE

It is every individual's right to advocate for policies that provide access and health benefits to patients through financial support to members of the Congress. To that end a CVC Political Action Committee (CVC PAC) was formed (see Fig. 37.7). The aim is to reduce disparities in care and continue to promote patient access and

CVCPAC

FIG. 37.7 Cardiovascular Coalition Political Action Committee.

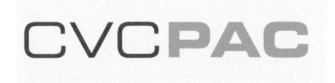

amputation prevention through coordinated care. The CVC is focused and dedicated to providing value for its members. This CVC PAC was created to be a "PAC with a Purpose" so that members will more directly understand and realize the value of advocacy to preserve patient access to receive high-quality healthcare in an office-based site of service.

SUMMARY

Advocacy is a vital function offered on behalf of patients and the medical community. We first and foremost advocate to ensure patients have access to lifesaving and lifestyle, improving interventions and specialists that provide this CV care. The office-based procedures are cost-effective and safe and provide a high degree of patient satisfaction. A unified voice is needed to further educate policymakers and payers to continue to advance patient-friendly, evidence-based, and efficient healthcare delivery models. We should all ensure that safe, appropriate, effective, and cost-efficient procedures are always available to our patients. If we do not advocate for our patients, who will? Advocacy works!

REFERENCES

1. American Health Care: Health Spending and the Federal Budget | Committee for a Responsible Federal Budget. https://www.crfb.org/papers/american-health-care-health-spending-and-federal-budget. Accessed June 19, 2019.
2. Fetter RB, Shin Y, Freeman JL, Averill RF, Thompson JD. Case mix definition by diagnosis-related groups. *Med Care*. 1980;18(2 Suppl):1–53. iii http://www.ncbi.nlm.nih.gov/pubmed/7188781.
3. Baadh A, Peterkin Y, Wegener M, Flug J, Katz D, Hoffmann JC. The relative value unit: history, current use, and controversies. *Curr Probl Diagn Radiol*. 2016; 45(2):128–132. https://doi.org/10.1067/j.cpradiol.2015.09.006.
4. FY 2018 Budget in Brief – CMS – Medicare | HHS.gov. https://www.hhs.gov/about/budget/fy2018/budget-in-brief/cms/medicare/index.html. Accessed June 19, 2019.
5. Burgess MC. H.R.2 – 114th Congress (2015–2016). *Medicare Access and CHIP Reauthorization Act of 2015*; 2015. https://www.congress.gov/bill/114th-congress/house-bill/2.
6. Sklar DP. Why effective health advocacy is so important today. *Acad Med*. 2016;91(10):1325–1328. https://doi.org/10.1097/ACM.0000000000001338.
7. Huddle TS. Perspective: medical professionalism and medical education should not involve commitments to political advocacy. *Acad Med*. 2011;86(3):378–383. https://doi.org/10.1097/ACM.0b013e3182086efe.
8. Sherbino J, Bonnycastle D, Côté B, et al. *CanMEDS: Health Advocate*. Ottawa, Ontario, Canada: Royal College of Physicians and Surgeons of Canada - Google Search; 2015. https://www.google.com/search?client=safari&rls=en&q=Sherbino+J,+Bonnycastle+D,+Côté+B,+et+al.+CanMEDS:+Health+Advocate.+2015.Ottawa,+Ontario,+Canada:+Royal+College+of+Physicians+and+Surgeons+of+Canada&ie=UTF-8&oe=UTF-8.
9. Goodney PP, Holman K, Henke PK, et al. Regional intensity of vascular care and lower extremity amputation rates, 1480.e1-3; discussion 1479-80 *J Vasc Surg*. June 2013; 57(6):1471–1479. https://doi.org/10.1016/j.jvs.2012.11.068. Epub 2013 Feb 1.
10. Goodney PP, Tarulli M, Faerber AE, Schanzer A, Zwolak RM. Fifteen-year trends in lower limb amputation, revascularization, and preventive measures among Medicare patients. *JAMA Surg*. 2015;150(1):84. https://doi.org/10.1001/jamasurg.2014.1007.
11. Leg Amputations per 1,000 Medicare Enrollees, by Race – Dartmouth Atlas of Health Care. http://archive.dartmouthatlas.org/data/table.aspx?ind=158. Accessed June 19, 2019.
12. Dillingham TR, Pezzin LE, MacKenzie EJ. Limb amputation and limb deficiency: epidemiology and recent trends in the United States. *South Med J*. 2002;95:875–883.
13. Uccioli L, Meloni M, Izzo V, Giurato L, Merolla S, Gandini R. Critical limb ischemia: current challenges and future prospects. *Vasc Health Risk Manag*. 2018;14:63–74. https://doi.org/10.2147/VHRM.S125065.
14. Vemulapalli S, Greiner MA, Jones WS, Patel MR, Hernandez AF, Curtis LH. Peripheral arterial testing before lower extremity amputation among medicare beneficiaries, 2000 to 2010. *Circ Cardiovasc Qual Outcomes*. 2014;7(1):142–150. https://doi.org/10.1161/CIRCOUTCOMES.113.000376.
15. Sheehan TP, Gondo GC. Impact of limb loss in the United States. *Phys Med Rehabil Clin N Am*. 2014;25(1):9–28. https://doi.org/10.1016/j.pmr.2013.09.007.
16. Healthcare Cost and Utilization Project (HCUP) | Agency for Healthcare Research & Quality. https://www.ahrq.gov/data/hcup/index.html. Accessed June 19, 2019.
17. federalregister.gov/d/2019-24138.

CHAPTER 38

Conducting Research in an Office Endovascular Center

LAURA D. BAULER, PHD

Research is essential to the success of the office-based endovascular center (OEC) because research solves problems. Without research the safety and efficacy of procedures performed in an OEC will not be proven, and these data provide the evidence needed to convince the Centers for Medicare and Medicaid Services (CMS) and insurance companies to continue to reimburse and expand the number of procedures that can be performed in an OEC. Quality improvement research allows you to track the success of your OEC and identify areas in your practice that could be improved upon. Both success rates and continued improvement of your practice will correlate directly to the recruitment and retention of patients. For clinicians who are associated with a medical school, research provides an opportunity to mentor students and residents, as well as advance your academic career. Most importantly, research is the key to advance the field of endovascular medicine, by testing new techniques, medications, and equipment, to identify tools that can be used to improve the health of patients.

Research develops the evidence needed for evidence-based medicine. Currently, the field of translational medicine, which moves research from the bench to the bedside, is rapidly growing. Basic scientists identify a multitude of treatments that could benefit patients; however, they do not have the clinical knowledge and expertise needed to transition those treatments to the bedside. As few as one in five basic research discoveries lead to a clinical trial.[1] By partnering with academic institutions, an OEC can provide a venue to bridge basic science research into the clinic.

This chapter will provide the foundational knowledge needed to initiate medical research from developing a research question to publishing the findings. Aspects such as defining a study team, project design, literature searches, regulatory oversight, and resources will also be addressed. When initiating research for the first time, we strongly advise identifying a mentor who can guide, train, and advise you as you develop your research project. However, even seasoned investigators should consider identifying collaborators who have expertise in areas beneficial to the project.

RESEARCH PROCESS

The strength of our knowledge depends upon the quality of the research that supports it. Research is a systematic process that starts with a question. The question is answered by a carefully designed study with appropriate controls to ensure the answer is valid. The best studies build off the work of others to expand the knowledge of the field; a literature review is key in identifying this foundational knowledge. Recruitment of a study team will enable the work to be dispersed and provides the expertise needed for each component. The project protocol should be designed using the most appropriate methodology to accurately answer the research question. For any project involving human participants or data, the study must be approved by an institutional review board (IRB) to ensure the protection of the rights and safety of participants. After IRB approval the data collection can begin, followed by data analysis, and presentation of the results. This process is outlined in Fig. 38.1.

RESEARCH QUESTIONS

The research process starts with a problem that forces you to begin asking questions. This may involve an aspect of medicine that does not make sense or a problem within the OEC practice itself that cannot be answered without collecting data. A research question guides a project like a map, directing what information needs to be obtained to answer the question. If the question is too broad or vague, the study will be

Office-Based Endovascular Centers. https://doi.org/10.1016/B978-0-323-67969-5.00038-1
Copyright © 2020 Elsevier Inc. All rights reserved.

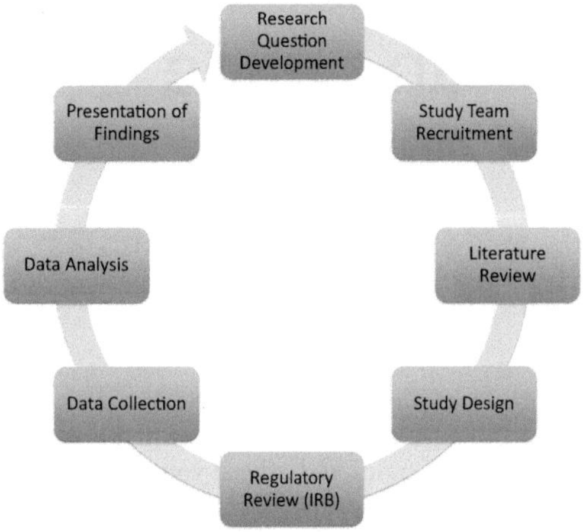

FIG. 38.1 The research process.

equally ambiguous and difficult to address; much like trying to use a map of the United States to direct patients to the location of your OEC. There are two types of questions, research questions and regular questions. A regular question can be easily answered, the information is already available, it just may take a bit of searching to find. A research question on the other hand has an answer that is unknown; it is a novel question that, when answered, will provide additional knowledge to the field. Good research starts with unanswered questions triggered by a curiosity that cannot be satisfied with a thorough literature search.

The development of a solid research question requires knowledge of the field. Initial questions are commonly generated during the practice of evidence-based medicine following a literature search that reveals insufficient evidence to address the question. Conferences, field-specific journals, and conversations with colleagues can also serve as a source of questions. Above all, the researcher must be interested in the answer to the question; without this investment, the project will not be propelled forward.[2] For research in an OEC, an important factor to consider is the feasibility of the question; can it be addressed by investigating the patients in your practice, with data from a registry that you participate in, or by collaborating on projects initiated by other centers.

The best research questions are very specific and significant. If we think back to the map analogy, good research questions are focused or "zoomed in" to the street level of your city, this provides a much better guide to reach your destination. The answer to the question should be significant, meaning that the problem that you are faced with needs to be solved. To publish, the problem and solution must be relevant and important to physicians and scientists beyond your practice.

One method of developing a clinical research question is based upon the acronym PICO, which stands for patient/problem, intervention, control/comparison group, and outcome.[3] The PICO method, commonly used in evidence-based medicine to guide development of a targeted literature search, provides a research question that is specific and answerable. It also enables easy searching of the literature to identify what studies have already been completed, and what questions are left unanswered. Regardless of the method used to develop your question, a good research question guides the project and has been developed with the desired outcomes in mind (Table 38.1).

THE STUDY TEAM

Following the development of a good research question, a study team should be recruited to conduct and support the research. The principal investigator is in charge of the project and responsible for recruiting the study team. Team members may include colleagues and collaborators, mentees (residents and medical students), and research support personnel.

Principal investigator (PI): The principal investigator is responsible for guiding the research team,

TABLE 38.1
Good Research Question Characteristics.

1. Addresses a Problem
2. The answer is unknown
3. Topic is interesting and significant
4. Specific enough to be answered

providing research expertise, topic-specific knowledge, and funding the project. Ultimately the PI is responsible for all aspects of the project. In order to conduct research and successfully complete the project, someone must lead the project and direct the team.

Project manager: The project manager is responsible for coordinating all aspects of a project including personnel, timelines, resources, and budget. This team member is often the "second-in-command" and can move the project forward when the PI is busy with other roles. A project manager can manage several projects at once but would need to have protected time dedicated to the project. This job may fall to an office manager, administrative staff within the OEC, or the PI. Due to the time and effort required to direct a research project, having the PI also be the project manager is not ideal.

Information technology/electronic health record (EHR) personnel: These personnel are responsible for mining the EHR to obtain the data needed to answer the question. They may also be involved in ensuring that any patient personal identifying information (PII) is safely protected. A full-time individual in this role is likely not required; another member of the team may fulfill this role including an office manager, administrative staff, residents, or students.

Research coordinator: This member is responsible for patient recruitment, documentation, and compliance with the clinical protocol. A research coordinator is especially important for participation in a clinical trial; however, a project manager may also fill this role. The need for a research coordinator depends upon the size and nature of the project, as well as the PI's ability to dedicate time to research. For a retrospective study examining OEC patient records, this role is likely not needed.

Data managers: This member of the team assembles the data collection tools and ensures the data are accurate, carefully documented, organized, and stored appropriately. They often work closely with the statisticians. A data manager is not a required role, as other team members may fulfill these tasks.

Statisticians: For a clinical research project, a statistician is essential. They contribute several important components to the study, including determining the sample size needed to adequately power the study, determining which statistical tests are required to answer the research question, and performing the final analysis. There are multiple options for statistical support: (1) collaborate or hire a statistician, (2) recruit a team member with appropriate statistical knowledge, (3) obtain the necessary training for personnel to fulfill this role.

Medical librarian: A medical librarian can assist with the literature search to ensure that all relevant literature is identified. They provide knowledge of keywords and databases available as well as access to the medical literature. While not a required team member, a literature search is extremely important aspect of research to ensure that the project is novel and will add new knowledge to the field.

Medical editor: This member provides knowledge of the publication process and editorial guidance on disseminating the project findings. They may identify journals as well as help with writing and revising the manuscript. They may also serve as a peer-reviewer of any manuscripts and abstracts that are generated. A formal medical editor is certainly not required to be a team member, a colleague with scholarly expertise and willingness to help would suffice.

Residents and student trainees: A trainee can fulfill almost any role within the project other than the PI. Mentoring a trainee during a research project can also have benefits for the mentor and project. Trainees are often very motivated and bring new ideas to the project. Trainees can also provide assistance with any aspect of the project, lightening the load of a research project from senior team members and increasing the productivity of the team.[4] Participation in research is a good learning opportunity for trainees who may want to pursue research in their future careers.[5] It helps to build their CVs with research experiences, presentations, and publications. Research also provides trainees with an opportunity to learn more about the specialty while gaining experience and insight about the medical field. Research also provides trainees with an opportunity to collaborate with mentors and colleagues, they may call upon for support of their future careers with recommendation letters or connections. While a trainee is not a required part of a research project, trainees are often extremely useful members of the team.

LITERATURE REVIEW

To develop a good specific research question, you need to have a thorough understanding of the current knowledge in the field: what research has been conducted, what is known, and what questions still remain. While the literature search typically comes after an initial research question has been developed, it serves to further shape and refine the research question into a specific and significant question. The literature review should be comprehensive, identifying all possible literature that has been conducted on a topic so that the research team can become experts in the field and identify the gap in the literature that could be addressed by their research.

For an OEC, physicians may not have ready access to the literature; obtaining privileges at a local hospital that has a library, collaborating with colleagues at an academic institution, or partnering with an academic institution as community or adjunct faculty member can provide access to the medical literature.

A number of databases are available to identify medical literature including PubMed, CINAHL, Scopus, Embase, Google Scholar, or the Web of Science. These databases can be searched by keyword, subject, or author to identify relevant literature. Developing a search string to identify relevant literature may help you focus your results. As discussed above, PICO is a common tool used to generate a patient-centered medical search string (Fig. 38.2).[6]

As an example, if you were interested in determining what factors put patients with critical limb ischemia undergoing an endovascular intervention at risk for bleeding, you may use the following PICO keywords: P: critical limb ischemia, I: endovascular, O: bleeding. The C: comparison/control is often difficult to determine before the literature search, as you may not know what control group was used in a particular study. While a PICO-based search string will provide focused results, it will be limited by the search terms used, thus may not be entirely encompassing of all relevant literature. Relevant literature may be found through a variety of means including multiple searches with different keywords, similar articles recommended by the search tool, from the reference list of key papers, or from manuscripts that have cited your key articles.

DESIGN OF THE STUDY AND RESEARCH PLAN

The design of the study is critical in determining the value of the research. A well-designed study is constructed in a manner that avoids all possible bias, and controls for as many factors as possible, to ensure the conclusions drawn from the data are valid. It is best to consult with a statistician during the study design phase to determine the sample size and ensure that the data collected can be analyzed in a manner that addresses the research question. A vitally important aspect of a research study is the control group, as without appropriate controls you cannot determine with any

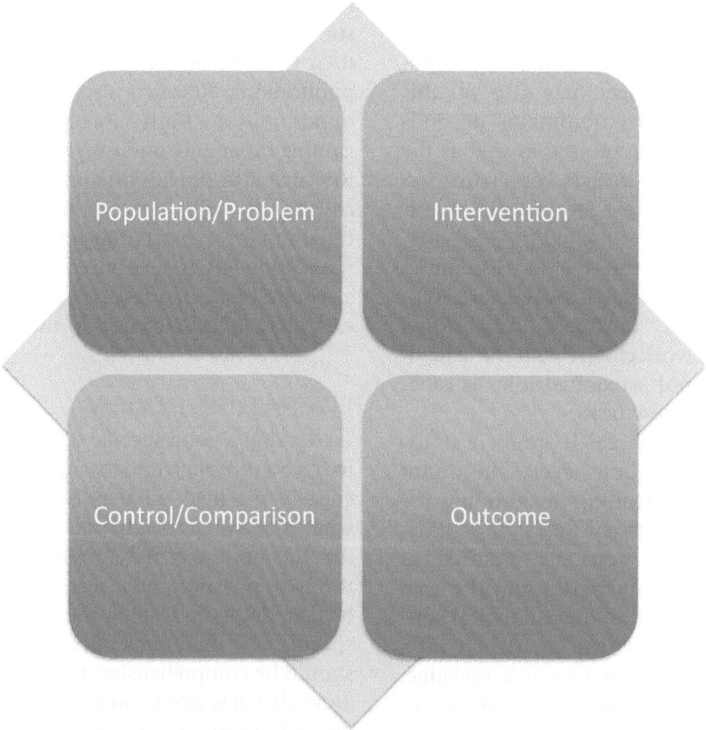

FIG. 38.2 PICO question components.

certainty that a particular variable had an impact on the outcome. For clinical research the gold standard study type is a randomized controlled trial (RCT); however, this type of study is not always feasible or appropriate to address the research question.

Clinical research can be divided into two categories: experimental research or observational research (Fig. 38.3). Experimental research involves the direct testing of a hypothesis or intervention, while observational research involves examination of the natural features of a study group without direct intervention.[7] The best study design is determined by the research question and the desired outcomes of the project. Each study design has strengths and weaknesses that should be considered.

Experimental Research

Experimental or interventional studies are often prospective and are designed to evaluate the direct impacts of a treatment on a specific disease outcome.

Randomized controlled trial (RCT): RCTs are the gold standard of clinical research; because of their design these studies can provide evidence for a causal relationship between an intervention and an outcome.[8] Due to the careful enrollment of participants who are randomly assigned into the control or experimental group, the only anticipated difference between these groups is the intervention.[7] These types of studies are extremely expensive, and recruitment is restricted resulting in problematic generalizability. For some studies, it would be unethical to conduct an RCT because when treatments are shown to improve the health of patients, it becomes unethical to maintain a control group. This is especially problematic for surgical interventions, as randomizing patients to a control group may result in irreparable consequences.

Quasi-experimental, pre-/poststudy or nonrandomized controlled trial: These trials are similar to RCTs, in that an intervention is tested in one group and compared with another group. In the absence of the randomization, these studies may lack internal validity, in that

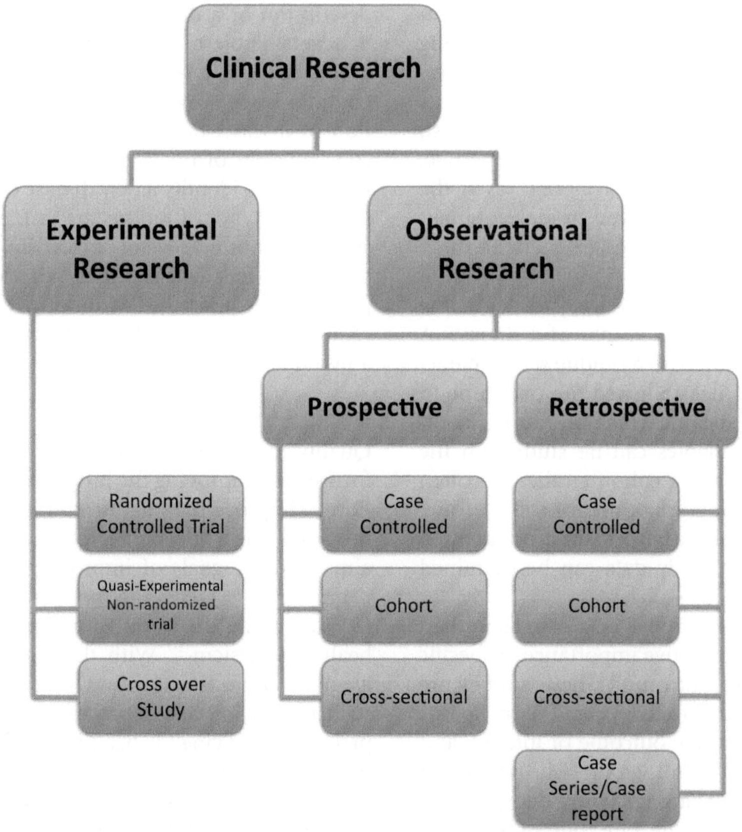

FIG. 38.3 Categories of research study design.

the treatment and control groups may not be comparable at baseline. Some of these biases can be overcome with careful statistical analysis, but others may not be overcome and may limit the generalizability of the results. Studies can be designed as single arm, which uses the same participant population as control and experimental subjects (as with pre-post studies), or as multiple arms where different groups are compared with each other.[7]

Crossover study: A crossover study is a type of interventional study where the study participants serve as both control and experimental group at different times during the study. Subjects are initially treated as experimental or control group in phase one, followed by a washout period where the treatment is stopped, and then in phase two the groups are swapped into the other condition. This crossover design demonstrates reversibility of a treatment and compensates for unsuccessful randomization, as subjects now become their own controls.[7]

Observational Research

Observational research studies examine the study and control groups to determine if they have different outcomes or risk factors that may be causal in determining those outcomes. Observational research can be prospective or retrospective depending upon the order of events within the project. When the project is designed first, and data collection follows, this is termed prospective. When the data have already been collected, as is the case of an EHR or registry, followed by development of a research question and study design, then the study is retrospective.

Cohort study: Cohort studies are used to determine the incidence rate and natural history of a disease. A study population or cohort with a unique set of characteristics is defined and then followed the over time to determine if a certain outcome develops. Multiple outcomes and exposure variables can be studied in the same population. Prospective cohort studies are often inefficient, as it may take a long time for the outcome to occur, and during that time participant dropout often occurs. However, cohort study data can be examined retrospectively to answer new questions.

Case-control study: The purpose of a case-controlled study is to determine the relative importance of specific factors in impacting an outcome.[9] These studies are typically conducted retrospectively, and participants are identified based upon the outcome of interest, and then matched with a control group who does not have the outcome.[8] This is a good study design if you are studying outcomes that are rare, but suffers from sampling bias in that you cannot control the selection of participants in your dataset. This type of study works well for secondary data analysis, such as that obtained from the EMR, and can be used to determine the relative odds of a certain surgical outcome such as mortality, 30-day readmission, or bleeding complication following a particular surgical intervention.

Cross-sectional study: Cross-sectional studies are used to determine prevalence of a specific outcome and exposure status simultaneously in a population.[8,9] Determining the prevalence of an outcome allows the physician to determine the likelihood of a particular diagnosis for a particular patient. These studies can be done prospectively or retrospectively, and their accuracy depends upon careful study group selection to avoid biasing the results. For an OEC, a cross-sectional study would be a good starting point to identify the baseline prevalence of certain conditions within your patient population that could be used as a basis for further intervention and research. This type of study is also useful for measuring the impact of quality improvement studies pre- and postintervention.

Case report or case series: A case report or series is a description of a disease process in a single individual or several subjects without a control group. The cases described are typically a variation from what is commonly seen in a disease, including unique presentation of disease, novel patient populations, or adverse consequences of treatment. Case reports are often the first report to identify a new disease or adverse health effect. These types of reports are fast, easy, and inexpensive. Describing several cases simultaneously with similar features increases the evidence available to support a hypothesis, but without a control group you cannot provide conclusive evidence to support or refute a hypothesis.

Quality Improvement

Quality improvement is a type of research that is focused on improving the processes within an organization to improve the quality, cost, and value of the care provided. The work is often focused on targeting a triple aim, with the goals of improving (1) the health of a community, (2) reducing the cost of medical care, and (3) improving the population's experience within the healthcare system.[10] With these goals in mind, there are many projects within an OEC that could be targeted, such as reducing cost of procedures for patients and the practice, improving the health outcomes of the community based upon preventative care, and improving the patient care experience while being treated at the OEC. Successful QI projects have a champion directing the project, who is invested in the outcomes. Thus, allowing operators or staff to identify areas they want to improve increases the success of QI projects. These concepts and methodology used in quality improvement are expanded further in Chapter 13.

Clinical Trials

Clinical trials provide the evidence needed by the Food and Drug Administration (FDA) to evaluate the benefits and risks of a new medication or medical treatment to determine if it is safe for patients. In order to obtain the necessary data, thousands of patients are enrolled in clinical trials, many more patients than can reasonably be identified from a single institution. Participation in a clinical trial has several benefits: (1) the patients in your practice may benefit from novel drugs, devices, and treatments currently being studied; (2) the medical protocols within your OEC may change based upon new clinical evidence identified in the clinical trial and; (3) participating in a clinical trial is a good way to develop research experience and skills.[11] Clinicians who have participated in clinical trials have also indicated that their clinic processes improved based upon documentation efforts required for the clinical trial, and that the profile of their practice has increased.[11] A list of clinical trials currently being conducted can be found on the NIH website https://clinicaltrials.gov.

Postmarket Studies

Postmarket studies are studies conducted after the FDA has approved a product for marketing. They are typically sponsored studies that serve to collect additional information about a product's safety, efficacy, and optimal use.[12] These may include RCTs, drug interaction studies, efficacy studies, pharmacokinetic and pharmacodynamic studies, or pediatric trials. Some device companies pay for data to be collected if the OEC is a participant in a national registry.

RESEARCH RESOURCES

Databases and Registries

Beyond conducting research using the medical records or patients within your own practice, a number of resources exist that can be utilized for research including databases and patient registries (see also Chapter 19). Clinical registries have increasingly been generated from existing practice data for use as patient safety improvement tools, but can also be used as an observational database to address clinical research questions.

The Healthcare Cost and Utilization Project (HCUP): A repository of longitudinal statewide inpatient data. HCUP is the largest collection of hospital care data in the United States that includes all payers, encounter-level data from 1988 to present.[13] HCUP consists of several different databases including the National Inpatient Sample (NIS), the State Inpatient Database (SID), and the State Ambulatory Surgery and Services Databases (SASD).

American College of Surgeons National Surgical Quality Improvement Program (ASC-NSQIP): A nationally validated, risk-adjusted, outcomes-based dataset that contains more than 28,000 cases with as many as 134 data points per patient tracked for 30 days after their operation. Currently, more than 710 individual hospitals have enrolled in this registry.[14]

Society of Vascular Surgery, Vascular Quality Initiative (VQI), and Patient Safety Organization (SVS-PSO): An aggregation and analysis of clinical data for patients undergoing specific vascular treatments designed to improve the quality, safety, effectiveness, and cost of vascular healthcare. Reports are generated twice per year to show trends, volume, process characteristics, and inhospital outcomes. The VQI consists of 12 registries with outcomes from more than 500,000 vascular procedures performed across the United States and Canada.[15] Centers that participate in the VQI can compare their performance with region and national benchmarks.

Medical Societies

Numerous medical societies exist that may serve to foster research in the field. They provide an environment for researchers to identify mentors and collaborators, discuss the latest advancements in clinical research, promote discussions that stimulate research questions, or may provide registries or grants to further research. Relevant societies include the Society for Vascular Surgery, the Society for Vascular Medicine, the Society for Vascular Ultrasound, the Vascular and Endovascular Surgery Society, the International Society of Endovascular Specialists, American College of Cardiologists, Society of Interventional Radiology, and the Outpatient Endovascular and Interventional Society.

Practice-Based Research Networks

Practice-based research networks (PBRN) are collaborations between clinical practice and academia designed to foster research.[16] PBRNs connect healthcare to research by providing support to clinicians throughout the research process. These networks serve to help clinicians develop specific impactful research questions, design and conduct studies, analyze data, and translate knowledge into practice. The PBRN network serves to better care for patients by conducting research in a patient population more representative of the general public, including patients with multiple comorbidities who are often excluded from RCTs. Additionally some diseases are only treated in certain settings making these topics more likely to be under represented in research studies.

Grants and Contracts

For more extensive research projects, the project may require funding support to pay for personnel, resources, or services. The National Institute of Health is the leading funding resource for medical research in the United States, supporting more than 44,000 research projects in 2017.[17] Starting in 2012, the National Center for Advancing Translational Sciences (NCATS) was established to fund translational research projects. Funding support for PBRNs can come from the Agency for Health Care Research and Quality (AHRQ). Funding may also come from local initiatives or societies as mentioned above. Many academic hospitals have award mechanisms that support the development of translational research or clinical trials. There are also nonprofit foundations, like the Kellogg Foundation, that support clinical research.

Regulations

To ensure patient consent and understanding of the research, an informed consent document is an important part of any research project. For research studies that involve human subjects there are a number of ethical considerations that need to be accounted for before the research is initiated, including review of the research protocol by an institutional review board (IRB). If the OEC does not have access to the local IRB at an academic institution, there are regional IRBs that can be utilized to get project approval.

Data obtained from medical records can be analyzed without informed consent as long as the findings of the project will not be published. For researchers interested in conducting quality improvement studies, this eases the burden of this hurdle, as long as they only report on the process utilized for improvement instead of the patient outcomes from the pre-post measures of their research.[18]

Institutional Review Board (IRB): The IRB is an ethical research committee, responsible for protecting the rights, welfare, and well-being of human research subjects.[19] Most academic institutions have an IRB, which is responsible for reviewing research protocols to ensure that the human subjects who will be asked to participate in that research are properly protected. Several factors are taken into consideration including the autonomy of the subject (their ability to opt in or out of the study), equitable selection of subjects, and the risk-benefits ratio of the study. Autonomy and consent are two of the cornerstone values in research ethics. The Declaration of Helsinki states that research "participants should be treated as autonomous beings capable of making an informed decision whether to participate in research."[20] In the case of database/EHR analysis at an OEC, individual patient consent can be obtained in their initial onboarding paperwork, or may be waived during the IRB review process if the research is determined to be of minimal risk to patients. The risk-benefit analysis helps the IRB determine how much risk the subjects will be exposed to in order to participate in the research, and what benefits will result from the study. The IRB reviews the research protocol including the scientific background of the project, rationale, objectives of the study, the study design, subject population (inclusion and exclusion criteria), subject recruitment, statistical analysis, expected results, study timeline, benefit and risk evaluation, dissemination plans, and any patient consent forms, surveys, or data collection forms that will be used in the study.

Ethical considerations: Of recent concern is the involvement of physicians in clinical trials, as they and their patients may both benefit financially from enrolling in the research. Patients can benefit from enrolling in clinical trials through limited financial compensation and receipt of free healthcare. Financial incentives are one of the most important factors motivating physician involvement in research.[21] Physicians are tasked with putting the concerns of their patient first above their own benefit, thus any incentives they receive must not influence their regard for their patients best interest.[22] The IRB protocol should include measures that will be taken to avoid bias or influence of any financial incentives to study participation.

DATA COLLECTION

Study Population

The degree that the study population accurately represents the overall population of patients suffering from a disease or variable of interest determines the value and generalizability of the results. In the ideal situation, the characteristics of the study sample will directly match the overall population. Random sampling is the simplest method to match populations; however, depending upon the source of your study participants the study may already be biased, thus you may need to carefully design your study sampling method to account for these biases as much as possible. Careful consideration of all the variables that may impact your outcome, and devising methods to overcome these hurdles, will ensure selection of a study population that best represents the general population.

Sample Size

The size of the study population should be predicted before the study begins. A statistician can use preexisting data about the outcome to help predict how many subjects need to be enrolled to adequately power the statistical analysis. Enrolling more subjects than is needed is costly and adds difficulty to the research project, but enrolling too few may mean the study fails to detect relationships that exist between variables and outcomes, and inadequately addresses the research question.[23] A statistical power analysis will determine the probability that the study can identify relationships that exist in the data.

Data Collection Tools

Care should be taken during the data collection phase to ensure that the data are accurate, complete, and organized. Missing values or duplication of records can cause problems down the road. A number of tools exist that can support the data collection process. For studies utilizing data in an EHR, the data can be obtained from an information technologist who can export a certain dataset with the variables of interest. However, not all EHRs are designed for research, thus the data may need to be abstracted from the medical record by study team members. Above all, the researchers must ensure that the subjects in their study are protected, this means developing a data management plan to protect any PII. Data may be collected into a simple password-protected database or into a tool designed for research data collection such as REDCap (Research Electronic Data Capture).[24] REDCap is a HIPAA-compliant data collection tool that enables academic researchers to develop surveys or data collection instruments.

DATA ANALYSIS

Analysis of the data is the most exciting aspect of the study, as you can finally begin to answer your question. With most medical questions the answer is rarely black or white, instead we are asking about the probability that a variable impacts an outcome. Statistics allows us to measure these probabilities. To get an accurate answer to the research question, an expert, typically a statistician, should conduct the analysis. Utilizing the appropriate data analysis method depends on the study design, variables collected, and desired outcome. Data analysis tools should be identified in the design phase of the study.

PRESENTING YOUR FINDINGS

Research findings should be disseminated beyond your group to maximize the benefits of conducting a project. Publication is the ultimate goal, creating a permanent record of the research and its findings. The work can also be disseminated at local, regional, or national conferences by submitting an abstract for presentation in a poster or oral format. While clinical research studies have clear value, quality improvement studies describing the process of improvement utilized to achieve your goals can also be published and are valuable to other groups who are attempting similar initiatives for improvement. To ease the burden of the presentation process, collaboration with an academic colleague or with a medical writer or editor can help by providing knowledge of the publication process.

PARTNERING WITH A MEDICAL SCHOOL

For many of the topics discussed above, access to resources and individuals who can collaborate on your project can be facilitated through partnering with a medical school. You can gain access to a number or resources including the library, students and residents, grants management, statisticians, medical editors, management of industry contracts, and colleagues. Due to the complexity and regulations surrounding a clinical trial, medical schools often have entire departments dedicated to ensuring compliance with FDA regulations.[25] Partnering with the medical school may be done through collaborations with medical school faculty or by joining a medical school as community faculty. At most medical schools, community faculty are volunteers who contribute to education, research, community engagement, and committees at the medical school. In return, community faculty gain access to the medical school resources described above in addition to opportunities for continuing education. For many medical schools their required commitment is minimal, often 25–50 h of service per year. For OECs looking to collaborate on research projects, committing to include students and residents on your research projects may satisfy these requirements.

FINAL CONSIDERATIONS

Conducting research requires an investment of time, resources, and effort toward a project. As research projects always take more time than anticipated, the research team must be fully invested and interested in the project to dedicate the time needed to move the project forward and successfully accomplish their goals. Numerous students and residents are interested in participating in research, but they often fail to realize the time commitment required. Setting clear expectations of time, investment, and quality is important to make sure the mentor-mentee relationship is built on common ground. Thus careful selection of students or residents is critical to both advance the project and generate a good mentor-mentee relationship that will be mutually beneficial. Similar care should be taken in identifying collaborators that have the needed skills for a project.

CONCLUSION

Research is essential to address questions that arise during the practice of medicine. While some questions can easily be addressed with a literature search, true research problems will have unanswerable questions that require research to solve. An OEC has a responsibility to provide the best patient care possible and to do this; research is a necessary aspect of patient care. Through contributing to registries, undertaking quality improvement studies, or answering unanswered questions, physicians of an OEC can make meaningful contributions to improving medical care provided. Not only does this research directly benefit the OEC, but it also can benefit the field of endovascular medicine.

REFERENCES

1. Cripe TP, Thomson B, Boat TF, Williams DA. Promoting translational research in academic health centers: navigating the "roadmap,". *Acad Med*. 2005. https://doi.org/10.1097/00001888-200511000-00008.
2. Alon U. How to choose a good scientific problem. *Mol Cell*. 2009;35:726–728. https://doi.org/10.1016/j.molcel.2009.09.013.
3. *Evidence-Based Medicine Resource Guide*. Georg. Univ. Dahlgren Meml. Libr.; 2019.
4. Morrison-Beedy D, Aronowitz T, Dyne J, Mkandawire L. Mentoring students and junior faculty in faculty research: a win-win scenario. *J Prof Nurs*. 2001. https://doi.org/10.1053/jpnu.2001.28184.
5. Mabvuure NT. Twelve tips for introducing students to research and publishing: a medical student's perspective. *Med Teach*. 2012;34:705–709. https://doi.org/10.3109/0142159X.2012.684915.
6. Richardson WS, et al. The well built clinical question: a key to evidence based decisions. *ACP J Club*. 1995. https://doi.org/10.7326/ACPJC-1995-123-3-A12.
7. Thiese MS. Observational and interventional study design types; an overview. *Biochem Medica*. 2014. https://doi.org/10.11613/BM.2014.022.
8. Noordzij M, Dekker FW, Zoccali C, Jager KJ. Study designs in clinical research. *Nephron Clin Pract*. 2009. https://doi.org/10.1159/000235610.
9. Mann C. Observational research methods. Research design II. *Emerg Med J*. 2003. https://doi.org/10.1136/emj.20.1.54.
10. *Triple Aim for Populations*. Inst. Healthc. Improv.; 2019. http://www.ihi.org/Topics/TripleAim/Pages/Overview.aspx.
11. Batchelor JM, Chapman A, Craig FE, et al. Generating new evidence, improving clinical practice and developing research capacity: the benefits of recruiting to the U.K. Dermatology Clinical Trials Network's STOP GAP and BLISTER trials. *Br J Dermatol*. 2017. https://doi.org/10.1111/bjd.15959.
12. *Postmarketing clinical trials, U.S. Food drug Adm*. 2018.
13. HCUP Overview. *Healthcare Cost and Utilization Project (HCUP)*. Agency Healthc. Res. Qual.; 2018. https://www.hcup-us.ahrq.gov/overview.jsp.
14. Ingraham AM, Richards KE, Hall BL, Ko CY. Quality improvement in surgery: the American College of Surgeons national surgical quality improvement program approach. *Adv Surg*. 2010. https://doi.org/10.1016/j.yasu.2010.05.003.
15. Vascular Quality Initiative, (2019). https://www.vqi.org/. Accessed October 18, 2019.
16. Pirotta M, Temple-Smith M. Practice-based research networks. *Aust Fam Physician*. 2017;46(10):793–795.
17. RePORT. *Funding Facts*. Natl. Institutes Heal.; 2018. https://report.nih.gov/fundingfacts/fundingfacts.aspx.
18. Feldman SR. Participating in trials can inform better clinical practice. *Br J Dermatol*. 2017;177:1148–1149. https://doi.org/10.1111/bjd.15946.
19. *Institutional Review Board Guidebook*. Off. Hum. Res. Prot.; 2019.
20. World Medical Association. Declaration of Helsinki world medical association declaration of Helsinki. *Bull World Heal Organ*. 2001. doi:S0042-96862001000400016 [pii].
21. Rahman S, Majumder A, Shaban S, Rahman N, Ahmed SM, Abdulrahman K, Dsouza UJ. Physician participation in clinical research and trials: issues and approaches. *Adv Med Educ Pract*. 2011. https://doi.org/10.2147/amep.s14103.
22. Fisher JA. Practicing research ethics: private-sector physicians & pharmaceutical clinical trials. *Soc Sci Med*. 2008. https://doi.org/10.1016/j.socscimed.2008.02.001.
23. Suresh G, Suresh K, Thomas S. Design, data analysis and sampling techniques for clinical research. *Ann Indian Acad Neurol*. 2011;14:287. https://doi.org/10.4103/0972-2327.91951.
24. REDCap: Research Electronic Data Capture, (n.d.). https://projectredcap.org/about/(accessed March 29, 2019).
25. Arbit HM, Paller MS. A program to provide regulatory support for investigator-initiated clinical research. *Acad Med*. 2006. https://doi.org/10.1097/00001888-200602000-00009.

Index

Note: Page numbers followed by "f" indicate figures and "t" indicates tables.

Printed and bound by CPI Group (UK) Ltd, Croydon, CR0 4YY

03/10/2024

01040300-0008